DATE DUE

DEC 2 7 2000	
APR 1 5 2003	
NOV 0 5 2009	
10/14/12	

GAYLORD   PRINTED IN U.S.A.

HANDBOOK ON
DRUG ABUSE
PREVENTION

HANDBOOK ON DRUG ABUSE PREVENTION

A Comprehensive Strategy to Prevent the Abuse of Alcohol and Other Drugs

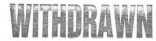

ROBERT H. COOMBS

University of California Los Angeles School of Medicine

DOUGLAS M. ZIEDONIS

Yale University School of Medicine

Editors

ALLYN AND BACON

Boston   London   Sydney   Toronto   Tokyo   Singapore

Vice President and Social Sciences Publisher: *Susan Badger*
Senior Acquisition Editor: *Susan Spivey*
Cover Administrator: *Linda Knowles*
Manufacturing Buyer: *Megan Cochran*
Editorial-Production Service: *Electronic Publishing Services Inc.*
Cover Designer: *Suzanne Harbison*

© 1995 by Allyn & Bacon
A Simon & Schuster Company
Needham Heights, Massachusetts 02194

Library of Congress Cataloging-in-Publication Data
Handbook on drug abuse prevention : a comprehensive strategy to
    prevent the abuse of alcohol and other drugs / Robert H. Coombs &
Douglas M. Ziedonis, editors.
        p.   cm.
    Includes bibliographical references and index.
    ISBN 0-13-377557-7
    1. Drug abuse—United States—Prevention.   2. Alcoholism—United
States—Prevention.   I. Coombs, Robert H.   II. Ziedonis, Douglas M.
HV5825.H219   1995
362.29'17'0973—dc20   94-45871
                                                 CIP

Printed in the United States of America

10 9 8 7 6 5 4 3 2 1   99 98 97 96 95

CONTENTS

FOREWORD

MATHEA FALCO

Most Americans are deeply concerned about drug abuse, and they strongly believe that prevention should be our top priority. According to a 1990 Gallup public opinion survey, 40% of all adults think that prevention deserves the most money and effort in the government's fight against drugs—compared with 23% who think arresting sellers and users should be the dominant strategy. Nonetheless, the federal government as well as most states and cities spend less than 15% of their total antidrug budgets on prevention. As John Haaga and Peter Reuter point out in this volume, prevention is the lauded orphan of drug policy whom everyone praises but no one adopts.

Since the early decades of this century, Americans have viewed the drug problem as essentially foreign, one that could be solved by cutting off supplies of drugs from other countries. The theory behind this supply-side approach is that reduced availability will drive up prices, discouraging new users and forcing addicts to seek treatment. In this view, prevention plays a modest supporting role by helping youngsters resist drugs.

The dominance of supply reduction efforts has been particularly pronounced since 1981, when Ronald Reagan was elected president. Virtually overnight, he shifted the federal spending away from prevention and treatment toward interdiction and enforcement, in the belief that he could effectively seal America's borders against drugs. Eighty percent of the federal drug budget was targeted at supply control, compared to 50% under President Carter and 40% under Presidents Nixon and Ford. Prevention was the biggest loser: From 1981 to 1986, only 1% of the national drug budget was allocated to prevention.

By 1986, with the crack cocaine epidemic spreading across the country, Congress recognized that supply control efforts were having a limited effect at best. The comprehensive Anti-Drug Abuse Act of October 1986 more than doubled money available for demand reduction, with a tenfold increase for prevention and education (from $24 million in 1986 to $249 million in 1987). Since then, funding for prevention has steadily increased, reaching $650 million in 1993. However, prevention remains by far the smallest portion of the $13 billion annual federal antidrug budget.

Why does prevention continue to be the orphan of drug policy? The failure to give prevention major priority is part of a larger pattern of neglect in America: We spend far less on our children than we do on any other age group. Countless studies have documented the cost-effectiveness of early prevention and education efforts, but we have not yet begun to act on this knowledge.

In addition, the impact of prevention is difficult to capture visually, particularly in 60-second reports on the evening news. The results of good programs are usually not instantly visible and may require several years to develop. Success is often measured in negative terms, when something bad (such as drug use, smoking, or drinking) *doesn't* happen. It is far easier and more dramatic to show seizures of cocaine on the high seas than a classroom of children learning resistance skills. To millions of Americans watching the television news, the small mountain of cocaine taken off a Colombian fishing trawler, for example, signals real progress in the war on drugs. They assume that such seizures must reduce the amount of cocaine on the streets of our cities and make drugs more difficult to obtain. Unfortunately, worldwide drug production is now so large that these seizures have no lasting impact. Heroin and cocaine are cheaper and more available in the United States than they were a decade ago. Meanwhile, the truly dramatic results of new prevention programs rarely appear in prime-time news.

Many Americans don't realize that prevention works. Much of the recent progress in combatting drug abuse, smoking, and drinking comes from reduced demand, not reduced supply. The decline in marijuana and cocaine use among better-educated Americans since 1987 reflects the power of health concerns and negative social attitudes toward drugs. Smoking has dropped by one-third since 1965, despite annual multibillion-dollar promotional campaigns by the tobacco industry. Hard liquor consumption has also declined, although more gradually, in the face of pervasive advertising, much of it aimed at minors for whom alcohol is illegal. Prevention and education are key to these fundamental changes in American behavior.

The public remains skeptical that prevention can really make a dent in substance abuse, even as they profess its importance. Part of the problem has been a dearth of reliable research, which has suffered from chronic neglect. Only recently have carefully structured evaluations begun illuminating effective approaches to prevention.

We are learning that prevention can be cost-effective, saving taxpayer dollars as well as children's lives. The Office of Management and Budget estimates that drug abuse costs our country $300 billion a year, including government antidrug programs as well as the costs of crime, healthcare, accidents, and lost productivity. Keeping 1.35 million Americans behind bars, for example—two-thirds of whom are there for drug-related reasons—costs more than $25 billion a year.

Many of the best prevention programs are not expensive compared to the costs of prison construction, high-tech interdiction equipment, and law enforcement hardware. For example, two of the most promising school programs, Life Skills Training (LST) and Students Taught Awareness and Resistance (STAR), cost about $15 to $25 per pupil, including classroom materials and teacher training. They reduce new smoking and marijuana use by half and drinking by one-third, and these results are sustained for at least three years.

Many school districts do not have access to research data and continue to pour federal dollars into curricula that have failed to produce proven results. One example is DARE (Drug Abuse Resistance Education), the most popular prevention curriculum in the country. Taught by uniformed police officers to middle school students, DARE has been evaluated extensively in its 10-year history. Repeated studies report no preventive effect on alcohol, drug or tobacco use; however, DARE does appear to improve students' perceptions of the police. This is a laudable goal but not the one school administrators are trying to achieve. In the meantime, millions of the nation's school children are not receiving effective prevention education.

Federal and state governments should provide current information and practical guidance to school districts on how their prevention dollars might most usefully be spent. For example, the social influences model, on which LST and STAR are based, teaches children to recognize the powerful influence advertising, peer pressure, and the desire to fit in socially have on their behavior. The programs help the children practice specific strategies for avoiding or leaving situations in which others are taking drugs, drinking, or smoking. The approach recognizes that young adolescents fear rejection from their peers and helps them understand that not everybody is taking illegal drugs.

For children who do not attend school regularly, prevention must be provided through community organizations, such as the Boys and Girls Clubs, which provide supervised recreation, education, and prevention training. But these programs reach only a tiny fraction of the children who are at very high risk of becoming drug abusers. Prevention funding should be provided directly to local communities to develop their own programs and strategies through their churches, clubs, and other organizations.

We know prevention must begin early, before children become involved with drugs. We know that they must be taught skills to resist social pressures. We also know that even the best school programs do not inoculate children against drugs for the rest of their lives. Thus, successful prevention efforts must expand beyond the classroom to include the larger environment that shapes our attitudes toward drugs—families, neighborhoods, businesses, and the media.

The national advertising campaign launched by the Partnership for a Drug-Free America in 1987 has shown positive results in changing attitudes about marijuana and cocaine, particularly in locations where the ads are seen often. The Partnership has recently developed local efforts that rely largely on donated time to reinforce school and community prevention programs. The power of advertising is also reflected in California's major antismoking campaign, supported by cigarette taxes. In 1991, smoking in that state dropped by 17%, more than twice the national average decline. As many communities have discovered, the media can play a key role in extending the reach of prevention efforts.

This volume provides a comprehensive review of the most promising approaches to prevention—the best of what we have learned in recent years. Alcohol and drugs account for one-fourth of healthcare costs, which now exceed $1 trillion annually, according to a 1993 study by the Institute for Health Policy of Brandeis University. We cannot afford the continued human and economic toll of our chronic neglect of prevention. It is time to act on what the American public has long believed and to make prevention the heart of our national drug strategy.

PREFACE

Substance abuse, the nation's number-one preventable health problem, places an enormous burden on American society, harming health, family life, the economy, and public safety, and threatening many other aspects of life (Robert Wood Johnson Foundation, 1993). Rather than developing a comprehensive plan to prevent drug problems in America, however, the government has instituted a punishment-oriented drug control policy that has been a national disaster. Based on mistaken premises, it has squandered enormous financial resources, provided criminal opportunities, undermined families, and devastated individuals and communities.

A sensible and comprehensive approach to drug abuse prevention is long overdue. Drug control policies must deal with *all* drugs, including alcohol and other legal substances, and must address the psychosocial dynamics that underlie their use. Drug policy has relied primarily on the criminal justice system to control the supply of illicit drugs among high-profile segments of society, such as inner-city residents. But the nation's drug problem is far broader than commonly perceived and requires the implementation of a comparably broad policy. An enlightened policy would recognize the impact of abused substances on *all* segments of society and would seek to marshall the resources of multiple societal sectors to reduce the demand for drugs.

Despite recurring presidential declarations of war on drug abuse, the destructive use of licit and illicit drugs in America continues unabated. Posturing as valiant warriors, politicians compete to appear toughest on drug users. Their theme: Catch the bad guys—the distributors and users of certain drugs—and punish them.

The first drug war in the late 1960s involved only two federal agencies with a budget of less than $10 million. By 1993, this number had grown to 54 agencies (including every branch of the armed forces) with an overall budget of $13 billion. The Drug Enforcement Agency alone spent more than $8 billion. In the past decade, taxpayers have spent $120 billion to combat illicit drug use, with no noticeable impact on drug importation, distribution, or consumption.

Drug war policy has focused primarily on reducing drug supplies by sealing the nation's borders from drug imports and rounding up drug dealers and users at home. Despite financial expenditures of about $50 billion on drug interdiction, drug offenses in the nation have more than doubled in the past 20 years and illegal drugs are cheaper and more plentiful today than they were even a decade ago. One expert compared the futility of these programs with trying to dig a hole in the ocean's bottom.

Since President Nixon created the Drug Enforcement Agency in 1973 and declared "all-out global war on drugs," property crime rates have tripled and violent crime rates doubled (Duke, 1993). The more extensively these law enforcement schemes have been implemented against drug distribution, the more costly the drugs have become to their consumers. Marijuana, cocaine, and heroin costs in America are about 100 times what they would be in a free market.

Federal drug policy has also created incentives for drug users and dealers to steal and rob. Murder and assault become the means of protecting or acquiring drug-selling turf and settling disputes among drug dealers and their customers (Duke, 1993). Said Paul Roberts, former assistant secretary of the Treasury, "The laws against drugs have created a profitable way of life for people who don't flinch at violence. In trying to protect society from drug use, we have created an alternative career pattern for people averse to formal education and regular work hours" (Roberts, 1993).

The police and Coast Guard approach has contributed to the costly doubling of the U.S. prison population during the past decade. Heavy drug abusers, a constantly rising crime-prone population, are now estimated at 5.5 million (Lacayo, 1992). Despite these dismal results, our government has allocated most of its drug budget to enforcement.

Caught in the frenzy of the latest drug war, Congress enacted dozens of tough federal drug laws in the early 1980s, each bearing a heavy sentence. By the late 1980s and early 1990s, federal district judges were drowning in drug cases. From 1982 to 1992, criminal drug cases in the federal courts increased 197%—from 4,218 in 1982 to 12,512 in 1992, an increase of 8,294 drug trials. By 1992, drug cases represented more than 26% of the criminal cases in federal courts. During this 10-year period, the civil case load increased by 10%. Overwhelmed with drug cases, district courts delay other important cases. Civil cases languish at the clerk's desk an average of nine months, creating needless expense and personal anguish for those awaiting judicial action. In some geographic areas, civil cases must wait three years for attention.

Senior judges complain that the mandatory minimum sentencing laws take away their judicial discretion and force them to impose harsh prison sentences that ignore mitigating circumstances. Some federal judges are distressed to imprison for years first-time, nonviolent offenders who could probably be rehabilitated with less Draconian measures.

There is no more room in our prisons. Crowding at federal prisons, currently bulging at 143% of capacity, is creating nearly unmanageable conditions. "Congress must act soon or the damage to the once-great federal judiciary system will be irreparable," said Don Edwards, vice-chair of the House Judiciary Committee (Edwards, 1993).

National drug policy affects ethnic communities unjustly, especially those of our inner cities, and particularly young African-American men. Incarcerating them for life actually perpetuates the very problems the justice system seeks to ameliorate. In 1989, for example, a 22-year old African American was sentenced to life in prison for distributing crack cocaine. Unlike chemically dependent professionals who are diverted to treatment programs (see Chapter 14), he has no chance to recover from his chemical dependence and no chance to become a productive member of his family or community. Taxpayers will assume the burden of housing him for the next fifty years or so.

History clearly demonstrates, with some exceptions (see Chapter 3), that most punitive approaches to drug problems are misguided, ineffective, or even counterproductive. Incarcerating drug users rarely, if ever, deters drug use. Instead, it reinforces drug careers by extending users' drug connections, makes them more familiar and comfortable with the illicit drug world, alienates them from conventional society, and hardens their attitudes against civil authorities.

More simple and inexpensive approaches are possible. For example, consider the inner-city liquor store. A fixture in the modern ghetto, these stores not only sell alcoholic beverages, they often become hangouts for distributors of illegal drugs. However, grass-roots efforts to limit liquor stores in high-risk neighborhoods have met with little success. When African-American activists in South Central Los Angeles energetically campaigned for city officials to rid their neighborhoods of liquor stores, their cries fell on deaf ears. When the city exploded in flames during the 1992 riots, there was a liquor outlet at virtually every major intersection—728 licensed liquor outlets, or thirteen per square mile. Roughly half were convenience stores that sold beer and wine; the rest sold hard liquor as well. South Central Los Angeles had more stores selling hard liquor than thirteen entire states combined (Whitman & Bowermaster, 1993).

A landmark study by the Federal Office of Disease Prevention (McGinnis & Foege, 1993), analyzing 1990 death certificates, found that tobacco was the number-one killer. It contributed to the deaths of 400,000 people, 19% of all deaths in the nation during 1990. This is more than the total deaths caused by illegal drug use, firearms, irresponsible sexual behavior, and other causes.

Despite this finding, no major tobacco control legislation was enacted by Congress between 1989 and 1992. It is significant that during the last two years of this period (1991–1992), the tobacco industry donated nearly $2.5 million to lawmakers, amounting to only .004% of the $60 billion in tobacco-related sales (*Public Citizen*, 1994).

Misuse of alcohol contributed to the deaths of 100,000 persons and the abuse of other drugs accounted for 20,000 deaths. Use of firearms resulted in 36,000 deaths, including 16,000 murders, 19,000 suicides, and 1,400 accidental killings. "People may not realize the extent [to] which deaths among Americans are preventable," the investigators concluded "If we want to get serious about controlling premature and unnecessary and costly death and illness, we need to . . . invest heavily in health promotion and disease prevention" (McGinnis & Foege, 1993).

About half of all traffic fatalities can be traced to drunk driving. Studies indicate that 54–74% of those convicted of drunk driving are alcoholics or problem drinkers. Someone is killed by a drunk driver every 24 minutes, and more than 540,000 people are injured in alcohol-related traffic accidents yearly.

Despite these shocking statistics, the federal government spends only about $50 per capita each year on prevention and treatment (including $3.7 billion to state and local governments). In contrast, the government estimates that the nation will spend $900 billion on healthcare this year—about $14,000 for a family of four. Only 5% of this amount is devoted to prevention. However, in 1993, the Surgeon General of the U.S. Public Health Service said, "If we are to succeed [in achieving our nation's health goals], all policy makers, opinion leaders, the media, the public, and leaders of Federal, State, and Local health, welfare, and education agencies must get informed and stay informed about the value of prevention" (address at the National Prevention Conference sponsored by the Center for Substance Abuse Prevention, *Prevention Pipeline*, 1993a).

As several chapters clarify (see Chapters 13 and 14 on college students and professionals),

most Americans are at risk for substance abuse, not just a deficient segment. Giant corporations annually spend billions of dollars to make gateway drugs—tobacco and alcohol—enticing and available. The alcohol industry spends at least $2 billion a year on advertising and promotion and beer companies alone budget more than $675 million annually, most of it for television advertisements that appear during sporting events. This is eight times the current total budget of the federal government's drug prevention agency, the Center for Substance Abuse Prevention. Last year, alcohol cost each of us $479, even if we didn't buy any, through lost work time, lower productivity, higher healthcare expenses, and extra hospitalization. We all pay for alcohol use and abuse—about $119 billion a year (*Prevention Pipeline*, 1993b).

Before the age of 21, the typical person has seen thousands of seductive beer commercials. The underground drug paraphernalia industry offers trendy items that glamorize drug use as "cool" and "hip" and the mass media glamorizes this lifestyle. Pharmaceutical companies, developers and purveyors of legal drugs, seek to persuade health professionals and their patients that drugs provide solutions to all physical and emotional problems. "Feel better fast; I haven't got time for the pain," has become a pervasive theme in American society. Is it any wonder that drug demand overwhelmed efforts to control supply and that, despite widely publicized drug busts, the illicit drug industry has little trouble making drugs easily accessible?

APPROACH

The conceptual basis for this book originated in 1985, when one of us (RHC), a member of the California Commission for the Prevention of Drug and Alcohol Abuse, developed the framework that guided the commission's activities (*Final Report*, 1986). This framework assumes the following: Drugs are used by average people, not just a deficient, disordered, or morally flawed segment of American society; people use drugs because it is socially and psychologically rewarding to do so; and the most effective way to prevent drug use at any level is to help potential users obtain highs in healthy ways—through personally rewarding encounters with their families and communities.

In our view, the prevention challenge is to help high-risk individuals of all ages and social circumstances to achieve psychological rewards by succeeding at home, school, and work. The task is to enlist all societal sectors—including the schools, mass media, and sports organizations—to affect high-risk individuals in health-enhancing ways. This approach assumes that individuals are best served by viable families and that such families are most likely to flourish in stable neighborhoods, supported by a feeling of community provided by healthy ethnic affiliations, religious groups, and other voluntary associations. Small wonder that the United States, lacking a coherent family policy, leads the world in illicit drug use.

Figure 1, "A Conceptual Model to Prevent the Abuse of Alcohol and Other Drugs," graphically illustrates this book's conceptual approach. It assumes that drug abuse is a symptom of lives that are emotionally and spiritually malnourished. High-risk individuals are subject to unique biopsychosocial influences that increase their propensity to abuse drugs or decrease their association with positive social networks that oppose drug abuse. This model includes systems-oriented and client-oriented approaches and includes both general and individualized prevention strategies. The prevention challenge, we propose, is to marshall the resources of each societal sector to help those they affect achieve healthy and psychologically rewarding lifestyles free from drugs.

ORGANIZATION

The book is organized in four parts. Part I, *Introduction,* begins with two insightful chapters. John G. Haaga and Peter H. Reuter first discuss prevention as a neglected area of drug control policy. Then Gilbert J. Botvin, explaining principles of prevention, defines basic terms, offers an empirical, conceptual foundation, and suggests issues in implementing and evaluating prevention programs.

Part II, *Systems-Oriented Prevention Strategies and Programs,* suggests how significant societal sectors can intervene to prevent substance abuse. We asked each author to clarify who is at risk and why, and to propose prevention strategies at the primary, secondary, and tertiary levels. Primary prevention aims to keep the uninitiated from drug experimentation; secondary prevention discourages those at early stages of drug involvement from escalating into more extensive drug involvement; and tertiary (relapse) prevention promotes ways to help addicts enter treatment and remain permanently free from their substance-abusing lifestyles.

These societal sectors are discussed: law enforcement and regulatory agencies (Chapter 3 by Roger L. Conner and Patrick Burns), local government and community organizations (Chapter 4 by Mary Ann Pentz), schools (Chapter 5 by Phyllis L. Ellickson), healthcare providers (Chapter 6 by J. Thomas Ungerleider, Naomi J. Siegel, and Bernard B. Virshup), employers (Chapter 7 by Paul J. Roman and Terry C. Blum), religious organizations (Chapter 8 by Stephen J. Bahr and Ricky D. Hawks), voluntary organizations (Chapter 9 by Sue Rusche), sports organizations (Chapter 10 by Gary I. Wadler and Eric D. Zemper), the advertising industry (Chapter 11 by Roger G. Pisani), and the mass media (Chapter 12 by Thomas E. Backer).

Part III deals with *Client-Oriented Prevention Strategies and Programs.* Effective prevention programs must identify those at high risk for the abuse of alcohol and other drugs and then develop appropriate interventions. It is unlikely that a single prevention approach will be effective for all groups. Those particularly vulnerable include college students (Chapter 13 by Lewis D. Eigen), helping professionals (Chapter 14 by Robert H. Coombs and Bernard B. Virshup), children and adolescents (Chapter 15 by Christoph M. Heinicke

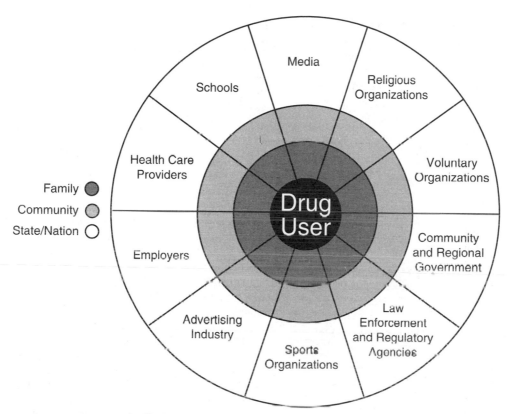

Family ●
Community ◐
State/Nation ○

FIGURE 1. A Conceptual Model to Prevent Alcohol and Drug Abuse

and Shirah Vollmer), pregnant women and their newborns (Chapter 16 by Judy Howard), the off-spring of alcoholics and other addicts (Chapter 17 by Timmen L. Cermak and Walter Beckman), ethnic minorities (Chapter 18 by Joseph E. Trimble), inner-city youth (Chapter 19 by Wade W. Nobles, Amado M. Padilla, and David Duran), the elderly (Chapter 20 by Meyer D. Glantz and Zili Sloboda), and psychiatric patients (Chapter 21 by Douglas M. Ziedonis).

We asked our authors, all experts on their assigned topics, to review past and current prevention programs and, based on personal and professional experience, to present their best prevention ideas. This was a challenging request because drug abuse prevention is still in an embryonic stage. There are relatively few systematic evaluation data.

Authors were asked to discuss prevention strategies and programs in the context of the graphic model (Figure 1). We encouraged them, when possible, to address the prevention programs aimed at the *individual level* (what programs and strategies best affect individuals directly?), the *family level* (what helps parents, spouses, and other family members mitigate or prevent drug use among family members?), the *community level* (what programs and strategies can be implemented in neighborhoods, ethnic groups, and other support networks to strengthen individuals and families?), and the *state and national level* (what programs would help develop and support healthy communities, families, and individuals?).

Part IV reviews *Controversial Prevention Issues.* Drug testing (Chapter 22) is discussed by

Deborah L. Ackerman, user accountability (Chapter 23) by John R. Hepburn, and legalization and decriminalization of drug use (Chapter 24) by Richard S. Sandor.

The authors differ in background and perspective, and their chapters vary in style and approach. Sometimes their concepts and data overlap, reinforcing their combined message.

Our hope is that this book will stimulate debate, innovations, and enlightened policies to prevent substance abuse and reduce its individually defeating and socially impoverishing impact.

ACKNOWLEDGMENTS

We would like to thank the following reviewers for their feedback and guidance: Charlene Agne-Traub, formerly affiliated with Harvard University; David Anderson, George Mason University; Mathea Falco, affiliated with Carnegie Mellon University; Ray Goldberg, State University College at Cortland; Dennis Gorman, Rutgers University; Howard Liddle, Temple University; Rita Myers, Kent State University; Alan Poling, Western Michigan University; Stephen Roberts, The University of Toledo; and Martin Turnauer, Radford University.

REFERENCES

Duke, S. B. (1993). How legalization would cut crime. *Los Angeles Times,* Dec. 21.

Edwards, D. (1993). Federal courts are causalities in war on drugs. (Federal drug laws enacted in 1980s bog down federal courts with minor cases.) *Los Angeles Times, 112,* Oct. 25, B7.

Final Report: California Attorney General's Commission on the Prevention of Drug and Alcohol Abuse, 1986, p. 147.

Lacayo, R. (1992). What would it take to get America off drugs? *Time,* Nov. 9, 36.

McGinnis, J. M., & Foege, W. H. (1993). Actual causes of death in the United States. *Journal of the American Medical Association, 270* (18), 2207–2212.

Prevention Pipeline, 6 (3), May/June 1993a, 3.

Prevention Pipeline, 6 (6), Nov./Dec. 1993b, 34.

Public Citizen (1994). Report shows tobacco's choke hold on Congress. Jan./Feb., 8.

Robert Wood Johnson Foundation (Oct. 1993). Substance abuse: The nation's number one health problem. Report prepared by the Institute for Health Policy, Brandeis University.

Roberts, P. C. (1993). Drug laws aid and abet crime wave. *Los Angeles Times,* Nov. 14, M5.

Whitman, D., & Bowermaster, D. (1993). A potent brew: Booze and crime. *U.S. News & World Report, 114* (21), 57–59.

CONTRIBUTORS

Deborah L. Ackerman, Ph.D., is a research associate in the Department of Psychiatry and Biobehavioral Sciences, UCLA School of Medicine. She has a M.S. degree in pharmacology and a Ph.D. in epidemiology.

Thomas E. Backer, Ph.D., is president of the Human Interaction Research Institute, a Los Angeles-based nonprofit center for research on organizational change in healthcare and human resources, and associate clinical professor of medical psychology at the UCLA School of Medicine.

Stephen J. Bahr, Ph.D., is professor of sociology and past director of the Family and Demographic Research Institute at Brigham Young University.

Walter Beckman, Ph.D., is a clinical psychologist in San Francisco and an adjunct faculty member at the California School of Professional Psychology, Berkeley. He has taught at the Stanford University Medical School and the Center for Psychological Studies in Albany, California.

Terry C. Blum, Ph.D., is professor of organizational behavior at Georgia Institute of Technology and principal investigator of a five-year NIDA grant to study employer and employee reactions to drug abuse.

Gilbert J. Botvin, Ph.D., is professor at the Cornell University Medical Center Department of Public Health and director of the Institute for Prevention Research, The New York Hospital Medical Center.

Patrick Burns, director of communications for the National Council for Senior Citizens, was formerly assistant director of the American Alliance for Rights and Responsibilities.

Timmen Lee Cermak, M.D., is clinical director of Genesis, a group psychotherapy practice specializing in treating chemically dependent families.

Roger L. Conner, J.D., is founder and director of the American Alliance for Rights and Responsibilities, a group providing legal support to grass-roots organizations that try to rid streets of drug dealing.

Robert H. Coombs, Ph.D., is professor of biobehavioral sciences at the UCLA School of Medicine.

David Duran is a graduate student in psychological studies at the School of Education, Stanford University.

Lewis D. Eigen, Ed.D., is president and chief executive officer of Social and Health Services, Ltd., a health education and promotion organization. Formerly he was director of the federal government's National Clearinghouse for Alcohol and Drug Information and Director of the National School Resource Network.

Phyllis L. Ellickson, Ph.D., is a senior behavioral scientist and resident scholar at RAND.

Mathea Falco, J.D., is president of Drug Strategies, a nonprofit initiative in Washington, D.C. to identify effective approaches to substance abuse. Formerly she was director of health policy, Department of Public Health, Cornell University Medical College and from 1977 to 1981, she was assistant secretary of state for international narcotics matters.

Meyer D. Glantz, Ph.D., is acting chief of the epidemiology research branch and chief of etiology research section at the National Institute on Drug Abuse.

John G. Haaga, Ph.D., is an associate of the Population Council, serving as director of a family planning and health services research project in Bangladesh. Formerly he was a policy Analyst at the Drug Policy Research Center at RAND.

Ricky D. Hawks, Ed.D., is a Clinical Psychologist with the Weber County Human Services Division of the Utah Department of Substance Abuse.

Christoph M. Heinicke, Ph.D., is professor of biobehavioral sciences at the UCLA School of Medicine and is on the faculty of the Los Angeles Psychoanalytic Society and Institute.

John R. Hepburn, Ph.D., is professor of justice studies at Arizona State University.

Judy Howard, M.D., is professor of clinical pediatrics, UCLA School of Medicine, and director of the UCLA Intervention Program for Handicapped Children.

Herbert Kleber, M.D., is professor of psychiatry at Columbia University, College of Physicians and Surgeons and the director, Division on Substance Abuse at the New York State Psychiatric Institute. Formerly he was deputy director for demand reduction at the White House Office of National Drug Control Policy.

Wade W. Nobles, Ph.D., is professor in the department of black studies, the School of Ethnic Studies at San Francisco State University and founder and executive director of the Institute for the Advanced Study of Black Family Life and Culture, Inc.

Amado M. Padilla, Ph.D., is professor of education, psychological studies in education, Stanford University.

Mary Ann Pentz, Ph.D., is associate professor and director of community prevention research at the Institute for Health Promotion and Disease Prevention Research, Department of Preventive Medicine, University of Southern California.

Roger G. Pisani, a media consultant in private practice, was formerly executive vice president and director of creative development and research for the Partnership for a Drug-Free America.

Peter Reuter, Ph.D., is professor and director of the social policy specialization in the School of Public Affairs at the University of Maryland. Formerly he headed RAND's Drug Research Center.

Paul M. Roman, Ph.D., is research professor of sociology and director, Center for Research on Deviance and Behavioral Health, Institute for Behavioral Research at the University of Georgia.

Sue Rusche is co-founder and executive director of National Families in Action, Atlanta, Georgia.

Richard S. Sandor, M.D., is medical director of the Chemical Dependence Center at Saint John's Hospital in Santa Monica, California and president of the California Society of Addiction Medicine.

Naomi Siegel, L.C.S.W., B.C.D., is a lecturer at the UCLA Neuropsychiatric Institute and Hospital and former director of psychiatric social work and the Outpatient Mental Health Center of St. John's Hospital in Santa Monica, California.

Zili Sloboda, Sc.D., is acting director of the Division of Epidemiology and Prevention Research of the National Institute on Drug Abuse. Her training is in medical sociology and epidemiology.

Joseph E. Trimble, Ph.D., is professor of psychology/educational administration and foundations and research associate in the Center for Cross-Cultural Research at Western Washington University.

J. Thomas Ungerleider, M.D., is emeritus professor of psychiatry at the UCLA School of Medicine.

Shirah Vollmer, M.D., is assistant clinical professor of family medicine and former medical director of the Children's Inpatient Psychiatric Unit and the Drug Treatment Program at the UCLA School of Medicine.

Bernard B. Virshup, M.D., is clinical professor of biobehavioral sciences at the UCLA School of Medicine.

Gary I. Wadler, M.D., is clinical associate professor of medicine at Cornell University Medical College, an attending physician at North Shore University Hospital in Manhasset, New York, and a fellow and trustee of the American College of Sports Medicine.

Eric D. Zemper, Ph.D., is president and director of research, Exercise Research Associates of Oregon. Formerly he was research coordinator for the National College Athletic Association.

Douglas M. Ziedonis, M.D., is assistant professor of psychiatry at Yale University and director of the Connecticut Mental Health Center's Dual Diagnosis Treatment and Research Program, and associate medical director of the Substance Abuse Treatment Unit.

HANDBOOK ON DRUG ABUSE PREVENTION

PART ONE

INTRODUCTION

CHAPTER 1

PREVENTION:
THE (LAUDED) ORPHAN
OF DRUG POLICY

JOHN G. HAAGA
PETER H. REUTER

The primary purpose of this chapter is to provide a historical and analytic account of how drug prevention fits into U.S. efforts to control problems related to illicit drugs. The usual division of drug policy is into enforcement, treatment, and prevention programs. Despite a long-standing and pervasive belief that prevention is the most effective long term program for reducing drug use, enforcement has received the lion's share of government expenditures for at least two decades. This may reflect the lack of credible evidence that systematic prevention programs had any discernible effect on drug use by adolescents. Since 1985, the emergence of some promising new prevention programs, together with a general despair about the effectiveness of enforcement, as well as the American predilections for solutions that go to the root of the problem, have led to growth in the share of federal drug expenditures going to prevention. Some of the difficulty in obtaining more financial support for prevention may lie in the institutional arrangements and the fact that the products of enforcement are far more tangible than those of prevention.

INTRODUCTION: THE PARADOX
OF PREVENTION

And as for drink, I believe in no Parliamentary restraint; but I do believe in the gradual effect of moral teaching and education.

Anthony Trollope, *An Autobiography*

There can be few sentiments so widely shared by policy makers, researchers, and the lay public as the belief that prevention of drug abuse is a good idea.[1] The alternative instruments of drug policy engender far more controversy; reliance on treatment seems ineffective to many and law enforcement, even if effective, is highly intrusive and coercive. This paper explores why the enthusiasm has not been translated into a programmatic emphasis on prevention.

The appeal of drug prevention is straightforward, as has been pointed out for health policy in general: "It is better not to suffer a disease than to have it and try to repair the damage afterward" (Russell, 1986, p. 2). Prevention is particularly attractive when treatments for the disease are expensive and uncertain, as is the case for drug dependence. However, drug prevention programs

The preparation of this paper was supported by RAND's Drug Policy Research Center, with funding from the Ford and Weingart Foundations. Joel Feinleib provided valuable research assistance. The paper covers the period to late 1990, with only limited updating for later events.

have always received far less public funding than have drug law enforcement and usually less than treatment programs. Prevention funding has increased considerably in absolute terms in recent years, and the share of the drug control budget devoted to prevention has started to grow from its very low base. But prevention still does not receive public funding in the proportions one would expect if it were really believed, as was claimed in a 1975 report from the Office of the President, that "ultimately the drug problem can only be contained through effective education and prevention efforts" (Domestic Council, 1975, p. 65).

It is not just a matter of policy catching up to a recent discovery. On the contrary, as this quotation from a 1975 "Drug Strategy" suggests, the low status of prevention among drug policy instruments antedates the current epidemic of cocaine use and renewed interest in drug policy. Even a 1972 report on drug problems to the Ford Foundation claimed that "[E]veryone now talks of pouring money into education to stop the problem before it begins," because of the general dissatisfaction with the results of overseas programs, law enforcement, and treatment (Wald & Abrams, 1972, p. 123). In that same report, "Prevention, education, and training" were estimated to account for only 10% of all drug-related federal expenditures in fiscal year 1972 (See Table 1.1). This included supplemental appropriations resulting from a major expansion of demand-reduction programs as part of the Nixon administration's "War on Drugs." In 1981, the last Carter administration budget (and the last fiscal year before the consolidation of prevention programs into block grants to the states), the Office of Management and Budget estimates that prevention activities accounted for 11% of drug-related budget authority at the federal level. This percentage shrank somewhat during the early years of the Reagan administration, and grew significantly only after passage of the 1986 Anti-Drug Abuse Act (Table 1.1). The shortchanging of prevention thus lasted through at least one "issue-attention cycle" (from Drug War to low priority to Drug War again) and through presidential administrations with very different styles of discourse on drug policy.

TABLE 1.1   Federal Government Expenditures on Drug Prevention—Selected Years, 1971–91

FISCAL YEAR	PREVENTION BUDGET AUTHORITY		
	(current $, millions)	*(constant 1987 $)*	*As percentage of total Federal Drug Expenditures*
1971	42	113	10
1981	125	158	11
1982	127	152	10
1983	143	164	9
1984	158	173	9
1985	184	195	9
1986	201	207	9
1987	533	553	13
1988	605	582	16
1989	758	699	12
1990	1,366	1,210	13
1991	1,633	1,387	13

Sources: 1972, Goldberg and DeLong; 1990b, Office of National Drug Control Policy, 1990–1992, Office of National Drug Control Policy, 1992.

Similar proportions can be found in drug-related expenditures of state and local governments. State and local governments in the aggregate spend more on public drug and alcohol programs (and on law enforcement) than does the federal government. Prevention has received considerably less public funding than treatment in every single state during the period (1984 to the present) covered by the annual surveys of the National Association of State Alcohol and Drug Abuse Directors (NASADAD). In fiscal year 1991, prevention received 16% of the combined local, state, and federal funding for publicly supported drug and alcohol programs, compared to 75% for treatment[2] (Butynski, Canova, & Reds, 1992.) As with federal expenditures alone, this represents an increase from the mid-1980s from an even lower percentage base.

Nor is this situation unique to the United States. A recent report of the Royal College of Psychiatrists in the United Kingdom puts the case in terms that would be familiar to any of the American drug policy reformers of the last two decades: "Prevention is more often neglected at every level and despite all the fine talk remains nobody's business at all. It is a responsibility always left to someone else. The community will leave it to the Government, while the Government suddenly discovers an enormous faith in the virtue of each person's captaincy of his own soul" (Royal College of Psychiatrists, 1987, p. 179).

Clearly something more fundamental is involved in the relative neglect of prevention than the misplaced preferences of one administration or a temporary enforcement frenzy induced by the latest drug epidemic. Everyone is for it; no one spends much on it, at least not in relative terms. In the rest of this chapter, we attempt to elucidate this paradox. We discuss the place of prevention in drug control policy and health policy in general, the recent history of public policy concerning drug prevention, and current problems in prevention policy. Along the way, we deal with the confusing issues of what constitutes prevention and whose job it should be.

HOW PREVENTION IS RELATED TO DRUG CONTROL POLICY

At least since the early 1970s, it has become customary to distinguish two basic categories of efforts to control the use of illicit drugs and associated problems: so-called supply-side and demand-side programs. Drug enforcement, carried out by all levels of government and coming in many forms, constitutes the supply-side effort. It aims either to reduce the availability of drugs to users or to raise the prices users must pay to obtain drugs. That enforcement can also have important demand-side effects has been given attention only lately and is still not a primary consideration for enforcement, particularly at the federal level.

The demand-side efforts consist of prevention and treatment programs. Prevention attempts to reduce the number of persons becoming first-time regular users of drugs in a particular time period; these programs aim primarily at adolescents. Treatment aims at reducing drug use among those who have a history of regular use, generally heavy use; the great majority of persons in drug treatment are adults.

The division between treatment and prevention is not always so clear-cut. Prevention efforts can be divided into primary, secondary, and tertiary programs, depending on whether the targets are persons who used no more than a few times or have used regularly but not heavily (Polich, Ellickson, Reuter, & Kahan, 1984). Tertiary prevention shades over into relapse prevention following treatment. We focus here on primary prevention.[3]

Drug policy debates of the 1980s have generally been about the balance of emphasis between supply- and demand-side programs.[4] The major criticism of the Bush administration's *National Drug Control Strategy* (Office of National Drug Control Policy, 1989, 1990a) has been its supposed overemphasis of enforcement, in terms both of budget allocations (particularly underinvestment in treatment and prevention programs) and the harshness of sanctions (Skolnick, 1990). In particular, increased emphasis on prevention has been a slogan for drug policy reform during the second half of the 1980s, following years of malign neglect.

More recently, this simple taxonomy of drug policy instruments has been attacked as unhelpful. The first *National Drug Control Strategy* produced by the Office of National Drug Control Policy (ONDCP), significantly, did not have *Prevention* in a chapter title: It started with "The Criminal Justice System," "The Drug Treatment System," and then "Education, Community Action, and the Workplace," wherein the activities usually grouped together as prevention are discussed along with others (Office of National Drug Control Policy, 1989, 1990a). This choice of headings accorded with William Bennett's determination to transcend the supply-side versus demand-side distinction.[5] The Strategy downplayed the distinction between enforcement and prevention, for example, arguing that enforcement of drug laws at every level is designed to discourage use by making it awkward and expensive to obtain illegal drugs and by expressing society's disapproval of drug use.[6] Likewise, drug education and early intervention in schools and workplaces were discussed in the same sections of the Strategy as the less formal enforcement of policies against drug use by these institutions.

Except at the rhetorical and moral level, the direct effect of drug law enforcement on demand is restricted to policing at the retail level. As Moore (1973) first observed, such policing adds to the nonmonetary costs of obtaining drugs such as the time, risks, and dangers that users must incur to find a willing seller. Other kinds of enforcement raise prices but do not directly affect demand.[7] In particular, the federal enforcement effort, aimed principally at smugglers and high-level dealers, has only modest effects on demand.

In many ways, this blurring of old distinctions between control measures and prevention is analogous to recent trends in policy toward the major legal drug, alcohol. As Mosher and Jernigan have explained, a change in emphasis has come about through "application of the familiar epidemiologic triad of environment–agent–host to alcohol-related problems":

> *In addition to strategies already in place targeting the host—i.e., the individual drinker—with education, deterrence, treatment, and so on, this "public health model" of alcohol-related problems calls attention to the role of environmental factors (the social and physical structures within which alcohol problems occur) and agent factors (the presentation of alcohol, including alcohol packaging, labeling and price) in the spread of alcohol problems. (Mosher & Jernigan, 1989, p. 248)*

The legal status of the drug in question does matter in the choice of policy instruments, of course. The retail price of alcoholic beverages and tobacco could be increased by taxation (or simply raising the price of beverages, because local governments are the sellers in many parts of the country);[8] the effective price of illegal drugs is raised instead by law enforcement.[9] The messages in the mass media concerning use of the legally available drugs are at best mixed; health promotion is outweighed by promotion of consumption (of alcohol in broadcast media and of tobacco and alcohol in the print media), whereas for marijuana, cocaine, and heroin, the "antis" have the field mostly to themselves.

An Analytic Framework

To sort out the various goals for drug policy and the relation of different instruments of policy, it may be useful to work backward from the set of interrelated problems with which the public is concerned. These include the extraordinary violence surrounding drug distribution in Washington, New York, and other big cities; drug-exposed babies; and the continued spread of AIDS among IV drug users. Many have concluded that the nation is suffering from a drug use epidemic, requiring drastic—even repressive—measures to contain it.

In fact, what concerns society under the rubric of "the drug problem" is more than just one problem, and more complex than just drug use. The classification shown in Table 1.2 suggests that there are at least eight different problems, separable in the sense that specific programs generally address only a subset of them, and have no effect—or even adverse effects—on the others. For example, we might be able to reduce the adverse effects of illicit heroin use on the health of users by ending enforcement of laws that prohibit the nonprescription possession of hypodermic needles in some states; however, that would not lower the crime rate and might increase the number of persons recruited into regular heroin use (Kleiman & Mockler, 1988). The problems are also separable in that each of them may respond differently to social and demographic trends.

Some of the problems in the list are related not so much to the consequences of drug use itself as to initiation of the young into drug use. It is the involvement of young people in the subculture surrounding illicit drugs or with the routine violation of law, and their possible progression to drug dependence, that are the central concerns. Another set of problems is caused by the dependence on or abuse of drugs (the spread of AIDS and crimes committed to support expensive illicit drug use), which are sometimes caused by the conditions of use society has created.[10] Others, such as the murder of rival sellers for increased market share, are directly related not to drug use but to the distribution of drugs.

Other problems—the distortion of social and political institutions in Bolivia, Colombia, and Peru—are a function of the production of the drugs themselves.

If it were possible to eliminate illicit drug use altogether, all of these problems would either vanish or be much ameliorated. Because different elements of the problems have different sources, however, lowering drug consumption does not necessarily have the desired effect on the other dimensions. For example, we may be able to reduce cocaine use through more stringent enforcement against dealers but suffer, at least in the short run, a worsening of related crime[11] and health problems.

Matching Programs and Problems

The traditional classification of programs dealing with drug problems has been enforcement, treatment, and prevention. If we further divide enforcement into the categories of source country control (such as crop eradication and refinery destruction) and domestic enforcement (including interdiction of smuggled drugs), we can match program types and the dimensions of the drug problem schematized in Table 1.2. That matching is presented in Table 1.3.

Programs are usually evaluated in terms of the targets suggested by this mapping. Thus, primary prevention programs are evaluated mostly

TABLE 1.2   Elements of the Drug Problem

ELEMENTS	SOURCE
Adolescents dropping out of school Gateway to other behavioral problems	Initiation
High mortality among users Crime by users	Drug dependence
Large criminal incomes Violence in competition	Drug distribution
Distortion of source country societies Strains on U.S. foreign policy	Drug production

TABLE 1.3   Program Targets

Prevention	→	Initiation
Treatment	→	Drug use
Enforcement	→	Drug distribution
Source country controls	→	Drug production

in terms of their effect on initiation into drug use; successful prevention efforts reduce the percentage of nonusers or experimental users who become regular users. Similarly, treatment programs are evaluated in terms of reducing the number of drug-dependent persons and associated harms.

Interactions among programs can actually be negative. Increasingly effective treatment may actually worsen initiation problems by removing the most visible and striking negative role models of addicted drug users. That is not a reason for failing to provide funding for drug treatment; it merely points to the difficulty of doing only good.

Program effects can be very complex indeed. For example, enforcement is now principally intended to control distribution-related problems, but it should also affect rates of initiation and drug dependence. By making it more difficult for users to find sellers or making the drug more expensive, enforcement should deter some of the curious or experimental from becoming regular users and persuade some regular users to desist or to enter treatment programs.

This matching of program types against goals provides a framework for systematic comparative assessment of programs and policies. We must ask of particular policies not simply how they will affect levels of drug use, but also what their consequences will be for other dimensions of the drug problem. For example, evaluations of street crackdowns should determine their effect on the crime rate and on recruitment rates. Similarly, in allocating resources between prevention and treatment, we must compare the benefits of reduced recruitment now with those of reduced heavy use now; the flow of benefits over time may be very different for the two kinds of programs.

THE RECENT HISTORY OF PREVENTION IN DRUG POLICY

The government agencies involved in prevention have changed over the years: Responsibilities have shifted, some agencies involved early on dropped out and then rejoined the cast in 1986, and in 1986, for the first time, a sole-purpose prevention agency has been created at the federal level. More continuity is apparent at the state and local levels, but even there, the recent creation of new "drug czar" offices may have had the effect of giving new prominence to prevention as a policy tool.

In 1972 (the first year of funding for many of the new demand-side programs of the Nixon administration), the largest appropriation for prevention was for the Law Enforcement Assistance Agency in the Department of Justice, which had $20 million in budget authority for a program for concerned communities, with four components: coordination of local and state information programs; implementation of health-information programs in every school at the earliest feasible grade level; development of programs to provide accurate information for adults; and predelinquent counseling services (see Goldberg & DeLong, 1972, for description). It is a measure of the subordination of prevention to law enforcement that a justice agency was expected to bring about sweeping change in every school and implement counseling services. The Office of Education had a continuing appropriation of $6 million for various programs to train teachers in drug education and to assist 26 community programs and 11 projects of individual school districts. This was augmented by a supplemental appropriation of $13 million for a program called "Help Communities to Help Themselves." The other federal agencies involved in drug prevention at that time were the National Institute of Mental Health, which dealt mainly with research and dissemination of results ($7 million) and the Department of Housing and Urban Development ($3 million for 37 programs in its Model Cities).

Evaluations of the early efforts at drug education (both in the schools and in mass media) were scarce. When they existed, they were hardly encouraging. The National Commission on Marihuana and Drug Abuse, appointed by the president and Congress, actually recommended in its second report of 1973 a moratorium on drug education efforts (National Commission on Marihuana and Drug Abuse, 1973, pp. 346–347). "Sentiment had been growing among drug experts that these efforts were a waste of federal money" (Musto, 1987, p. 262). Prevention survived, though, not because of any demonstrated success, but simply because the alternatives did not seem so promising for the long term either. The Domestic Council report of 1975 summarized the record. Despite efforts to reduce the supply of imported drugs, "[i]llicit drugs are likely to remain available for a long time" (p. 64). Despite some innovations in treatment methods, notably the spread of methadone maintenance programs for heroin users to all the major cities, "[w]e now understand that once a person begins to abuse drugs, long-term rehabilitation is both expensive and difficult" (Domestic Council, 1975, p. 64). The Task Force concluded that "greater emphasis must be placed on education and prevention efforts that promote the healthy growth of individuals and discourage the use of drugs as a way to solve (or avoid) problems" (p. 64). It lacked specificity on how this was to be done, however.

Most drug treatment, prevention, and research programs were consolidated within the federal government and assigned to a new institute, the National Institute on Drug Abuse (NIDA). A similar institute, the National Institute on Alcohol Abuse and Alcoholism, was created by the same 1972 legislation (Drug Abuse Office and Treatment Act of 1972). NIDA gradually replaced the older policy of funding treatment

and prevention programs directly or through local agencies and began to make large grants to single state agencies for alcohol and drug problems. Most of the state agencies were created around this time to meet the requirements for receiving and distributing the federal grants, as well as to channel state funds to localities and programs. States varied (and still vary) in the status of these agencies within their governmental structure: Many are relatively autonomous units within health agencies or health and welfare superagencies; others are connected more closely to mental health agencies.

During the Carter administration, drug policy generally occupied a lower spot in the federal agenda (reflecting the end of the heroin epidemic and the reduced fears about the consequences of marijuana use), and there was a retreat at all levels of government from the harsher enforcement policies of the previous decade. The institutional and funding changes brought about in the early 1980s by the Reagan administration were basic. All drug, alcohol, and mental health categorical programs were consolidated by the 1981 Omnibus Budget Reconciliation Act into an Alcohol, Drug, and Mental Health (ADM) block grant to be handled by the single state agencies. Total funding was cut at the same time. The separate reporting requirements and allocation criteria were reduced in number and simplified. For our purposes, the most important change was that states had to spend at least 20% of their total grant for drug and alcohol programs on prevention activities.

Few states spent more on prevention than was required. Often the prevention funding went for statewide programs (such as teacher or youth worker training); the prevention requirement was not handed down to lower-level jurisdictions and few counties or city governments had full-time prevention specialists. Especially in the big cities and urbanized states, the drug agencies were stretched to cover for the loss of federal funds to keep treatment programs going, and the early 1980s were not a period of innovation in prevention by the public sector.

Federal enforcement agencies that had been involved in drug prevention either disappeared (the LEAA) or dropped their demand-side work (the Drug Enforcement Administration) in these years.[12] Policy coordination at the federal level was the responsibility of the National Drug Enforcement Policy Board, composed of representatives of all the supply-side agencies and chaired by the Attorney General.

Prevention did receive emphasis in the public pronouncements of administration officials, but it was considered a private-sector responsibility. The most important role for the public sector was to be moral suasion by elected officials and their families. The best-known initiative was Nancy Reagan's "Just Say No" campaign. Besides calling attention to individual responsibilities, the "Just Say No" approach accorded with the exclusive emphasis on primary prevention and with the refusal to discriminate between "soft" and "hard" drugs, which had been promoted since the late 1970s by the increasingly powerful parents' movement, some of whose leaders were appointed as drug policy advisers or officials (Musto, 1987).

The sudden increase in cocaine use associated with the introduction of a cheap smokable form (crack), along with well-publicized deaths of popular athletes, led to renewed concern with drug issues in 1985 and 1986. The administration resisted congressional calls for appointment of a "drug czar" to take control of the situation and coordinate what were perceived as fragmented and ineffective drug programs. A common complaint was that "Just Say No" is not enough, especially in communities devastated by the drug trade, violence, and widespread use by young people. The administration did agree to promote demand-side policies by widening the membership of the Policy Board to include health and education agencies and changing its name to the National Drug Policy Board; the secretary for Health and Human Services became the vice-chair of the board.

Congressional initiatives brought about a more far-reaching change in the salience of prevention policy, however. The 1986 Anti-Drug Abuse Act created for the first time a federal agency with exclusive responsibility for drug prevention. This was the Office of Substance Abuse Prevention (OSAP), set up within the Alcohol, Drug Abuse and Mental Health Administration (ADAMHA) of the Department of Health and Human Services at a level equivalent to that of NIDA and NIAAA. OSAP is mainly engaged in making demonstration grants for drug and alcohol prevention among groups that previous efforts were considered to have neglected: high-risk youth, racial and ethnic minorities, and women of child-bearing age. In 1992, OSAP was renamed the Center for Substance Abuse Prevention (CSAP), within the newly organized Substance Abuse and Mental Health Services Administration (SAMHSA).

Table 1.4 presents data on prevention expenditures by various federal agencies. ADAMHA still handles the ADM block grants to the state agencies, which constitute the largest source of prevention funding for programs outside the schools. The largest federal prevention programs, though, are those of the Department of Education. These consist mainly of federal grants to the states under the Drug-Free Schools and Communities Act (part of the 1986 Act); 70% of these grants is designated for the state education agencies, and the remaining 30% is for allocation at the governor's discretion. (The practice varies among states, but the most common choices are for this money to be handled either by the state alcohol and drug agency that handles the ADM block grant funds or by the state education agency.)

The Department of Housing and Urban Development, like the Department of Education, has been brought back into the drug prevention field. Various programs support efforts of local public housing authorities and tenants to end the drug trade and discourage drug use within housing projects, usually as adjuncts to enforcement efforts directed at drug trafficking in housing projects. (What has changed since 1972 is that no one refers to "Model Cities" anymore.)

TABLE 1.4   Federal Funding for Prevention Programs, Fiscal Year 1992

BUDGET AUTHORITY	($ MILLIONS)
Department of Health and Human Services	697
ADAMHA other than OSAP (includes block grant to states)	304
OSAP	285
Department of Education	627
Other departments (Defense, Labor, etc.)	383
Total	1,707

Source: ONDCP, 1992.

PROBLEMS OF PREVENTION POLICY

Lack of a Research Base and Evidence of Success

One of the explanations for the paradox of rhetorical support for prevention not translating into high spending levels has no doubt been the lack of detailed knowledge about what works. As the later chapters in this book make clear, our knowledge about the effects of programs and the replicability of small-scale successes is very incomplete, and of recent vintage. This is partly a recursive explanation, however, because a major reason so little is now known is that there was little funding for research into prevention until very recently, and that forms part of the larger question of why there was so little public funding for anything connected with prevention.

Lack of systematic knowledge is also rather a technocratic explanation. After all, evaluations of the effectiveness of drug enforcement are almost as scanty and unconvincing. More important may be that the federal government does have agencies directly involved in drug enforcement, providing a very visible product. More money for the Customs Service generates what is colloquially referred to as "powder on the table": tangible, short-term evidence that the federal expenditures have accomplished something.

The closest equivalent to "powder on the table" for prevention programs would be clear evidence linking particular measures to subsequent reductions in drug use among target populations, but this is hard to obtain, especially when programs operate outside the relatively controlled environment of schools. Again, the problem is partly the scarcity and methodological weakness of research in this field,[13] but there are also problems intrinsic to the nature of prevention. Prevention works, if it works at all, by hastening and reinforcing changes in the social environment of drug use and in the attitudes of potential drug users. Such changes can never easily be ascribed to single acts of the authorities or of private organizations, but such acts may cumulatively have a large effect on them.

Lack of an Institutional Home

Although there is now a prevention agency at the federal level, it is not responsible for the largest portion of prevention funding. Before the creation of OSAP, prevention had always been a shared, usually secondary, concern of agencies at the federal level. NIDA was more interested in basic research and treatment (being traditionally dominated by the "bench scientists" rather than social scientists or policy entrepreneurs). The Department of Education, other social policy agencies, and the law enforcement agencies had their own core tasks, and drug prevention would never occupy much of their budgets or high-level attention.[14] At the state and local levels, drug prevention in the public sector is still the responsibility of the education agency and school districts and of the alcohol and drug agencies. The schools, of course, have a great deal besides drug prevention on their agenda. They are under pressure to improve performance in teaching the basic subjects.

The competition may be fiercer for class time than for money, though the popularity of programs like Project DARE, which bring police into classrooms to conduct drug education and teach resistance skills, may have something to do with the fact that they are usually funded out of law enforcement budgets. This is because one of the most consistent research findings underlying current reform efforts is that student performance in the basic subjects is related to time on task. Time spent on administrative minutiae, disciplinary measures, moving around, getting ready for activities, and drug prevention, however necessary, is time not spent learning mathematics. Under rising pressure to improve the workforce skills of their graduates, schools are reluctant to allocate more time to "life skills" courses. Pressure for increasing prevention funding may well decline in the near future as middle-class parents see diminishing risk of their children becoming seriously involved with drugs.

The alcohol and drug agencies are responsible for treatment, which has always occupied more of their funding and staff time than prevention. Here the problem may be that treatment, as well as law enforcement, is demand- or incident-driven. Public agencies are ultimately responsible for providing treatment to the large numbers of indigent clients and those referred by the criminal justice system. Treatment budgets have been growing. But the task imposed on agencies by the recent cocaine epidemic is much greater than that posed by the heroin epidemics of the late 1960s and 1970s. Several million persons, by most estimates, are dependent on cocaine;[15] many lack adequate health insurance to cover private treatment; many others will run through the coverage they have and show up in the public system for future treatment episodes. A repetition of the experience of the early 1980s, when agencies were fully occupied providing treatment to the stable population of heroin addicts left over years after the growth phase of the epidemic, seems likely. Moreover, the task will be a harder

one for the lack of any counterpart to methadone for cocaine addicts.

As drug problems have changed and proliferated and efforts to control them have rapidly increased, allocation of responsibility has shifted without much attention being given to the appropriate roles of different institutions. For example, Congress has enacted a law to withhold various federal privileges such as student loans for persons convicted of drug possession offenses; this represents an effort by the federal government to extend its reach beyond the higher levels of trafficking to the punishment of users, a traditional state role (Anti-Drug Abuse Act of 1988, Title V, Subtitle G). The federal government is also under pressure to increase its funding and regulation of public treatment programs, traditionally a state responsibility. Private–public boundaries are also being redefined as the pressure for workplace testing programs rises (Anti-Drug Abuse Act of 1988, Title V, Subtitle D; ONDCP, 1989, 1990a).

The involvement of many players in the drug policy process is appropriate. However, it exacerbates the problem of formulating policy. The new federal strategy may have redirected federal efforts and reduced friction among federal agencies. However, it cannot, except through exhortation, impose a strategy on the nonfederal actors, who are responsible for most drug policy decisions and program implementation. Prevention is a program area whose implementation is primarily determined by autonomous school districts and by voluntary groups, ranging from the Partnership for a Drug Free America to local church groups trying to prevent drug use in high-risk adolescents in inner-city communities.

Fragmentation of Programs

At least since the publication of the Drug Abuse Council's Final Report in 1980, observers have recognized the problems caused by the sharp barriers between the various agencies and professions involved in controlling drug problems. Enforcement officials are now rhetorical enthusiasts for increased prevention, but never at the expense of their own budgets. Moreover, notwithstanding the use of police officers in classrooms (as in Project DARE), the barriers that divide enforcement, treatment, and prevention are not noticeably lower than in the past.

To some extent, this division reflects the different backgrounds and orientations of professionals in the different kinds of agencies. Police and doctors are not natural allies; they speak different languages, they have different constituencies and different goals. The alliances between schools and police departments are not much easier to create.

Agencies also fail to take into account (and often have no incentive to do so) the interdependence of their individual actions. The crackdowns on street markets by big-city police departments have flooded treatment systems with criminal justice referrals; yet rarely if ever is an effort made to coordinate the treatment and enforcement efforts. At the federal level, the fact that more intense interdiction is likely to exacerbate source country drug problems is an important interaction that has never been considered in discussions of the appropriate allocation of efforts among different programs (Reuter, 1988). For prevention, which works on a much larger time scale, interdependence is less striking. Note, however, the difficulties of mounting effective prevention programs in inner-city schools whose students daily confront the availability of both drugs and drug selling opportunities, absent an effective police effort aimed at reducing visible drug trafficking.

Mix of Public and Private Sector Responsibilities

A larger concern may be that the government at any level is very limited in its ability to induce changes in behavior. The tasks entailed by drug prevention may just be more suited to private than to public action, and within the public sphere, to local rather than to central government. An official of NASADAD put this point

well, claiming that "prevention is not so much a service you deliver as a movement you support." How does the government support a nongovernmental movement?

Values are transmitted from generation to generation mainly through what Berger and Neuhaus (1977) termed the "mediating structures" of family, church, school, and neighborhood. The ability of the central government, in particular, to affect the content of what is transmitted, or the intensity of concern with different topics, is very limited. There has always been, for example, great suspicion in the United States of any attempts to introduce a national curriculum into the schools; states and local school districts jealously guard their control over the content of education in the public system. (The Model Drug Curriculum issued by OSAP and the Department of Education in 1990 does not yet have counterparts in mathematics or any of the core subjects.) Most of the money spent on schooling is raised locally; the federal contribution consists largely of funding for some special efforts such as Head Start programs, as well as research and dissemination.

It is even more firmly regarded as none of the government's business what the churches do and say. At a local level, especially in the inner cities, churches often form the nucleus around which community prevention activities are organized. None of the grantees in the first round of OSAP demonstration grants included church affiliates, and no religious groups were listed in the *Citizen's Alcohol and Other Drug Prevention Directory: Resources for Getting Involved,* published by OSAP.

Nonetheless, the idea of the government promoting behavioral change through its research and dissemination, through the schools, and in cooperation with voluntary community efforts is in accord with a larger trend in public health policy; it is not idiosyncratic to the drug field. An influential report from the Surgeon General in 1979 distinguished the older tasks of "disease prevention" from the newer requirements of "health promotion" (Surgeon General, 1979).

The former includes programs and campaigns mainly directed at controlling infectious diseases such as immunization, vector control, surveillance, and contact tracing. The latter includes efforts aimed mainly at reducing chronic diseases through inducing changes in lifestyles;[16] the preeminent example cited in the 1979 report was the MRFIT program to reduce hypertension. Chronic diseases for which personal behaviors are the major risk factors have become the major killers in the United States, and there is little dispute about the legitimacy (as opposed to the effectiveness) of government programs aimed at modifying a range of behaviors, many perfectly legal, in the interests of public health.

Long Time Horizons

Primary prevention is at best a long-term proposition: If large-scale school-based programs aimed at early adolescents have as much effect on initiation of drug use as some experimental programs have shown, and if the reductions persist through adolescence and young adulthood, then we should see a substantial reduction in the numbers of persons requiring treatment for drug dependence some time after the year 2000, because the peak ages for treatment admissions are in the twenties and thirties. A comparable time perspective can be used to judge the effects of the sustained campaign against tobacco use. After decades of a buildup of scientific evidence of its dangers, which had passed into folk wisdom about tobacco, the visible public-sector effort to discourage use can be said to have begun in 1965 with the publication of the first Surgeon General's report. Subsequent declines in tobacco use are now just beginning to show up in lower prevalence of lung cancer and other diseases. The pace of these profound behavioral changes is thus brisker—but not much more so—than that envisioned a half-century ago by W. R. Inge, who wrote that "the best time to influence a child is 100 years before he is born" (Marchant, 1968, p. 78).

Such a long time horizon is a serious defect for a program in the domestic policy arena. When budgets must be cut, it is always least painful to cut the budget of the program of which the effects will not be felt immediately.[17]

The "Drug War" metaphor itself shows some of the impatience surrounding drug policy: Nobody wants, nor at their beginning expects, wars to drag on for too long. Inge's time scale seems geologic compared to that Congress adopted in the 1988 Anti-Drug Abuse Act, which declared a national policy to achieve a "Drug-Free America" by 1995. No one, probably not even the authors of this section of the Act, takes such pronouncements too seriously. After all, there has never before been a Drug-Free America, nor a Drug-Free Anywhere Else, a point sensibly made by the 1989 ONDCP *Strategy*. But constant repetition of such phrases may have an unintended harmful effect, setting up public opinion for disappointment and premature disillusion. Prevention campaigns aimed at deadly chronic diseases have managed to win support without promising a "Heart-Disease-Free America" or a "Cancer-Free America," certainly not within the next decade. Drug policy would probably benefit at this point from the long-term commitment, rational setting of targets, and evaluation of alternative policy instruments that have (sometimes) characterized policy in other public health areas.

THE FUTURE OF PREVENTION POLICY

A variety of indicators point to a decline in rates of initiation into drug use by adolescents. Indeed, data from the two major surveys, the High School Senior Survey (HSSS) (Johnston, O'Malley, & Bachman, 1992) and the National Household Survey (NHS) (NIDA, 1993), suggest that these rates began to decline by the mid-1980s at the latest. This has important implications for prevention as a component of drug control efforts.

The decline seems to have its origins in changing attitudes toward health and an increased belief in the dangerousness of drug use. The percentages reporting in the HSSS that the regular use of marijuana or occasional use of cocaine will lead to adverse affects has been rising steadily even as the perceived availability of drugs has either been constant or has risen. The decline is not a consequence of tough enforcement making drugs more difficult to obtain.

The role of prevention programs in the decline in reported drug use is difficult to determine. There are no data on the exposure of adolescents to drug prevention messages, even in schools. It is impossible to determine whether the respondents in the HSSS of 1989 received more such messages than those of 1979. Our impression is that large-scale systematic prevention efforts did not take hold until at least the mid-1980s and were aimed primarily at junior high and elementary school students. The senior class of 1989, for example, already in ninth grade by 1985, may not have had much more exposure to drug prevention programs in their classes than did their 1979 counterparts.

Of course, they did have considerable exposure to the mass media reporting of the drug problem, such a staple of the nightly news and front pages in the second half of the 1980s. Whether reports of deaths and violence associated with drug use and trafficking affect adolescent behavior is uncertain. At least one recent survey of teen attitudes correlated declining prevalence with exposure to mass media messages as well as other community and school efforts (Black, 1990). Analyses of time devoted to drug stories in prime time television news show that very little of that time goes to coverage of prevention or treatment programs. Similarly, it is impossible to say much about the impact of the government's use of the mass media, such as Nancy Reagan's "Just Say No" campaign.

Our own view is that the change in adolescent behavior is largely a change in social attitudes toward health, accelerated by the spread of knowledge about the health consequences of drug use.[18] Continued progress will probably require more experimentation with ways to deliver the messages and more creative efforts by the public sector to support the social institutions through which the most powerful communication takes place. As the drug epidemic fades from public prominence, the task of the prevention community will be to maintain the funding levels for their programs as the more visible and intrusive enforcement efforts take their cuts. In an environment of concern for cost-effectiveness and long time horizons, prevention may finally play the dominant role.

NOTES

1. We deal here mainly with programs aimed at use of illegal drugs. The distinction between drugs that are illegal (except for very limited research uses) and those that are legal, at least for adults or for medical use, is often artificial but important for many aspects of policy. The school-based prevention programs typically concern alcohol and tobacco use and prescription drug misuse as well as use of illegal drugs. Mass media campaigns and other community-based prevention efforts are often more narrowly focused on the illegal drugs.

2. Another 9% was uncategorized.

3. In doing so, we hesitantly follow the conventional path that gives little systematic attention to prevention programs aimed at those who are regular users but have not yet experienced serious problems related to that use. The numbers of such persons are a great deal smaller than those targeted by primary prevention efforts and it may be that, with appropriate outreach efforts (such as Student Assistance Programs), expansion of secondary prevention programs could be an efficient use of resources.

4. We put to one side the entertaining but so far inconsequential debate about changing the legal status of drugs; see Nadelmann (1989) and Wilson (1990a), for statements of the basic positions in this debate.

5. However, the distinction lives on in the very structure and organization of the ONDCP, which was required by its authorizing legislation to have one deputy for supply reduction and one deputy for demand reduction.

6. See Wilson (1990b) for similar arguments.

7. Reuter and Kleiman (1986) present a framework for analyzing the varieties of drug enforcement programs.

8. Proponents of the federal subsidies to tobacco farmers have occasionally argued that they help keep prices high and thus hold consumption down. More commonly, the tobacco lobby ignores the health issues with one voice. No one, to our knowledge, has proposed on public health grounds similar price supports for domestic growers of marijuana or manufacturers of other drugs.

9. That intensified enforcement will raise prices is an article of faith, not yet tested in any systematic empirical study.

10. Cocaine sells in illegal markets for about 20 times its legal price; use of dirty needles by heroin addicts is largely a function of the prohibition on unauthorized possession of hypodermic needles.

11. Indeed, drug-related homicide appeared to rise in 1990, despite evidence of reduced drug consumption. See ONDCP (1990c).

12. The DEA resumed its demand reduction activity in the late 1980s; it now consists primarily of a speakers program wherein its agents give talks to youth and community groups.

13. Tonry (1990) makes similar points about the weakness and fragmentation of drug policy research in general. A recent conference considered the narrower issues of federal data needs (Haaga & Reuter, 1990a), pointing to how little is currently well-measured in the drug policy field.

14. A partial exception to this rule was the Department of Education under Secretary Bennett, later the first head of ONDCP.

15. There are no estimates of the cocaine-dependent population as such. The closest available estimate is of the number of current weekly users of cocaine (U.S. Senate, 1990).

16. The identification of health promotion with modification of individual behavior has been criticized as being too narrow because many efforts to improve the environment and living standards could also be regarded as health promotion, yet did not easily fit into the report's other categories of health programs, "medical care" and "disease prevention" (Terris, 1986, p. 149). A larger concern is the degree to which all the health problems of poor people and ethnic minorities will be misleadingly ascribed simply to their presumed greater prevalence of substance abuse, which can then be dismissed as something for which the government is not responsible.

17. This is the converse of what Charles Peters, editor of the *Washington Monthly,* has termed the "Firemen First Rule": When policymakers want to pretend to cut budgets, they announce cutbacks in visible and vital services whose beneficiaries can bring overwhelming pressure to bear. Despite the active interest of the parents' movement in the last decade, there is no such powerful lobby speaking for the presumed beneficiaries of prevention programs.

18. Evidence to support this conclusion can be found in the attitudinal data from the Monitoring the Future project, (Bachman, Johnston, & O'Malley, 1990a, 1990b).

REFERENCES

Anti-Drug Abuse Act of 1988, Title V, Subtitle D, Drug-free workplace act, PL 100-960.

Anti-Drug Abuse Act of 1988, Title V, Subtitle G, Denial of federal benefits to drug traffickers and possessors, PL 100-960.

Bachman, J. G., Johnston, L. D., & O'Malley, P. M. (1990a). Explaining the recent decline in cocaine use among young adults: Further evidence that perceived risks and disapproval lead to reduced drug use. *Journal of Health and Social Behavior, 31* (June).

Bachman, J. G., Johnston, L. D., & O'Malley, P. M. (1990b). Explaining the recent decline in marijuana use: Differentiating the effects of perceived risks, disapproval, and general lifestyle factors. *Journal of Health and Social Behavior, 29* (April).

Berger, P., & Neuhaus, R. (1977). *To empower people: The role of mediating structures in public policy.* Washington, DC: American Enterprise Institute.

Black, G. S. (1990). The partnership for a drug-free America attitude tracking study. Rochester, NY: Gordon S. Black Corp.

Butynski, W., Canova, D., & Reds, J. L. (1992). *State resources and services related to alcohol and other drug abuse problems, fiscal year 1989.* Washington, DC: National Association of State Alcohol and Drug Abuse Directors, Inc.

Domestic Council Drug Abuse Task Force (Sept. 1975). *White paper on drug abuse.* Washington, DC: The White House.

Drug Abuse Council (1980). *The "facts" about drug abuse.* New York: Free Press.

Drug Abuse Office and Treatment Act of 1972, PL 92-255.

Goldberg, P. B., & DeLong, J. V. (1972). Federal expenditures on drug-abuse control. In *Dealing with drug abuse: A report to the Ford Foundation.* New York: Praeger, pp. 300–328.

Haaga, J., & Reuter, P. (1990a). The limits of the czar's ukase: Drug policy at the local level. *Yale Law and Policy Review, 8,* pp. 36–74.

Haaga, J., & Reuter, P. (Eds.) (1990b). *Improving data collection in support of federal drug policy.* Santa Monica, CA: RAND Corporation.

Johnston, L., O'Malley, P., & Bachman, J. (1992). *Monitoring the future.* Rockville, MD: National Institute on Drug Abuse.

Kleiman, M., & Mockler, R. (1988). *Heroin and AIDS strategies.* Washington, DC: The Urban Institute.

Marchant, Sir J. (1968). *The wit and wisdom of Dean Inge.* New York: Books for Libraries Press.

Moore, M. (May 1973). Achieving discrimination in the effective price of heroin. *American Economic Review, 63.*

Mosher, J. F., & Jernigan, D. H. (1989). New directions in alcohol policy. *Annual Review of Public Health, 10,* pp. 243–279.

Musto, D. F. (1987). *The American disease: Origins of narcotic control,* expanded edition. New York: Oxford University Press.

Nadelmann, E. (1989). Drug prohibition in the United States: Costs, consequences, and alternatives. *Science, 245.*

National Commission on Marihuana and Drug Abuse (1973). *Drug use in America: Problem and perspective.* Washington, DC: U.S. Government Printing Office, pp. 346–367.

National Institute on Drug Abuse (1993). *National household survey of drug abuse.* Washington, DC: U.S. Dept. of Health and Human Services.

Office of National Drug Control Policy (1989, 1990a). *National drug control strategy.* Washington, DC: U.S. Government Printing Office.

Office of National Drug Control Policy (1990b, 1992). *National drug control strategy: Budget summaries.* Washington, DC: U.S. Government Printing Office.

Office of National Drug Control Policy (1990c). *Leading drug indicators.* Washington, DC: U.S. Government Printing Office.

Polich, J. M., Ellickson, P. L., Reuter, P., & Kahan, J. L. (1984). *Strategies for controlling adolescent drug use.* Santa Monica, CA: RAND Corporation.

Reuter, P. (1988). Can the borders be sealed? *The Public Interest, 92.*

Reuter, P., & Kleiman, M. (1986). Risks and prices: An economic analysis of drug enforcement. In M. Tonry & N. Morris (Eds.), *Crime and justice: An annual review of research,* vol. 7. Chicago: University of Chicago Press.

Royal College of Psychiatrists, Special Committee on Drugs and Drug Dependence (1987). *Drug scenes.* London: Gaskell.

Russell, L. B. (1986). *Is prevention better than cure?* Washington, DC: Brookings Institution.

Skolnick, J. (1990). A critical look at the national drug control strategy. *Yale Law and Policy Review, 8* (1).

Surgeon General of the United States (1979). *Healthy people: The surgeon general's report on health promotion and disease prevention.* Washington, DC: U.S. Dept. of Health, Education, and Welfare.

Terris, M. (1986). What is health promotion? *Journal of Public Health Policy, 7* (2).

Tonry, M. (1990). Research on drugs and crime. In M. Tonry & J. Q. Wilson (Eds.) *Drugs and crime.* Chicago: University of Chicago Press.

U.S. Senate, Committee on the Judiciary (May 10, 1990). *Hard-core cocaine addicts: Measuring and fighting the epidemic.* Washington, DC: U.S. Government Printing Office.

Wald, P. M., & Abrams, A. (1972). Drug education. In *Dealing with drug abuse: A report to the Ford Foundation.* New York: Praeger, pp. 123–172.

Wilson, J. Q. (Jan. 1990a). Against legalization. *Commentary, 79* (1).

Wilson, J. Q. (1990b). Drugs and crime. In M. Tonry & J. Q. Wilson (Eds.), *Drugs and crime.* Chicago: University of Chicago Press.

CHAPTER 2

PRINCIPLES OF PREVENTION

GILBERT J. BOTVIN

INTRODUCTION

Recent years have witnessed a dramatic change in the stature of drug abuse as a national problem. According to countless public opinion surveys, drug abuse is widely viewed as one of the most important problems facing this country. Although the ascendancy of drug abuse to the top of the national agenda is a relatively recent phenomenon, drug abuse has been a source of concern to schools, community organizations, health professionals, and law enforcement agencies for more than two decades. Efforts to reduce drug abuse that began toward the end of the psychedelic '60s have intensified in recent years with the active involvement of both public and private agencies.

The Need for New Solutions

According to recent survey data, the United States has the highest rate of drug use in the industrialized world (Johnston, Bachman, & O'Malley, 1988). As drug-related crime has soared, the American public—along with community leaders, health professionals, and policymakers—has become increasingly concerned about finding effective solutions. In recent years, this concern has grown into a sense of urgency due to the role intravenous drug use plays in the transmission of AIDS, a fatal disease for which no known cure exists.

Past efforts to reduce demand for drugs through treatment or prevention approaches have produced disappointing results. Drug abusers often possess a knowledge of drugs that may be daunting to even the most experienced practi-

tioner. Although there are a number of effective treatment models, treatment gains are often eroded by recidivism unless ongoing support is provided. Moreover, the availability of drugs and a network of friends who use drugs promote continued drug use and can undermine progress made by individuals trying to kick the habit. A related problem that has hindered efforts to decrease drug abuse is that there are many more individuals in need of treatment for drug dependence than there are available treatment slots. At the same time, prevention approaches based on information about the adverse consequences of drug use, personal development, and alternatives to drug use have had little measurable impact on drug use. Finally, law enforcement (supply reduction) efforts have done little to reduce the flow of drugs or disrupt distribution systems; most drugs continue to be widely available.

The Quest for Effective Prevention Strategies

The magnitude of the drug problem and the disappointing results of past treatment and prevention approaches provide a powerful dual impetus for developing new intervention strategies. Unfortunately, finding more powerful approaches to the drug abuse problem has been far more difficult than was initially imagined. For example, only in the past decade has evidence demonstrating the potential of drug abuse prevention approaches gradually emerged. This evidence comes from studies testing the efficacy of primary prevention strategies designed to affect the social and psychological factors believed to promote initial use and later abuse. The earliest studies were small-scale pilot studies that focused on cigarette smoking. More recent studies have been not only larger but better designed and more methodologically sophisticated, and have focused on multiple substances. Together, the existing literature of evaluation studies ranging from small-scale pilot studies to large-scale randomized prevention trials now provides substantial evidence for the effectiveness of prevention approaches that target the social and psychological factors believed to promote the onset and early stages of drug abuse.

Thus, despite the conventional wisdom that drug abuse prevention does not work and criticism of the past prevention studies, there is considerable evidence supporting the efficacy of contemporary prevention approaches. This evidence is much stronger and more impressive than the evidence that drug abuse can be reduced using supply reduction strategies, but prevention still receives a disproportionately small amount of federal funding. Although additional research is clearly needed to refine existing prevention models, enough is known at this time to delineate some general prevention principles.

In this chapter, we shall begin with a general consideration of prevention issues and discuss the empirical and conceptual foundations of contemporary drug abuse prevention strategies. Next, we specify the objectives that should guide prevention research and serve as a standard against which to assess the success of prevention approaches. The key ingredients of effective prevention approaches are then summarized along with a description of the target population, program providers, program parameters, and implementation issues. The final section provides an overview of critical evaluation issues.

UNDERSTANDING THE CONCEPT OF PREVENTION

Many different approaches to drug abuse are routinely included under the general classification of prevention. Some of these approaches may involve law enforcement activities such as arresting drug kingpins and stopping the flow of drugs both across and within the borders of our country. Others consist of providing educational programs to elementary and secondary school students. Still others attempt to involve adolescents in sports and other activities viewed as either being inconsistent with drug use or possibly serving as alternatives to drug use. These programs involve a diversity of individuals, including those who have never used drugs, those identified as being at risk for becoming drug abusers, and those who already are using drugs. Thus, it is readily apparent that some clarification is necessary to better understand what prevention is.

Defining Prevention

Prevention is a broad concept that has frequently included a wide range of approaches. Three types of prevention have been defined: primary prevention, secondary prevention, and tertiary prevention. *Primary prevention* is activities designed to *prevent* a disease, disorder, or condition from ever developing by intervening before any manifestations of that disease, disorder, or condition are present. Targets of primary prevention may, however, be at high risk for the disorder. To the prevention purist, only primary prevention is prevention in its truest sense.

The objective of *secondary prevention,* on the other hand, is to *treat* individuals who have been identified as having some disorder or disease as early as possible in order to reduce the length and severity of the disorder or disease, and to return individuals to their previous level of functioning as quickly as possible. Another way of conceptualizing secondary prevention is as early intervention.

The objective of *tertiary prevention* is to reduce the degree of impairment and suffering once a disorder or disease has developed, in order to minimize the long-term consequences. Thus, tertiary prevention is more correctly understood as *rehabilitation.*

Interventions fall along a continuum ranging from primary prevention to treatment. To
some extent, the tripartite conceptualization of
prevention used in public health has blurred the
lines separating prevention and treatment, and
has created ambiguity concerning what is meant
by prevention and confusion over precisely where
one draws the line between prevention and treatment. The definition of prevention has important
implications for defining the goals of prevention
activities and for determining the most appropriate intervention strategies. Although this chapter
has been written largely from the perspective of
primary prevention, the principles articulated
have applicability to a wide range of prevention
activities.

Prevention and Physical Health

In public health terminology, primary prevention
works to reduce incidence of disease by neutralizing or eliminating the noxious agent in the environment, strengthening the host, or preventing
the transmission of the noxious agent to the host
There are many examples of the success of primary prevention in the field of public health.
When chlorine was added to water supplies, the
incidence of cholera declined; the noxious agent
had been neutralized. Vaccinations have reduced
the incidence of polio, smallpox, and tetanus by
strengthening the resistance of the host. Controlling the mosquito population has prevented the
transmission of malaria and yellow fever.

In the field of medicine, prevention has been
responsible for a much greater proportion of the
historic improvements in the health and
longevity of the general public than all of the
treatment modalities put together, including the
most dazzling developments of modern high-tech
medicine. Infectious diseases such as measles
and cholera were clearly identifiable by the presence of a germ. With the eradication of many
sources of infection in the United States, however, and the development of safe inoculations,
the leading cause of death and morbidity has
largely shifted from infectious diseases to diseases caused by unhealthy lifestyle patterns or
health-compromising behaviors.

Cigarette smoking, for instance, is the leading preventable cause of death and disability in
the United States today. Alcohol and other forms
of drug use also account for a high incidence of
death and disability. However, unlike traditional
illnesses such as cholera and measles, it is not always clear exactly when a behavioral disorder
begins. For example, experts disagree about the
precise point along the drug use–abuse continuum at which use becomes abuse. Moreover, the
definition of abuse often varies by substance and
population.

Prevention and Mental Health

Albee (1984) has used prevention strategies in
public health to organize prevention activities in
the field of psychology. Specifically, Albee observes that the incidence of mental disorders or
problem behaviors can be reduced by decreasing
the noxious agent or by increasing the resistance
of the host. Noxious agents related to problem
behaviors include organic factors such as brain
damage or lead poisoning, stress, and exploitation, which includes poverty and oppression. The
resistance of the host includes personal and social competence, coping skills, self-esteem, and
social support—factors that protect an individual
from stress and disruption.

Prevention and Drug Abuse

The official definition of drug abuse used by the
American Psychiatric Association (DSM-III;
APA, 1987) is based on the following criteria: a
pathological pattern of use, impairment of functioning in work and social relationships, and a duration of at least a month. However, many experts
believe that to wait to intervene until this point
with adolescents would be irresponsible (Semlitz
& Gold, 1986). There is no widely accepted consensus as to when drug use becomes abuse, and
for children and adolescents—especially young

adolescents—any degree of drug use is often viewed as abuse.

Although national drug abuse policy goals correctly address reducing the prevalence of drug abuse, the appropriate goal of prevention efforts should be defined in terms of reducing the *incidence* of drug abuse (the number or percentage of new cases) rather than in terms of overall prevalence (the total number or percentage of existing cases, combining both old and new cases). The implication for the development, implementation, and evaluation of individual preventive interventions is that they should focus on preventing the onset of drug use.

With respect to drug abuse prevention, then, prevention strategies should target a general population of individuals who, for the most part, have not yet begun using tobacco, alcohol, or other drugs. Moreover, preventive interventions should target individual and environmental factors viewed as promoting or supporting the initiation of drug use and subsequent patterns of drug abuse.

THE EMPIRICAL FOUNDATION FOR PREVENTION

The development of effective drug abuse prevention approaches logically presupposes an understanding of the causes of drug abuse. The natural foundation on which to build successful prevention strategies, therefore, is one that takes into account the existing empirical evidence concerning the etiology of drug abuse. In addition to understanding the causes of drug abuse, it is also important to know something about the age of onset and the developmental course. These are summarized in the next section to provide a context for understanding contemporary drug abuse prevention approaches.

Onset and Early Stages of Drug Use

Most efforts to prevent drug abuse have targeted adolescents because drug use typically begins during the adolescent years. Drug use follows a predictable developmental progression beginning initially with experimentation and the recreational use of alcohol and cigarettes (Hamburg, Braemer, & Jahnke, 1975; Kandel, 1978). The individual may then progress to the use of marijuana. Only later is the individual likely to use other illicit drugs, with opiates and hallucinogens coming late in the sequence (Yamaguchi & Kandel, 1984).

During experimentation and recreational use, drugs are associated with pleasure and euphoria, and are not perceived to have negative effects. With more regular use, however, tolerance and need for the drug begins to develop; the individual becomes increasingly involved with drugs, and may begin using every day. Often at this stage more than one drug is being used. Performance and functioning begin to decline and the reason for using drugs shifts from using the drug for pleasure to avoiding negative feelings or withdrawal. Both psychological and physical addiction or dependence may follow the stage of regular use (Czechowikz, 1988; Millman & Botvin, 1992).

The existence of this sequence does not necessarily mean that an individual who begins using drugs occasionally will necessarily progress beyond that stage or that individuals who use one or more of the so-called gateway substances of tobacco, alcohol, or marijuana will necessarily progress to the use of other drugs (Yamaguchi & Kandel, 1984). In fact, most people use alcohol and other drugs without ever developing compulsive habits and loss of control.

Risk for drug use (legal and illicit) peaks between 18 and 22, with the exception of cocaine use, and risk for using drugs besides cocaine and prescription psychoactive drugs appears to decline after age 25 (Kandel & Logan, 1984). *The greatest risk that an individual will develop long-lasting or lifelong patterns of abuse occurs in individuals who begin using drugs before the age of 15* (Robins & Przybeck, 1985). For these reasons, then, the most natural target population for drug abuse prevention efforts is middle school and junior high students. However, as is noted in other chapters in this volume, prevention efforts can also be targeted at other populations, such as college students (Chapter 13), pregnant women (Chapter 16), and even the elderly (Chapter 20).

Etiologic Factors and Drug Abuse Risk

A large body of research suggests that a number of factors contribute to the initiation and early stages of drug use, including social influences and expectations, personality characteristics, pharmacological effects, and developmental factors of adolescence (Blum & Richards, 1979; Braucht, Follingstad, Brakrash, & Berry, 1973; Jessor, 1976; Meyer & Mirin, 1979; Ray, 1974; Wechsler, 1976).

Social influences play a powerful role in promoting and maintaining drug use. The single most important factor promoting drug use is whether parents, older siblings, and friends engage in drug use, and individuals whose friends or family members smoke, drink, or use other drugs are significantly more likely to become drug users than individuals whose family members or friends do not. Another important social influence to engage in drug use comes from the popular media, which all too often portray drug use as something that leads to increased popularity, sex appeal, sophistication, success, and good times.

Individual personality characteristics have also been found to be associated with drug use (Millman & Botvin, 1992). These include psychological characteristics, health knowledge, and attitudes. Some of the psychological characteristics associated with drug use and abuse include low self-esteem, low self-confidence, low self-satisfaction, greater need for social approval, low social confidence, high anxiety, low assertiveness, greater impulsivity, rebelliousness, a low sense of personal control, and an impatience to acquire adult status. Furthermore, individuals who know about the adverse consequences of tobacco, alcohol, and drug use as well as those who have negative attitudes toward drug use are less likely to become drug users.

Drug use and abuse have also been found to be highly correlated with a variety of other "problem behaviors." First, the use of one psychoactive drug is highly correlated with the use of other drugs. Second, individuals who smoke, drink, or use drugs also tend to get lower grades in school, are not generally involved in socially approved activities such as sports and clubs, and are also more likely than nonusers to exhibit antisocial patterns of behavior, including lying, stealing, and cheating (Demone, 1973; Jessor, Collins, & Jessor, 1972; Wechsler & Thum, 1973). Finally, drug use has also been found to be related to premature sexual activity, truancy, and delinquency.

Developmental factors associated with the adolescent period appear to increase risk for drug use and abuse. Adolescence is characterized by dramatic change and readjustment (Mussen, Conger, & Kagan, 1974), which often results in new stresses and anxieties and may increase vulnerability to peer pressure. Puberty, for example, is characterized by striking and rapid physical changes that can often disrupt self-image and self-esteem.

Changes occurring immediately before or during the beginning of adolescence that are part of the normal process of psychosocial development increase the likelihood that an individual will experiment with one or more psychoactive drugs. One way in which these developmental changes affect drug use risk is that they increase adolescents' susceptibility to direct and indirect social influences to smoke, drink, or use drugs. If drug use is consistent with the norms of their friends or the reference group with which they identify, the decline in parental influence with respect to lifestyle matters, the increased reliance on the peer group, and the increased tendency to conform to peer group norms will increase the probability that adolescents will use one or more drugs.

Furthermore, cognitive developmental changes can undermine previously acquired knowledge of the potential risks of using these drugs. Adolescents may notice inconsistencies between adult warnings and behavior or discover logical flaws in the arguments being advanced by adults against drug use. Finally, issues relating to identity and public image may substantially increase general susceptibility to advertising appeals and other social influences promoting drug use.

THE CONCEPTUAL FOUNDATION FOR PREVENTION

In order to develop effective prevention approaches, it is necessary not only to understand the causes of the disease, disorder, or condition to be prevented, but also to organize this information according to some theoretical or conceptual framework. In the case of drug abuse prevention, it is insufficient to simply catalogue the various factors researchers have identified as correlates or predictors of drug abuse. It is necessary to have some sense of how the various factors fit together and which factors are potentially amenable to intervention, and to design an intervention based on a comprehensive understanding of these different elements.

Two theories that provide the basis for developing a useful conceptual framework for both understanding the etiology of drug abuse and developing potentially effective prevention strategies are social learning theory (Bandura, 1977) and problem behavior theory (Jessor & Jessor, 1977). The central features of each of these theories are summarized here in terms of their importance for drug abuse prevention.

Social Learning Theory

According to social learning theory (Bandura, 1977), individuals learn how to behave through a process of modeling and reinforcement. This not only includes the imitation of specific observed behaviors and the direct reinforcement of those behaviors; it also includes vicarious observation of other individuals who engage in those behaviors and the consequence models they experience as a result of their behavior. Repeated exposure

to successful, high-status role models who use drugs—whether these role models are figures in the media, peers, or older siblings—are likely to influence adolescents.

Similarly, the perception that smoking, drinking, or the use of other drugs is standard practice among peers also serves to promote drug use through the establishment of normative beliefs supportive of drug use. These influences may suggest to adolescents that drug use is not only socially acceptable, but perhaps even necessary if they are to become popular, cool, sexy, grown up, sophisticated, macho, or tough. This perceived social payoff for drug use is likely to increase adolescents' susceptibility to peer pressure.

Susceptibility or vulnerability to social influences that promote drug use is affected by knowledge, attitudes, and beliefs. Because individuals can establish goals for the future, social learning theory recognizes the importance of self-regulation and self-control. Individuals who have goals for the future that are inconsistent with drug use and who are aware of the negative consequences of drug use are expected to be less likely to smoke, drink, or use drugs.

Personality characteristics also help determine susceptibility to social influence in general (Bandura, 1966; Rotter, 1972) and to drug use influences in particular (Demone, 1973; Jessor, Collins, & Jessor 1972; Wechsler & Thum, 1973). High susceptibility to these influences has been found to be related to low self-esteem, low self-satisfaction, low self-confidence, greater need for social approval, low sense of personal control, low assertiveness, greater impulsivity, and impatience to assume adult roles or appear grown-up. Thus, one strategy for promoting resistance to social influence might be to foster the development of characteristics associated with low susceptibility to such influence.

Problem Behavior Theory

Jessor's problem behavior theory (Jessor & Jessor, 1977) was developed to explain the development of problems occurring during adolescence such as drug use, precocious sexual behavior, delinquency, and truancy. The theory derives from a social psychological framework and recognizes the complex interaction of personal factors (cognitions, attitudes, beliefs), physiological and genetic factors, and perceived environmental factors.

Problem behaviors, as defined by Jessor, typically elicit a social response designed to control them. The social response may be informal and may merely involve disapproval. On the other hand, this response may be both formal and substantial, as in the case of incarceration. Many behaviors that are permissible for members of an older age group are viewed as problems for younger ones (such as smoking, drinking, and sexual involvement); for these, age norms may serve as the defining characteristic.

The reason adolescents engage in problem behaviors such as drug use and premature sexual behavior, according to problem behavior theory, is that these behaviors help the adolescent achieve desired personal goals. To the extent that adolescents perceive these behaviors as functional, they are motivated to engage in them. For example, problem behaviors may serve as a way of coping with real or anticipated failure, boredom, social anxiety, unhappiness, rejection, social isolation, low self-esteem, and lack of self-efficacy. These behaviors may also serve as a way of gaining admission to a particular peer group.

For adolescents who are not achieving academically, the use of psychoactive drugs may provide a way of achieving social status. Adolescents may believe that smoking, drinking, or using drugs will enhance their public image by making them look cool or by demonstrating independence from authority figures. Adolescents at the greatest risk of becoming drug users are those who perceive that alternative ways of achieving these same goals are unavailable.

Vulnerability to peer pressure is greater for adolescents who have fewer effective coping strategies in their repertoire, fewer skills for handling social situations, and greater anxiety about social situations. For these adolescents, the range of options for achieving personal goals is restricted at the same time that discomfort in interpersonal situations is high, motivating them to take some action in an effort to alleviate that discomfort.

Consistent with this pattern, one obvious and immediate way to delay drug use would be to make adolescents realize that it is a misperception to believe that the benefits of drug use outweigh the risks. However, unless adolescents believe that there are alternative ways of coping with anxiety, establishing effective interpersonal relationships, or achieving any other desired goal, they may be unwilling to forgo the perceived benefits of drug use.

Translating Theory into Practice

Consideration of the factors promoting drug use and abuse within the framework of these theoretical perspectives described provides general guidance concerning the type of prevention strategy that might be optimally effective. First, drug abuse prevention should eliminate, or at least reduce to the greatest extent possible, environmental influences promoting or facilitating the use of tobacco, alcohol, or drugs. This might be accomplished through measures that decrease the availability of these drugs (either directly or indirectly), by decreasing the visibility of negative (drug-using) role models, by increasing the visibility of attractive, high-status positive (non–drug using) role models, by altering attitudes and social norms concerning the acceptability of drug use and abuse, and by eliminating the promotion of drug use through the media (banning the advertisement of tobacco products and alcoholic beverages) or presenting drug use in a less exciting and glamorous way in movies and TV shows.

Such changes, however, are extremely difficult and expensive, and may take years to achieve. Moreover, because drug abuse occurs as a result of both environmental and individual factors, it is unlikely that drug abuse could be entirely prevented using this strategy, even in the rare event that substantial environmental changes were achieved.

Second, drug abuse prevention efforts should involve the development of preventive interventions designed to reduce susceptibility or vulnerability to the various environmental factors promoting drug use while attempting to reduce potential motivations to use drugs. One strategy for decreasing susceptibility to pro-drug environmental influences might involve the teaching of specific skills designed to resist social influences to smoke, drink, or use drugs. Two types of resistance skills should be taught: One involves teaching adolescents techniques for resisting peer pressure, and the other involves the teaching of skills designed to increase resistance to persuasive appeals from advertisers. Thus, adolescents' ability to deal with environmental influences promoting drug use might be increased by making adolescents aware of these sources of influence and by teaching them specific skills for countering them.

Susceptibility to negative environmental influences might also be reduced by increasing self-esteem, perceived control, self-confidence, self-satisfaction, and assertiveness. It is also important to teach adolescents the requisite life skills (decision making, goal setting, social skills, assertiveness) for increasing their likelihood of achieving desired goals and to provide them with an array of general coping skills (anxiety reduction and problem solving).

SPECIFICATION OF PREVENTION OBJECTIVES

In order to develop effective prevention programs and move the field of prevention forward, it is important to specify a set of clear and well-defined objectives. These objectives can be used both as targets to guide prevention efforts and as a means of assessing success. Eight general prevention objectives have been specified (Botvin, 1988). These objectives have been ordered in a hierarchical fashion and can be used to guide a logical and sequential approach to prevention research.

According to these objectives, prevention research should identify interventions that are feasible and acceptable to the target populations; can affect variables associated with drug abuse or drug abuse risk; can reduce the use or abuse of at least one drug; can reduce the use or abuse of multiple drugs; can produce lasting effects; are effective with several different populations; are adaptable to different conditions, providers, and delivery methods; and are exportable and easy to disseminate.

Feasibility and Acceptability

The first objective concerns determining whether promising prevention models are feasible and acceptable to both the target population and the program providers. Interventions that are too complex, require skills that program providers are unlikely to possess, have goals that are inconsistent with the norms of the community, or are mandated by overly zealous administrators may not be implemented at all or may be implemented with an inadequate degree of fidelity. Under these circumstances, even the most effective prevention approach will fail.

Impact on Drug Abuse Risk Factors

A second objective to be met in developing effective prevention approaches is to demonstrate that interventions affect variables associated with drug use and abuse. These variables might include knowledge of the deleterious effects of drug use, attitudes toward drug use, perceptions of the prevalence of drug use by peers or adults, behavioral intentions, self-efficacy, self-esteem, and locus of control. However, it is important to point out that many studies have been published that have produced significant knowledge or attitude changes, but have not produced changes on drug use behavior. Consequently, affecting variables associated with drug use and abuse, in the absence of any demonstrated impact on drug use, must be regarded as a low level of evidence for the effectiveness of a particular prevention approach.

Although the ultimate test of the effectiveness of a particular prevention program is the extent to which it reduces drug use, it may not be possible to collect behavioral data in some circumstances or with certain populations. Some school administrators or parents may refuse to permit the collection of data on drug use, particularly illicit drug use. As a result, the only means of evaluating program outcome may be measures of variables associated with drug use and abuse. Similarly, studies evaluating preventive interventions conducted with elementary school children cannot use behavioral variables because the prevalence of drug use is too low in most instances to permit meaningful statistical comparisons among individuals this young.

Interventions that can demonstrate an impact on variables that might be considered either risk factors for drug use and abuse or proxy measures of drug use behavior (such as behavior intention) can at least be viewed as demonstrating the *potential* of being effective prevention approaches. Clearly this kind of evidence alone does not indicate that a particular approach is effective, but it is a step in the right direction and does provide at least some basis for claiming a modicum of success.

Impact on a Single Type of Drug Behavior

A third and critically important objective in drug abuse prevention is to produce evidence indicating that a given prevention approach can prevent or delay at least one form of drug-taking behavior. Typically, drug involvement is measured by assessing the frequency or amount of use, patterns of use, and use associated with negative consequences. Outcome evaluation can be conceived of in terms of drug use status or scales of drug involvement. At the extreme end of both kinds of measures should be the inclusion of behavior that would be defined as drug abuse.

Although the overall goal of drug abuse prevention is, by definition, to prevent (or at least delay) the onset of drug abuse, in actuality the goals of preventive interventions are generally operationalized in terms of the wider continuum of drug use. Indeed, for both ideological and re-

search reasons, the goals of prevention programs targeted at youth tend to be defined in terms of the prevention of relatively low levels of drug use rather than in terms of drug abuse as it might be defined clinically. A reasonable expectation of prevention programs targeted at students during the beginning of junior high school would be that significant and meaningful reductions in the incidence of new drug use (i.e., the transition from nonuse to use) could be demonstrated using a standard 30-day current use variable. With somewhat older populations, where overall drug rates are typically higher, a reasonable expectation would be that prevention programs be able to demonstrate an impact on higher levels of drug involvement (weekly or daily use) that approach what might be defined as abuse.

Because primary prevention programs must be implemented before individuals are likely to become drug abusers, this generally means conducting preventive interventions during or before the junior high school years (the beginning of adolescence). However, among individuals in this age group, the base rates of drug abuse are so low that unless sample sizes are extremely large, statistical power is generally too low to identify real program effects. Hence, although the ultimate goal of drug abuse prevention efforts is to decrease the incidence of drug abuse, the most appropriate outcome variable for most preventive interventions targeted at individuals during the early adolescent years is *use* rather than *abuse*. Reducing drug use, then, is viewed not only as a legitimate goal of prevention approaches, but also as presumptive evidence of the efficacy of an intervention for preventing drug abuse. Still, if drug use is the outcome variable, then the burden must fall on researchers to demonstrate that interventions found to reduce drug use do result in reductions of drug abuse incidence.

Furthermore, the efficacy of preventive interventions targeted at adolescents can most reasonably be judged in terms of their impact on the use of tobacco (nicotine), alcohol, or marijuana because their use occurs toward the beginning of the developmental progression of drug abuse

(Kandel, 1978). In addition, because these are the three most prevalent drugs in our society, their base rates are higher than for other drugs. Consequently, statistical power for data analyses is higher for these drugs than for drugs with lower base rates, increasing the potential for detecting prevention effects. Thus, one of the most significant drug abuse prevention objectives is the ability of interventions to produce measurable effects on at least one of these three gateway drugs.

Impact on Multiple Types of Drug Behavior

Assuming that it is possible to demonstrate an impact on the use or abuse of one drug, a problem that must be confronted when attempting to develop effective preventive interventions is the extent to which prevention programs designed to affect one drug can also affect others—that is, the issue of generalization. If a particular intervention designed to prevent the use of drug X is found through evaluation research to be effective with X, what kinds of intervention modifications might be necessary to render it generalizable to drug Y and other drugs? Thus, a fourth objective is to demonstrate that a given preventive intervention can reduce the use of more than one drug. For example, interventions may be demonstrated to reduce all three gateway drugs.

A potential problem confronting prevention researchers is that they may need to develop specific interventions for different drugs or at least for different classes of drugs. If this turned out to be the case, then it would not bode well for the future of prevention in the real world. Interventionists would be overwhelmed by the complexity of a multitude of different interventions, each tailored for a specific drug or class of drugs. School schedules would buckle under the sheer weight of the number of interventions that would need to fit into an already crowded academic calendar. The best hope is that the causes of the various forms of drug use and abuse are similar enough that a generic intervention can be developed that is reasonably effective with all—or at least most—forms of drug abuse.

Durability of Prevention Effects

Demonstrating that prevention approaches can reduce drug use to any extent is a significant accomplishment, particularly in view of the fact that few prevention programs have been able to affect drug-taking behavior. Still, although it is certainly of theoretical significance that a particular prevention approach is capable of reducing drug use based on comparisons conducted immediately after its conclusion, it is of limited practical significance. If preventive interventions are to ultimately result in reductions in the incidence of drug abuse, they must produce effects that are reasonably long-lasting. Thus, the next major objective is to develop prevention approaches that produce durable effects.

Determining the durability of observed program effects requires longitudinal evaluation studies. Such studies are fraught with difficulties relating to tracking individual participants over the course of the study, differential attrition, the flagging enthusiasm of institutional support personnel (administrators and teachers in school-based studies), and resistance on the part of participants, who quickly lose interest in answering the same questions year after year.

Beyond the arduous task of conducting longitudinal drug abuse prevention research, it may be unrealistic to expect that any short-term intervention will produce a lasting impact on behavior. Rather, in order to achieve long-term effects, it may be necessary to implement long-term preventive interventions. For example, in school-based prevention, it may be unrealistic to expect that a single prevention unit conducted at the beginning of junior high school will produce lasting reductions in drug abuse incidence without ongoing interventions throughout junior and senior high school. If it is necessary to conduct interventions over an extended period of time, with different age groups as they move through different developmental stages, it is also necessary to determine the most effective interventions for each of these developmental stages as well as the most effective combination of intervention components.

Effectiveness with Multiple Populations

Another important issue concerns the generalizability of prevention effects from one population to another or, alternatively, the development of interventions that can be tailored to specific populations. Thus, a major prevention objective is to demonstrate the efficacy of one or more prevention approaches to several different populations. Because interventions are likely to be developed and initially tested on a particular population, a basic question that must be answered concerns the extent to which interventions developed and proven effective with one population will work with other populations. These different populations can be defined in various ways: in terms of race or ethnicity, socioeconomic status, age group, or drug abuse risk, for example.

Based on the fact that these populations are different, it might be argued that different preventive interventions are necessary. Different interventions might be necessary, for example, because the causes of drug abuse might differ in some fundamental way. Alternatively, the causes of drug abuse may be similar enough to warrant the application of a given prevention approach to several populations, but aspects of the intervention may need modification to render it more suitable to other populations. For example, interventions targeted at minority populations must be designed to be culturally sensitive. Some modifications might simply involve the kind of translation that can be accomplished by a skilled provider familiar with the population being targeted. Other modifications might need to be more extensive.

Adaptability

To be effective in the real world, preventive interventions must be adaptable to a variety of intervention conditions, providers, and delivery systems. Different conditions may require interventions that can be effective when implemented under different scheduling formats, to different group sizes, or in different types of institutions (schools or community agencies, for example). These interventions must be flexible and adaptable. They must be capable of being effective when implemented by more than one type of provider (by health professionals, teachers, or older peers, for example). Moreover, they must be adaptable to different delivery systems, such as those targeting individual students, schools, parents, and the larger community. Another prevention objective, therefore, is to determine the extent to which interventions that have been demonstrated to be effective under certain conditions, with certain providers, or using certain delivery systems are effective when adapted to other conditions, providers, and delivery systems.

Exportability and Ease of Dissemination

Related to adaptability are the issues of exportability and ease of dissemination. It may be quite difficult to transplant interventions found to be effective in one kind of environment to another. For example, interventions found to be effective in a nurturing research environment may be ineffective in a less nurturing environment where there is tremendous competition for time and resources. Some interventions may require specific intervention conditions that rarely exist or that are relatively unique to a particular situation. Such interventions, even if highly effective, are difficult to disseminate and consequently are of minimal value in achieving national reductions in the incidence of drug abuse. Thus, important considerations are the nature and structure of particular interventions as well as the resources needed to successfully implement them. For these reasons, a final objective in drug abuse prevention concerns developing interventions that are not only effective, but are also exportable and have a high potential for widespread dissemination.

COMPONENTS OF CONTEMPORARY PREVENTION PROGRAMS

Taking into account what is currently known about the etiology of drug abuse, relevant theories, reasonable drug abuse prevention objectives, and the results of evaluation studies, what kind of preventive intervention is likely to be effective? Based on existing knowledge, it is clear that the most effective prevention strategy would be one that has multiple components, uses program providers and delivery channels that efficiently reach the target population, and provides ongoing intervention throughout the critical period for the initiation of drug use.

Role of Information Concerning Drugs and Drug Use

In the past 25 years, schools across the United States have provided their students with tobacco, alcohol, and drug education courses. Most of these curricula are fragmented and poorly conceived, and are all too often taught by individuals with little or no expertise in the subject area. More recently, researchers have explored newer models of prevention based on a more complete understanding of the reasons why individuals become involved with one or more psychoactive drugs. Virtually all of the earlier approaches to drug education were based on the implicit assumption that adolescents behave in a logical and rational matter and that the solution to the problem of drug abuse was simply a matter of education (Goodstadt, 1978). The most common traditional approach involved providing adolescents with the facts about drugs and the risks of drug use.

Information alone does not work. Despite the ubiquity of traditional prevention approaches, the results from numerous evaluation studies have made it is abundantly clear that these approaches are not effective. Although approaches that rely exclusively on providing factual information about drugs have generally increased awareness of the negative consequences of drug use and occasionally have even had an impact on attitudes towards drug use, they have rarely been able to demonstrate an impact on actual drug use behavior (Berberian, Gross, Lovejoy, & Paparella, 1970; Braucht, Follingstad, Brakrash, & Berry, 1973; Goodstadt, 1974; Schaps et al., 1981; Swisher & Hoffman, 1975).

Information may increase drug use. Caution must be exercised in the type of information provided to adolescents in drug abuse prevention programs. Some information may be counterproductive: Instead of preventing or decreasing drug use, it may actually increase it. First, programs that emphasize the dangers of drug use may attract individuals who like to take risks because they find it exciting. Second, programs that provide specific information about the pharmacologic effects of drugs may arouse the curiosity of individuals who may wish to experience the psychoactive effects of these drugs first-hand. Finally, prevention programs that include information concerning modes of administration and other detailed information about drug use may inadvertently be providing a brief course in how to use drugs rather than in preventing use.

Information should address adverse consequences. Notwithstanding the fact that traditional information-based prevention approaches are either ineffective or in some cases even potentially harmful, some information may contribute to the impact of a prevention program. Although factual information about the adverse consequences of drug use is clearly not sufficient to deter use, it seems reasonable to assume that individuals should be provided with enough basic information to be aware of these consequences.

An awareness of the hazards of using drugs may serve as a deterrent for many individuals. However, the level of information necessary to accomplish this goal may be relatively low and may be acquired by most individuals before they reach middle or junior high school. In the case of cigarette smoking, for example, surveys have consistently demonstrated that by the time students reach junior high school, they are fully cognizant of the adverse health consequences of smoking. Providing individuals with a level of information beyond the minimum needed to know that using drugs may lead to health or legal problems probably does not lead to any meaningful decrease in drug abuse risk and may simply be a waste of time.

Information should be developmentally appropriate. For example, programs targeting adolescents should be guided by an understanding of how adolescents think and the major sources of concern for them. Because adolescents tend to be more concerned with the present than with the future, less emphasis should be place on information about long-term consequences of drug use than on more immediate ones.

Similarly, it is important to take into account the basic concerns of adolescents when discussing the adverse consequences of drug use. A major driving force in all adolescent activities concerns interpersonal relationships and group acceptance. Any perceived social benefits of using drugs may override concerns about long term consequences of drug use. On the other hand, the kind of negative consequences that may be the most salient for them are those that adolescents might view as social liabilities. Thus, instead of focusing on the adverse long-term health effects of cigarette smoking, for example, prevention programs should include information on more immediate consequences of smoking, such as nicotine stains on teeth and fingers, bad breath, the smell of smoke on clothes, and decreased endurance when participating in sports or other strenuous physical activities.

For young populations, information concerning drug dependence may be of little value. Adolescents are not only impervious to arguments concerning the adverse consequences of drug use, but labor under the illusion of control and invulnerability. They do not fully understand the subtle and seductive process that leads from initial experimentation and casual use to addictive patterns of use. Prevention programs should provide some information concerning the development of drug dependence to counteract the natural tendency of adolescents to believe that they can use drugs without succumbing to psychological or physical dependence.

Psychosocial risk factors should be addressed. Many prevention programs have included information on the psychosocial factors that promote and sustain drug use. This is an explicit or implicit objective of most effective contemporary approaches to drug abuse prevention. If they are aware of the predominantly social reasons why individuals initially become involved with drugs, adolescents may be less susceptible to those influences. To some extent, this is similar to the psychological inoculation approach initially advocated by Richard Evans and his colleagues in the area of smoking prevention (Evans et al., 1978). Information was included in the prevention approach developed by Evans to inoculate students against common social influences to smoke by gradually exposing them to those influences in progressively more intense amounts. Although most current prevention programs do not gradually expose participants to prodrug social influences, there does appear to be a general consensus that making individuals aware of the important role that social factors play in promoting drug use makes them more vigilant.

Attitudes, Beliefs, and Normative Expectations

A stated objective of many prevention programs (and an unstated one in others) is to change existing attitudes, beliefs, and norms concerning drug use in the target population. Evidence suggests that adolescents generally overestimate the prevalence of drug use among both peers and adults. Moreover, individuals who overestimate the prevalence of drug use tend to be at higher risk for becoming drug users themselves. The result of this misperception of drug use prevalence, particularly concerning peer use, is to provide individuals with the mistaken impression that everyone uses drugs, that it is both normal and acceptable.

Prevention programs endeavor to change normative expectations in one or more ways. First, information may be included that directly challenges the common belief that drug use is widespread. This information takes the form of facts concerning the actual prevalence rates of drug use among peers and adults. Second, the belief that drug use is widespread may be challenged through several class activities in school-based programs. For example, students may be asked to conduct their own survey of drug use in the school using an anonymous survey that can then be published in the school paper. Alternatively, program providers can simply conduct an informal poll of how many students currently smoke, drink, or use drugs. Third, even if the question is not addressed directly, prevention programs that use peer leaders may produce a change in normative expectations by actually changing school norms. Fourth, media campaigns or other community approaches to drug abuse prevention may include messages and images designed to modify attitudes, beliefs, and normative expectations.

Resistance Skills

The prevention model originally developed and tested by Evans and his colleagues (Evans et al., 1978) has been revised and refined by a host of other investigators (Arkin et al., 1981; Hurd et al., 1980; Johnson, Hansen, Collins, & Graham, 1986; Luepker, Johnson, Murray, & Pechacek, 1983; McAlister, Perry & Maccoby, 1979; McAlister et al., 1980; Murray, Johnson, Luepker, & Mittelmark, 1984; Perry, Killen, Slinkard, & McAlister, 1980; Telch et al., 1982) who were quick to see the potential in a prevention strategy that focused on social and psychological factors. A point of departure with Evans that has gradually become more evident over the past few years is a decreased reliance on psychological inoculation and an increased emphasis on training students to deal with both peer and media pressures.

Two distinctive features of these expanded approaches are the use of peer leaders (either older or same-age) to deliver some or all of the program and the use of role playing and social reinforcement techniques for teaching students skills for resisting offers to smoke cigarettes. Some studies have also included a public commitment component in which students were asked to publicly state that they would not smoke cigarettes. The hallmark of the resistance skills training approach is teaching adolescents specific skills or tactics for resisting influences from the media, friends, and family members to engage in drug use as well as skills for refusing explicit offers to use drugs or for dealing with direct coercive pressure from other individuals.

One aspect of resistance skills training involves making adolescents aware of the techniques used by advertisers to promote the sale of their products. Adolescents learn how to identify specific advertising techniques, analyze ads and their messages, and formulate counterarguments to common advertising appeals. Teaching these skills to adolescents is intended to increase their resistance to advertisements promoting cigarette smoking and alcohol use.

Another aspect of resistance skills training involves teaching adolescents how to refuse offers to smoke, drink, or use drugs. This includes teaching them what to say when they are invited or even pressured to engage in some form of drug use. It also includes teaching them how to say it in the most effective way possible. Adolescents are also taught to identify high-risk situations and to develop action plans for handling pressure in such situations.

The main objective of resistance skills training is to provide adolescents with a repertoire of verbal and nonverbal skills that they can call on when confronted by pressure to use drugs in a variety of situations. These skills are generally taught in the classroom (for school programs) through instruction or demonstration and practice (role playing). Extended practice outside the classroom to promote generalization and application to real-life situations is usually encouraged through behavioral homework assignments. A secondary objective of teaching and practicing these skills is to increase adolescents' confidence (self-efficacy) in their ability to handle difficult situations involving drug offers.

Personal and Social Skills

A second psychosocial approach to drug abuse prevention was designed to address the factors promoting drug use in a more comprehensive way (Botvin & Eng, 1982; Botvin et al., 1984; Botvin et al., 1990; Botvin, Renick, & Baker, 1983; Gilchrist & Schinke, 1985; Pentz, 1983;

Schinke & Blythe, 1981; Schinke & Gilchrist, 1983, 1984). The purpose of this approach is to teach a variety of personal and social skills in order to promote general competence and there by reduce motivations to smoke, drink or use drugs. This approach emphasizes generic skills including some combination of general problem-solving and decision-making skills, cognitive skills for resisting interpersonal and media influences, skills for increasing self-control and self-esteem, skills for coping effectively with anxiety or stress, general social skills, and general assertive skills. This type of generic skills training and competence enhancement approach can be used either alone or in combination with other prevention components.

Research conducted by Botvin and his colleagues at Cornell University has tested the efficacy of a prevention strategy called Life Skills Training (LST) that involves conducting resistance skills training within the context of a program focusing primary attention on teaching generic personal and social skills. This combined resistance skills and competence enhancement approach includes features of both types of preventive interventions. A brief description of the pertinent components of the LST program provides an example of the skills included in an intervention emphasizing personal and social skills training.

Personal Skills

Three types of personal self-management skills are taught in the LST program: self-appraisal, goal setting, and self-directed behavior change; decision making and independent thinking; and anxiety management. Students are taught how to assess their strengths and weaknesses and to identify specific aspects of themselves that they would like to improve, and learn principles of goal setting and self-directed behavior change.

Participants are taught a five-step formula for making decisions systematically, along with an abbreviated three-step formula. They are also taught how to identify and analyze the techniques used by advertisers to influence consumer

decisions to buy their products, and to formulate counterarguments.

Anxiety-management skills are taught through a combination of instruction, demonstration, practice, and reinforcement. The first is a self-directed relaxation technique similar to progressive relaxation, which involves systematically relaxing all the muscles in the body starting with the toes and gradually progressing through each of the muscle groups up to the forehead. The second is a deep breathing technique that involves breathing slowly and deeply into the diaphragm, holding the breath, and then slowly breathing out. The final skill is mental rehearsal. This involves imagining oneself in a situation that produces anxiety and mentally practicing how to handle the situation calmly and effectively.

Social Skills

The final component of the LST curriculum focuses on the development of several important social skills. Participants are taught communication skills such as how to communicate clearly by being specific, asking questions, and paraphrasing. They are also taught social skills such as overcoming shyness, making conversation, complimenting, and asking someone out for a date. Verbal and nonverbal assertive skills are also taught, as well as application of these skills to situations in which there is peer pressure to smoke, drink, or use drugs.

POPULATION AND PROVIDERS

Target Population

As is evident from what is now known about the development of drug abuse and the factors promoting it, adolescence is a time of increased risk for drug involvement. However, adolescence is also a time when health habits and future patterns of behavior are still being formed, a time when many of the lifetime strategies for coping with stress and peer pressure are developed (Jessor, 1991). As such, adolescence and the years immediately before it represent an important window of opportunity for prevention. In more concrete terms, this generally translates into targeting preventive interventions at middle school or junior high school students (grades 6 through 9) who are typically between 11 and 14 years old.

Most prevention efforts have involved predominantly white, middle class, suburban adolescents. This has been particularly true for evaluation studies testing the efficacy of contemporary prevention approaches. More recently, however, there has been a substantial increase in the amount of work being done with minority populations including inner-city, disadvantaged adolescents. There is at least preliminary evidence indicating that the newer prevention approaches are effective with minority populations (Botvin, Batson, et al., 1989; Botvin, Dusenbury, et al., 1989; Botvin et al., 1992; Ellickson and Bell, 1990; Schinke et al., 1988). These studies suggest that essentially the same prevention approaches are effective with widely differing ethnic or racial groups. Despite the generalizability of current prevention approaches, it is important to pay considerable attention to issues of cultural appropriateness and cultural sensitivity in order for these prevention programs to be both acceptable to the target population and optimally effective.

An issue that must be resolved through additional research concerns whether prevention programs should take the form of universal interventions targeted at all available individuals (for example, all the students in the seventh grade) or should only be targeted at high-risk populations (for example, a subgroup of seventh graders identified using established criteria of risk). One obvious difficulty is the definition of risk. Another is that little is known about the potential of even the most effective contemporary prevention approaches with high-risk individuals. Because researchers have generally not attempted to identify individuals who are the most likely to become drug abusers and examine the relative effectiveness of existing prevention approaches with different risk groups, it is difficult to determine the extent to which these interventions would be effective with high-risk individuals. Thus, although

it might be a more efficient use of resources to target prevention interventions at high-risk adolescents, the most prudent strategy at this point is to include everyone.

Program Providers

A variety of providers have been involved in conducting drug abuse prevention programs. These include peer leaders, regular teachers, health professionals, and police officers. Some providers are clearly more effective than others. They should be capable, motivated, and highly committed. In addition, they should be good role models who have high credibility with the target population. Similarly, actors or models used in media campaigns should be attractive, high status, credible individuals who are also good role models.

Moreover, there should be an appropriate match between the type of provider selected and the nature of the prevention program. Programs conducted by police officers and other traditional authority figures that use moralistic appeals may propel rebellious individuals toward drug use rather than away from it. Peer leaders are generally believed to have higher credibility with adolescents about lifestyle issues such as clothes, music, and drug use than adults. Therefore, prevention components involving the discussion of these issues may be more effectively conducted by peer leaders.

Programs using peer leaders have involved both older peer leaders and same-age peer leaders. Nearly all peer-leader programs are organized and conducted by adults with the assistance of peer leaders; few programs have given peer leaders total responsibility for implementation. One reason for this is that students do not have good teaching or classroom management skills. Whatever benefit they may offer in terms of credibility may well be offset by their lack of training and experience. A natural combination is to include both adult and peer providers with each having specifically defined responsibilities commensurate with their strengths.

PROGRAM PARAMETERS AND IMPLEMENTATION ISSUES

Program Length

A basic practical consideration in developing preventive interventions is the amount of time necessary for implementation. At this point, it is difficult to specify how long prevention programs should be. The evaluation literature contains programs ranging from as few as three or four sessions to as many as twenty. A consensus meeting of smoking prevention experts convened by the National Cancer Institute concluded that the minimum program length for smoking prevention programs should be five sessions (Glynn, 1990).

Several factors may affect program length. It is natural to expect that prevention programs targeting more than one substance would require more time than those targeting one substance. Another factor affecting program length is the type of prevention program. Prevention programs teaching domain-specific skills (that is, skills specific to resisting social influences to use drugs) require less time to implement than programs teaching generic personal and social skills (that is, competence enhancement skills not related exclusively to drug use). Programs that combine both specific and generic skills training approaches are longer still. Although there is some evidence to suggest that longer programs are more effective, it is not yet clear what the optimal program length is for producing a meaningful and lasting reduction in drug use.

Booster Sessions

Examination of follow-up data from individuals involved in prevention evaluation studies indicates quite clearly that prevention effects tend to erode over time without additional intervention. When booster sessions or ongoing preventive interventions are provided, preventive gains are generally maintained and, in some instances, even enhanced (Botvin, Renick, & Baker, 1983; Botvin et al., 1990).

For prevention programs targeted at adolescents, booster sessions should be implemented throughout middle or junior high school. It may also be necessary to provide preventive interventions throughout high school. The same is true for prevention programs targeting other populations. Booster sessions generally build on the material covered previously in the prevention program, providing both a review of program content and an opportunity to practice the skills taught in the program. The developmental appropriateness of the material taught in the various years of the prevention program may warrant the introduction of new material in one or more of the booster years. Typically, booster sessions require fewer prevention sessions than those involved in the primary intervention.

Delivery Channels

Prevention programs may be conducted through several different delivery channels. The principal delivery channels are school, family, community organizations, and the media. Interventions delivered through these channels may affect individuals in the target population directly or indirectly by modifying the environment in which they live. Some delivery channels (such as school) offer greater potential for affecting adolescents directly, whereas others (such as the media) offer greater potential for affecting the environment as well as populations not attending school.

School

The most obvious delivery channel for reaching adolescents in the 11- to 14-year-old age group is school. For this reason, most prevention programs targeting adolescents have been school-based (see Chapter 5). Many schools have preexisting slots that make the scheduling of drug abuse prevention programs relative easy. Prevention programs can either be schoolwide interventions such as assembly programs or classroom-based prevention curricula. Prevention curricula can be taught through any major subject area where all students can be reached. Prevention programs have been implemented through health, physical education, science, and social studies. Some schools have even allocated curriculum time specifically for tobacco, alcohol, and drug education.

Family

The family is another logical channel for drug abuse prevention. Parents play an important role in establishing core values and beliefs. They also serve as significant role models. Research studies have consistently demonstrated that adolescents whose parents or siblings do not use drugs are significantly less likely to use drugs themselves. Similarly, adolescents whose parents have communicated strong antidrug sentiments are less likely to use drugs. Adolescents whose parents are involved and interested in what they do and monitor their behavior are also less likely to become drug abusers. Therefore, prevention programs involving the family can help make parents aware of the causes of drug abuse, their importance as role models, the need to clearly and consistently communicate antidrug values, the importance of active involvement in their children's lives, and the need to appropriately monitor and supervise their children. Parents can be taught an array of parenting skills, including how to help their children deal with social pressure. However, despite the importance of family prevention approaches, most attempts have been disappointing because it is generally difficult to get a high degree of parental participation.

Media

It has long been recognized that the media have a powerful influence on attitudes, beliefs, norms, and behavior. A number of mass media campaigns (see Chapter 12) concerning health promotion and drug abuse prevention have been developed and implemented. These campaigns have typically taken the form of public service announcements (PSAs). Unfortunately, PSAs designed to prevent drug abuse typically run during times of low viewership and are infinitesimal compared with ads promoting tobacco, alcohol, and drug products. A notable exception is the media campaign sponsored by the Partnership for a Drug-Free America, which runs its PSAs during prime time. Most mass media campaigns rely on information dissemination or fear-arousal strategies and, like traditional school-based prevention approaches, they have produced disappointing results. Some campaigns have increased knowledge and changed attitudes in the desired direction; others have had no effects; still others have produced negative effects (Flay & Sobel, 1983). Still, this is not surprising when one recognizes that most PSA campaigns fail to reach the intended audience.

The one major exception was the counteradvertising campaign mounted against cigarette smoking in the late 1960s, when there was approximately one counterad for every four or five cigarette ads. It is often said that the effectiveness of that particular PSA campaign was the single most important factor in obtaining the cooperation of the tobacco industry concerning the elimination of cigarette ads on television.

Despite the general lack of efficacy of mass media campaigns and the paucity of high-quality evaluation research, the possibility remains for the mass media to be a powerful weapon in the war against drug abuse. However, to do so, media campaigns must overcome the deficiencies of past campaigns. It is axiomatic that mass media campaigns must reach their target audience if they are to be effective. That clearly means PSAs must be aired during prime time or other high-viewership periods. Furthermore, media campaigns must deemphasize information dissemination and fear-arousal strategies and place greater emphasis on strategies designed to combat the powerful social influences to smoke, drink, or use drugs. Finally, high-quality evaluation research is needed to develop and refine the most effective prevention-oriented mass media campaigns.

Community

Community-based approaches (see Chapter 4), although difficult to evaluate, may provide a supportive context for other prevention efforts. It may be difficult to sustain the preventive gains that the newer psychosocial approaches have demonstrated without affecting the larger social environment of the community. Although organizing a community and raising awareness of severity of the drug abuse problem are important objectives, they are only the vehicles for initiating the types of changes needed to prevent drug abuse. Unfortunately, even if the need for drug abuse prevention is recognized in a community, it might not be entirely clear how these communities should proceed. For the most part, communities have continued to rely on prevention approaches that have previously been demonstrated to be ineffective.

Community-based prevention approaches should use state-of-the-art primary prevention strategies derived largely from school-based drug abuse prevention and community-based heart disease prevention. Community-based prevention approaches should include three levels of intervention based on the principles of social learning theory: direct training of youth to promote drug resistance skills; indirect training of youth through continued provision of program implementation skills to teachers, parents, and other providers; and support for the continued practice of resistance skills through reinforcement (Pentz et al., 1986). Intervention modalities should be designed to increase individual self-efficacy and skills, apply resistance skills to specific interpersonal situations involving drug offers or drug availability, and promote social norms consistent with lower levels of drug use.

Implementation Fidelity

Assuming that one is using an intervention approach with the ability to prevent or reduce drug abuse, the success of that intervention is directly related to implementation fidelity. Two important dimensions of implementation fidelity are quality and completeness. The most effective drug abuse prevention strategy will not be effective if it is only partially implemented. Similarly, if a pre-

vention program is implemented with a high degree of completeness but poor quality, then it is also less likely to produce the desired results. This is not only a logical assumption, but has already been empirically demonstrated in drug abuse prevention research. For example, in our own work (Botvin, Schinke, & Orlandi, 1989; Botvin et al., 1990), we have demonstrated a strong relationship between implementation fidelity and prevention program effectiveness (based on level of drug use). In a study of smoking prevention among inner-city minority students, strong prevention effects were observed for the high-implementation group, no prevention effects were observed for the controls, and the low-implementation group was between the high-implementation group and the control group. Similarly, the strongest prevention effects emerging in a long-term follow-up conducted nearly six years after the initial baseline assessment were found among individuals who received at least 60% of the prevention program (Botvin et al., 1993).

EVALUATION ISSUES

In drawing conclusions about the effectiveness of existing prevention approaches and designing new experimental studies, it is essential that due consideration be given to issues of assessment, evaluation, and methodology. Recent reviews (Biglan & Ary, 1985, Botvin, 1986; Flay, 1985) have identified a number of critical issues that require careful consideration by prevention researchers. These issues include the validity of self-report data, the appropriateness of research designs, the unit of assignment, the unit of analysis, the pretest equivalence of experimental groups, and the potential impact of attrition on internal and external validity.

Validity of Self-Report Data

Nearly all of the research that has been done on the etiology of drug use, surveys assessing the prevalence of drug use trends, and the evaluation of prevention approaches has relied on self-report data. A fundamental question concerns the veracity of self-report data from a given individual regarding drug-taking behavior. Because it is reasonable to assume that many individuals may be less than truthful because drug use is perceived to be undesirable (resulting in underreporting) or desirable (resulting in overreporting), it has been argued that procedures should be adopted to either provide an objective method of determining drug use status or reduce the motivation to lie.

Although methods exist for objectively determining whether individuals are using one or more psychoactive substances, for a variety of reasons, they may be neither practical nor acceptable to the target population. Therefore, data should be collected in a manner designed to reduce as much as possible the potential motivations to under- or overreport. For the most part, this involves either collecting data anonymously or using an ID coding system and stressing the importance of being truthful and emphasizing the fact that all data collected will be viewed only by the members of the research staff.

Research Design

The area of research design is complex; entire textbooks are devoted to it. However, several fundamental issues of prevention research can be briefly summarized. First, prevention studies must include control or comparison groups; only by comparing individuals receiving a given preventive intervention with those receiving either nothing (a no-contact control group) or some other intervention (a placebo control group or comparison control group) can useful results be obtained. Second, in order to avoid contamination across conditions, it is generally advisable to assign entire units (such as schools) to a particular condition. Third, degrees of freedom for statistical analyses should be based on the number of units (rather than individuals) assigned to each condition, if practical; a more recently developed approach that seems to be gaining some degree

of acceptance is to statistically adjust for any resulting intracluster correlations that might inflate the type I error rate (i.e., increase the probability of finding effects that are not real). Fourth, a cardinal rule of experimental research is standardization as a means of controlling extraneous variance. Preventive interventions and data collection procedures should be put in the form of a written protocol and individuals involved in both data collection and intervention should be given adequate training to ensure standardization. Fifth, although it may be necessary to use quasi-experimental designs if experimental units cannot be randomly assigned to conditions, randomization of units or individuals (if appropriate) is the preferable strategy.

Comparability of Groups

A number of factors can affect the comparability of experimental groups in prevention research studies. Preexisting differences (based on a comparison of groups at the initial pretest or over a series of pretests or baseline assessments) may either mask significant prevention effects or lead one to conclude erroneously that a particular prevention approach reduced drug use incidence or prevalence. Although it is possible in many studies to control for the lack of comparability (using tests of difference scores or analysis of covariance techniques, for example), large differences in pretest drug use rates may produce misleading results. In general, groups with high initial drug use rates do not only continue to remain high relative to other groups, but may actually increase over time at a very different rate.

Random assignment typically eliminates most sources of sample or selection bias, but may not necessarily result in highly comparable groups. If a small number of units (schools, classes, or individuals) is to be assigned to experimental conditions, a matching strategy would be preferable to random assignment and in most circumstances provides more comparable groups. On the other hand, one method of maximizing comparability of groups when using random assignment is a blocking strategy that involves dividing all units into homogeneous blocks using one or more variables and then assigning these units randomly to prevention and control conditions.

Regardless of the method used, however, an essential first step in making a convincing argument for the presence of prevention effects in an evaluation study is demonstrating the initial comparability of experimental and control groups. Thus, an effort should be made from the outset to form experimental groups that are as comparable as possible and then to provide evidence of that comparability as part of the process of presenting prevention effects.

Minimizing and Assessing Attrition

Another potential flaw in prevention research studies affecting the comparability of experimental groups arises from attrition. As with groups that lack comparability because of preexisting differences, noncomparability resulting from differential attrition can also lead to erroneous conclusions in a drug abuse prevention study. In this case, groups may start out being highly comparable, but differential attrition across groups may occur over the course of a study, producing noncomparable groups. Groups that appear to be comparable in all relevant respects may end up being quite different.

Depending on the direction of the differential attrition (that is, the manner in which groups end up being different), prevention effects may appear to be stronger or weaker than they actually are. For example, if the prevention group suffers a higher rate of attrition than the control group and the individuals being lost to follow-up are disproportionately drug users or high-risk individuals, the presence of prevention effects may be largely the result of attrition. Conversely, differential attrition resulting in the disproportionate loss of drug users or high-risk individuals from the control group may mask the presence of real prevention effects. It should be pointed out that virtually all prevention studies conducted with junior and senior high school students have at least one type of differential attrition—more drug users are lost to follow-up. This is the result of higher-than-normal absenteeism, dropouts, or noncompliance in completing evaluation questionnaires. Although this type of attrition affects the external validity (generalizability) of prevention studies, it does not undermine the internal validity, which is the most serious threat to the integrity of any prevention study. Internal validity would be affected if there were a differential loss of drug users between the prevention and control groups.

In view of the serious problems accruing from differential attrition, aggressive follow-up of absentees and dropouts should be used to minimize attrition to the greatest extent possible. Moreover, an important step in the analysis and presentation of drug abuse prevention results is to determine whether any attrition has occurred, how extensive it was, and the degree to which it may have had a differential impact on experimental groups. At the same time, the ability to demonstrate that no differential attrition occurred clearly strengthens the argument that a particular prevention is effective if effects are found.

Process and Outcome Evaluation

The evaluation of drug abuse prevention approaches should proceed on two levels: process and outcome evaluation. The collection and evaluation of process data are important because they provide information on the implementation of the preventive intervention. It is very important to know whether the prevention program being evaluated was actually implemented, the degree to which it was implemented, and with whom and by whom it was implemented. If a prevention program is evaluated without the inclusion of process data and no effects accrue, it is not possible to know whether the lack of effects was the result of an ineffective approach or of poor implementation. Moreover, if a prevention approach is implemented with fidelity by some providers and not others, the efficacy of the prevention approach can be examined more accurately by focusing on the individuals who received it.

Outcome evaluation data should be collected to determine the extent to which the prevention program affected relevant variables. This should include a mix of variables derived from an underlying theoretical model or conceptual framework. Previous prevention evaluation studies have focused on knowledge, attitudes, and beliefs with little attention being given to behavioral variables (determining whether the prevention approach affected drug use). More recent studies have focused almost exclusively on drug use behavior, failing to include potential mediating variables. Both types of outcome evaluation data are important. Although it is essential that preventive interventions be evaluated in terms of the target behaviors (tobacco, alcohol, and drug use), age and developmental factors must be taken into consideration. Because of the age of onset and the normal developmental progression of drug use in this country, the most appropriate age for evaluating drug abuse prevention programs targeting adolescents is during or after the early adolescent years. Before that, the prevalence of drug use is too low to determine statistically significant difference except in very large studies because of problems related to statistical power. For studies conducted with populations younger than this, it is generally necessary to rely on proxy measures of drug use.

The measures that might be used as reasonable proxies for drug use behavior depend on one's theoretical formulation of drug use onset and the accuracy of such a formulation. Put more broadly, for very young populations, it is necessary to rely on variables that are associated with risk (such as behavioral intention, self-esteem, knowledge, attitudes, beliefs, and refusal assertiveness).

SUMMARY

Considerable effort has been expended in an attempt to develop new solutions to the problem of drug abuse. One major area of interest is prevention. Many different types of programs have been included under the general rubric of prevention, including primary, secondary, and tertiary prevention.

The appropriate population for primary prevention efforts is adolescents and pre-adolescents (roughly between the ages of 11 and 14). Preventive interventions should include components that focus on the individual or environmental factors that promote the onset and early stages of drug use and abuse.

Prevention approaches must be feasible and acceptable to the target population and affect both the risk factors associated with drug use and drug use itself. Prevention programs must affect one or more gateway substances and produce effects that are reasonably durable and effective with the broadest possible range of individuals. To be effective in the real world, they must be adaptable to a variety of conditions, providers, and delivery systems; they must also be easily exportable to different intervention sites.

The current state of the art in prevention suggests that to be effective, programs must go beyond providing factual information about the adverse consequences of drug abuse. Although some information may contribute to the effectiveness of prevention programs, the type of information provided should be selected with care in order to be developmentally appropriate, relevant to the target population, and not likely to inadvertently increase drug abuse risk. Prevention programs must include components designed to change perceived drug use norms and teach social resistance skills, either alone or in combination with general personal and social skills.

A variety of program providers appear capable of effectively implementing contemporary prevention programs. Providers should be carefully selected and trained to conduct the program. Where feasible, an implementation model should be used that combines the strengths of adult and peer providers. Program length varies considerably depending on the nature of the program, with resistance skills programs requiring less time than combined resistance skills and competence enhancement approaches. To be maximally effective, prevention programs should be implemented over several years and use multiple delivery channels. Moreover, because effectiveness is directly related to implementation fidelity, it is critically important that preventive interventions be properly implemented.

Finally, preventive interventions must be carefully evaluated. Attention must be paid to the way in which self-report data are collected, the appropriateness of the research design selected, and the comparability of experimental and control groups. Attention must also be given to minimizing attrition over the course of a study, as differential attrition may undermine the initial comparability of groups. Although the emphasis in evaluation should be on behavioral outcome measures, the collection of process data is important for increasing our understanding of why current interventions do or do not work and for providing feedback useful in further refining existing prevention methods.

A great deal of progress has been made in the past decade. More is known about the causes of drug abuse. More is also known about what kinds of prevention approaches work and under what conditions. Evaluation research methodology has improved significantly. Although the field of drug abuse prevention is still in its infancy, a number of promising prevention methods are currently available along with well-developed evaluation methods. Understanding those methods and the principles on which they are based should prove useful in further refining existing prevention approaches and in developing new ones.

REFERENCES

Albee, G. W. (1984). Prologue: A model for classifying prevention programs. In J. M. Joffe, G. W. Albee, & L. D. Kelly (Eds.), *Readings in primary prevention of psychopathology: Basic concepts.* Hanover, MA: University Press of New England.

American Psychiatric Association (1987). *Diagnostic and statistical manual of mental disorders,* 3rd ed. Washington, DC: American Psychiatric Association.

Arkin, R. M., Roemhild, H. J., Johnson, C. A., Luepker, R. V., & Murray, D. M. (1981). The Minnesota smoking prevention program: A seventh grade health curriculum supplement. *Journal of School Health, 51,* 616–661.

Bandura, A. (1966). *Principles of behavior modification.* New York: Holt, Rinehart and Winston.

Bandura, A. (1977) *Social learning theory.* Englewood Cliffs, NJ: Prentice Hall.

Berberian, R. M., Gross, C., Lovejoy, J., & Paparella, S. (1976). The effectiveness of drug education programs: A critical review. *Health Education Monographs, 4,* 377–398.

Biglan, A., & Ary, D. V. (1985). Current methodological issues in research on smoking prevention. In C. Bell & R. Battjes, (Eds.), *Prevention research: Deterring drug abuse among children and adolescents.* Washington DC: National Institute on Drug Abuse Research Monograph.

Blum, R., & Richards, L. (1979). Youthful drug use. In R. I. Dupont, A. Goldstein, & J. O'Donnell (Eds.), *Handbook on drug abuse.* Washington, DC: U.S. Department of Health Education and Welfare and Office of Drug Abuse Policy, Executive Office of the President, National Institute on Drug Abuse, pp. 257–267.

Botvin, G. J. (1986). Substance abuse prevention research: Recent developments and future directions. *Journal of School Health, 56,* 369–386.

Botvin, G. J. (1988). Defining "success" in substance abuse prevention. In L. Harris (Ed.), *Problems of Drug Dependence.* NIDA Research Monograph Series, USPHS, 90, 203–212.

Botvin, G. J., Baker, E., Botvin, E. M., Dusenbury, L., Cardwell, J. & Diaz, T. (1993). Factors promoting cigarette smoking among black youth: A causal modeling approach. *Addictive Behaviors, 18,* 397–405.

Botvin, G. J., Baker, E., Botvin, E. M., Filazzola, A., & Millman, R. (1984). Alcohol abuse prevention through the development of personal and social competence: A pilot study. *Journal of Studies on Alcohol, 45,* 550–552.

Botvin, G. J., Baker, E., Dusenbury, L., Tortu, S., & Botvin, E. M. (1990). Preventing adolescent drug abuse through a multimodal cognitive-behavioral approach: Results of a three-year study. *Journal of Consulting and Clinical Psychology, 58,* 437–446.

Botvin, G. J., Batson, H., Witts-Vitale, S., Bess, V., Baker, V., & Dusenbury, L. (1989). A psychosocial approach to smoking prevention for urban black youth. *Public Health Reports, 104,* 573–582.

Botvin, G. J., Dusenbury, L., Baker, E., James-Ortiz, S., Botvin, E. M., & Kerner, J. (1992). Smoking prevention among urban minority youth: Assessing effects on outcome and mediating variables. *Health Psychology, 11* (5), 290–299.

Botvin, G. J., Dusenbury, L., Baker, E., James-Ortiz, S., & Kerner, J. (1989). A skills training approach to smoking prevention among Hispanic youth. *Journal of Behavioral Medicine, 12,* 279–296.

Botvin, G. J., & Eng, A. (1982). The efficacy of a multicomponent approach to the prevention of cigarette smoking. *Preventive Medicine, 11,* 199–211.

Botvin, G. J., Renick, N., & Baker, E. (1983). The effects of scheduling format and booster sessions on a broad spectrum psychosocial approach to smoking prevention. *Journal of Behavioral Medicine, 6,* 359–379.

Botvin, G. J., Schinke, S. P., & Orlandi, M. A. (1989). Psychosocial approaches to substance abuse prevention: Theoretical foundations and empirical findings. *Crisis, 10,* 62–77.

Braucht, G. N., Follingstad, D., Brakrash, D., & Berry, K. L. (1973). Drug education: A review of goals, approaches and effectiveness, and a paradigm for evaluation. *Quarterly Journal of Studies on Alcohol, 34,* 1279–1292.

Czechowikz, D. (1988). Adolescent alcohol and drug abuse and its consequences—An overview. *American Journal of Drug & Alcohol Abuse, 14,* 189–197.

Demone, H. W. (1973). The nonuse and abuse of alcohol by the male adolescent. In M. Chafetz (Ed.), *Proceedings of the second annual alcoholism conference,* DHEW Publication no. HSM 73-9083. Washington, DC: U.S. Government Printing Office, pp. 24–32.

Ellickson, P. L., & Bell, R. M. (1990). Drug prevention in junior high: A multi-site longitudinal test." *Science, 247,* 1299–1305.

Evans, R. I., Rozelle, R. M., Mittlemark, M. B., Hansen, W. B., Bane, A. L., & Havis, J. (1978). Deterring the onset of smoking in children: Knowledge of immediate physiological effects and coping with peer pressure, media pressure, and parent modeling. *Journal of Applied Social Psychology, 8,* 126–135.

Flay, B. R. (1985). Psychosocial approaches to smoking prevention: A review of findings. *Health Psychology, 4,* 449–488.

Flay, B. R., & Sobel, J. (1983). The role of the mass media in preventing adolescent substance abuse.

In T. Glynn, C. Luekefeld, & J. Ludford (Eds.), *Preventing adolescent drug abuse: Intervention strategies* (47th ed.). Washington, DC: National Institute on Drug Abuse Research Monograph, pp. 83–1280.

Gilchrist, L. D., & Schinke, S. P. (Eds.) (1985). *Preventing social and health problems through life skills training.* Seattle: University of Washington.

Glynn, T. (1990). *School programs to prevent smoking: The National Cancer Institute guide to strategies that succeed.* NIH Publication (90-500). Washington, DC: National Cancer Institute.

Goodstadt, M. S. (1974). Myths and methodology in drug education: A critical review of the research evidence." In M. S. Goodstadt (Ed.), *Research on methods and programs of drug education.* Toronto: Addiction Research Foundation.

Goodstadt, M. S. (1978). Alcohol and drug education. *Health Education Monographs, 6* (3), 263–279.

Hamburg, B. A., Braemer, H. C., & Jahnke, W. A. (1975). Hierarchy of drug use in adolescence: Behavioral and attitudinal correlates of substantial drug use. *American Journal of Psychiatry, 132,* 1155–1167.

Hurd, P., Johnson, C. A., Pechacek, T., Bast, C. P., Jacobs, D., & Luepker, R. (1980). Prevention of cigarette smoking in 7th grade students. *Journal of Behavioral Medicine, 3,* 15–28.

Jessor, R. (1976). Predicting time of onset of marijuana use: A developmental study of high school youth. In D. J. Lettieri (Ed.), *Predicting adolescent drug abuse: A review of issues, methods and correlates.* Research Issues 11, DHEW Publication no. (ADM) 77-299. Washington, DC: Superintendent of Documents, U.S. Government Printing Office. Rockville, MD: National Institute on Drug Abuse.

Jessor, R. (1991). Risk behavior in adolescence: A psychosocial framework for understanding and action. *Journal of Adolescent Health, 12,* 597–605.

Jessor, R., Collins, M. I., & Jessor, S. L. (1972). On becoming a drinker: Social-psychological aspects of an adolescent transition. *Annual of the New York Academy of Sciences, 197,* 199–213.

Jessor, R., & Jessor, S. L. (1977). *Problem behavior and psychosocial development: A longitudinal study of youth.* New York: Academic Press.

Johnson, C. A., Hansen, W. B., Collins, L. M., & Graham, J. W. (1986). High school smoking prevention: Results of a three-year longitudinal study. *Journal of Behavioral Medicine, 9,* 439–452.

Johnston, L. D., Bachman, J. G., & O'Malley, P. M. (1988). Summary of 1987 drug study results. Ann Arbor: University of Michigan News and Information Service press release.

Kandel, D. B. (1978). Convergences in prospective longitudinal surveys of drug use in normal populations. In D. B. Kandel (Ed.), *Longitudinal research on drug use: Empirical findings and methodological issues.* Washington, DC: Hemisphere (Halsted-Wiley), pp. 3–38.

Kandel, D. B., & Logan, S. A. (1984). Problems of drug use from adolescence to young adulthood. I: Periods of risk for initiation, continued use, and discontinuation. *American Journal of Public Health, 74,* 660–666.

Luepker, R. V., Johnson, C. A., Murray, D. M., & Pechacek, T. F. (1983). Prevention of cigarette smoking: Three year follow-up of educational programs for youth. *Journal of Behavioral Medicine, 6,* 53–61.

McAlister, A., Perry, C. L., Killen, J., Slinkard, L. A., & Maccoby, N. (1980). Pilot study of smoking, alcohol, and drug abuse prevention. *American Journal of Public Health, 70,* 719–721.

McAlister, A. L., Perry, C. L., & Maccoby N. (1979). Adolescent smoking: Onset and prevention. *Pediatrics, 63,* 650–658.

Meyer, R. E., & Mirin, S. M. (1979). *The heroin stimulus. Implications for a theory of addiction.* New York: Plenum, p. 276.

Millman, R. B., & Botvin, G. J. (1992). Substance use, abuse, and dependence. In M. Levine, N. B. Carey, A. C. Crocker, & R. T. Gross (Eds.), *Developmental–behavioral pediatrics* (2nd ed.). New York: W.B. Saunders, pp. 451–467.

Murray, D. M., Johnson, C. A., Luepker, R. V., & Mittlemark, M. B. (1984). The prevention of cigarette smoking in children: A comparison of four strategies. *Journal of Applied Social Psychology, 14* (3), 274–288.

Mussen, P., Conger, J., & Kagan, J. (1974). *Child development and personality,* 4th ed. New York: Harper and Row.

Pentz, M. A. (1983). Prevention of adolescent substance abuse through social skill development. In T. J. Glynn, C. G. Leukfeld, & J. P. Ludford (Eds.), *Preventing adolescent drug abuse: Intervention strategies.* Washington, DC: National Institute on Drug Abuse Research Monograph no. 47, pp. 195–232.

Pentz, M. A., Cormack, C., Flay, B., Hanson, W., & Johnson, C. A. (1986). Balancing program and research integrity in community drug abuse prevention: Project STAR approach. *Journal of School Health, 56,* 389–393.

Perry, C. L., Killen, J., Slinkard, L. A., & McAlister, A. L. (1980). Peer teaching and smoking prevention among junior high students. *Adolescence, 9* (58), 277–281.

Ray, O. S. (1974). *Drugs, society, and human behavior.* St. Louis: C.V. Mosby.

Robins, L. N., & Przybeck, T. R. (1985). Age of onset of drug use as a factor in drug and other disorders. In C. L. Jones & R. J. Battjes (Eds.), *Etiology of drug use: Implications for prevention.* National Institute on Drug Abuse Research Monograph #56, DHHS Publication no. (ADM) 85-1335, Washington, DC: U.S. Government Printing Office.

Rotter, J. B. (1972). Generalized expectancies for internal versus external control of reinforcement. In J. B. Rotter, J. E. Chance, & E. J. Phares (Eds.), *Applications of a Social Learning Theory of Personality.* New York: Holt, Rinehart and Winston, pp. 260–295.

Schaps, E., Bartolo, R. D., Moskowitz, J., Palley, C. S., & Churgin, S. (Winter 1981). A review of 127 drug abuse prevention program evaluations. *Journal of Drug Issues,* 17–43.

Schinke, S. P., & Blythe, B. J. (1981). Cognitive-behavioral prevention of children's smoking. *Child Behavior Therapy, 3,* 25–42.

Schinke, S. P., & Gilchrist, L. D. (1983). Primary prevention of tobacco smoking. *Journal of School Health, 53,* 416–419.

Schinke, S. P., & Gilchrist, L. D. (1984). Preventing cigarette smoking with youth. *Journal of Primary Prevention, 5,* 48–56.

Schinke, S. P., Orlandi, M. A., Botvin, G. J., Gilchrist, L. D., Trimble, J. E., & Locklear, V. S. (1988). Preventing substance abuse among American Indian adolescents: A bicultural competence skills approach. *Journal of Counseling Psychology, 35,* 87–90.

Semlitz, L., & Gold, M. S. (1986). Adolescent drug abuse: diagnosis, treatment and prevention. *Psychiatric Clinics of North America, 9,* 455–473.

Swisher, J. D., & Hoffman, A. (1975). Information: The irrelevant variable in drug education. In B. W. Corder, R. A. Smith, & J. D. Swisher (Eds.), *Drug Abuse Prevention: Perspectives and*

Approaches for Educators. Dubuque, IA: William C. Brown, pp. 49–62.

Telch, M. J., Killen, J. D., McAlister, A. L., Perry, C. L., & Maccoby, N. (1982). Long-term follow-up of a pilot project on smoking prevention with adolescents. *Journal of Behavioral Medicine, 5,* 1–8.

Wechsler, H. (1976). Alcohol intoxication and drug use among teenagers. *Journal of Studies in Alcohol, 37,* 1672–1677.

Wechsler, H., & Thum, D. (1973). Alcohol and drug use among teenagers: A questionnaire study. In M. Chafetz (Ed.), *Proceedings of the Second Annual Alcoholism Conference,* DHEW Publication no. HSM 73-9083. Washington, DC: U.S. Government Printing Office, pp. 33–46.

Yamaguchi, K., & Kandel, D. B. (1984). Patterns of drug use from adolescence to young adulthood, II. Sequences of progression. *American Journal of Public Health, 74,* 668–672.

PART TWO

SYSTEMS-ORIENTED PREVENTION STRATEGIES AND PROGRAMS

CHAPTER 3

LAW ENFORCEMENT AND
REGULATORY AGENCIES

ROGER L. CONNER
PATRICK BURNS

In recent years, the role and rhetoric of drug and alcohol abuse prevention programs has become increasingly tortured. On one side are those who note that alcohol is a drug and who caution against its use. On the other are those who advertise, promote, or wink at alcohol use even they vigorously condemn illegal drugs. A great deal of the confusion in the current debate comes from the almost fluid movement between different paradigms: law enforcement, sociohistorical, and medical, to name just three.

This chapter deals with law enforcement and regulation in drug and alcohol abuse prevention. Because the role of law enforcement in drug abuse prevention is different from the social, legal, and administrative obstacles encountered in alcohol abuse prevention, these two substances will be dealt with separately using a parallel analytical structure that looks at the harms of abuse, the history of legal control and prevention, and suggestions for a law enforcement-based policy response to the current problem of alcohol and other kinds of drug abuse. Law enforcement and regulation has an important role in drug and alcohol abuse prevention, but its role is slightly different for each of these substances.

Alcohol is a legal product for people over age 21 and has a long tradition of use in Judeo-Christian culture. Other psychoactive drugs are not legal, are far less widely used than alcohol, and are relatively new arrivals, being identified as a significant social problem only in the last 30 years.

ALCOHOL

The Problem

Alcohol is the most widely used and abused drug in the United States, with approximately 65% of all adults drinking alcoholic beverages and 35% abstaining for moral, religious, or personal reasons (NIAAA, 1990). No other powerfully psychoactive drug is so commonly used, sold, and advertised in the United States.

Although alcohol is used by most Americans, most Americans are not regular problem drinkers. The vast majority of Americans seem to be able to get by with one or two beers at a sitting, rarely, if ever, getting drunk or allowing alcohol to impair their work, home, or social life.

Although chronic drinkers represent a minority of U.S. society, they are the cornerstone of alcohol sales, with just 10% of consumers consuming approximately 70% of all alcoholic beverages (Moore & Gerstein, 1981). This population of problem drinkers is closely correlated with the estimated 10.5 million alcoholics in the nation (NIAAA, 1990).

Most of the toll alcohol abuse exacts on society is not sanctionable by law. This toll includes alcohol-fueled divorce, which in turn begets child poverty and an increase in the welfare rolls. Add to this lost productivity, cirrhosis, increases in cancer deaths due to alcohol consumption, the psychological pain of seeing parents and children destroying themselves, and the numerous cancers and other diseases caused by alcohol use and

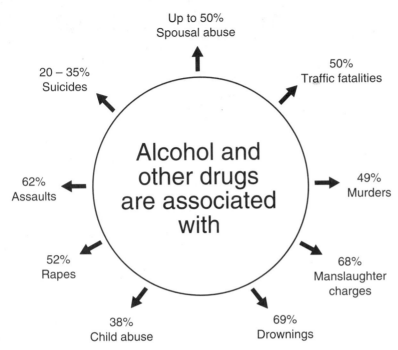

FIGURE 3.1. Relationship of Alcohol Abuse and Crime
Spousal abuse figures reported in the *NIAAA Special Report to Congress,* 1983;
all other figures reported in the *NIAAA Sixth Special Report to Congress,* 1987.

abuse, and it is easy to see that widespread use of alcohol is a serious public health problem. This alone might be reason enough to argue for its restricted use and sales.

But alcohol abuse is also a causal factor in a great deal of criminally sanctionable crime (see Figure 3.1). The Office of Substance Abuse Prevention (OSAP) estimates that alcohol is involved in 49% of murders, 52% of rapes, 62% of assaults, 50% of traffic fatalities, 38% of child abuse cases, 69% of drownings, 20–35% of suicides, 68% of manslaughters, and up to 50% of spousal abuse cases (OSAP, 1989). Approximately 40% of people now in prison were alcohol-intoxicated at the time of their offense. Half of this population committed their crimes while intoxicated only on alcohol, the other half were inebriated on a mixture of alcohol and other drugs (Kleiman, 1992). It can be argued that a

significant percentage of this crime might have occurred even without alcohol intoxication, but even a 20% reduction in alcohol-associated crime would result in a significant decrease in overall crime.

Clearly, prevention of alcohol abuse is in society's best interest. But how best to achieve this goal? This question has haunted American policymakers for more than two hundred years.

America's 200-Year War on Drunks

The 200-year history of alcohol control in the United States can be divided into three eras: the era of alcoholic laissez-faire that existed before 1830, when there were no laws and per capita alcohol consumption was twice current levels; the period stretching from 1830 to 1933, when the problem was defined as a demon that could best be combated by exorcising the product from the marketplace; and the medical paradigm of the post-Prohibition era in which the solution to the national alcohol problem has been to discourage and sanction drunk driving and to encourage chronic abusers to voluntarily seek treatment.

Alcohol Laissez-Faire before 1830

During the colonial period and stretching into the first several decades after the American Revolution, there was little or no control over alcohol use and sales in the United States.

In 1770, the per capita absolute alcohol consumption for all adults over age 15 was approximately 5.1 gallons per annum (Rorabaugh, 1979) and by 1800 it had topped 6.6 gallons. The effect of this high level of inebriation was not lost on policymakers concerned about the effects of alcohol intoxication on health, production, and child welfare. In 1785, Benjamin Rush, the first Surgeon General of the United States (and a signatory to the Declaration of Independence), put out a pamphlet on alcohol consumption titled "An Inquiry into the Effects of Ardent Spirits" that noted the health effects of rampant alcohol abuse in the new country and called for repeal of the rum ration. Between 1800 and 1830, more than 200,000 copies of this pamphlet were printed, and calls for alcohol control became common as the ravages of alcoholic excess became increasingly self-evident (Tischler, 1986). In response to a perception of rampant alcohol abuse, the alcohol reform movement was born in Boston in 1825 as the American Society for the Promotion of Temperance.

The Rise of Alcohol Restriction and Prohibition, 1830–1933

Almost from the beginning, the alcohol restrictionist movement focused on "demon rum" and the elimination of alcohol from the national marketplace.

From the restrictionist point of view, alcohol was a corrupting influence, changing responsible men into irresponsible social scourges. If alcohol were removed, otherwise good men would return to family, jobs, and a regimen of responsible behavior.

The alcohol restrictionist movement began to pick up speed in the early part of the nineteenth century as first Maine and then 11 other states followed with short-lived prohibition laws. With a massive wave of Irish and German immigration beginning in the mid-1840s, however, alcohol consumption escalated and the temperance movement made relatively little headway.

In 1872, in Hillsboro, Ohio, a more direct and local approach to alcohol control was inaugurated when sixty women dressed in their Sunday best began singing church hymns at the top of their lungs in front of the local saloon, forcing it to shut down. Thus was born the Women's Christian Temperance Movement. In 1893, the temperance movement gave birth to the Anti-Saloon League, which was formed to apply direct political pressure on candidates to pass legislation curbing and eliminating alcohol sales. By 1907, seven states had statewide prohibition laws on the books, and by 1917, some 26 states were dry (American Alliance for Right and Responsibilities, 1991).

In December 1917, partly as a response to anti-German sentiment generated by World War I, Congress passed national Prohibition legislation slated to take effect beginning in January 1920.

Contrary to popular wisdom, nation alcohol prohibition sharply reduced per capita alcohol use. Per capita alcohol consumption was 2.4 gallons of absolute alcohol per year before Prohibition; it dropped to an estimated 0.9 gallons per year between 1920 and 1933, and was only 1.5 gallons the year after Prohibition was repealed. Most experts agree that per capita alcohol consumption declined 40 to 60% during the Prohibition years (Moore, 1989; Moore & Gerstein, 1981). Not until 1970 did per-capita alcohol consumption reach pre-Prohibition levels.

This is not to say that Prohibition was a complete public policy success. Prohibition resulted in a rapid rise in organized crime and bootleg alcohol poisonings remained a serious problem throughout the era. In addition, Prohibition had a profoundly negative impact on the administration of the criminal justice system.

With criminalization of alcohol manufacture, sales, and use, otherwise law-abiding members of society now faced arrest, fines, and jail for drinking beverages most had grown up with. With millions unwilling to let go of the old alcohol convention, police and courts quickly found that alcohol offenders outmatched apprehension and detention resources. Courts and jails filled to overflowing. By 1930, it was common to hear even the most staid policymakers argue for alcohol legalization as a way of relieving court and jail overcrowding.

In the end, the real problems of law enforcement administration, combined with the real and perceived problems of organized crime and continuing alcohol consumption, conspired to make Prohibition politically untenable. By December 1933, 36 states had ratified the Twenty-First Amendment, and national Prohibition was repealed.

The Rise of the Medical-Treatment Paradigm

The end of national Prohibition remanded responsibility for alcohol control back to the individual states. The alcohol problem, which had never really gone away, was now back on the table. But if making the manufacture, sale, possession, and use of alcohol illegal was not a politically viable solution, what was?

The answer was found in 1935 in Akron, Ohio with the beginning of Alcoholics Anonymous (AA). The AA program of personal recovery is centered around treating alcoholism as a medical and spiritual illness. Whereas Prohibition sought to control the drinking of all persons, AA seeks to treat individual alcoholics through a program of voluntary personal abstinence.

Unlike other treatment programs that preceded it, AA worked for a significant percentage of alcoholics. Relapse was high, but those who stuck with the program often got sober and remained sober for an extended period of time. The

most obvious reason for AA's success was that it treated alcoholism as a disease that required ongoing therapy rather than a one-time "dry out," as many past programs had offered.

As AA grew from a few hundred members to many thousands, it drew the attention of policymakers from all walks of life. Here, at last, was a "solution" to America's alcohol problem that involved no government expense and no government legislation!

AA, of course, never claimed that the medical paradigm of alcohol abuse was a solution for *generalized* alcohol abuse. AA claimed only that it could help *individuals* who had a desire to get sober. But with public policymakers less than enthusiastic about controlling alcohol sales and distribution and unable to lock up everyone who abused alcohol, the treatment paradigm was quickly embraced as a politically viable solution to America's alcohol problem.

Aside from alcohol abuse associated with alcoholism and alcoholics, policymakers have focused on only one other kind of alcohol-related harm: drunk driving.

Since the late 1970s, Mothers Against Drunk Driving (MADD), Remove Intoxicated Drivers (RID), and other organizations have launched a full-court press to change laws and attitudes about drinking and driving. As a consequence, increasingly tough drunk driving laws and enforcement practices are being adopted and alcohol-related traffic deaths have steadily declined over the last 10 years.

The Need for an Expanded Debate and a New Paradigm

Since the end of Prohibition, and throughout the reign of the medical-treatment paradigm, America's per capita alcohol consumption rate has climbed. Today, per capita alcohol consumption in the United States is higher than it was just before Prohibition.

Although treatment and AA have provided solace and freedom for hundreds of thousands of alcoholics across the nation, the medical paradigm is probably an inappropriate policy response to problems caused by millions of people who only rarely or occasionally get drunk. This population has none of the physical characteristics normally associated with alcoholism, such as dependence, enlarged livers, routine drunkenness, and delirium tremens. However, a person who drinks to excess only one or twice in his or her life can—and too often does—inflict real damage to self, community, and family. A single incident of alcoholic excess can result in acquaintance rape, a fire started by a lit cigarette, a child drowned due to neglect by a drunken caregiver, a case of AIDS gotten during unprotected sex, and myriad other social harms. Across the nation, alcohol is the catalyst for thousands of such occurrences every day.

One of the lessons of Prohibition is that regulation and enforcement *can* reduce the damage alcohol inflicts on society. Between the extremes of authoritarian prohibitionism, which is not politically tenable, and libertarian bacchanalia, which is not morally tenable, lies a vast middle way of regulation, law enforcement, and general denormalization that can ameliorate a great deal of the social harms now associated with alcoholic excess.

By making alcohol use less socially rewarding and more difficult, and by penalizing drunkenness and irresponsible use and sales of alcoholic products, a program of regulation and law enforcement offers the chance for Americans to embrace an alcohol control paradigm that guarantees maximum liberty interests while sharply discouraging behavior that has a known, quantifiable, and predictable index of harms associated with it. Everyone would retain a *right* to drink, but society would encourage and enable responsible drinking and sharply discourage and sanction irresponsible use and sales.

The Role of Regulation and Law Enforcement in Combating Drunkenness

Regulation and law enforcement are the most direct ways of changing social behavior. In the field of alcohol policy, use and abuse of alcoholic beverages can best be mitigated by focusing on three overarching objectives:

- Increasing the barriers to routine and ritual alcohol use
- Changing the social cues we get and receive about drinking and drunkenness
- Penalizing antisocial drinking and antisocial alcohol sales

Increasing Barriers to Use

Alcohol is a powerful psychoactive substance that is sold as a cheap, convenience store item. At the low end of its price range, it is cheaper than Coca-Cola and, even for persons under age 21, not much more difficult to purchase.

The predictable outcome of such ubiquitous distribution and loose control is that alcohol has become an integral part of America's social fabric, with very little or no incentive for hosts to promote soft drinks over beer, or for thirsty people to drink pop rather than Coors.

By increasing the barriers to use, including price, availability, and ability to purchase, alcohol consumption can be discouraged and a reduction in routine and ritual drunkenness can be expected.

Step One: Increase the Price of Alcohol through Taxation and Use the Revenue for Anti-Drinking Ads.

The federal tax on beer and wine has not increased since 1951 and the federal tax on distilled spirits was increased only slightly in 1985 after remaining unchanged for the previous 35 years. In real terms, this means that, between 1950 and 1988, the tax on beer, wine, and liquor fell between 71 and 75% (Kleiman, 1992).

The low price of alcoholic beverages is a direct encouragement to consumption. If current alcohol taxation rates were indexed to the 1951 rate, the average price of a six pack of beer would climb from less than $5 to more than $7.50, and the price of a bottle of scotch would jump by approximately $5.50 (Grossman, 1991). There is little question that the alcohol industry can survive such a large tax increase because this same relative tax burden was borne by the industry in the early 1950s.

According to research by Michael Grossman of New York City University, such a price increase would have the effect of reducing heavy drinking across the population, and would especially reduce underage drinking by youths with less discretionary income. Grossman estimates, for instance, that if beer taxes were indexed to the 1951 rate, 32% of heavy-drinking youths between the ages of 16 and 21 would cut their drinking from four to seven times per week to one to three times per week (Grossman, 1991).

Another benefit of higher alcohol prices would be fewer cirrhosis deaths. Cook found that cirrhosis rates were lower in states that had higher taxes for distilled spirits, and calculates a 20% increase in the current tax on distilled spirits would reduce cirrhosis mortality by about 20% nationwide (Cook, 1981).

An additional benefit to indexing alcohol taxes to the 1951 tax rate is that such a program would bring in billions of dollars at a time of real fiscal constraint. An appropriate use for at least some of this revenue would be to allocate it to underwrite the cost of an anti-alcohol advertising campaign similar to those seen on television for smoking and illegal drugs.

Step Two: Reduce the Number of Alcohol Sales Establishments.   In most states, alcohol can be bought at bars, restaurants, liquor stores, grocery stores, convenience stores, bait shops, gas stations, marinas, ball parks, and even some movie theaters. Few products are as easy to purchase as alcohol, and none have such obvious social consequences if abused. Guns, for example, are typically sold only in gun stores, hardware stores, and some sports shops. No one would think of selling ammunition in as broad an array of stores and locations as alcohol, even though most ammunition, like most alcohol, is legally and responsibly used.

Studies examining the relationship between drunk driving and alcohol sales have found that the more establishments selling alcohol in a given area, the greater the frequency of alcohol-related traffic accidents. In North Carolina, for example, a 250% increase in the number of establishments selling liquor by the drink resulted in a 6–7.4% increase in distilled spirit sales and a 16–24% increase in alcohol-related traffic deaths (Blose & Holder, 1987). Conversely, it can be expected that a decrease in the number of alcohol sales establishments in a given area would reduce overall alcohol sales and incidents of drunk driving in particular.

One of the most obvious places to eliminate alcohol sales is where cars and alcohol are closely associated, such as at gas stations, mini-marts, and convenience stores. Research conducted in Orange and San Diego Counties, California, shows that 8.5% of persons who bought gasoline and alcohol at the same outlet consumed the product in their car (Ryan & Segars, 1987). Alcohol sold at grocery stores was less likely to be consumed while driving—just 2.8% of all sales were consumed in cars. Moreover, although gas station mini-marts represent just 6% of alcohol outlets in San Diego County, they were the source of 15% of the alcohol sold. Clearly, making alcohol less readily available to drivers is a promising way of reducing overall drunk driving deaths.

Step Three: Mandate Secure Identification for All Alcohol Purchases.   Under current law, it is illegal for persons under age 21 to purchase alcohol. It is also illegal for a significant percentage of adult parolees to drink alcohol or even enter a bar. For both groups, enforcement of an absolute ban on alcohol use should be a prime public policy and law enforcement objective.

Yet, under the current regime of lax control and enforcement, underage drinkers and persons specifically banned from drinking face few, if any, obstacles to intoxication. A study of alcohol sales establishments in Washington, D.C. by the Insurance Institute for Highway Safety, for example, found that 97 of 100 stores surveyed readily sold alcohol to underage buyers without asking for identification. For parolees and others whose alcohol intake is court-restricted, there is currently no way to verify or enforce a sobriety sentence short of catching the person while drunk and knowing he or she is alcohol-restricted.

One of the surest ways of changing this equation is to mandate that all persons buying alcoholic beverages show a valid, state-approved picture ID card such as a driver's license. Such a license would indicate, through use of a differently colored photo background or other indelible marking, whether the license holder was legally able to buy and consume alcoholic beverages.

Mandating that *all* alcohol sales be dependent on proof of legal age and a legal right to drink would eliminate a large number of problem drinkers from the drinking population. Although some leakage would occur as the result of fraudulent identification and proxy-buying of alcohol for others, such activity could be sharply discouraged by making such violation punishable by mandatory jail time or by revocation of the offending party's license to drink.

Step Four: Ban Certain Kinds of Alcohol Products.
The function of high-alcohol beer, wine, and liquor is to enable people to get plastered at the lowest possible price. The most direct approach to high-content alcohol products is to ban them from the marketplace. In the case of beer and wine, such a ban could be achieved by narrowing the acceptable variance in alcohol content. Grain alcohol should be totally banned at the retail level and should be made available only to cordial manufacturers granted a special license by the state.

Changing the Social Cues
Most people begin drinking because they are curious about a substance that television, radio, and their peers have told them is closely identified with companionship, sex, status, sophistication, and liberation. From the age of three or four, children are socialized to identify drink as a central icon around which most social discourse surrounds. Television, for instance, shows characters drinking alcohol or ordering and serving

alcohol an average of 10 times per hour (Wallack, Breed, & Cruz, 1987), or about five times the rate for all other beverages *combined,* even though, in real life, alcoholic beverages represent just one-sixth of all drinks consumed. Clearly, changing the social cues we send and receive about alcohol in society is an important and necessary step to normalizing sobriety and denormalizing drunkenness.

Step One: Mandate an Array of Comprehensive Health Warnings.
Mandating health warnings on all alcohol beverages and in all alcohol advertising would curb drinking in general and abusive drinking in particular. Such health warnings should go beyond the current notice to not drink if pregnant and embrace a full panoply of health warnings that spell out the predictable outcomes of widespread alcohol intoxication: assault, drunk driving, rape, murder, and spousal abuse.

Step Two: Mandate Server Training Programs.
Beyond the social cues we receive on television are the social cues we receive in other settings such as restaurants, bars, and the workplace. In the area of alcohol control policy, the most obvious set of social cues amenable to regulation are those emanating from serving professionals in bars and restaurants. These professionals can play a critical role in reducing collateral harms associated with alcohol abuse if for no other reason than they are the last dispensers of alcohol to about half of all drunk drivers on the road (Center for Injury Prevention, 1991).

Thirty-five states currently have dram shop laws that allow the victims of drunk driving to sue establishments that "over serve" their patrons. These laws are designed to encourage bars and restaurants to closely patrol their client base and cut off consumption to obviously intoxicated patrons.

In order to reduce liability and establish a positive defense against dram shop liability claims, some bars and restaurants are now requiring their bartenders and waiters to take alcohol server training courses.

Server training programs teach bar personnel how to gauge the alcohol intake of patrons and how to respond to alcohol requests from intoxicated guests. By serving more food, slowing down service, and simply refusing to serve patrons beyond a certain point, trained waiters and bartenders are able to dramatically reduce the incidents of drunk driving associated with their establishments. Saltz found that when trained personnel served patrons, the incident of bar and restaurant intoxication was reduced by as much as half (Saltz, 1989).

Although server training programs are a voluntary outgrowth of dram shop laws, there is no reason graduation from such a course should not be a mandatory requirement for all persons serving alcohol at restaurants and bars. Irresponsible bartending, after all, creates far more serious problems than irresponsible barbering, which requires a license and hundreds of hours of in-class training.

Step Three: Ban Open Alcohol Containers in All Vehicles.

Thirty-two states currently allow people to drive with open containers of alcohol in their car. In these states, the overt message is that drinking and driving is O.K. provided you do not legally cross the magic line of a .10% blood alcohol content (BAC) level. Any serious effort to control alcohol abuse must broadcast the message that *any* alcohol use is incompatible with certain kinds of potentially dangerous activity, such as driving. States that allow open alcohol containers in moving vehicles are winking at drinking and driving and are overtly condoning irresponsible behavior that leads to death and destruction.

Penalizing Antisocial Sales and Use

One of the quickest ways of encouraging people to change their thinking about drinking is to sanction inappropriate alcohol sales and use. Under the current paradigm, however, alcohol sales are barely regulated and violations are frequent and penalties light. As for drunkenness, it is not a crime at all unless you are in public, extremely intoxicated, and usually engaging in some other kind of antisocial conduct (such as screaming at passersby or urinating on the sidewalk).

What is needed, but is currently lacking, are sanctions on alcohol offenders, short of jail or liquor license revocation, that can be triggered at lower levels of abuse. By discouraging and preventing inappropriate behavior *before* it reaches a critical threshold, a community can safeguard its interests while at the same time permitting responsible use and sales of alcoholic beverages.

Step One: Revoke an Individual's License to Drink.

One possible sanction, frequently levied by judges but not yet codified and operationalized at the state level, is to ban certain individuals from drinking alcohol altogether. As previously mentioned, such a sanction could be implemented by mandating that all alcohol sales be dependent on display of a state-issued driver's license or ID card that would note whether an individual was legally able to purchase and consume alcohol.

Step Two: Close or Suspend the Licenses of Irresponsible Alcohol Vendors.

Under the current paradigm, alcohol sales offenders rarely lose their alcohol sales license due to the paucity of alcohol license investigators and the natural reticence of Alcohol Beverage Control Board's to inflict economic capital punishment on bars, restaurants, and liquor stores.

The most obvious solution to this problem is to mandate intermediate sanctions that would allow an offending establishment to keep its liquor license but to force it to close for a period of time as a penalty for each offense.

There is clear precedent for such a law. In Boston, Baltimore, Tampa, New York City, and myriad other locations across the country, the police routinely close or padlock establishments where illegal drugs are routinely sold. The presence of a similar Alcohol Nuisance Abatement Board would encourage all liquor establishments in a given area to listen more closely to community and police complaints about patterns of alcohol intoxication and illegal sales from the establishment.

Step Three: Pass Administrative License Revocation Laws.   Perhaps the single most effective law to curb drunk driving is an administrative license revocation (ALR) law. ALR laws empower police to revoke an individual's driver license if his or her blood alcohol level is greater than the state minimum (generally 0.10%) or if he or she refuses a breathalyzer or other blood alcohol concentration test. Twenty-two states currently have ALR laws on the books and their enforcement has, as a rule, resulted in an 8 to 12% decline in fatal drunk driving incidents in these states (Ross, 1987).

Step Four: Seize the Cars of Repeat Drunk Drivers or Drunk Drivers with Revoked, Suspended or No Licenses.   ALR laws work when drunk drivers stop driving, but many drunk drivers continue to get behind the wheel despite license revocation. One way to rectify this situation is to seize, subject to forfeiture, cars used by repeat drunk drivers. Such a program has precedent: If you use your car to buy drugs, it is subject to seizure and forfeiture as an instrument in the crime of drug possession and sales. Current law allows police to similarly seize the car of repeat or unlicensed drunk drivers if they so wish.

Step Five: Set Up Sobriety Checkpoints.   Sobriety checkpoints are a way of indicating to the public that drunk driving laws are being enforced and that there is a level of certainty to being caught if driving drunk. Although sobriety checkpoints typically turn up only a small percentage of drunk drivers, checkpoints can serve as a powerful deterrent to driving drunk. Surveys indicate that up to 13% of adults think they may have driven drunk during the past month (NIAAA, 1990). To put this another way, more than one out of every seven drivers going through a sobriety checkpoint is breathing a sigh of relief that due to God and good timing, they are not going directly to jail or court.

There is little question that sobriety checkpoints, if widely used and publicized, can reduce drunk driving. Research in New South Wales, Australia (Homel, 1986) found that when one-third of all drivers passed through a sobriety checkpoint during a one-year period, total traffic deaths declined by 23%.

Although sobriety checkpoints are currently being used in all but a few states, their presence is sporadic and publicity relatively sparse. In order to be more effective, checkpoints must be considered a routine part of preventive law enforcement and their presence unremarkable.

OTHER DRUGS

The Problem

Although drug abuse routinely ranks among the top concerns of rank-and-file Americans, surveys indicate that illegal drug use of all kinds is far less common than routine alcohol abuse. According to the 1990 National Household Survey conducted by the National Institute on Drug Abuse (NIDA), the most commonly used illegal drug, marijuana, has been smoked by just 5.1% of Americans over age 12 in the past month, whereas alcohol is used by more than 50% of this same population and is routinely abused, according to the Secretary of Health and Human Services, by more than 10% of adults over age 18 (NIAAA, 1990).[1]

Marijuana use is half as common as routine alcohol abuse, but monthly use of other illegal drugs is even less common. Just 0.2% of persons over age 12, for instance, report having smoked crack in the last month, just 0.8% report snorting or shooting cocaine, 0.6% report snorting inhalants such as glue, paint thinner, or gasoline, and just 0.3% report using hallucinogens such as LSD, mescaline, and psilocybin. Other psychotherapeutics (methamphetamine, barbiturates, analgesics) are illegally used by just 1.4% of the population, and only 0.8% of Americans over age 12 admits to ever having used heroin (NIDA, 1991).

If we set aside marijuana use, we find that monthly alcohol abuse by chronic problem drinkers is about five times more common than illegal drug use and 50 times more common than crack cocaine use.

Drug use figures for the general population, however, obscure an important point: A tremendous number of young adults are using illegal drugs on a regular basis. NIDA data (1991) show, for instance, that nearly 20% of males and more than 10% of females age 18–25 report some kind of illegal drug use during the preceding month. Clearly, drug use and abuse among the young is a serious national problem, rivaling if not exceeding chronic alcohol abuse among young adults.

The Commotion over Crack

From these statistics, it is clear that crack cocaine represents only a fraction of illegal drug use. Even young Americans make scant use of this drug. Just 0.7% of adults age 18 to 25, for example, report having used crack in the preceding month (NIDA, 1991). Why then are press, public, and politicians so obsessed with this narrow aspect of the national drug problem?

One answer is that crack, more than other drugs, tends to externalize damage to nonusers and communities. Due to its highly addictive nature, crack users, like heroin addicts, often engage in theft and prostitution to support their habits, and commonly buy and sell drugs in open-air drug markets, crack houses, and "shooting galleries," which are the source of frequent violence and community disorder.

In addition, unlike other drugs, as much as 30% or more of crack addicts are women whose drug use directly impinges on the health and welfare of millions of American children. More than 100,000 children a year are now born with cocaine in their bloodstream, and our neonatal wards are filled with abandoned babies struggling with crack-induced brain damage and physical problems ranging from retinal damage to spinal curvature and renal failure (Dorris, 1990).

In contrast to crack cocaine and heroin, LSD, mescaline, and psilocybin are not addictive and tend to be used only episodically. Although marijuana and PCP appear to foster a kind of psycho-logical dependence, they are not physically addictive in the traditional sense of the word, and marijuana appears to have relatively few harmful health effects beyond lung damage and memory impairment. Highly addictive pharmaceutical drugs such as Valium and prescription tranquilizers are generally obtained from pharmacists and doctors or from networks of underground suppliers. As a consequence, the use and sale of these drugs is largely invisible and they are only rarely associated with the violence and crime commonly associated with street drug markets.

Legal and Nonlegal Problems Associated with Drug Use

From the perspective of law enforcement, all illegal drug use is a crime and therefore bad. But both law enforcement and the law recognize that some drugs are worse than others. Addictive drugs such as heroin, crack, methamphetamine, and barbiturates, for example, tend to fuel a tremendous amount of prostitution, theft, burglary, robbery, and embezzlement above and beyond the crime of drug use and sales itself. Drugs such as PCP tend to induce psychosis, and troubled persons on LSD and other hallucinogens occasionally harm themselves and others. Compared with these drugs, marijuana use is considered relatively benign by law enforcement officials and, as a consequence, penalties for possession and use of marijuana in small amounts is usually relatively light.

Along with property crimes fueled by addiction and very occasional acts of violence fueled by drug use, drugs are also implicated in most of the same problems associated with alcohol abuse: fatal auto crashes, child abuse, spousal battery, divorce, and poverty.

In addition to these social ills, illegal drugs foster a tremendous amount of violence and community damage directly attributable to illegal drug sales. From Boston to Los Angeles, and from Miami to Anchorage, the explosive combination of drugs, gangs, and guns is responsible for scores of thousands of bone and life-shattering acts of violence every year, most of them associated with street and crack house drug sales. It is this collateral damage resulting from street drug markets that is at the heart of law enforcement's current obsession with eradicating crack cocaine.

America's One-Hundred-Year War on Drugs

America's one-hundred-year war on drugs can be divided into three eras: the patent medicine and immigrant era, stretching from the Civil War to 1960, the counterculture period, stretching from 1960 to 1980, and the post-counterculture era of today.

The Patent Medicine and Immigrant Era, 1865–1960

Beginning with the Civil War and continuing until the 1960s, drug use other than alcohol was extremely rare among the general population and was largely confined to immigrant populations and those taking patent medicines.

Immediately following the Civil War, and beginning with the importation of Chinese laborers to build railroads, opium use on the West Coast became established, was then outlawed, and largely evaporated.

After the Civil War and continuing until World War I, cocaine and opiate derivatives were common legal additives to a wide variety of patent medicines, where their pain-killing and antidiarrheal properties were appreciated. During this period, laudanum was commonly prescribed for "female problems" and dependency on opiate and cocaine solutions was observed among a narrow spectrum of the general population. With passage of the Harrison Narcotics Control Act of 1914 and creation of the Federal Narcotics Board in 1922, however, narcotics use fell precipitously and most cocaine and opiate abuse disappeared.

With the Mexican Revolution of 1923, and a subsequent rise in illegal immigration from Mexico, marijuana use in the southwestern United States began to increase at a significant rate. In order to put a crimp on the spread of marijuana, and to facilitate the deportation of unwanted Mexican nationals during the Depression, marijuana was made illegal in the late 1930s and from then on was largely confined to occasional use by jazz musicians, immigrants, and isolated social experimenters.

Throughout the 1940s, '50s, and very early '60s, drug use in the United States remained at low levels. Beginning in the late 1950s, however, a few psychologists, biologists, and writers began experimenting with drugs being used as therapeutic agents in the treatment of depression, mania, and other mental illness. New drugs, such as LSD, were synthesized and showed promise in the treatment of alcoholism, and the chemistry behind such other drugs as amphetamines and barbiturates became increasingly widespread. Doctors and pharmacists soon found that there was money to be made by overprescribing certain kinds of medication and diverting some legal drugs to the illegal marketplace. As the late 1950s faded into the early 1960s, a small group of influential writers, led by Aldous Huxley and Timothy Leary, began writing about the personal enlightenment to be had by using LSD and marijuana. With the message "turn on, tune in, and drop out" ringing in their ears, drug use among the college-age population began to accelerate.

The Counterculture Era, 1960–1980

As the Baby Boom generation swelled the ranks of students on college campuses and the Civil Rights movement bloomed full flower, young college students became increasingly eager to break the bonds of convention they associated with parents, "the establishment," and the Cold War. A new music—rock and roll—came to campus and a new issue—the war in Southeast Asia—became a new organizing political force. The watchwords were free speech, free sex, and free drugs. As drug use became increasingly normalized on campus, images of freedom, music, sex, and drugs became so intertwined that it was difficult to tell where one started and the other stopped.

In response to widespread flouting of drug laws, schools and parents began early antidrug education efforts, which were designed to demonize illegal drug use. In their zeal to insulate children from the effects of drugs, these early antidrug campaigns inadvertently glamorized drug use by associating it with opposition to such authority figures as teachers, parents, and "the system" that was supporting the war in Vietnam. In addition, by failing to differentiate between the dangers and effects of different drugs, early antidrug programs sowed the seeds of future ridicule. As more and more young Americans experimented with marijuana and discovered that it did not inexorably lead to "reefer madness," other, more appropriate warnings about LSD, methamphetamine, heroin, and barbiturates were treated as factually incredible.

By the mid-1970s, marijuana use had become so endemic that it was now one of California's top cash crops and LSD, psilocybin, and cocaine could be found on most college campuses. Marijuana was openly smoked in parks and on street corners, and the National Organization for the Reform of Marijuana Laws (NORML) was considered a powerful, if somewhat underfunded, political force. Drug laws, though still on the books, were increasingly seen by the young as little more than a nod to an outdated social convention. Cheech and Chong movies, *High Times* magazine, and drug paraphernalia became cultural icons of the decade.

By the late 1970s and early 1980s, cocaine was a rising star in the drug trade, with its use and sales commonly associated with discos, high-fashion models, money, glamour, and sex. The height of young yuppie decadence was to snort cocaine through a rolled-up one-hundred-dollar bill, and such scenes were commonly played out in the bathrooms of trendy bars from coast to coast. This was the high-water point of drug use in America, and cocaine was the newest, most popular game in town.

The Post-Counterculture Period, 1980–Today

As the late 1970s faded into the early 1980s, a new drug appeared on the scene: phencyclidine, or PCP.

PCP, originally used as an analgesic for racing horses, proved to be a cheap but explosive drug, and horror stories about its use quickly began to circulate among the drug community. Tales of suicide, murder, animal mutilation, and total and permanent insanity deterred a great deal of potential users from ever trying this drug. But PCP was astonishingly cheap and its markup high, making its use and sales attractive to low-income teenagers anxious to try this "poor man's cocaine" sold under the street moniker "Love Boat."

As PCP use became increasingly widespread, the long shadow of PCP-induced psychosis began to cast itself over the drug culture. Conventional methods of police restraint seemed to have little or no effect on users of this body-numbing drug, and stories about police shootings of crazed, knife-wielding PCP users became routine in most big cities. The Faustian bargain of normalizing drug abuse was at last coming home to roost. Here was a drug every bit as evil and dangerous as anything ever described by the shrillest antidrug proponents.

The death knell for the drug culture came in the early 1980s with the arrival of freebase and crack cocaine. The public initially treated crack and freebase cocaine as little more than a variation on coke-snorting. Cocaine, after all, was a drug everyone thought they knew. What was overlooked, however, was that when cocaine was rendered into a smokable form, the body was able to ingest and release a tremendous amount of cocaine in a very short period of time. With nasal ingestion, cocaine entered the bloodstream very slowly though the relatively sparse cocaine-constricted capillaries lining the inside of the nose. When smoked, however, cocaine was absorbed through the much larger net of capillaries lining the lungs; absorption was complete and very nearly immediate. The result: Cocaine smokers very rapidly became addicts.

From a dealer's perspective, crack was the ultimate seller's drug, with a tremendous markup and almost instantaneous addiction for a large segment of first-time users. Crack carried the sexual mystique of powdered cocaine at a fraction of the cost: $5 a rock rather than $100 a gram. In addition, like marijuana, crack was easily smoked, easily divided, and required no needle to use. Finally, right from the start, a significant portion of crack users were women, a phenomenon that inflated the crack market by 30% and helped forge a complete culture around crack use and sales.

The arrival of crack cocaine and PCP changed the American drug culture forever. Drug use was no longer being treated as a mildly illegal social vice. Now it was the scourge of the nation. Cheech and Chong movies were no longer funny, *High Times* was no longer found on magazine racks, and drug paraphernalia was summarily banned in most states. Where once it was "hip" to be stoned, it was now considered pathetic and profoundly antisocial to be seen using drugs of any kind.

Throughout the 1980s, a full-court press was initiated to criminalize and stigmatize drug use. Congress and state legislatures embraced a host of mandatory drug penalties and new nonincarceration sanctions for illegal drug use began to be explored. Old-style drug education programs were replaced by more realistic programs designed to give students the tools to "just say no." Finally, antidrug ads on television, coupled with news stories about drug deaths (John Belushi and Len Bias) and career destruction (Richard Pryor and John DeLorean) worked to hammer home the message that drug use was both stupid and personally dangerous.

The Role of Regulation and Law Enforcement in Combating Drug Abuse

Education, criminalization, and stigmatization, coupled with crop eradication and antismuggling efforts, have worked, over the course of the last 10 years, to dramatically decrease the number of casual drug users in the United States. In 1985, for example, the National Institute for Drug Abuse reported that 12% of the population over age 12 had used illegal drugs in the one-month period before the National Household Survey. By 1990, this number had declined to just 6.4%, a decline of nearly 50% in just five years.

Although casual drug use appears to be going down across the United States, more Americans than ever say they feel threatened by drugs and drug-related violence. Murder rates are up. Burglaries are up. Neonatal drug abuse rates have reached astounding levels. In many residential neighborhoods, our parents and our children no longer feel safe on the street. How could we be winning the war on drugs when we are so obviously losing the war on violence, fear, intimidation, and disorder in our streets?

The answer appears to be that, though we have diligently focused on interdicting drugs and apprehending major drug dealers, we have ignored the explosive growth of street drug markets. With the introduction of PCP and crack cocaine in the early and mid-1980s, and with the entry of new ethnic and youth gangs in the drug trade, these street drug markets have become pervasive, unstable, and violent. In addition, though overall drug use has declined significantly since 1985, chronic cocaine use has been rapidly on the rise.

The lesson to be learned is not that the "war on drugs" has been a failure, or that drug use has declined to a point where it is no longer a problem. Rather, the lesson is that we should continue to focus on reducing overall drug use through education, stigmatization, and apprehension of major drug shipments, but we also need to concentrate on reducing the collateral damage that street drug trafficking is inflicting on our communities.

The Private Referral and Public Anonymous Markets

Drugs are sold in every community in the United States, from small towns with feed stores and single stop lights to large cities with underground subways and dance halls that never close. The product may be the same everywhere, but the manner in which drugs are sold varies from one location to another.

In general, it can be said there are two kinds of retail drug markets in the United States: the private marketplace and the flagrant drug market. Drug sales that occur in the private marketplace are those that occur between people who formally or informally know each other—college students who attend the same school, people who work in the same business, or patrons of the same bar or club.

Because parties in private drug transactions are familiar with each other or are referral customers, there is generally a minimum level of public exposure and violence. Because both dealers and buyers want to discourage the amount of traffic coming to their homes or businesses, sales in the private marketplace tend to involve larger quantities of drugs than those in street transactions. For instance, whereas $10 envelopes of marijuana or vials of crack are commonly sold on the street, most private transactions involve larger quantities of drugs costing $50 or more.

Because private transactions occur behind closed doors on private property, there is a high degree of impermeability to the dealer–customer relationship. As a consequence, police find it much more difficult to make arrests in this market than with street drug sales.

The private marketplace is amenable to middle-class and well-to-do customers who use drugs recreationally (i.e., they are not addicted), but it is generally inappropriate for poor drug users, addicts, and persons who only rarely or very occasionally use illegal drugs. The reason for this is that drug purchases in the private marketplace generally require five to fifteen times more capital than street drug purchases and the drug lots sold in these private transaction tend to be significantly larger than those sold on the street. On a practical level, this means that a person who wants to buy a single joint or half gram of cocaine finds he must buy an entire ounce of marijuana or several grams of cocaine to satisfy what is essentially a modest urge. Like the occasional drinker forced to buy a case of gin when all he really wants is a gimlet, the occasional drug user tends to defer his desire for the product more or less permanently.

The same is true for the poor buyer who finds it hard to save the money needed to make a bulk drug buy. As for the addict, a large drug purchase is fundamentally incompatible with their basic nature. Addicts know that a large drug buy will inevitably result in a short, unsustainable splurge that will deepen the addiction and worsen the withdrawal. Rather than "shoot the works" on a single party, an addict will usually opt to make smaller buys as a way of controlling the addiction.

For all of the reasons described above, eradicating street drug markets is a direct way of changing the economics of addiction and discouraging casual drug use. If street drug markets are systematically eradicated, addicts will find it harder to sustain their habits and casual drug users will be economically discouraged from recreational use.

Is it possible to eradicate street drug markets? Most assuredly. In Tampa, Florida, a concerted drug market eradication campaign successfully wiped out 95% of that city's drug markets in just two years.[2] Other successful community-based antidrug efforts in New York City, Chicago, Washington, D.C., and Charleston, South Carolina have shown that *no* community need suffer the burden of having street drug markets destroy property values, terrorize law-abiding residents, and undermine the antidrug messages being taught to children in school and at home.

Permanent eradication of entrenched street drug markets is not easy, however. In general, it requires crippling the basic marketing *systems* employed in street drug sales. A thorough understanding of the mechanics of street drug markets, then, is a precondition of any successful anti–drug market effort.

The Mechanics of the Street Drug Market

From a market perspective, open-air drug markets and crack houses can be thought of as the 7-Elevens of the drug trade, making up in number of sales transactions what they lack in individual sale size.

In general, street drug markets are dependent on large numbers of customers coming to a known and stable location in order to buy one or more packets or vials of a particular type of drug.

In this sense, drug markets can be seen as emulating Arab bazaars where whole sections are devoted exclusively to one product, and where local prices and quality are generally uniform.

Drug markets follow the bazaar model because this model is conducive to the rapid sale of illegal drugs. Because drug customers know where to go to get their drug of choice, and because customers already know the unit price of the product sold, sales can occur in just a few seconds and change rarely needs to be made.

Like other businessmen, drug dealers look for likely locations in which to set up shop and avoid certain kinds of venues. In practice, this means that drug markets tend to thrive in locations that exhibit four basic characteristics that suggest maximum profit and minimal social and legal sanction:

- *A sense of disorder and community abandonment:* Drug dealers know that communities with well-maintained yards, clean streets, and strong community associations will not tolerate their activities. Instead, dealers gravitate to neighborhoods with overgrown yards, abandoned cars, litter-strewn lots, and poor lighting.
- *Legitimate cover:* Drug dealers need a legitimate source of social disorder to help shield their activities. Bars, restaurants, dance clubs, and housing developments provide such a cover and offer dealers a legitimate excuse for being in an area.
- *A recruitable labor force:* Drug dealers are naturally drawn to poor communities that have large numbers of poorly supervised children. These children are easily recruited as lookouts and street drug sellers. If arrested, juveniles are likely to receive only probation.
- *Easy access and escape:* Drug markets are dependent on a steady stream of customers. As a consequence, street drug markets tend to be located in areas accessible by cars where approaching police can be seen from some distance away. In order to avoid apprehension, dealers prefer locations where they can flee into housing developments, bars, and other hard-to-access hiding areas.

By focusing enforcement and regulatory efforts on removing as many of the above market criteria as possible, communities can force street drug markets to stay on the move, thereby decreasing market efficiency and increasing the time costs associated with illegal drug acquisition. Once the time costs of sales and acquisition are increased, casual customers tend to drop off and addicts begin to find it harder and harder to make a drug purchase. In Lynn, Massachusetts, for example, eradication of the local heroin markets in 1983–1984 resulted in an 85% increase in the demand for drug treatment, as well as a 37% decline in burglaries and 66% decline in crimes against persons (BOTEC Analysis Corporation, 1990).

How to Break the Back of Street Drug Markets

Street drug markets can be eradicated by focusing on three basic objectives designed to reduce the volume of customer traffic coming to a particular site. These objectives are broadcasting community intolerance for street drug activity, removing marketing space, and removing the sense of impunity that currently surrounds street drug activity.

Broadcast a Sense of Community Intolerance for Drug Activity.

Communities must broadcast a sense of intolerance for street drug activity if they are to prevent dealers from colonizing their neighborhoods and discourage them from returning once they have been driven out. Two ways of achieving this objective are to create organized citizen patrols and to launch an aggressive community clean-up program.

Step One: Create citizen patrols. Community patrols use the moral presence of law-abiding members of the community to drive off dealers and their customers and to encourage an increased police presence in an area. By walking in groups identified by a common hat or t-shirt, and by equipping themselves with video cameras, walkie-talkies, clipboards, and whistles, citizen patrols are actively reclaiming the streets of Philadelphia, New York City, Washington, D.C., and dozens of other cities across the country.

Citizen patrols work because they turn the table on drug dealers by using the same techniques the dealers themselves use to gain territory:

banding together as a group, intimidating people in order to carve out space, and broadcasting individual membership in a highly organized group that can cause trouble for those who oppose it. The overall effect of citizen patrols is to throw an element of uncertainty into the drug marketplace; to keep the marketplace off balance and increase the element of distrust already present in the drug dealer–buyer relationship.

Citizen patrols do more than just discourage drug dealing. They also change how the police view the entire community. A common police response to the creation of a citizen patrol is to renew interest in the neighborhood and to dramatically increase police patrols within the community. With increased police presence and improved information provided by citizen patrols, a synergistic effect often results that leads to a rapid decline in drug-related activity.

Experience in communities across the country suggests that violence by dealers against citizen patrols is extremely rare. Dealers are loath to draw attention to themselves, and recognize that assaulting a citizen patrol member will be considered by press, public, police, and potential jurors as being just one step removed from assaulting a police officer.

Step Two: Clean up the neighborhood. In addition to citizen patrols, community clean-up programs are an integral part of most successful anti–drug market initiatives. By removing abandoned cars, installing street lights, painting over graffiti, clearing abandoned lots, and sweeping streets and alleys, communities can signal that they are willing to defend their space. In Tampa Florida, more than 80 tons of trash was hauled out of a community in one day. With abandoned cars and trash removed, dealers found it harder to stash drug caches in the neighborhood. Noted one community member, "If you see rats running around a neighborhood, you know it's because there's garbage and trash in the street. It's the same with drug dealers. If you clean up a neighborhood and haul away the garbage and trash, both the rats and dealers move on. Vermin can't last long in a community that respects itself."

Seize Marketing Space.   Street drug markets and crack houses depend on location stability to maintain their customer base. If a crack house or street sales operation is forced to move, it cannot easily advertise its new location. The more frequently a drug market is forced to move, the less likely it is to return a profit and stay in business.

As many as four separate steps may be necessary to reclaim marketing space and force dealers to change their sales location.

Step One: Abolish site-specific locations. When drug sales become closely identified with a particular location, such as a house, an apartment, a bar, a store, or an abandoned building, the drug dealers who occupy these places must be summarily routed. In practice, four possible options can be exercised:

- *The drug dealers or users can be evicted.* This is easier now than it used to be, due to expedited eviction procedures for drug dealers living in public housing.
- *The property can be seized and sold* if multiple drug transactions have occurred at the property or if the property was bought with drug money. Though used less frequently than it should, the threat of seizure and forfeiture is often enough to force a landlord to evict his tenants, for an owner to throw out his or her drug-using adult children, and for a bank to call in the note on a property.
- *The property can be bricked up or, if in a serious state of disrepair, razed to the ground.* In Tampa, Florida, for example, 50 buildings used as "crash pads" by local addicts were bulldozed to the ground in one day. Similar programs have been embraced in Dallas, Detroit, and many other major cities.

Step Two: Cut off dealer escape routes and discourage customer access. The second step to removing marketing space is to examine customer and dealer entrance and escape routes. If drug dealers cannot easily evade the police, or if drug customers are discouraged from entering a particular sales area, the market will generally relocate to a more hospitable venue.

In practice, different techniques are appropriate for different market settings. If the local drug problem is centered around a public housing development, for example, nonresident dealers and customers can be discouraged from entering the building by requiring all residents to sign the lease and carry a resident photo-ID card as condition of entrance. In Chicago, such a program is now used to control drug dealing in high-rise low-income developments previously terrorized by gang activity. For other market locations, a more appropriate response might be strategic fencing around parks, playgrounds, and housing developments, or the closing of certain building entrances and exits. In Charleston, South Carolina, routine driver's license checkpoints are set up to discourage drive-through drug sales in certain locations. In suburban Washington, D.C, and in Brooklyn, New York, street banners and signs warn of police and community drug enforcement efforts ("We Spy: Don't Buy Drugs Here"). Other possible techniques: making the street one way, closing off alleys to vehicular traffic, and installing remote video monitoring equipment.

Step Three: Increase penalties for dealing in certain venues. One way to reclaim marketing space is to outlaw the choreography of street drug sales and to increase the penalty for selling drugs in certain venues. In Tacoma, Washington and Tampa, Florida, loitering laws proscribe a narrow band of activity common to street drug markets: loitering in a drug market area, waving to passing cars, engaging in multiple brief meetings with passing motorists and cars, and covertly exchanging small packages and money. When these activities are seen together, police can enforce local legislation that makes it a crime to loiter with the intent to sell drugs. Another commonly used anti–drug market technique is the creation of Drug-Free School Zones, which assign additional penalties for sale or possession of illegal drugs within 1,000 feet of a school, church, or youth center.

Step Four: Remove drug market enablers. The final step in reclaiming marketing space is to examine whether it may be necessary to remove existing drug market "enablers." These enablers may range from public telephones used by dealers to conduct business, to bars, dance clubs, and convenience stores that serve as a restocking and meeting place for drug market activity. Pay telephones can be removed or altered so they cannot receive incoming calls. Bars, dance clubs, convenience stores, and liquor stores can be forced to change their operations through use of pickets and rallies, and through threatened or actual liquor and business license revocation. In New York City, Tampa, Boston, and many other cities, businesses that serve as the hub of drug market activity can be closed for up to a year if they fail to take action to discourage drug dealing on, in, and near their premises. Under Boston's padlock law, the police, the District Attorney, or any ten registered voters can force a business to close for up to a year if three prior arrests and convictions for drug activity have occurred at that address. In Tampa, a Drug-Related Public Nuisance Abatement Board routinely meets to decide the fate of properties where at least two previous drug convictions have been won. At the board's discretion, an establishment can be closed and padlocked for up to one year. As one community activist put it, "The city closes down a restaurant that sells poisonous food fast enough. Why can't it do the same with a bar that creates a dangerous and poisonous environment?"

Among the greatest enablers of street drug markets are physicians and pharmacists who divert controlled pharmaceuticals into the illegal drug trade. No single measure is likely to reduce such abuse as quickly as than widespread adoption of triple-prescription legislation such as that used in New York and 10 other states.

Triple-prescription laws require doctors prescribing commonly abused drugs (such as Valium, Percadan, Dilaudid, quaaludes, and phenobarbital) to fill out triplicate, sequentially numbered forms that have the doctor's DEA registration number preprinted on them. When prescribing a listed, potentially abused drug, the doctor keeps one copy of the prescription for his or her files and gives the patient the other two copies to take to the pharmacy. After filling the prescription, the pharmacist sends one copy of the prescription form to the state pharmaceutical regulatory agency and keeps the other for his or her files. The state pharmaceutical agency enters the prescription into a computer database. Patterns of abuse by a doctor, a patient, or a pharmacy can be exposed by analyzing the data.

Physicians and pharmacists who violate triple-prescription laws face jail and loss of medical license, a compound threat that sharply discourages abuse of prescription pharmaceuticals. In New York State, passage of triple-prescription legislation resulted in an immediate 65% decline in Valium (diazepam) prescriptions paid for by Medicaid. Clearly, triple-prescription legislation is one of the single fastest ways of curbing drug abuse in America.

Remove the Sense of Impunity Surrounding Drug Markets

In order to combat flagrant drug markets successfully, the sense of impunity that currently surrounds most open-air drug markets and crack houses must removed. In practice, three steps have been found most effective at achieving this goal: increasing police presence, improving police efficiency, and increasing the probability and severity of penalties levied against drug buyers and sellers.

Step One: Increase Police Presence.

The first step in removing the sense of impunity surrounding flagrant drug markets is to increase the visible police presence within the neighborhood in general and around the drug market in particular. The simplest and most effective way of doing this is to assign uniformed beat officers to stand in front of a crack house or in the middle of a drug market area where the officer can be seen by potential customers. If a dealer moves a few blocks up the street to avoid an officer's presence, the uniformed patrol member is authorized to move with him. A drug dealer who moves more than a block or two in either direction quickly finds that if the market moves too far, it loses contact with its customer base or runs into the turf of a competing drug enterprise.

This technique was pioneered by police chief Reuben Greenberg of Charleston, South Carolina, who notes that it is particularly successful when uniformed officers are provided Polaroid cameras with which to snap pictures of dealers and customers loitering on the street. Another favorite technique: knocking on the door of suspected crack houses "to inquire whether the residents are O.K." Notes Chief Greenberg, "[Y]ou get all sorts of interesting reactions [when you knock on a drug suspect's door], such as the sound of toilets being flushed furiously. There goes the dealer's supply of drugs for the night. Sometimes the dealer won't open the door at all. Alarm and uncertainty have descended on that dealer."

Step Two: Increase Police Efficiency.

The second step to removing the sense of impunity surrounding drug market areas is to increase the efficiency of police patrols in the neighborhood. In Tampa, this has been done by giving telephone beepers to special anti–drug market officers and giving these in-field beeper numbers to local citizens. When citizens page anti–drug market officers, they receive a call back, on a cellular phone, from the officer in their neighborhood. An immediate response is guaranteed if street sales are in progress. The result: improved citizen–police cooperation and a dramatic decline in street drug activity across the city.

Another anti–drug market technique that has proven successful is to mail postcard warnings to owners of cars seen cruising in drug market areas. Postcard warnings note that a vehicle (license plate number XYZ-1234) was spotted in an area known to be frequented by drug dealers or prostitutes and that "frequenting the area during certain hours can be a health risk." Postcard health warnings sharply reduce drive-through drug traffic by making customers fearful their spouses, parents, employers, or children will find out about their activities.

Because 40 states are currently under court order to reduce prison overcrowding, fewer and fewer first-time drug offenders are now being incarcerated. With the majority of first-time drug offenders given no punishment more serious than probation, drug dealers now believe they have at least two or three "bites at the apple" before receiving substantial jail time. In almost every case, they are right.

In order to deter both adolescents and adults from selling drugs, and in order to change current marketing strategies, state and local law enforcement officials must create nonincarceration penalties that can be used against all convicted drug dealers and buyers. Such alternative sentencing might include mandatory loss of driving privileges, mandatory public service work, regular urinalysis, daily participation in Alcoholics Anonymous and Narcotics Anonymous meetings, participation in self-funding drug treatment, and asset seizure of cars, bars, apartments, houses, and leases.

Car seizures are a particularly effective, low-cost way of penalizing buyers in street drug markets. Because cars can be seized under a civil preponderance-of-the-evidence standard rather than the more stringent beyond-a-reasonable-doubt standard of the criminal code, cars may be legally seized even in cases where a defendant is not charged or convicted in court. Persons who believe that their vehicles have been seized unfairly—such as a person who unknowingly lends a car to a drug user—have two avenues of appeal under the civil statute used in vehicle seizures. They can request nonreviewable summary judgment by a Justice Department hearing officer, or they can post a bond of $2,500 or 10% of the car's value (whichever is less) and take the case to federal court for adjudication.

Properly publicized, car seizures can have a deeply chilling effect on drug sales across an entire city, especially among suburban drug buyers traveling to the city to make drug purchases. Notes the special narcotics prosecutor for New York City, "When (one of these suburban kids) comes home without momma's car or without daddy's, the criminal-justice system is often the least of their worries."

Why Most Anti–Drug Market Efforts Are Now Failing

The most common way of combating street drug markets is to use undercover police officers to pose as drug buyers or dealers. These buy-and-bust programs are the cornerstone of most local anti–drug market programs. Sadly, however, experience has shown that these programs are only rarely successful in eradicating entrenched urban drug markets.

The reason for this is that although buy-and-bust operations generally result in a large number of arrests, they also tend to result in relatively few convictions leading to lengthy jail sentences. In many cases, street dealers are out and on the street even before the police have finished processing the paperwork. During New York City's Operation Pressure Point, for example, the police made 19,600 drug arrests and seized $4.9 million in drugs and 314 guns. Although 88% of Operation Pressure Point misdemeanor arrests resulted in convictions, the median jail sentence was just seven days—even though half of all defendants had prior misdemeanor convictions. Half of the people convicted in Operation Pressure Point did not receive any jail time at all beyond the day to day-and-a-half between arrest and arraignment. A similar story is true for Operation Clean Sweep in Washington, D.C., and other massive buy-and-bust operations in other major cities. In almost every case, jail space and money were in short supply and court dockets were already overflowing.

Although these operations were designed to send the message that drug dealers would be arrested and dealt with harshly, the message received in the street was entirely different. Instead of being wary and impressed with the efficiency of the criminal justice systems, most street dealers learned that, even if apprehended, they would not go to jail. Massive numbers of arrests resulted only in massive numbers of probations, routine sentence reductions, and early inmate releases for drug offenders.

Despite the failure of buy-and-bust operations, these operations continue to be the cornerstone of most local anti–drug market efforts. Instead of trying to collapse and cripple the mechanics of street drug markets, most police departments continue to embrace a "body count" mentality in the war against drugs. The end result has been increased crowding in court and in jail and the rapid release of most apprehended drug offenders.

This is not to say that street sweeps do not have an important role to play in the destruction of open-air drug markets. It does mean, however, that if street sweeps are the first and only technique employed by the police, they are likely to fail in their ultimate mission of wiping out the street drug trade.

SUMMARY

Successful prevention of alcohol and drug abuse depends on embracing a three-legged program of education, stigmatization, and criminalization. In the arena of alcohol control, mass education is being conducted only in the arena of drunk driving, and there is almost no effort at all to stigmatize drunkenness or to criminalize abusive drinking or improper alcohol sales.

In the arena of drug abuse prevention, a full-tilt program of education, stigmatization, and criminalization is successfully working to reduce illegal drug use. Because of the arrival of crack cocaine, however, and a generalized failure to focus on the nature of the harms drug use and sales inflict on nonusers in the community, drug abuse continues to have a profoundly negative impact on U.S. society.

Policymakers intent on using law and regulation to control alcohol and other kinds of drug abuse must reexamine the real problems caused by these drugs. Alcohol policymakers must embrace a definition of the problem that goes beyond drunk driving and alcoholism and that recognizes the vast array of social harms caused by nonalcoholic, situational, periodic, routine, and ritual drunkenness. A full accounting of the true nature of America's alcohol problem is a necessary first step toward adopting the regulations and laws necessary to denormalize drunkenness

and normalize sobriety and abstinence. Only when we recognize that drunkenness is drug abuse can we progress to the next stage of examining the possible legal and regulatory mechanisms that could work to discourage drunkenness and encourage sobriety and abstinence.

In examining possible alcohol control mechanisms, the war on drugs and the campaign against tobacco have much to teach us. Both efforts show the power education and stigmatization can have in reducing product use and abuse. A war on *drunkenness* would necessarily embrace some of the techniques used to control tobacco (such as health warnings and increased taxation) and some of the techniques used to control drug abuse (nonincarceration penalties for abuse and illegal sales, a licensing regime for all users, and complete prohibition of certain kinds of products). In addition, a successful program of alcohol control would embrace certain techniques used against both tobacco and illegal drugs (such as anti-alcohol ads on radio and television and a reduction in the number of market venues).

In the arena of drug control policy, we must stay on course while adding a new item to the list of current policy objectives: abolition of street drug markets and crack houses.

By focusing very specifically on the eradication of street drug markets, we can ameliorate much of the collateral harm drug abuse currently inflicts on the non-drug-using community. In addition, by eradicating street drug markets, we can further discourage casual drug use and make it more difficult for addicts to sustain their habits. Finally, eradication of street drug markets promises to eliminate an area of the drug trade that draws children in at an early age and undermines every antidrug message currently being taught in school, at home, and in our places of worship.

NOTES

1. The NIDA data undoubtedly underrepresent drug use in America. A doubling of NIDA-reported use patterns for such drugs as crack, heroin, and ampheta-

mines, however, does not appreciably change any of the basic points made here.

2. Tampa had 154 drug markets in the summer of 1989 and just 4 in the summer of 1991.

REFERENCES

American Alliance for Right and Responsibilities (1991). *Prohibition and the misuses of history in the drug legalization debate: An information backgrounder.* Washington, DC: AARR.

Blose, J. O., & Holder, H. D. (July 1987). Public availability of distilled spirits: Structural and reported consumption changes associated with liquor-by-the-drink sales. *Journal of Studies on Alcohol, 48.*

BOTEC Analysis Corporation (Dec. 1990). Drug abuse in Jackson County, Missouri: Problems and recommendations. Cambridge, MA: Botec Analysis Corporation, Appendix B.

Center for Injury Prevention (Fall 1991). Spinning the bottle: The role of alcohol in injuries not caused by car crashes. *Injury Prevention Network Newsletter,* San Francisco General Hospital.

Cook, P. (1981). The effect of liquor taxes on drinking, cirrhosis and auto accidents. In *Alcohol and public policy: Beyond the shadow of prohibition.* Washington, DC: National Academy Press.

Dorris, M. (1990). My Turn. *Newsweek,* June 25.

Grossman, M. (May 1991). Rational addiction and the effect of price on consumption. *American Economics Review, 81.*

Homel, R. (1986). *Policing the drinking driver: Random breath testing and the process of deterrence.* Sydney, Australia: Federal Office of Road Safety.

Kleiman, M. (1992). *Against excess: Drug policy for results.* New York: Basic Books, p. 193.

Moore, H. H., & Gerstein, D. R. (Eds.) (1981). *Alcohol and public policy: Beyond the shadow of prohibition.* Washington, DC: National Academy Press.

Moore, M. (1989). Actually prohibition was a success. *New York Times,* October 12.

National Institute on Alcohol Abuse and Alcoholism, U.S. Department of Health and Human Services (1990). *Seventh special report to the U.S. Congress on alcohol and health.* Alexandria, VA: Editorial Experts.

National Institute for Drug Abuse (1991). *National household survey on drug abuse, population estimates, 1990.* Rockville, MD: Division of Epidemiology and Prevention Research.

National Institute on Alcohol Abuse and Alcoholism Special Report to Congress on Alcohol and Health (1983). Rockville, MD: U.S. Department of Health and Human Services.

National Institute on Alcohol Abuse and Alcoholism Special Report to Congress on Alcohol and Health (1987). Rockville, MD: U.S. Department of Health and Human Services.

Office of Substance Abuse Prevention (1989). *Prevention plus II: Tools for creating and sustaining drug-free communities.* Rockville, MD: National Clearinghouse for Drug and Alcohol Information.

Rorabaugh, W .J. (1979). *The alcoholic republic: An American tradition.* New York: Oxford University Press.

Ross, H. L. (1987). Administrative license revocation in New Mexico: An evaluation. *Public Health Reports, 102.*

Ryan, B. E., & Segars, L. (1987). Mini marts and maxi-problems: The relationship between purchase and consumption location. *Alcohol Health and Research World, 1* (12).

Saltz, R. F. (1989). Server intervention and responsible beverage service programs. In *Surgeon General's workshop on drunk driving.* Washington, DC: U.S. Dept. of Health and Human Services.

Tischler, B. (1986). *Alcohol use and abuse: The social and health effects: Report and recommendations by the Presbyterian Church (U.S.A.).* New York: The Program Agency.

Wallack, L., Breed, W., & Cruz, J. (1987). Alcohol on prime time television. *Journal of Studies in Alcohol, 48.*

CHAPTER 4

LOCAL GOVERNMENT AND COMMUNITY ORGANIZATION

MARY ANN PENTZ

INTRODUCTION

Drug Abuse in the United States

In the last decade, epidemiological research has shown several changes in patterns of drug use among the U.S. population. Among adults, tobacco use has continued a steady decline for more than two decades (Pierce et al., 1989). Marijuana and heroin use have shown declines of 1–3% since 1978 (NIDA, 1991). Alcohol, cocaine, and other substance use have shown similar declines since the late 1980s (Adams et al., 1990; Adams, 1990). Among high school seniors, college students, and young adults, declines in illicit drug use have mirrored adult declines (Johnston, O'Malley, & Bachman, 1993). On the other hand, eighth grade adolescents, who showed some decrease in rates of tobacco, alcohol, and cocaine use in the late 1980s, began to increase their rates of illicit drug use in the 1990s (Johnston, O'Malley, & Bachman, 1993).

The slight declines of use among adults and youth in the 1980s prompted U.S. Cabinet member William Bennett to conclude in late 1989 that the drug war was being won in America, through the combined efforts of interdiction, deterrence, and prevention (Bennett, 1990). This statement was countered by several research reports and at least one congressional report that showed continuing increases in rates of cocaine use among prison populations and emergency room admissions through 1989 and early 1990 (Biden, 1990; Adams, 1990). It was only in the second and third quarters of 1990 that use rates among these high-risk populations showed declines consistent with general adult and youth populations (Adams, 1990; Adams et al., 1990). Some researchers attributed this apparent lag to the longer length of time required for effects of prevention programs to filter down to high-risk populations, who are assumed to be out of the loop for direct participation in prevention programs and may be affected later and indirectly through diffusion and social normative change issuing from the general population (Hawkins, Lishner, Catalano, & Howard, 1985). Others hypothesize a maturation effect, whereby cohorts of youth exposed to prevention programs will not be represented among prison and emergency room admission populations until early adulthood (Johnson, 1986).

Do these trends signal an end to the drug abuse problem in the United States? Obviously not, for several reasons.

First, anthropological research suggests that drug abuse may be cyclic, following patterns that may peak every 16 years or more (Musto, 1989). Because few epidemiological studies and no prevention or treatment studies have followed subjects for this length of time, there is little evidence to indicate that the United States is as yet out of the woods in terms of controlling drug abuse. A related issue is the limited scope of most prevention and treatment interventions, which are designed for implementation within small social units such as schools, hospitals, and service agencies (Biglan, Glasgow, & Singer, 1990). Unless systematically replicated across 10% or more of the universe of units, these interventions are unlikely to be adopted and maintained by the U.S. population for long periods of time (Rogers, 1987).

Second, despite the declines in use prevalence rates, the social, health, and economic costs of drug abuse continue to rise, particularly costs associated with violent crimes (Goldstein & Kalant, 1990). These costs are not amenable to change at the local school level, where most prevention efforts have been focused. They are, however, a daily concern of communities, and within the purview of communities and community-level governments to change.

Third, most prevention programs to which drug use decreases have been attributed are school-based (Battjes, 1985). School programs do not reach youth who are generally acknowledged to be at high risk for drug abuse in adulthood, including school dropouts and chronic absentees, runaways, gang members, and youth who are otherwise isolated from prevention and treatment support services offered through schools (Battjes, 1985). Reaching these high-risk groups requires intervention that is sufficiently broad-based to include at least one setting that youths attend regularly, and comprehensive enough to affect youth with very little direct participation.

Special Problems Facing Communities

In addition to general problems of drug abuse on the national scale, there are several specific drug abuse problems facing local communities across the United States. These problems can be roughly categorized as psychosocial and organizational.

Psychosocial Problems

Consistently, epidemiological and etiological research have shown that psychosocial influences are the most significant predictors of drug use and drug abuse development in individuals (Kandel, Kessler, & Margulies, 1978; Newcomb & Bentler, 1988). These individual influences include, but are not limited to: negative social behavior such as delinquent, unassertive, or aggressive behavior; early drug use onset relative to peers; peer and parent use; lack of social support for alternative nondrug activities; a social norm of drug use acceptance; and exposure to situations and environments in which drugs are readily available and accessible (Jessor, 1982). It is not surprising that these influences are visibly multiplied at the community level. The reputation of a community as a good or bad place to live often rests on the prevalence rates of antisocial behavior, including drug use and social influences on drug use. Communities—not counties, states, or the federal government—are faced daily with the responsibility for reducing or, at worst, accommodating these social influences and the individuals, groups, and environments that spawn them. Finally, although larger demographic units such as counties may provide funding, local communities are expected to serve homeless and unemployed individuals, transient families, youth who are bused to schools out of their neighborhoods, and other potentially disaffected groups who are likely to fall through the prevention service net.

Although the mantle of responsibility for controlling social influences on drug use and potentially high-risk groups appears to fall squarely on communities, community is not well-defined in the United States. Demographic or physical boundaries are insufficient criteria for defining a community in areas that are expected to fill or lose census tracts rapidly, include populations that commute regularly over these boundaries for work or school, or that have no local town governing structure (Pentz, 1986). They also do not apply to metropolitan areas, which are typically too large and diverse for local residents to relate to as a whole. Social and cultural population boundaries might appear to be more appropriate for defining communities, especially for the purpose of delivering drug abuse prevention programs designed to identify and counteract social influences. Unfortunately, units formed by social and cultural boundaries tend to represent population subgroups that relate to members on individual and familial levels, but have little tolerance or interest in other groups that occupy the same area and are subject to the same social influences. The result is isolation and diminution of potential communications and resources for drug prevention. Sarason has proposed an alternative configuration of community, one that includes demographic or physical boundaries insofar as they include governing structures and services that contribute to prevention intervention at the local level; social and cultural factors to the extent that they contribute to the identification of population groups with special needs and resources and motivation of these groups to participate in prevention; and psychological and behavioral factors that represent identity and affiliation with an area (Sarason, 1983).

Defining a community for prevention intervention based on physical, social, and psychological factors requires extended study and planning before program delivery can actually occur. Estimates have ranged from two months under conditions of preexisting planning, organizational cooperation, and population interest, to more than two years with no preexisting planning (Pentz & Valente, 1993; Bracht, 1988; Lefebvre, Lasater, Carleton, & Peterson, 1987). To schools and demographic areas faced with immediate loss of Drug Free Schools and Communities money—an annual "use it or lose it" process—and a barrage of popular programs and mass media material, a purposive planning period in which to define community may be a luxury they cannot afford.

Organizational Problems

Several problems impede the efficient and effective delivery of drug prevention programs in communities. These problems involve organizational structure, process, and communication.

First, all but the most isolated communities in the United States have been saturated with popular prevention programs, mass media, and community events since the mid-1980s, coincident with Reagan's Just Say No campaign and national media coverage of the drug abuse problems of several prominent athletes. The programs, materials, and events are typically structured for implementation at the local school, school district, or community level. Few communities have a formal structure or procedures for monitoring programs and materials that are introduced at these levels, evaluating whether they are likely to be effective in changing youth drug use behavior, and determining the extent to which they can be integrated to reduce overlap and competition for time and resources. For example, the majority of communities and schools in the United States have participated in at least one of the following popular programs or events for drug abuse prevention: Here's Looking At You, QUEST, DARE, Just Say No Clubs, Red Ribbon Days, Mothers Against Drunk Driving (MADD), Chemical People Task Forces, Students Against Driving Drunk (SADD), or PRIDE. With few exceptions, these activities have not been evaluated for their effects on changing drug use behavior. Recent studies that constitute the exceptions have shown some short-term effects on changing individual and community attitudes toward drug use and rates of program participation, but little evidence thus far for changing drug use (Rogers, Howard-Pitney, & Bruce, 1989; Hopkins, Mauss, Kearney, & Weisheit, 1988; Clayton, 1990; Ungerleider & Bloch, 1987; Flay, Pentz, Johnson, et. al., 1985). Furthermore, there is little published information available to assist communities in deciding if and how these activities should be implemented and integrated into a comprehensive communitywide drug abuse prevention strategy (Giesbrecht et al., 1990; Pentz, 1992; Pentz, Alexander, Cormack, & Light, 1990).

A second problem involves the lack of cooperative linkages, and thus the potential for territorial competition between prevention and treatment services in communities. At least five factors contribute to this competition: appropriations of Drug Free Schools and Communities monies that do not distinguish between prevention, early intervention, and treatment; limited state bloc grant monies that do not distinguish between primary prevention and long-term prevention; a lack of formal communication channels (such as professional conferences and meetings) through which prevention and intervention specialists can share knowledge and resources; weak or unspecified services that should logically represent referral links between prevention and treatment, such as generic or on-paper-only student assistance programs (SAPs) in schools that do not include procedures for referring at-risk students for early intervention; and lack of formal training of primary care physicians to identify and refer at-risk students to appropriate prevention or treatment.

The third problem is the lack of formalized local government involvement in most community-based drug prevention efforts. As with prevention and treatment services, this problem represents a weakness in linkages between systems, although the contributing factors are different.

One factor is that prevention programs are not yet an institutionalized part of communities and local government budgets. For example, the United Way system of organizations and campaign budgets, an institutionalized part of community services, a civic service complement to local Chambers of Commerce, and an annual complement to local government budgets for services does not typically include formal organizations that are specifically mandated for drug abuse prevention. The lack of institutionalized budgets for prevention also extends to federal Drug Free Schools and Communities monies, which are appropriated to states for direct allocation to school districts and communities. Local governments are not involved, or at most peripherally, if individual government leaders are represented on school boards or in community prevention coalitions.

Another factor is the apparent schism between grass-roots groups for drug prevention, often initiated by parents in reaction to drug abuse events in the community, and formal organizations that participate in drug prevention activities as part of a broader mandate for services, such as schools providing a drug prevention curriculum as part of health education for youth. Although there are few systematic comparisons of grass-roots groups and formal organizations for drug abuse prevention, numerous examples of conflicts between the two, impeding or completely terminating efforts to develop comprehensive community-based prevention programming, have been described at recent professional conferences and meetings (Pentz et al., 1985; Pentz, Alexander, Cormack, & Light, 1990; Pentz, 1990). Ever sensitive to public opinion and short election terms, government leaders may be reluctant to commit the local government system to a controversial area of community service or to make a partisan commitment to one group or organization.

An additional difficulty involves the distinction between demand and supply approaches to drug abuse control. Educators usually have been involved in demand reduction, focusing on training individuals to resist pressures to use drugs. Law enforcement personnel have been involved in supply reduction, focusing on drug trafficking interdiction and legal and physical deterrence. Historically, these approaches have been considered antithetical, the former associated with drug prevention, the latter with drug control. The U.S. Office of National Drug Control Policy (ONDCP) still considers demand and supply interventions separate, with separate budgets for operation. Recently, a few school and community-based programs have attempted to blur these distinctions by involving educators and parents in supply reduction activities and law enforcement personnel in demand reduction programs. For example, the school-based program DARE uses uniformed police to train students how to resist drug use pressures (Clayton, 1990). Parents Who

Care and the National Federation of Parents for Drug Free Youth include parents in local government initiatives to control the sale of alcohol (Pentz et al., 1985). However, local governments, with a structure that almost always includes police departments and the judiciary, are more familiar with and equipped to fund deterrence and control efforts rather than education and prevention programs.

The final factor contributing to a failure of local government involvement in community drug abuse prevention may be the reluctance of nongovernment community leaders and prevention specialists to include government in their planning activities. A seminal self-study of health planning by 22 major U.S. cities showed that community leaders were inclined to include the business sector first, to generate funding and increase public motivation to participate in programs; health professionals and educators second, to develop and implement the specific health programs and services; and government last, if at all, because of concerns about political favoritism toward individual health organizations or groups and the lack of longevity of political leaders (Wilson, 1970)

Local Government and Community Organization Integration Needs

The special drug abuse problems facing communities may appear insurmountable, particularly the lack of integration of local government and community organization efforts. If school, parent, mass media, and community organization programs alone have shown promise in preventing youth drug use, as the next section of this chapter describes, why include local government? Why should local government be an integral part of community organization?

The social influences on adult and youth drug use extend to any near or salient figures who serve as models for drug use behavior. The models can include prominent local government leaders as well as government employees who are visible to the public. As a social influence, local government can be mobilized to model and disseminate drug prevention messages that are consistent with other prevention programs operating in a community.

Adults, and particularly youth, are more likely to adopt drug prevention behavior and a community social norm of nondrug use if multiple channels for prevention program delivery are used simultaneously or at least consistently. The effect is a dose-response or exposure effect of prevention (Farquhar, 1978). Based on social learning and other behavior change theories, the choice of program channels should be determined by whether the channel is a social influence on community behavior and whether it is structured to and expected by the community to disseminate programs or information (Bandura, 1977; Watzlawick, Weakland, & Fisch, 1974). A local community government meets both of these criteria. It also represents a formal structure for relating to community organizations, both directly through its service mandate (police assistance in monitoring school grounds as part of a drug-free school prevention program) and indirectly through endorsements (community drug prevention rallies cosponsored by the mayor's office).

Prospective prevention program channels with the greatest probability of institutionalizing prevention may be those that the community expects to set policy and mandate services. No prospective program channel is more equipped or expected to provide policies and mandates than local government. Because of its structure and community expectations regarding its policy-setting role, local government may have the greatest potential for institutionalizing drug prevention in the community. Ironically, community organizations have been reluctant to engage local governments in drug prevention for fear that political biases and changing political agendas may result in less than comprehensive prevention plans and in disrupted intervention (Wilson, 1970).

Local governments disseminate policies and service information by making public proclamations. Public proclamations are perceived by community organizations and residents as statements of public commitment to act on an issue or a set of issues. Social learning theory and research have suggested that public commitment statements by individuals to avoid drug use and to practice prevention skills may increase their subsequent prevention intentions and behavior (Johnson, 1986; Bandura, 1977). Public commitment by a local government to prevent drug use could increase the entire community's prevention intentions and behavior, particularly if existing community organizations make the same public commitment.

Currently, funding for drug prevention programs in schools depends on the ability of school districts to shift existing funds for health curriculum instruction and on new funds distributed through state governor's offices and school districts or other local education agencies (LEAs) from Drug Free Schools and Communities monies. Similarly, funding for existing community organizations and service agencies depends on agency ability to shift existing funds from drug treatment to prevention, and on new Drug Free Schools and Communities monies distributed through state governor's offices and state agencies (Single State Agencies or SSAs) and county agencies (LEAs). The proposed 1990 Anti-Drug Abuse Act was designed to distribute funds directly to community consortia or community councils as well as to governor's offices, SSAs, and LEAs (U.S. Senate, 1990). The language of the proposed Act assumed that these community consortia represent an integration of local community governments and agencies for the express purpose of planning and implementing communitywide drug prevention programs.

Subsequent sections of this chapter address mechanisms by which local governments can contribute to prevention of drug use that also serve as points of integration with existing community organizations. Two primary mechanisms are participation of government leaders in the development of a special community organization specifically directed at drug prevention and control, and government development or refinement of community policies restricting drug use, including smoking ordinances, restriction of alcohol outlets or server policies, and monitoring of neighborhoods and public areas to maintain drug-free zones.

PREVENTION PROGRAMS INVOLVING COMMUNITIES

Theory

Several theoretical perspectives first proposed in the 1960s were applied to the understanding of adolescent drug use development and prevention in the late 1970s. They continue to predominate drug prevention research today. The theories are loosely referred to as social influences theories and include but are not limited to psychological inoculation, social learning, and problem behavior theories (Evans, 1976; Jessor, 1982; Bandura, 1977; Hansen, 1988; Kellam et al., 1989). As a group, these theories were intended to focus on individual behavior change and are based on epidemiological research findings that, next to prior drug use, the most significant predictors of subsequent drug use in children and adolescents are perceived peer use, parent use, availability and access to drugs, approval or tolerance of others' drug use, perceived tolerance of own use by others, low social expectations, poor social skills, and poor parent–child communication (Hawkins, Lishner, Catalano, & Howard, 1985; Botvin, 1986; Hansen, 1988; Kellam et al., 1989; Pentz, 1985a). The predictors are assumed to represent social pressures to use drugs. Thus, prevention programs aimed at social skills building have been developed to counteract these social pressures. According to social influences theories, drug prevention programs are assumed to work through the use of active learning methods that include modeling, rehearsal (or role-playing), feedback and Socratic discussion, public commitment statements, and extended practice in real-life settings. The progression of change is hypothesized as knowledge–attitudes or social normative beliefs–self-efficacy–resistance or other social competency skills–intentions–behavior.

The social influences theories aimed at individual behavior change may not be sufficient for understanding how whole populations and social units such as communities change their drug use behavior. Consistent with the U.S. Surgeon General's report "Healthy People" (1979) and similar subsequent reports, theorists and researchers have attempted to model drug use change on a sufficiently large scale to promote significant changes in the U.S. population's health by the turn of the century (Department of Health and Human Services, 1979). This larger conceptualization of behavior change requires an understanding of environment-level social influences that shape youth drug use behavior, including school climate or environment, mass media, informal and formal community organizations, and public policies that represent social norms for drug use in a community (Pentz, 1986; Sarason, 1983; Farquhar, 1978).

Organization development models, communications theories, diffusion, and ecological theories focusing on person–situation–environment relationships have been applied increasingly to the development and implementation of drug prevention strategies on a scale larger than the classroom, including school, school district, and community (Biglan, Glasgow, & Singer, 1990; Rogers, 1987; Pentz, 1986; Farquhar, 1978; Watzlawick, Weakland, & Fisch, 1974). According to these theories, drug use behavior change may occur in at least one of two sequences. If a large-scale prevention program is designed to affect community systems first, such as a health services policy designed to change how agencies refer youth for prevention services, then the drug use behavior change sequence could be conceptualized as policy awareness–social normative beliefs–acceptance–compliance–drug use behavior. This type of program can be considered a health protection or systems-level health promotion approach (Wallack & Corbett, 1987). On the other hand, a program designed to change the drug use

resistance skills of all youth in a community simultaneously might be expected to yield a change sequence of social norms–social normative beliefs–behavior. This type of program can be considered a mass health education approach to drug prevention (Wallack & Corbett, 1987).

Social influences theories that encompass both individual and environmental change show the most promise for explaining drug use development and prevention over the long term. When translated to prevention strategies, these theories assume that drug use behavior change occurs as a result of two factors: a dose-response relationship whereby magnitude and maintenance of change is directly related to how many program channels are used in the intervention (school plus mass media versus school alone) and how often and how much they deliver drug prevention messages; and the synergistic interaction of individuals and program channels within a community, such as the development of a new community organization for drug prevention from the combined efforts of existing agencies, community leaders, and parents who are participating with their children in a school or parent program (Becker et al., 1989).

Application

Current drug prevention programs can be roughly classified by the main channel or channels used for program delivery within a community. These include school, parents and family, mass media, community organization, and local government.

School Programs

School programs continue to dominate the field of drug prevention, and as noted earlier, most of these continue to focus on drug education, decision making, and affect management rather than counteracting social influences to use drugs. Reviews and meta-analyses of the effects of social influence programs have shown consistent changes in attitudes toward drug use and in cigarette smoking behavior, and some changes in short-term alcohol and marijuana use for some subgroups of youth (Sarason, 1983; Hopkins, Mauss, Kearney, & Weisheit, 1988; Botvin, 1986; Perry, 1987; Pentz, 1985a; Department of Health and Human Services, 1979).

Most school programs have shown effects in delaying onset of use rather than reducing overall prevalence rates (Battjes, 1985; Tobler, 1986; Botvin, 1986; Ellickson & Bell, 1990; Flay, 1985; Hansen et al., 1988). Few studies have evaluated maintenance of program effects for more than two or three years. Two recent smoking prevention studies have followed seventh grade youth through high school (Murray et al., 1988; Flay, Ryan, Best, et al., 1985). Both of these showed some maintenance of program effects until twelfth grade, after which effects disappeared. The failure of these studies to demonstrate significant long-term reductions in adolescent drug use suggests that school programs may not be sufficient to change drug use behavior patterns. However, evaluations have been based on school programs that were typically implemented in only one school year. Little is known about the potential effectiveness of school programs that continue implementation over several years. One such school program is Know Your Body, which is designed for implementation in grades K through 12. A recent six-year follow-up showed significant reductions in cigarette smoking in one of the school districts included in the original study; earlier program effects in all districts were mixed across years (Walter, Vaughan, & Wynder, 1989). With these equivocal findings, the question of long-term effectiveness of school-based programs still remains.

Compared to earlier school-based studies, evaluations of social influences programs represent a marked improvement in research and measurement design. Several if not most studies have randomized schools to conditions to match the unit of assignment, and have included pipeline or bogus pipeline biochemical measures of cigarette smoking to increase the validity of self-reported drug use (Biglan, Glasgow, & Singer, 1990; Flay, 1985). Despite these improvements, multiple pro-

grammatic and methodologic issues continue to characterize most school-based prevention studies. Schools tend to reinvent or modify drug prevention over time, and program deliverers—usually teachers—change (Rogers, 1987). A national study of health education showed that reinvention by teachers may be associated with more efficient program delivery and better student behavioral outcomes, although little is known about the conditions under which reinvention is helpful (Connell & Turner, 1985). It is not surprising that at least two studies have shown that the magnitude of prevention effect on student health behavior is directly related to the amount and quality of program implementation (Connell & Turner, 1985; Pentz, Trebow, Hansen, et al., 1990). However, few drug prevention programs systematically monitor program implementation or control for differences in implementation in the estimation of program effect. Also, relatively little is known about whether social influences programs operate to change behavior as theorized. Studies of social influence mediator effects are few and not altogether clear in their conclusions (Hopkins, Mauss, Kearney, & Weisheit, 1988; Connell & Turner, 1985; MacKinnon et al., 1991).

Parent Programs

Few drug prevention programs have been conducted that focus specifically on parents; most are school-based programs that attempt to involve parents through parent–child homework activities (Perry, 1987; Hansen, 1988). A major factor prohibiting widespread use of parent programs is the difficulty in getting large numbers of parents to participate on a regular basis (Glynn, 1989). Compared to school programs, which have a captive audience on a regular basis and built-in incentives for participation (typically grades or course credit), parent programs are subject to scheduling problems and lack of interest by parents whose children are not having academic or social problems.

There are a few exceptions. A review of parent-based programs revealed several studies that attempted to teach parents prevention, communication, or support skills; however, data on behavioral outcomes were largely missing from these studies (Glynn, 1989). A study conducted in the early 1980s was one of the first to evaluate the effects of a parent drug prevention counseling program using a quasi-experimental design (Gersick, Grady, & Boratynski, 1983). Results showed some change in parent attitudes toward drug prevention and variables related to positive communication and support; however, interpretation of results was hampered by severe attrition after the first few sessions. Another study showed that parents' involvement in homework and viewing of a mass media smoking prevention program could be enhanced through student encouragement or cuing, as part of a school-based program (Flay, Hansen, Johnson, & Collins, 1987). Although based on student self-reports of parent behavior, results of this study suggested that parent smoking rates declined after the program. Currently, a parent program that is promoted through elementary schools shows promise for changing developmental antecedents to child drug use and other problem behavior; the program teaches parents communication, support, and child-rearing skills (Hawkins, Lishner, Catalano, & Howard, 1985). However, published data are not available. Finally, there is some evidence to suggest that the effects of school-based social influences programs are enhanced by high rates of parent participation in homework activities that require active parent–child discussion (Perry, 1987; Flay, Hansen, Johnson, & Collins, 1987).

Collectively, these studies suggest that parent programs may contribute to the effectiveness of school programs; increased parent–child communication about drug use prevention and family rules prohibiting drug use may be the mechanisms through which parents contribute to decreased drug use in their children; and a secondary benefit of parent programs may be decreased parent drug use behavior. Unfortunately, these conclusions are based on a few studies with limited or selective samples and limited measures.

Mass Media Programs

Mass media campaigns and programs are receiving increasing attention as a potential means to decrease youth drug use on a population-wide scale. Several national campaigns have been disseminated since the early 1980s, including Chemical People, Just Say No, the National Institute on Drug Use ads, and messages sponsored by the Partnership for a Drug Free America. Several studies of current campaigns are underway. Results of previous studies are mixed. An early mass media plus school program, Feeling Fine, suggested effects on decreasing parent smoking rates; a later version of this program showed no effects (Flay, Hansen, Johnson, & Collins, 1987). An evaluation of Chemical People suggested that involvement of parents and community leaders in this campaign depended more on personalized letters of invitation from school principals than on national or local advertising of the campaign (Flay, Pentz, Johnson, et. al., 1985). A recent qualitative analysis of Project DARE, a school-based drug prevention program conducted by police and a campaign including widespread national and local news coverage, posters, and logos, suggests that the campaign has resulted in rapid and widespread adoption of the school program nationally (Rogers, 1990). An evaluation of community agency leader perceptions of the efficacy of MADD suggests that the small and mass media promotion of this grass-roots effort may contribute to community acceptance of more stringent laws regarding alcohol use (Ungerleider & Bloch, 1987).

These studies have used a range of experimental, quasi-experimental, and "natural" experimental (opportunistic, nonequivalent group) designs to assess the effects of mass media programs on drug use behavior. Collectively, the results suggest that the most significant contributions of mass media programs are community agenda-setting (making the issue of drug abuse prevention salient and worthy of public attention) (McGuire, 1984); increasing the motivation of nontarget or hard-to-reach populations to participate in available programs (Flay, Hansen,

Johnson, & Collins, 1987); and cuing recall of prevention messages and skills that are delivered through other program channels that provide face-to-face instruction (Farquhar, 1978).

Community Organization

This type of programming focuses on organizing community leaders for the express purpose of planning and implementing communitywide campaigns or programs. Leaders also may receive special education in drug abuse epidemiology and prevention, or skills training for demonstrating prevention techniques to agency staff members, clients, or the general public.

In studies of the effects of community organization, large social units such as community or county serve as the unit of assignment and analysis, and research designs are typically quasi-experimental, with units assigned to intervention or control conditions on the basis of demographic matching, readiness for intervention, or availability (Biglan, Glasgow, & Singer, 1990). Most of the published studies concern community organization for heart disease prevention, including the Stanford Three and Five City Projects, the Minnesota Heart Health Project, and the North Karelia and Pawtucket Projects (Bracht, 1988; Lefebvre, Lasater, Carleton, & Peterson, 1987; Farquhar, 1978; Perry, 1987). The significant effects of these programs on reducing cigarette smoking in adults and adolescents may be generalizable to community drug abuse prevention programs with youth. However, the heart disease prevention programs have included multiple program components in addition to and simultaneous with community organization; thus interpretation of the independent effects of community organization to reduced smoking is difficult. More recent are studies of community organization for alcohol abuse and drunk driving prevention, including a study in New Zealand (Casswell & Gilmore, 1989) and an evaluation of the grass-roots community organization efforts of MADD (Ungerleider & Bloch, 1987). Both of these studies suggested effects on perceived efficacy and acceptance of community interventions

for alcohol abuse prevention; however, neither study reported effects on alcohol use behavior.

Local Government Programs

With the exception of employee assistance (EAP) programs and health maintenance organization (HMO) services for adults, local government programs for drug abuse prevention consist of smoking, alcohol, or other drug use policy change. Policy strategies pertinent to youth drug use have been limited to pricing, availability, and age increase policies for alcohol use. Reviews of these policies indicate that they can reduce drunk driving and consumption in older adolescents, at least for short periods of time (Wallack & Corbett, 1987; Moskowitz, 1989). A recent study of school government smoking policies showed similar results for cigarette smoking in adolescents (Pentz, Brannon, Charlin, et al., 1989). With the exception of the school smoking policy study, in which schools were preassigned randomly to receive a smoking prevention program, most policy studies are natural experiments that use time-series designs and analysis methods to evaluate effects of policies initiated by local governments in response to public pressure rather than as a systematically planned part of a community drug prevention program.

ILLUSTRATION OF A COMPREHENSIVE COMMUNITY-BASED PREVENTION PROGRAM: THE MIDWESTERN PREVENTION PROJECT

Multiple community influences affect youth drug use, including school, mass media, home, and community organizations (Johnson, 1986). Thus, single prevention programs or programs using a single channel for delivery may not have a sustained impact on drug use in youth. Collectively, results of the current studies just described suggest that comprehensive or multichannel community-based interventions may have a larger and more sustained impact on cigarette smoking, alcohol use, and other drug use in diverse populations of adolescents than single programs alone.

The Midwestern Prevention Project (MPP) is a large multicommunity trial for drug abuse prevention with adolescents and, secondarily, their parents and other community residents. The MPP evaluates the effects of five program components that are introduced in sequence into the schools and communities that comprise the Kansas City and Indianapolis metropolitan areas: mass media programming, a school program, parent organization and education, community organization, and health policy change. Components are introduced at the rate of six months to one year apart, with the exception of mass media programming, which is initiated with the school program. Once initiated, the programs are continuously implemented in both sites.

The mass media component consists of approximately 31 television, radio, and print broadcasts per year about the intervention. The broadcasts range from hour long talk shows and press conferences to 15-second commercials and public service announcements. Mass media broadcasts are designed initially by project staff and their communications link with the mass media (Marion Laboratories Communications Department or Goldsmith Marketing) and then refined by mass media producers and writers who are familiar with drug abuse prevention theory and behavior-change principles. Each year, mass media broadcasts introduce the purpose and content of that year's new program component to the community, illustrate individuals' use of drug abuse prevention skills, and reinforce participation in each program component by featuring examples of individual, family, school, and community level program implementation.

The school program component is delivered by trained teachers, and includes 10–13 classroom sessions in grade 6 or 7 (the transition year to middle or junior high school), a 5-session booster in the following year, and peer counseling and support activities in high school. The school program focuses on increasing skills to resist and counteract pressures to use drugs and to change the social climate of the school to accepting a drug-free norm.

The parent program component is delivered by a trained core group of the principal, four to six parents, and two student peer leaders from each school. The parent program includes regular meetings throughout each school year to plan and implement an annual parent skills night for all parents, focusing on parent–child communication and prevention support skills; conduct monitoring activities to keep the school grounds and surrounding neighborhood drug-free; and refine school policy to institutionalize prevention programming in the school. The focus is to develop family support for drug abuse prevention and a drug-free norm in school neighborhoods.

The community organization component involves the identification, commitment, and training of existing city leaders to plan and implement drug abuse prevention services, funds and other resources, and activities that complement the other program components. The focus is on networking agencies and facilitating referrals for services across agencies. The resulting community organization structure and process is used to plan and direct the intervention in its early phases, facilitate intervention dissemination to the population, and institutionalize the intervention after the research phase is completed.

The health policy change component is implemented by a subcommittee of the community organization and other local government leaders. This component focuses on changing local ordinances restricting cigarette smoking in public settings, increasing alcohol pricing and limiting availability, and including prevention and support provisions to drug policies aimed at deterrence.

The overall intervention varies program channels, messages, and time of message delivery in order to saturate the community with intervention without sacrificing novelty or salience of the drug prevention message (Farquhar, 1978). Models of the intervention have been published previously to illustrate the organizational structure and process of program component implementation (Pentz, 1986; Pentz & Valente, 1993). Communitywide organization and implementation of the program differs from several other health protection and health promotion programs, such as antismoking campaigns and programs, on two major points. The intervention is organized from the top down, from school and community leaders organizing the initial program components with relatively little input from program deliverers and consumers, to deliverers and consumers providing more feedback, refinement, and modification to the intervention over time. Prevention messages are organized from the bottom up, from an initial focus on individual change in drug use resistance skills and drug use behavior to interpersonal or situation-level change in communications supportive of abstinence, to social normative or environmental-level change in policies supportive of abstinence (Bracht, 1988; Pentz, Alexander, Cormack, & Light, 1990; Farquhar, 1978).

The top-down model follows recommendations by Wilson for citywide health interventions (Wilson, 1970). Prominent business leaders were approached first for early sanction of the project and assistance in networking, followed by educators and health professionals and their organizations for implementation, and finally, late-stage incorporation of local government leaders for assistance in policy change. The juxtaposition of a top-down organizational model with a bottom-up drug use change model required that leaders receive introductory training in individual drug resistance skills and behavior change principles in order to make informed decisions about how to facilitate community adoption of the proposed intervention in the absence of lay public input.

Existing organizations were identified to assist in the overall intervention based on three sets of criteria: Wilson's recommendations to include organizations that represent business, education and health professions, and government sectors of a city (Wilson, 1970); indirect or direct capacity to deliver, or to influence delivery of, drug abuse prevention services to youth; and recognition by community leaders as a credible civic-service organization (Sarason, 1983; Bracht, 1988; Pentz, Alexander, Cormack, & Light, 1990). As post-hoc verification of the validity of the third criterion, all health organizations that

were nominated by community leaders were endorsed by the United Way.

The structure of the organization was hierarchical, following several community heart health programs (Bracht, 1988; Farquhar, 1978). The structure consisted of a steering committee of 6 to 8 individuals, mostly drawn from businesses; a community task force or council with total memberships varying from 50 to 100, and active memberships of 25 (members with responsibility for chairing or cochairing various subcommittees); and 9 subcommittees with 10 or more members each. In contrast to heart health campaigns, however, the subcommittees were structured according to function or youth service area rather than disease risk factor.

In its most basic form, effectiveness of the intervention is evaluated in a two-group research design by comparing drug use and use-related behaviors of adolescents in schools assigned to receive direct intervention with adolescents in schools assigned to a control condition. The measurement design is longitudinal, with samples of adolescents, their parents, school staff, adult community residents, and community leaders assessed annually through self-report surveys, phone surveys, observations, archival records, and—for adolescents—a biochemical measure of cigarette smoking.

Effects of the MPP on adolescent drug use through the first four years in Kansas City, and at baseline in Indianapolis, have been described elsewhere (Pentz, Trebow, Hansen, et al., 1990; MacKinnon et al., 1991; Pentz, Dwyer, MacKinnon, et al., 1989; Pentz, Johnson, Dwyer, et al., 1989; Pentz, MacKinnon, Dwyer, et al., 1989; Pentz, MacKinnon, Flay, et al., 1989; Dwyer et al., 1989; Johnson et al., 1990). Briefly, adolescents in schools assigned to the intervention condition show consistently lower prevalence rates of cigarette, alcohol, and marijuana use than adolescents in schools assigned to the control condition; by the fourth year in Kansas City (grades 9 and 10), adolescents in intervention schools also show less cocaine and crack use compared with adolescents in control schools. Analyses of the first two years of follow-up data in Kansas City have also shown decreased alcohol and marijuana use among parents of adolescents in intervention compared with control schools, and increased parent–child communication about drug abuse prevention.

Analyses have also been conducted on secondary outcomes of the program. An early analysis of program diffusion among a general population-based sample of community residents one year after program initiation in Kansas City showed that 11% of the population was aware of the project and showed knowledge of its content (Pentz et al., 1985). Analysis of spontaneous mass media coverage of drug abuse topics in the first two years in Kansas City suggested that the first two components of the intervention (planned mass media and the school program) may have increased reporting of drug abuse prevention topics relative to drug abuse, drug-related crime, and treatment topics in the metropolitan area (Johnson et al., 1988). The community organization component of the intervention was analyzed 1.5 years after initiation in Kansas City compared with baseline in Indianapolis. Results showed that the special community organization effected increases in personal participation of community leaders in drug abuse prevention, support for drug abuse prevention from existing organizations, and collaboration with existing organizations. Kansas City leaders also showed more centralized (efficient) networking for drug abuse prevention among individuals from existing organizations.

The demonstration of program effects on secondary as well as primary outcomes supports the hypothesis that the MPP is operating as a comprehensive, communitywide intervention. However, a confirmation of this omnibus hypothesis is subject to several other tests, including analyses of program implementation, components, and mediators that are hypothesized to operate within the overall intervention, as well as assessment of whether the intervention is effective with various subgroups that comprise the community population. Recent MPP studies have shown the following. The magnitude of program effects on

adolescent drug use are directly related to the quantity and quality of program implementation as measured on the school program component through first year follow-up, with the largest effect in schools with high implementation scores on teacher self-report and staff observation, smaller effect in schools with low implementation scores, and no effect in schools with no implementation (Pentz, Trebow, Hansen, et al., 1990). Preliminary analyses have been conducted on the first two components of the intervention: the school program introduced in the first year and the parent program introduced midway through the second year. Results show significant effects of the school program at one-year follow-up; significant, smaller effects of the school program and nonsignificant, positive effects of the parent program at two-year follow-up; and significant, smaller effects of the school program and significant, larger effects of the parent program at three-year follow-up. Analyses of program mediators through four-year follow-up show that perceived social norms for drug use—including perceived parent and peer acceptance of drug use, apathy about others' drug use, and perceived proportion of users—decreased significantly over time in program compared with control groups, and that these social normative variables mediated the effect of the intervention on later adolescent drug use (MacKinnon et al., 1991). Finally, analyses have been conducted through four-year follow-up on different demographic subgroups within communities and different risk groups defined by baseline use, parent use, and social skills and normative variables (Johnson et al., 1990). Results indicate that the MPP intervention has a significant effect on the program compared with control groups, regardless of demographic group or risk status.

Collectively, the results of the MPP thus far suggest that a comprehensive community intervention for drug abuse prevention can effectively reduce drug use prevalence among youth, that these effects can be maintained over the long term with the various groups that comprise a community, and that, for the sake of internal validity and replication, the intervention is operating as was theoretically intended. However, the MPP, like other community interventions, does not clearly differentiate or integrate the roles of local government and community organizations in prevention. Local government leaders are subsumed within the community organization specially developed for the MPP, and policy change—typically a local government responsibility—evolves from the work of the community organization in the late phase of the intervention.

PROPOSAL FOR AN INTEGRATED COMMUNITY PROGRAM

Based on findings from epidemiological and prevention research and on the evolution of prevention theory and intervention methods, an ideal community drug prevention program is proposed. The program would retain the MPP focus on primary prevention initiated with early adolescents and the multiple sequenced components that represent community influences on drug use (as have been used in the MPP and in several of the heart health programs). The development of a community organization with local government involvement in a later stage of the intervention also would be retained from the MPP, based on research suggesting that communities require sufficient time to institutionalize a program after initial adoption (Sarason, 1983). However, several modifications are proposed in the theoretical basis of the intervention, the structure and process of integrating local government and community organization resources for the planning and implementation. In addition, a typology of communities is proposed that would match community readiness for intervention with appropriate strategies for initial community organization.

Theoretical Model of Local Government and Community Organization Integration

The modifications in theory are shown in Figure 4.1. This theoretical model assumes that certain influences interact to affect community drug use. For example, prevention advocates on a local city council or school board may vote to reappropriate funds or other resources to improve the coordination of prevention service delivery across existing agencies; effective coordination then renders council members more likely to continue to support prevention efforts. The model adds to previous theoretical formulations of community drug use behavior change by elucidating specific points of integration of local government, existing community organizations, and a new community organization developed for drug abuse prevention. It also addresses several of the needs and gaps in government–organization integration described earlier in this chapter.

First, the model assumes an improvement in the flow of communication about prevention activities between local government and existing community organizations, and that prevention messages will be disseminated through internal media (government departmental memos), local small media (community calendars and brochures about jointly sponsored government and community organization meetings and activities), and local mass media channels (television news coverage of a city council meeting to determine funding allocations for a special community organization for drug abuse prevention). It also assumes that local government and existing community organizations have or will develop sufficient newsworthiness about their joint activities to stimulate media agenda-setting during the initial stages of integration, and to maintain community interest by regularly linking interpersonal communications by prominent government and organizational leaders, to small media communications aimed at neighborhoods and schools, and to local mass media communications aimed at the general public (Pentz, 1985b).

Second, the model assumes that funding for drug abuse prevention can be developed by reallocating existing resources. Thus, the model does not depend on new or external funding from philanthropic organizations or corporations, such

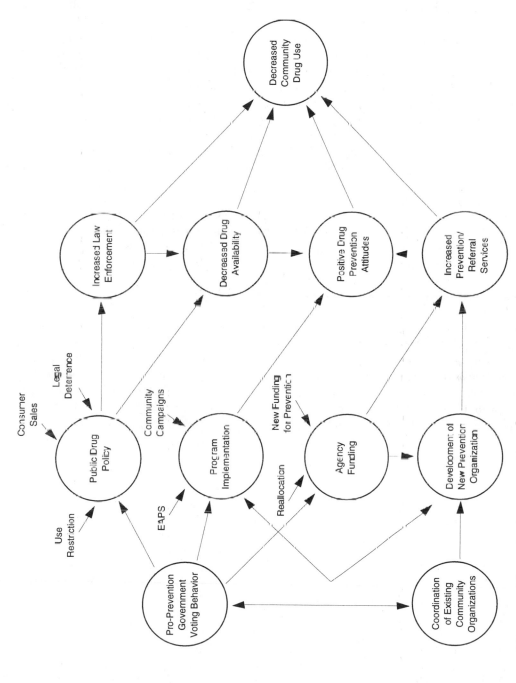

FIGURE 4.1 Theoretical Model of Local Government and Community Organization Influences on Changes in Community Drug Use

83

as have been used in the MPP, and is likely to be generalizable to small communities that do not have access to external funds.

Third, the model requires that a local government recognize its direct relevance to and need for participation in drug prevention. Direct participation is achieved by modeling drug-free behaviors and messages in community campaigns and by implementing in-house EAPs for drug prevention. The model assumes that government leaders most skilled in organizational development and management will apply these skills to gaining agency cooperation to consolidate and share resources.

Fourth, the model is structured to provide local government with the major responsibility for initiating community policies for drug abuse prevention. Thus, policy change is proactive rather than reactive to community pressure. Policy change is assumed to be in the direction of providing environmental and social support for a drug-free norm in the community, including the supportive rather than punitive use of law enforcement agencies. Further, the model assumes that policy will incorporate, if not eliminate the distinctions between, supply and demand reduction approaches to drug prevention. Both approaches would be aimed at changing social norms for drug use in the community, and consequently, decreasing community drug use behavior.

Delineation of Structure and Process of Integration

Discrete steps or stages of integrating local government and community organizations for drug abuse prevention are shown in Figure 4.2. The figure is adapted from the general stepwise model for community organization used in the MPP (Pentz, 1986). A new community organization for drug abuse prevention is created out of existing local government and agencies by Step 3 (left-hand column of Figure 4.2). Subsequent steps are devoted to creating viable working groups that design and implement observable prevention activities and programs in the com-munity. Each step includes evaluation of progress and completion (the right-hand column of Figure 4.2) before the next step is initiated. Thus, the participating members generate their own feedback to determine whether community organization is proceeding effectively, and if not, which steps require repetition or modification.

Ideally, one of the tasks achieved by the community organization in following these steps is the development of a review board or clearing-house to monitor prevention activities and materials that are incoming or available to the community over the long term. The MPP and most of the heart health studies have included this function in their respective community organizations. The result is increased quality control over program content and delivery, and regular (usually annual) updating of prevention materials.

Identification of Community Readiness and Organizational Strategies

Although the general theoretical causal sequence and structure just described are intended to generalize across most communities, regardless of demographic characteristics, communities are expected to vary in their readiness to organize for comprehensive drug abuse prevention. They are also expected to vary in terms of specific types of existing agencies to include in a community organization for drug abuse prevention, the focus of the community organization on prevention, early intervention, or treatment, and the timing of local government involvement. Identifying community readiness and tailoring organizational strategies to fit community needs may be expressed roughly as a function of community type. Based on community psychology and organization development literature, a typology of communities is proposed based on three criteria: whether a community is defined as a recognizable geographic, social, and psychological unit (Pentz, 1986; Sarason, 1983); whether the perceived empowerment of community and government leaders to effect drug prevention is high or low (Wallerstein & Bernstein, 1988); and whether

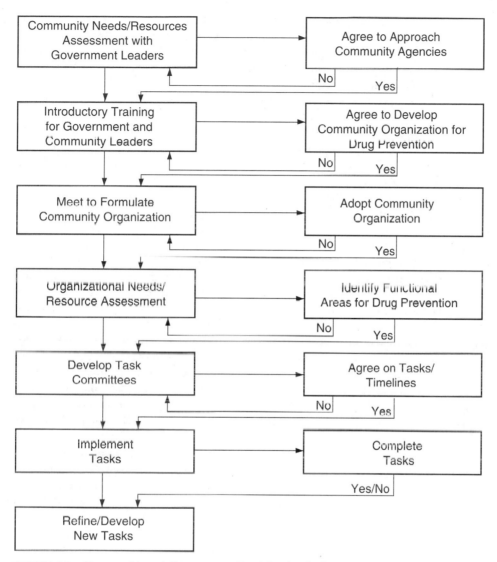

FIGURE 4.2   Stages of Local Government Participation in Community Organization for Drug Abuse Prevention

formal groups or agencies for drug prevention exist before the development of an integrated community organization for drug abuse prevention (Pentz, 1986; Wandersman, 1981). Crossing the three criteria yields eight categories or types of communities. In general, communities that are well-defined, with empowered leaders and existing structures for drug prevention, could be expected to organize most quickly, incorporate more types of agencies with less threat of territoriality, focus on primary prevention as a major objective but have sufficient resources to include early intervention and treatment, and manage without local government involvement until later phases of intervention focus on policy change. This type of community (Table 4.1) is most similar in the MPP to Kansas City, which organized initially within 2.5 months and has included prevention, early intervention, and treatment as part of its community organization mandate. In contrast, Indianapolis is most similar to the type of community that is well-defined, with empowered leaders, but with no preexisting structures for drug prevention (see Table 4.1). However, in the MPP, the definition of the community unit was modified to constrain intervention to the Marion County portion of the Indianapolis area; the redefinition may have been partially responsible for the longer length of time (2.5 years) to develop the community organization structure.

The typology has not been evaluated experimentally; thus, typing criteria, time periods, and organizational strategies are approximate. As the relationships between community characteristics and organizational capacities are evaluated systematically in future research, the typology can be expected to shift and expand. Also, changes in secular trends in drug use and acceptance of drug abuse prevention strategies nationally can be expected to contribute to changes in conceptualizing the typology.

SUMMARY

Epidemiological and prevention research point to the need for a more comprehensive approach to changing the social influences on drug use than is currently possible with school, parent, or mass media programs. Comprehensive prevention programs that have been developed at the level of community are too few in number to generalize from, particularly concerning strategies or models by which to organize the multiple program channels and interest groups that comprise communities. Even less is known about how to involve local government in community organization for drug abuse prevention, an increasing necessity if the proposed 1990 Anti-Drug Abuse Act is enacted. A theoretical model of community influences on drug use behavior and an applied model of stages of involvement are proposed for conceptualizing local government participation in community organization for drug abuse prevention. The theoretical model proposes to bridge the gap between supply (mostly law enforcement) and demand (mostly educational) efforts at drug abuse control in communities. The applied model provides definitive stages through which existing community agencies—or informally recognized community groups or leaders if formally organized community agencies with prevention interests do not operate within the boundaries of a local community or jurisdiction—and local government should develop a special nonpartisan community organization to plan and implement communitywide drug abuse prevention programming. Finally, because the models have been developed out of recent, limited research on communities that are well-defined and have extensive formal organizational resources for drug prevention and highly empowered leaders, a typology is recommended as an initial guide for communities to plan how and with which resources they may apply the theoretical and organizational models within their own boundaries.

Results of current research on community-based drug prevention appear promising. Despite the capacity to make direct comparisons that control for differences, research and measurement design, population, time of measurement, and cohort differences, results of community drug prevention programs also appear to have a similar or perhaps greater magnitude of effects than community-based heart disease prevention programs, on which several current drug prevention programs have been modeled. However, several issues remain to be addressed before community-based drug prevention strategies can be recommended to communities nationally, particularly strategies that promote the involvement of local governments. These issues can be classified roughly into three categories: organizational, implementation, and research.

Organizational Issues

A significant issue that precedes the actual organization of community agencies to prevent drug

TABLE 4.1 A Typology of Communities for Identifying Readiness and Organizational Strategies for Drug Abuse Prevention

COMMUNITY TYPE					ORGANIZATIONAL STRATEGIES	
Defined Unit	Level of Empowerment	Formal Organizations for Drug Prevention	Length of Time to Organize	Types of Agencies to Include	Focus of New Community Organization	Timing of Local Government Involvement
1. Yes	Mod–High	Present	2–6 mos.	Business, media, school, parent, youth groups, youth service, health/medical	Primary intervention + early intervention + treatment	Late
2. Yes	Mod–High	Absent	6 mos –1.5 yrs.	Business, media, school, parent	Primary intervention + early intervention[b]	Mid
3. Yes	None–Low	Present	2+ yrs.	Media, school, parent, youth group, youth service	Early intervention + treatment	Early–Mid
4. Yes	None–Low	Absent	2+ yrs.	School, youth group	Early intervention[b]	Early
5. No	Mod–High	Present[a]	1–1.5 yrs.	School, health/medical	Early intervention + treatment	Mid–Late
6. No	Mod–High	Absent	2+ yrs.	School, parent	Early intervention[b]	Early[c]
7. No	None–Low	Present[a]	2+ yrs.	School, youth group, youth service, health/medical	Treatment	Early–Mid[c]
8. No	None–Low	Absent	—	School	N/A	Late or Not at all[c]

[a]County-level organizations
[b]Early intervention limited to schools such as SAP and peer counseling groups
[c]County-level government

use is how to overcome political agendas of local governments that could bias, abbreviate, weaken, or disrupt an otherwise cohesive and cooperative community intervention plan. Given the modeling, funding, policy, and public commitment capabilities of local governments, their involvement, although not sufficient, is critical for institutionalizing community-based drug prevention programs. There are several potential methods for addressing this issue by neutralizing drug abuse as a political agenda in a community. For example, government representatives in a community organization for prevention (also referred to in recent research and congressional literature as a community partnership or consortium) could be selected on the basis of their political neutrality relative to the local party in power or on their relative longevity in office. Alternatively, as suggested by the typology in Table 4.1, the involvement of local governments might be delayed until a community organization for drug prevention is already mounted and operating with funds independent of local governments. Local government could be approached at this middle or late stage of community organization to coalesce local and media into presenting a message of the importance of continued community drug prevention. Broadcasting this message across multiple types of media is well within the purview of local government, and serves the purpose of agenda-setting, or increasing the public's perceived importance of maintaining attention to drug prevention as a high-priority area for discussion and intervention (McGuire, 1984).

A second major organizational issue is that little is known about whether top-down or bottom-up approaches to community organization are more or less effective for integrating local government and community agency efforts. A third issue is maintaining the function of local government as providing environmental support for a drug-free social norm in the community. Because local government oversees the use of law enforcement in the service of drug abuse prevention, it may be difficult to inhibit the development or perceived development of local government as a community watchdog of drug abuse, a function that could engender resentment rather than cooperation from community residents and agencies.

Implementation Issues

Previous research in drug abuse prevention clearly demonstrates that didactic instruction methods, testimonials, and mass media campaigns are ineffective for changing drug use behavior. However, raising the initial motivation of some communities to organize for drug prevention—especially communities that are ill-defined, perceive little empowerment, and have few organizational resources for drug prevention—may depend on the strategic use of instruction, testimonials, and campaigns. Little is currently known about whether, when, and how much to use these strategies in conjunction with other more proven methods of drug prevention to achieve community motivation to act. A second major issue is actual program delivery: research has shown that a prevention program is effective only insofar as it is implemented as designed. Furthermore, these findings suggest that sustained implementation may depend on reinforcing program deliverers and participants, providing periodic retraining of deliverers, and enabling deliverers to reinvent some aspects of a prevention program that result in more efficient or more tailored programming (Rogers, 1987; Botvin, 1986; Pentz, Trebow, Hansen, et al., 1990). However, research on these suspected implementation variables has not been sufficiently replicated to make definitive predictions about conditions for program maintenance.

Research Issues

A comprehensive community approach to drug abuse prevention looks promising. Unfortunately, conclusions about relatively larger effects to be derived from this approach versus single channel prevention approaches are still speculative. Most of the community prevention research conducted thus far has depended on natural experiments or quasi-experimental designs to evaluate program effects. Few studies and few research agencies can afford to operate and fund community-level research that randomizes a sufficient number of communities to experimental conditions to satisfy questions of statistical power, environmental confounds, and group equivalence. In addition, communities participating in a prevention research study can be expected to be affected by multiple historical events, changes in secular trends in drug use, and demographic shifts over time, all of which can jeopardize interpretations of program effect. Research and measurement design strategies and statistical methods for the special requirements of community-level research are still evolving (Biglan, Glasgow, & Singer, 1990; Johnson et al., 1990). It is hoped that these methodologies will yield more definitive conclusions about the efficacy of community drug prevention programs in the future.

REFERENCES

Adams, E. H. (June 1990). *Recent trends in cocaine use in the United States.* Paper presented at the 18th International Institute on the Prevention and Treatment of Drug Dependence, Berlin.

Adams, E. H., Blanken, A. J., Ferguson, L. D., et al (1990). *Overview of selected drug trends.* National Institute on Drug Abuse unpublished report.

Bandura, A. (1977). *Social learning theory.* Englewood Cliffs, NJ: Prentice Hall.

Battjes, R. J. (1985). Prevention of adolescent drug abuse. *International Journal of Addictions, 20,* 1113–1134.

Becker, S. L., Burke, J. A., Arbogast, R. A., Naughton, M. J., Bachman, I., & Spohn, E. (1989). Community programs to enhance in-school anti-tobacco efforts. *Preventive Medicine, 18,* 221–228.

Bennett, W. J. (1990). *National drug control strategy,* Washington, DC: U.S. Government Printing Office.

Biden, J. R. (Jan. 1990). Fighting drug abuse: A national survey, prepared by the Majority Staff of the Senate Judiciary Committee and the International Narcotics Control Caucus.

Biglan, A., Glasgow, R. E., & Singer, G. (1990) The need for a science of larger social units: A contextual approach. *Behavior Therapy, 21* (2), 195–215.

Botvin, G. J. (1986). Substance abuse prevention research: Recent developments and future directions. *Journal of School Health, 56* (9), 369–374.

Bracht, N. F. (1988). Use of community analysis methods on community-wide intervention programs. *Scandinavian Journal of Primary Health Care, 1,* 23–30.

Casswell, S., & Gilmore, L. (1989). An evaluated community action project on alcohol: Community organization and its evaluation. *Journal on Studies of Alcohol, 30* (4), 339–346.

Clayton, R. (Oct. 1990). The National Institute on Drug Abuse (NIDA) longitudinal DARE evaluation, presented at the Alcohol, Tobacco, and Other Drugs Conference, San Diego.

Connell, D. B., & Turner, R. R. (1985). The impact of instructional experience and the effects of cumulative instruction. *Journal of School Health, 55,* 324–331.

Department of Health & Human Services (1979). *Healthy people: The Surgeon General's report on health promotion and disease prevention.* Washington, DC: Department of Health & Human Services, Education and Welfare (PHS) Publication No. 79-55071.

Dwyer, J. H., MacKinnon, D. P., Pentz, M. A., Flay, B. R., Hansen, W. B., Wang, E. Y.I., & Johnson, C. A. (1989). Estimating intervention effects in longitudinal studies. *American Journal of Epidemiology, 130* (4), 781–795.

Ellickson, P. L., & Bell, R. M. (1990). Drug prevention in junior high: A multi-site longitudinal test. *Science, 247,* 1299–1305.

Evans, I. R. (1976). Smoking in children: Developing a social psychological strategy of deterrence. *Preventive Medicine, 5,* 12–127.

Farquhar, J. W. (1978). The community-based model of lifestyle intervention trials. *American Journal of Epidemiology, 108* (2), 103–111.

Flay, B. R. (1985). Psychosocial approaches to smoking prevention: A review of findings. *Health Psychology, 4,* 449–488.

Flay, B. R., Hansen, W. B., Johnson, C. A., & Collins, L. M. (1987). Implementation effectiveness trial of a social influences smoking prevention program using schools and television. *Health Education Research Theory and Practice, 2* (4), 385–400.

Flay, B. R., Pentz, M. A., Johnson, C. A., Sussman, S., Mestell, J., Scheier, L., Collins, L. M., & Hansen, W. B. (1985). Reaching children with mass media health promotion programs: The relative effectiveness of an advertising campaign, a community-based program, and a school-based program. In D. S. Leather (Ed.), *Health education and the media,* vol. 2. Oxford: Pergamon Press.

Flay, B. R., Ryan, K. B., Best, A. J., Brown, K. S., Kersell, M. W., d'Avernas, J. R., & Zanna, M. P. (1985). Are social-psychological smoking prevention programs effective? The Waterloo study. *Journal of Behavioral Medicine, 8* (1), 37–59.

Gersick, K. E., Grady, K., & Boratynski, M. (June 1983). Parent programs in conjunction with school programs, presented at the NIDA Technical Review on Community Prevention Research, Rockville, MD.

Giesbrecht, N., Consley, P., Denniston, R. W., et al. (Eds.) (1990). *Research, action, and the community: Experiences in the prevention of alcohol and other problems,* OSAP Prevention Monograph 4. U.S. Department of Health and Human Services.

Glynn, T. J. (1989). Essential elements of school-based smoking prevention programs. *Journal of School Health, 59* (52), 181–188.

Goldstein, A., & Kalant, H. (1990). Drug policy: Striking the right balance. *Science, 249,* 1513–1521.

Hansen, W. B. (1988). Theory and implementation of the social influence model of primary prevention. Paper presented at the First National Conference on Prevention Research Findings: Implications for Alcohol and Drug Abuse Program Planning, National Prevention Network, Kansas City, MO.

Hansen, W. B., Johnson, C. A., Flay, B. R., Graham, J. W., & Sobel, J. S. (1988). Affective and social influences approaches to the prevention of multiple substance abuse among seventh grade students: Results from Project SMART. *Preventive Medicine, 17,* 1–20.

Hawkins, J. D., Lishner, D. M., Catalano, R. F., & Howard, M. O. (1985). Childhood predictors of adolescent substance abuse: Toward an empirically grounded theory. *Journal of Children in Contemporary Society, 18* (1–2), 11–48.

Hopkins, R. H., Mauss, A. L., Kearney, K. A., & Weisheit, R. A. (1988). Comprehensive evaluation of a model alcohol education curriculum. *Journal of Studies on Alcohol, 49,* 38–50.

Jessor, R. (1982). Problem behavior and developmental transition in adolescence. *Journal of School Health, 52* (5), 295–300.

Johnson, C. A. (1986). Prevention and control of drug abuse. In J. M. Last (Ed.), *Maxcy-Rosenau: Public Health and Preventive Medicine,* 1075–1087.

Johnson, C. A., MacKinnon, D. P., Pentz, M. A., et al. (Dec. 1988). Which risks to communicate?: Lessons learned from drug abuse prevention campaigns. Paper presented at the Annenberg School of Communication Science Symposium.

Johnson, C. A., Pentz, M. A., Weber, M. D., Dwyer, J. H., MacKinnon, D. P., Flay, B. R., Baer, N. A., & Hansen, W. B. (1990). The relative effectiveness of comprehensive community programming for drug abuse prevention with risk and low risk adolescents. *Journal of Consulting and Clinical Psychology, 58* (4), 40047–40056.

Johnston, L. D., O'Malley, P. M., & Bachman, J. G. (1993). National survey results on drug use from Monitoring the Future Study, 1975–1992. *National Institute on Drug Abuse Publication no. (NIH)93-3597.* Washington, DC: Superintendent of Documents, U.S. Government Printing Office.

Kandel, D. B., Kessler, R. C., & Margulies, R. Z. (1978). Antecedents of adolescent initiation into stages of drug use: A developmental analysis. In D. B. Kandel (Ed.), *Longitudinal research and drug use: Empirical findings and methodological issues.* Washington, DC: Hemisphere, pp. 73–98.

Kellam, S., Ialongo, N., Brown, H., Laudolff, J., Mirsky, A., Anthony, B., Ahern, M., Anthony, J., Edelsohn, G., & Dolan, L. (1989). Attention problems in first grade and shy and aggressive behaviors as antecedents to later heavy or inhibited substance use. *NIDA Research Monograph 95,* 368–369.

Lefebvre, R. C., Lasater, T. M., Carleton, R., & Peterson, G. (1987). Theory and delivery of health programming in the community: The Pawtucket Heart Health Program. *Preventive Medicine, 16,* 80–95.

MacKinnon, D. P., Johnson, C. A., Pentz, M. A., Dwyer, J. H., Hansen, W. B., Flay, B. R., & Wang, E.Y.I., (1991). Mediating mechanisms in a school-based drug prevention program: First year effects of the Midwestern Prevention Project. *Health Psychology, 10* (3), 164–172.

McGuire, W. J. (1984). Public communications as a strategy for inducing health-promoting behavior. *Preventive Medicine, 13,* 299–319.

Moskowitz, J. M. (1989). The primary prevention of alcohol problems: A critical review of the research literature. *Journal of Studies on Alcohol, 50* (1), 54–88.

Murray, D. M., Davis-Hearn, M., Goldman, A. I., et al. (1988). Four and five year follow-up results from four seventh-grade smoking prevention strategies. *Journal of Behavioral Medicine, 11,* 396–405.

Musto, D. F. (1989). Evolution of American attitudes toward substance abuse. *Annals of the New York Academy of Sciences, 562,* 3–7.

National Institute on Drug Abuse (1991). *1990 national household survey on drug abuse.* Washington, DC: National Institute on Drug Abuse, Division of Epidemiology and Prevention Research.

Newcomb, M. D., & Bentler, P. M. (1988). *Consequences of adolescent drug use: Impact on the lives of young adults.* Newbury Park, CA: Sage.

Pentz, M. A. (1985a). Key integrative communication systems (KICS): The role of media in community approaches to alcohol prevention. In A. M. Mecca (Ed.), *Prevention action planning for alcohol-related problems.* Sacramento: California Health Research Foundation, pp. 85–91.

Pentz, M. A. (1985b). Social skills and self-efficacy in adolescent drug abuse prevention. In T. A. Wills & S. Shiffman (Eds.), *Coping and substance use.* New York: Academic Press, pp. 117–42.

Pentz, M. A. (1986). Community organization and school liaisons: How to get programs started. *Journal of School Health, 56* (9), 382–388.

Pentz, M. A. (Oct. 1990). A multi-community trial for primary prevention of adolescent drug abuse: Effects on drug use prevalence, presented at UCLA International Conference, What Do We Know About School-Based Prevention Strategies? Alcohol, Tobacco, and Other Drugs. San Diego, California.

Pentz, M. A. (1992). Integrated school and community programs. In G. S. Parcel, J. Igoe, H. M. Wallace, K. Patrick, G. S. Parcell, & J. B. Igoe (Eds.), *Principles and practices of student health.* Oakland, CA: Third Party Press.

Pentz, M. A., Alexander, P., Cormack, C. C., & Light (1990). Issues in the development and process of community-based alcohol and drug prevention: The

Midwestern Prevention Project (MPP). In N. Giesbrecht, P. Consley, R. W. Denniston, et al. (Eds.), *Research, action, and the community: Experiences in the prevention of alcohol and other drug problems,* OSAP Prevention Monograph 4. U.S. Department of Health & Human Services, pp. 136–143.

Pentz, M. A., Brannon, B. R., Charlin, V. L., Barrett, E. J., MacKinnon, D. P., & Flay, B. R. (1989). The power of policy: The relationship of smoking policy to adolescent smoking. *American Journal of Public Health, 79* (7), 857–862.

Pentz, M. A., Dwyer, J. H., MacKinnon, D. P., Flay, B. R., Hansen, W. B., Wang, E.Y.I., & Johnson, C. A. (1989). A multi-community trial for primary prevention of adolescent drug abuse: Effects on drug use prevalence. *Journal of the American Medical Association, 261* (22), 3259–3266.

Pentz, M. A., Johnson, C. A., Dwyer, J. H., MacKinnon, D. P., Hansen, W. B., & Flay, B. R. (1989). A comprehensive community approach to adolescent drug abuse prevention: Effects on cardiovascular disease risk behaviors. *Annals of Medicine, 21* (3), 219–222.

Pentz, M. A., Johnson, C. A., Flay, B. R., et al. (Aug. 1985). Community approaches to prevention and health promotion: Current directions. Presented at the American Psychological Association Meeting, Los Angeles.

Pentz, M. A., MacKinnon, D. P., Dwyer, J. H., Wang, E.Y.I., Hansen, W. B., Flay, B. R., & Johnson, C. A. (1989). Longitudinal effects of the Midwestern Prevention Project (MPP) on regular and experimental smoking in adolescents. *Preventive Medicine, 19,* 304–321.

Pentz, M. A., MacKinnon, D. P., Flay, B. R., Hansen, W. B., Johnson, C. A., & Dwyer, J. H. (1989). Primary prevention of chronic disease in adolescence: Effects of the Midwestern Prevention Project (MPP) on tobacco use. *American Journal of Epidemiology, 130* (4), 713–724.

Pentz M. A., Trebow, E., Hansen, W. B., MacKinnon, D. P., Dwyer, J. H., Flay, B. R., Daniels, S., Cormack, C., & Johnson, C. A. (1990). Effects of program implementation on adolescent drug use behavior: The Midwestern Prevention Project (MPP). *Evaluation Review, 14* (3), 264–289.

Pentz, M. A., & Valente, T. (1993). Effects of community organization on a drug abuse prevention campaign. In T. E. Backer, E. M. Rogers,

& R. Denniston (Eds.), *Impact of organizations on mass media health behavior campaigns.* Newbury Park, CA: Sage.

Perry, C. L. (1987). Results of prevention programs with adolescents. *Drug and Alcohol Dependence, 20* (1), 13–19.

Pierce, J., Fiore, M. C., Novotny, T. E., et al. (1989). Trends in cigarette smoking in the United States. Projections to the year 2000. *Journal of the American Medical Association, 261* (1), 61–65.

Rogers, E. M. (1987). The diffusion of innovations perspective. In N. D. Weinstein (Ed.), *Taking care: Understanding and encouraging self-protective behavior.* New York: Cambridge University Press, pp. 79–94.

Rogers, E. M. (April 1990). Cops, kids, and drugs: Organizational factors in the spontaneous diffusion of Project D.A.R.E. Presented at the Conference on Organizational Factors in Drug Abuse Prevention Campaigns, Bethesda, MD.

Rogers, T., Howard-Pitney, B., & Bruce, B. L. (Eds.) (1989). *What works? A guide to school-based alcohol and drug abuse prevention curricula.* Palo Alto, CA: Health Promotion Resource Center, Stanford Center for Research in Disease Prevention.

Sarason, S. (1983). Psychology and public policy: Missed opportunity. In R. E. Felner, L. A. Jason, J. M. Moritsugu, et al. (Eds.), *Preventive psychology: Theory, research, and practice.* New York: Pergamon Press.

Tobler, N. S. (1986). Meta-analyses of 143 adolescent drug prevention programs: Quantitative outcome results of program participants compared to a control or comparison group. *Journal of Drug Issues, 17,* 537–567.

Ungerleider, S., & Bloch, S. A. (1987). Perceived effectiveness of drinking–driving countermeasures: An evaluation of MADD. *Journal of Studies on Alcohol, 49* (2), 191–195.

United States Senate (1990). *U. S. Senate Bill No. 231011.097: 101st Congress, 1st Session.*

Wallack, L., & Corbett, K. (1987). Alcohol, tobacco and marijuana use among youth: An overview of epidemiological, program and policy trends. *Health Education Quarterly, 14* (2), 223–249.

Wallerstein, N., & Bernstein, E. (1988). Empowerment education: Friere's ideas adapted to health education. *Health Education Quarterly, 15* (4), 379–394.

Walter, H. J., Vaughan, R. D., & Wynder, E. L. (1989). Primary prevention of cancer among children: Changes in cigarette smoking and diet after six years of intervention. *Journal of the National Cancer Institute, 81* (13), 995–999.

Walter, H. J., & Wynder, E. L. (1989). The development, implementation, evaluation, and future directions of a chronic disease prevention program for children: The 'Know Your Body' studies. *Preventive Medicine, 18* (1), 59–71.

Wandersman, A. (1981). A framework of participation in community organizations. *Journal of Applied Behavioral Science, 17,* 27–58.

Watzlawick, P., Weakland, J. H., & Fisch, R. (1974). *Change: Principles of problem formation and problem resolution.* New York: W. W. Norton.

Wilson, R. N. (1970). Community structure and health action: A report on process analysis. Washington, DC: National Commission on Community Health Services, Public Affairs Press.

CHAPTER 5

SCHOOLS

PHYLLIS L. ELLICKSON

INTRODUCTION

School-based programs have constituted the bulk of prevention efforts in the past and are likely to do so in the foreseeable future. Although prevention experts increasingly advocate supplementing school programs with support from parents, community groups, and other societal institutions, few would replace broad-based school programs as the core of a prevention campaign. Schools have the advantage of providing a captive audience that encompasses nearly everyone in the appropriate age range for primary prevention. They offer more extensive coverage of the youthful population than churches and youth groups. Unlike the mass media, they also provide opportunities for face-to-face communication and feedback, both of which enhance the prospects for changing behavior (Maccoby & Farquhar, 1975).

This chapter examines what research can tell us about school-based prevention—what it should be doing and what it has accomplished. I define prevention as aimed at stopping the problem before it starts or, failing that, delaying onset and disrupting the transition from experimental to regular use. I begin by examining the data on which drugs are most frequently used by young people and when.

Drug Use Patterns

Statistics on the prevalence and sequencing of drug use suggest that prevention programs for children and young adolescents should target alcohol, cigarettes, and marijuana. These three substances are the drugs of choice among American young people. The most widely used drugs among adults as well, they have maintained that status for decades. They are also the drugs that most young people try first, and they pose serious health, safety, and developmental risks for growing children and adolescents.

In 1992, 51% of high school seniors had used alcohol in the last month, 28% had smoked cigarettes, and 12% had used marijuana (Johnston, O'Malley, & Bachman, 1993). In 1975, the corresponding figures were 68%, 37%, and 27%, respectively. Despite the media attention given to crack and cocaine, far fewer American teenagers use these substances or other hard drugs. Slightly more than 1% of high school seniors were current users of cocaine in 1992, substantially lower than the high of 7% in 1985. Stimulants (2.8%) were more popular than cocaine, followed by inhalants (2.5%), LSD, PCP, and other hallucinogens (2.3%) and sedatives (1.2%).

Alcohol, cigarettes, and marijuana are also known as the gateway drugs. Research has shown that young people are unlikely to use marijuana if they have not already used alcohol or cigarettes; they are even less likely to use the hard drugs if they have not already used marijuana (Kandel & Faust, 1975; Huba, Wingard, & Bentler, 1981). Furthermore, use of illicit drugs other than

The preparation of this paper was supported by Rand. Charlotte Cox provided valuable research assistance.

marijuana tends not to occur in the absence of problem drinking (Donovan & Jessor, 1983). Hence, focusing on the gateway drugs also offers the prospect of curbing use of hard drugs.

Targeting the gateway drugs makes sense from the public health perspective as well. Cigarettes and alcohol are responsible for more deaths than all other drugs combined. Although tobacco use has declined among adults and teenagers, it still accounts for approximately 400,000 deaths per year or one out of six preventable deaths in the United States (Office on Smoking and Health, 1990). Because nicotine is so addictive, the earlier one starts smoking the harder it is to stop and the longer the period during which one is exposed to tobacco's harmful effects (Office on Smoking and Health, 1987).

Drinking poses immediate life-endangering threats to teenagers: Alcohol-related accidents are the leading cause of death among young people between the ages of 15 and 19 (Statistical Abstracts, 1986). In addition, an alarming 30% of high school seniors have engaged in recent bouts of binge drinking (having five or more drinks in one sitting), which significantly heightens the likelihood of other high-risk behavior such as unprotected sexual intercourse or violent acts. Marijuana use presents risks for children in school because it causes short-term memory impairment, hinders learning capacity, and diminishes the ability to concentrate. Chronic use of marijuana and hard drugs has been linked to dropping out of school, delinquency, and other problems, including inability to hold a job, to maintain a stable marriage, or otherwise make a successful transition to adulthood (Elliott, Huizinga, & Ageton, 1985; Kandel, Davies, Karus, & Yamaguchi, 1986; Mensch & Kandel, 1988; Newcomb & Bentler, 1988).

Giving priority to the gateway drugs does not mean, however, that prevention programs should totally ignore other substances. Children who are likely to be exposed to cocaine, crack, or other hard drugs clearly need to know about their dangerous effects. As children mature, their likely exposure to hard drugs increases: Crack use is rare among seventh graders in California (2%), but it is twice as prevalent among eleventh graders (Skager & Austin, 1993). Regional data suggest that specific forms of hard drug use such as PCP are more common in some cities and neighborhoods than others (Reuter, Haaga, Murphy, & Praskac, 1988). Thus the drugs targeted by specific programs should vary by age, and sometimes by location. Data on use patterns for different age groups within localities can help practitioners tailor program goals to the particular circumstances in their communities.

National data also provide broad guidelines for decisions about when to provide prevention programs. They indicate that the middle or junior high school years represent a particularly vulnerable period for young people, a time when they are increasingly susceptible to pressures toward drug use.[1] Although current use of cigarettes by ages 12 and 13 is quite low (2%), it increases sevenfold by the time students enter high school (ages 14 to 15). Marijuana use jumps up by at least as much and alcohol use nearly quadruples by age 15 (NIDA, 1991). In addition, grades eight and nine appear to be peak years for conforming to antisocial behaviors such as using drugs (Berndt, 1979).

These statistics suggest that prevention programs for middle and junior high students have potential for reaching the great majority of young people before they can become regular users. However, disparities in age of initiation across substances have important implications for programs that focus on preventing *any* use. One study of eight California and Oregon communities found that nearly 80% of the students surveyed had tried alcohol by the time they were in grade seven, whereas only 20% had tried marijuana (Ellickson, Bell, Thomas, Robyn, and Zellman, 1988). Thus, preventing marijuana onset was a feasible goal for the vast majority of students, but preventing any alcohol use was not.[2]

If similar patterns occur in other communities, beginning prevention programs at grade seven would preclude the possibility of stopping alcohol use before it starts for most adolescents.

Given the prevalence of drinking in American society and alcohol's easy availability, preventing any use of it may not be a realistic goal, and would require prevention efforts during the elementary school years for most young people.

Risk and Protective Factors for Drug Use

Developing effective drug prevention also requires an understanding of how drug use begins and continues. Programs that fail to address major risk factors are unlikely to be effective; those that mitigate the factors promoting drug use and strengthen the factors that inhibit it have a greater chance of success. Research on drug use antecedents clarifies what these factors are.

Dominating early work in this area are studies conducted by Denise Kandel and her colleagues in New York, France, and Israel, and work carried out by Richard Jessor in Colorado and elsewhere. Each implies a different answer to the question of whether a single generic program can work for all substances. In Kandel's stage model of drug use, participation at the first level of use "puts adolescents at risk for progression to the next stage," and each prior stage is a necessary but not sufficient condition for movement to the next level (Kandel & Adler, 1982, p. 306). The stages of drug use that she initially identified were (1) drinking beer or wine, (2) smoking cigarettes or drinking hard liquor, (3) using marijuana, and (4) using hard drugs. Numerous other studies have found a similar sequence—legal drugs first, then marijuana, and then hard drugs (Ellickson, Hays, & Bell, 1992; Welte & Barnes, 1985). Of particular importance for prevention strategies is Kandel's proposition that different antecedent variables are associated with different stages of drug use. The stage model implies that prevention programs might have different components, depending on which stage they address.

Jessor's (1977) theory of problem behavior, on the other hand, implies that similar factors foster a wide range of adolescent problem behaviors (delinquency, early sexual experience, use of different drugs). In this system, three categories of precipitating factors work together to foster problem behavior susceptibility: the perceived environment system (peer approval, models for drug use), the behavior system (cutting school, delinquent acts), and the personality system (attitudes, values, expectations). Jessor also distinguishes between factors directly or obviously related to drug use (such as parental drug use) and those more remote in the causal chain (such as the relationship between parent and child). He postulates that the former (proximal variables) are more influential in the onset of drug use than the latter (distal variables). The emphasis, however, is on the generality of the theory—that adolescents can be classed along a dimension of deviance susceptibility that will predict their use of drugs.

Both models—the one implying different prevention strategies for different substances, the other implying similar strategies for all substances—have merit. As we show below, alcohol, cigarette, and marijuana use appear to share a similar set of psychosocial predictors, although different variables within that set play more important roles for some substances than for others, and for later stages of use. The variables are usually divided into sociodemographic factors, such as sex and race; environmental or situational variables, such as parental or peer approval and drug availability; intrapersonal characteristics, variously labeled personality attributes, attitudes, beliefs, or values; and actual behavior.

Sociodemographic Factors

Age is the most important demographic factor correlated with substance use. Prevalence rates for all drugs increase with age, tending to peak in the early to mid-20s for marijuana and alcohol (Kandel & Logan, 1984). Drug use initiation before age 15 increases the risk of dysfunctional use or abuse in later years (Robins & Przybeck, 1985). Researchers generally agree, however, that other sociodemographic variables add little predictive power to models of drug use. Although males typically use more than females, differences in drug use rates between the two sexes have declined over time and now appear "too small and subtle to justify differential interpretations or program design" (Gersick, Grady, Sexton, & Lyons, 1981, p. 43). Research on drug use rates and socioeconomic status supports similar conclusions (Bachman, Johnston, & O'Malley, 1981; Ellickson et al., submitted for publication; Maddahian, Newcomb, & Bentler, 1986).

Among students who are still in school, white and Hispanic adolescents report higher rates of experimentation with gateway and other drugs than black youth. Asian-Americans generally report the lowest initiation rates for all substances, and American Indians show the highest prevalence rates for most drugs (Bachman et al., 1991). For young adolescents, however, these differences are typically not substantial enough to support differences in program design.

The findings relating ethnicity and drugs are more ambiguous for substance abuse. Although black youth in New York reported more alcohol-related problems per ounce consumed than whites or other groups (Welte & Barnes, 1987), black Job Corps members in San Diego reported fewer problems than whites (Morgan, Wingard, & Felice, 1984). Hispanics and American Indians have been found to be at high risk for alcohol abuse (Bettes et al., 1990), and Hispanics are similar to white youth in the comparatively higher proportions classified as high-risk users and multiple substance users (Skager, Frith, & Maddahian, 1988; Maddahian, Newcomb, & Bentler, 1985). Thus, interventions designed for specific groups of high-risk youth may need to take ethnic differences into account.

Environmental Factors

Social Influences and Availability

Exposure to prodrug social influences (others who use drugs or approve of doing so) is consistently among the most important factors predicting initial and continued substance use (Kandel, Kessler, & Margulies, 1978; Chassin, 1984). Most adolescents first try drugs with someone else. It is usually a friend, although parents and other

relatives play a central role for alcohol use (Orive & Gerard, 1980; Friedman, Lichtenstein, & Biglan, 1985). These influences also tend to be drug-specific. Huba, Wingard, & Bentler (1979) argue that young adolescent drug users group themselves into "drug-specific interactional nets" composed of peer and adult users of the same substance.

Parents and peers are the dominant role models for initial use, although siblings and media images enter in as well. Which source has greater influence varies across substances. Peer use and approval of marijuana are the most important predictors of future marijuana use (Kandel, Kessler & Margulies, 1978), and peer smoking has been found to have more influence on adolescents than smoking by their parents (Krosnick & Judd, 1982). In contrast, parental drinking ranks close to or somewhat higher than peer drinking in promoting initial alcohol use (Ellickson & Hays, 1991a; Glynn, 1981). Heavy drinking, in particular, has been associated with parental misuse of alcohol (Zucker, 1976). Parental influences also weigh stronger in predicting use of harder drugs (Kandel, Kessler, & Margulies, 1978).

Peer and parental influences vary with a child's age as well. Before children reach adolescence, parents and peers wield equal influence on smoking. After age 11 or 12, peers become more influential than parents (Krosnick & Judd, 1982). The relatively greater influence of peers during adolescence also shows up in matters of language, dress, use of leisure time, and conformity to antisocial behavior (Berndt, 1979; Kandel, 1985).

The attitudes of those around them also affect adolescents' drug use. Peer acceptance of marijuana and alcohol use predicts their onset; peer beliefs in the harmlessness of marijuana promotes initiation into it and other illicit drugs (Jessor & Jessor, 1977; Kandel, 1978). Parental tolerance of smoking and drinking supports later experimentation (Ellickson & Hays, 1991a; Krosnick & Judd, 1982). On the other hand, strict parental rules against drug use or punitive measures have been associated with greater use of alcohol, marijuana, and hard drugs (Akers, Krohn, Lanza-Kaduce, & Radosevich, 1979; Kandel, Kessler, & Margulies, 1978).

Finally, whether drugs are available in the social setting affects adolescent drug use. Parents and friends who use drugs influence onset and maintenance because they are likely sources of supply as well as models for use. The comparatively high rates of adolescent drinking and smoking undoubtedly reflect the easy accessibility of legal substances. High school seniors also report that marijuana is more readily available than other illicit drugs, though there have been significant increases in the perceived availability of heroin, crack, LSD, and PCP (Johnston, O'Malley, & Bachman, 1993).

Familial and School Bonds

More general aspects of the child's environment, particularly family structure and quality of the parent–child relationship, affect drug use less strongly. For example, disruption of the family unit appears to influence initial use indirectly rather than directly (Oetting & Beauvais, 1987). Recent research among seventh graders found that being a member of a disrupted family (and having low academic orientation) increased the likelihood of exposure to drug offers, which then triggered initial use within three months (Ellickson & Hays, 1992). However, the strength of the parent–child relationship is clearly linked to more serious use. Weak or negative bonds with parents are associated with heavy drinking among adolescents, frequent marijuana use, use of harder drugs, and problems with drugs during adulthood (Newcomb & Bentler, 1988; Shedler & Block, 1990; Simcha-Fagan, Gersten, & Langner, 1986). Perceived closeness to parents, by contrast, appears to directly inhibit drug use (Dembo et al., 1981).

Weak bonds with school (usually indicated by frequent class cutting, absenteeism, or poor grades) show up in several studies, especially those that focus on cigarette and marijuana use among younger students (Skinner, Massey,

Krohn, & Lauer, 1985; Brunswick & Messeri, 1985). Poor high school grades have been correlated with use of several illicit drugs besides marijuana, but variations in academic performance are less likely to be associated with drug use among college students (Mills & Noyes, 1984; Newcomb, Maddahian, & Bentler, 1986). High school dropouts have much higher rates of use than those who stay in school (Mensch & Kandel, 1988).

Deviant Behavior

Behavior that indicates rebellion (prior substance use, delinquency, aggression, and truancy) foreshadows future use. Once a child has tried alcohol, for example, the likelihood of a repeat performance rises dramatically (Ellickson & Hays, 1991a). The same argument applies to cigarettes, marijuana, and other drugs. Indeed, the most powerful predictor of later use is prior experience with the specific substance (Bachman, O'Malley, & Johnston, 1984; Winfree, 1985). Further, trying a substance that precedes another in the use sequence heightens the probability of trying the next drug in the sequence (Yamaguchi & Kandel, 1984), hence the argument for delaying onset or stopping drug use before it occurs.

Numerous studies have also found a positive relationship between delinquency and drug use, with minor delinquent or deviant acts typically preceding drug use onset (Elliott & Morse, 1989). Jessor & Jessor (1977) found a positive relationship between general deviant behavior (lying, stealing, aggression) and subsequent marijuana use. Kandel (1978) found that minor delinquent acts (cheating, driving too fast) predicted hard liquor initiation in adolescents, both minor and major delinquency preceded marijuana onset and drug-dealing, and major delinquency (car theft, robbery) predicted initiation into other illicit drugs. Johnston, O'Malley, & Bachman (1978) singled out criminal activities involving property (vandalism, theft) as precursors of college and young adult use of marijuana, pills, and heroin.

The influence of antisocial behavior may begin much earlier than adolescence, at least for males. In a study of inner-city black children, Kellam & Brown (1982) found that aggression among first-grade boys predicted substance use 10 years later, and aggression combined with shyness was especially important for predicting cigarette and marijuana use.

Intrapersonal Characteristics

Given the relationship between deviant behavior and drug use, it is not surprising that a predisposition toward rebellion, independence, or nonconformity consistently stands out as a precursor of adolescent drug use. Among youth in Los Angeles, rebelliousness and low law-abidance preceded later use of both alcohol and marijuana (Huba & Bentler, 1984), and low levels of religious commitment predicted intentions to use cocaine (Newcomb & Bentler, 1986). In a five-year study of seventh and eighth graders, scoring low on obedience and law-abidance was an important predictor of adolescent marijuana use (Smith & Fogg, 1978). Rebellion, independence, and low conformity to adult expectations have also been associated with later use of illicit drugs (Kandel, Kessler, & Margulies, 1978).

The relationship between nonconformity and drug use takes on added significance for prevention programming because rebellious youth are likely to be particularly susceptible to peer values and models (Wingard, Huba, & Bentler, 1979). That argument applies to adolescent extroverts as well. Sensation-seeking and sociability have been linked to marijuana and other drug use (Brook, Whiteman, Brook, & Gordon, 1981; Clayton, Cattarello, & Walden, 1991; Kandel, 1978). These findings suggest that extroverts more readily find themselves in situations where peers are using drugs (Kaplan, 1980).

As for other personality traits, there is only weak or conflicting evidence supporting a relationship between onset of the gateway drugs and such characteristics as low self-esteem, external locus of control, alienation, and anomie (Kandel,

1978; Gersick et al., 1981; Orive & Gerard, 1980; Vicary & Lerner, 1983). However, emotional distress does appear to signal a shift to harder drugs or to problem use of a substance. Psychological distress, indicated by low self-acceptance and high self-derogation during high school, has predicted later problems with drugs and alcohol during young adulthood (Newcomb & Bentler, 1988). Prior depression heralded the onset of hard drug use in one study (Paton, Kessler, & Kandel, 1977) and predicted increased involvement with cocaine and other drugs in another (Newcomb & Bentler, 1989). Such findings are consistent with the notion that drug use after initiation may be reinforced by pharmacological effects—perceived reduction in stress, tension, or anxiety; improved mood; and enhanced sociability (Leventhal & Cleary, 1980).[3]

Several studies suggest that adolescents develop favorable attitudes or beliefs about drugs before starting to use them. However, recent work indicates that attitudes about drugs are more stable after onset and are more strongly related to continued use than to initiation (Chassin, 1984; Ellickson & Hays, 1991a). The relevant beliefs are typically drug-specific. They include expectations about whether one is likely to use a particular substance in the future, the consequences of using it, and the ability to resist pro-drug pressures (resistance self-efficacy).[4] Normative beliefs about whether important reference groups use drugs or approve of their use enter in as well, particularly for alcohol.

Summary of Research on Risk and Protective Factors

Research on drug use antecedents indicates that social influences play a dominant role in both initial and continued use. Peers, parents, siblings, and other admired role models who use drugs or approve of doing so all contribute to a prodrug climate in which models for use are plentiful, drugs are readily available, and social norms foster use. Peer influences attain increasing power as children mature, but parental drug use or acceptance of use by their children contributes to heavy use and progression through the drug use sequence.

The child's own beliefs and attitudes about drugs also promote drug use onset and maintenance. Favorable images of the benefits of use, beliefs that drugs cause little harm, and a perception that use is accepted behavior predict future drug involvement. Having confidence in one's ability to successfully resist prodrug pressures (resistance self-efficacy) inhibits use, as do beliefs about the negative consequences of using. The most relevant beliefs are usually drug-specific (the likely consequences of drinking or smoking, not of using drugs in general), but resistance self-efficacy appears to generalize across drugs (Hays & Ellickson, 1990).

By increasing the child's susceptibility to social influences and thus the likelihood of initial use, weak bonds with family and school set the stage for drug use. Impaired relationships with parents also presage more serious use, whereas closeness to parents inhibits it. Previous antisocial behavior (deviance, prior drug use) provides further information about who is the most likely to be susceptible to prodrug influences, as do predispositions toward unconventionality, rebellion, and sensation seeking. However, psychological variables that tap negative emotional states (depression, anxiety, self-derogation) fail to provide useful clues about gateway drug initiation. By contrast, emotional distress does predict hard drug use and drug abuse.

In general, similar antecedents promote initial use of the gateway drugs. However, specific variables within that set may have a greater impact on one substance than the others (for example, sociability and drinking, peer influences and marijuana use, beliefs about specific drugs and use of that drug).

Implications for Prevention

The research on how drug use begins and continues has clear implications for prevention program goals and strategies. Because most drug use occurs as a result of social influences, prevention programs must help young people identify and resist these sources of pressure. Teaching resistance skills and providing role models for successful resistance are essential components of prevention programs aimed at young adolescents.

Such programs also must combat motivational risk factors (beliefs about drugs and about oneself and others in relation to drugs). Appropriate techniques include helping young people to develop reasons not to use, to identify the benefits of nonuse, to recognize that most people do not use drugs or approve of doing so, and to believe that they can successfully resist. These techniques should be tailored to the specific beliefs and norms associated with each targeted drug. Telling children that smoking causes bad breath and that only a minority of teens use tobacco is unlikely to dissuade them from drinking. Because beliefs about drugs are more stable after drug use has begun, modifying them after initiation presents a challenge. Because such beliefs affect continued use, successfully doing so may also yield substantial payoffs.

Programs aimed at helping youngsters cope with social pressures to use drugs should be provided just before and during the period of greatest susceptibility to those influences. For most young people, this is typically early adolescence (grades six to eight). In some communities and neighborhoods, however, environmental pressures may put even younger children at risk.

Programs aimed at risk factors that heighten susceptibility to prodrug influences (weak bonds with family and school, impaired family relationships, poor school performance and attitudes, early antisocial behavior) should logically precede those designed to combat the more proximal causes of use (prodrug social influences and attitudes). Because these factors are linked with several other adolescent problem behaviors (pregnancy, dropping out, delinquency), addressing them during the elementary school years could yield multiple benefits.

The literature provides little support for promoting improved self-esteem as a way to keep children from trying drugs. However, the link between emotional distress and drug use escalation appears to be considerably stronger. More frequent use and abuse are also linked with impaired family relationships, serious delinquency, and dropping out of school. Thus, keeping children or adolescents who already use drugs from abusive patterns will probably require different and more intensive programs than those designed for the general population—programs that address their emotional problems and more general deviant behavior as well as their drug use.

CURRENT AND PAST PREVENTION PROGRAMS AND STRATEGIES

There are two broad approaches to prevention: helping children cope with the societal and personal forces that promote drug use, and changing the social institutions themselves. The vast majority of prevention programs has focused on the former, an emphasis this review will follow. Two of the leading institutionally oriented programs are discussed in the final section.

School-based programs, with their focus on helping the individual, have been the dominant prevention mode for adolescents and children. Districts have scrambled to adopt or design drug-prevention curricula, especially since Congress passed the 1986 Drug-Free Schools and Communities Act, designed to promote drug prevention across the country. Hundreds of drug education programs are now available. However, only a small number have been evaluated (U.S. General Accounting Office, 1993).

This review stresses programs designed for all children in a particular grade, and discusses only programs that have been tested and for which published evaluations exist. It focuses, in particular, on studies that have an experimental or quasi-experimental design. Other methodological strengths include controls for possible confounding variables, multiple posttests, assessment of attrition and data validity, adjustments

for within-school correlation (school effects) in individual level analyses, and the use of appropriate statistical tests of significance. However, very few studies meet all these criteria; thus, they did not constitute grounds for elimination.

Three approaches have dominated school-based drug programs in the United States—the information model, the affective model, and the social influence model. Only the latter, however, has shown promise in curbing actual drug use.

Information Model

Popular in the 1960s and early 1970s, the information model represents the traditional form of drug education. According to this model, providing students with the facts about drugs—their history, pharmacology, physical and psychological effects, and legal sanctions—is the solution to the problem of adolescent drug use. The underlying assumption is that adolescents use drugs because they do not understand the potential health hazards and social consequences; once students obtain knowledge about drugs, they will develop antidrug attitudes, and further, those negative attitudes will then deter them from using drugs, or at least decrease their drug use. In short, the information model posits a causal sequence leading from knowledge (about drugs) to attitude change (negative) to behavior change (nonuse).

Early drug information programs emphasized the harmful consequences of drugs, particularly the long-term effects of continued or heavy usage, often included exhortations against using drugs, and frequently used scare tactics. The delivery style was generally didactic, with limited classroom discussion. Although many of these programs enhanced students' knowledge about drugs, few led to antidrug attitudes, and none produced substantial reductions in drug use (Swisher, 1974; Goodstadt, 1978). Some programs actually increased it (Stuart, 1974; Blum, Blum, & Garfield, 1976). A meta-analysis of 143 drug prevention programs for adolescents (Tobler, 1986) found that the only measure affected by information-based programs was knowledge, with virtually no effects on other outcome measures (attitudes, skills, drug use, and other behavior).

Why did they fail? Experience tells us that millions of adults have continued to smoke more than 20 years after the Surgeon General's report about the damaging effects of tobacco. In other words, knowledge alone rarely changes behavior. Moreover, many early drug prevention efforts exaggerated the harmful effects of drugs and, not surprisingly, adolescents dismissed both the inaccurate appeals and those who articulated them as lacking in credibility (Kinder, Pape, & Walfish, 1980).

Affective Model

The affective model, which emerged in the early 1970s, shifted the focus of drug education efforts away from information about the substances themselves to the personality of the person using them. This model assumes that adolescents who turn to drugs do so because of problems within themselves—low self-esteem or inadequate personal skills in communication and decision making.

Programs based on the affective model include efforts to improve the affective skills (communication, decision making, self-assertion) hypothesized to be related to drug use (Kim, 1981). The goal is to improve a child's self-image, ability to interact within a group, and ability to solve problems. Focus is on feelings, values, and self-awareness, with little or no information provided about drugs per se. Other affective variants helped students clarify their personal values and the relationship between those values and choices about drugs (Carney, 1971, 1972).

These general skill programs have had inconclusive results. Among those that have been adequately evaluated, a few claim positive effects (Carney, 1975; D'Augelli, 1975), but the majority report conflicting, ambiguous, or zero effects.[5] Some observers have attributed the weak performance of the affective model to faulty implementation. However, a carefully implemented test of several affective programs did no better. The programs not only failed to inhibit drug use;

they also failed to produce the expected intervening effects of improved self-esteem and more positive attitudes toward school (Schaps, Moskowitz, Malvin, & Schaeffer, 1986).

The drawbacks of this model differ from those of the information approach. First, trying to raise a child's self-esteem is a complex task not likely to be accomplished in a short-term program. Second, as we noted earlier, the relationship between low self-esteem and drug use onset is weak. Third, little is known about the conditions under which value changes might lead to behavior change (Goodstadt, 1978). Fourth, early affective programs failed to link general skills in communication or decision making with specific drug situations, such as what to do about the offer of marijuana from a friend. Many teachers avoided any mention of drugs at all, not wanting to be associated with the propagandizing that had undermined earlier drug information programs. Finally, both the information and the affective education approaches failed to counter the single most important reason for beginning drug use—the influence of others who use drugs or approve of doing so. A more recent approach aimed at countering these influences has had more positive results.

Social Influence Model

The social influence model is the most recent, and most promising, approach to drug prevention. The original versions of the model focused on the external influences that push adolescents toward drug use, especially pressures from family, peers, and the media (Evans et al., 1978; McAlister, Perry, & Maccoby, 1979). Newer versions also stress internal pressures to use drugs—subtle influences of which an adolescent may not even be aware, such as the desire to be accepted, to look cool, and to be part of the crowd (Ellickson, 1984).

This model recognizes that adolescents are especially vulnerable to social pressures. In their desire to put childhood behind them and to appear grown up, they tend to emulate what they perceive as adult behavior, including drinking, smoking, and using drugs. Accordingly, drug education programs based on the social influence model seek to familiarize adolescents with the sources—both internal and external—of pressure to use drugs, to help them develop counters to prodrug arguments and to teach them techniques for saying no in pressure situations.

The social influence model explicitly recognizes that teaching children *how* to resist drugs is not enough—programs must also *motivate* them to resist (Ellickson & Robyn, 1987; Evans et al., 1978). Creating understanding of the consequences of drug use, undermining beliefs that "everyone uses," and reinforcing group norms against use are all ways in which social influence programs seek to motivate resistance against drugs. Because adolescents tend to be present-oriented and unconcerned about serious harm in the distant future, discussions focus on how drugs can affect them now, in their daily lives and social relationships.

The theoretical underpinnings of this model, as well as the methods used in programs based on it, derive primarily from William McGuire's (1964) social inoculation theory and Albert Bandura's theories of social learning (1977b) and self-efficacy (1977a). Social inoculation theory argues that exposure to persuasive arguments reduces susceptibility to subsequent persuasion. Social learning theory stresses the importance of modeling (imitation) and reinforcement (social approval or disapproval) on learning, with self-efficacy theory highlighting the importance of believing in one's capacity to accomplish a task. Most programs include several strategies for reinforcing resistance self-efficacy that are derived from Bandura's work: role modeling the desired behavior, repeated practice, reinforcement of successful performance, and statement of proximal goals.

Many social influence programs use peers (older or same-age) to help deliver the curriculum. Although it is widely believed that peers are more credible than teachers or parents,[6] research on their efficacy is inconclusive. Some studies have reported better results for students in peer-led (versus teacher-led) conditions (Botvin, 1987; Murray, Pirie, Luepker, & Pallonen, 1989; Perry & Grant, 1988); others have suggested that peer leaders may not be equally effective for all children (Fisher, Armstrong, & De Klerk, 1983), or have found no difference in effectiveness when older teenagers were involved in program delivery and when they were not (Ellickson & Bell, 1990a).

Model Applied to Smoking Prevention: "Pure" and Hybrid

The earliest research based on the social influence model applied it to smoking prevention among junior high students. The pioneering work was done during the late 1970s by Evans and his colleagues at the University of Houston (Evans et al., 1978). It was followed by research at Stanford and the University of Minnesota (McAlister, Perry, & Maccoby, 1979; Hurd et al., 1980; Murray, Johnson, Luepker, & Mittelmark, 1984).

Each of these early efforts targeted seventh graders and assigned a limited number of schools to experimental and control conditions. Each added different components to the curriculum: nonsmoking peers who demonstrated resistance techniques on film, and information about the short-term consequences of smoking (Houston); live high school role models, role playing practice, and a public commitment session (Stanford); and testing known and unknown peer role models on videotape and comparing the program when delivered by live same-age peers with one delivered by adults only (Minneapolis). A fourth research program, begun in Waterloo, Ontario, during the 1980s, broke new ground by beginning with sixth graders, adding a booster session in grades seven and eight, and recruiting 22 experimental and control schools (Best et al., 1988).

In 1984, the National Cancer Institute began funding a series of new school-based prevention trials while also providing support for long-term follow-up of the Minnesota and Waterloo programs (Glynn, 1989). Most of these trials, though still limited in the number of schools included, used more rigorous experimental designs and sophisticated analysis techniques than their predecessors.[7] As a stimulus to truth-telling, most also collected physiological samples before administering questionnaires about use.[8]

Two preexisting programs that combine elements of the social influence and affective models were included in this group—the Life Skills Training curriculum developed by Botvin and his colleagues at Cornell Medical School, and a similar approach developed by Steven Schinke in Washington State. Both incorporate strategies for improving general personal competence as well as the capacity to identify and resist social pressures (Botvin, Eng, & Williams, 1980; Schinke, Gilchrist, & Snow, 1985). As in earlier affective programs, the general skills components are designed to modify individual personality differences that the authors believe promote the onset of substance use—low self-esteem, low sense of personal control and assertiveness, high influenceability, and social anxiety. The general skills components typically include skills related to problem solving, self-control, communication, assertiveness, and coping; Botvin also includes interpersonal skills related to conversation and dating. His program is aimed at seventh graders, whereas Steven Schinke has tested his approach with fifth and sixth graders.

Results from these multiple prevention trials suggest that tobacco prevention programs based on the social influence model can produce modest but significant reductions in smoking behavior. Those reductions are typically realized for 5 to 8% of the targeted population (Cleary et al., 1988) and last for one to two years after initial program delivery. Follow-up booster lessons help to extend effects (Botvin, Renick, & Baker, 1983; Best et al., 1988), but few programs have included that feature. Follow-up lessons in high school are particularly rare. Not surprisingly, therefore, program effects have usually disappeared during high school (Flay et al., 1989; Murray et al., 1988; Murray, Pirie, Luepker, & Pallonen, 1989).

Overall, these studies provide cumulative evidence that programs based on the social influence

model can effectively deter or reduce adolescent smoking for at least one to two years. Smoking prevention programs have been "particularly effective in delaying the onset of tobacco use and less successful in targeting high-risk and minority youth" (Glynn, 1989). Because most of them have been tested in communities that are largely white and middle class, less evidence exists about their effectiveness with minorities and children of low socioeconomic status. However, two recent studies reported significant reductions in smoking behavior among urban black youth and Hispanic students (Botvin et al., 1989a, 1989b).

Even within the white middle-class context, there has been considerable variation in which types of children benefit from antismoking programs and when those benefits are realized. Some programs have produced results only for preprogram nonsmokers; others report positive results for baseline experimenters, but not for baseline smokers. Lagged effects, as well as erosion of early results, are common. In the Waterloo program, for example, no effects showed up among baseline experimenters until students had received follow-up booster lessons; those effects eroded once the booster lessons stopped (Best et al., 1988). In the Minnesota test of peer versus adult-led programs, one-year results for nonsmokers had dissipated a year later, whereas those for students who experimented with cigarettes showed up two years after program delivery (Murray, Johnson, Luepker, & Mittelmark, 1984). Several programs have also reported boomerang effects, wherein children exposed to the prevention program smoked more than those without it (Biglan et al., 1987; Murray et al., 1988). Thus, we still need to clarify precisely who benefits from these programs and for how long.

Model Extended to Other Substances

Given the success of the social influence approach to smoking prevention, a number of studies have investigated the applicability of the model to other substances, primarily alcohol and marijuana. The major work in broadening the focus of the social influence approach has been carried out at the University of Southern California (USC), the Rand Corporation, Cornell University Medical College, and the University of Michigan.

Researchers at USC have been responsible for several such projects. In 1981–1983, they tested the TAPP (Tobacco and Alcohol Prevention Program) curriculum, which featured resistance training, information, and decision-making training. The program yielded negative or no effects on alcohol use among sixth and seventh graders (at 6, 18, and 30 months after the pretest), and it had only a minor effect on tobacco use (Hansen, Malotte, & Fielding, 1988). The authors suggest that the results may reflect faulty implementation by poorly motivated classroom teachers.

Project SMART (Self-Management and Resistance Training) was a USC research demonstration project conducted in Los Angeles between 1982 and 1985. The project's purpose was to test the effectiveness of a curriculum based on the social influence model against one based on the affective education approach. The study targeted all three gateway drugs and provided nondidactic instruction in resisting peer, media, and parental pressures. The results clearly favored the social influence approach. Among the first cohort of seventh graders to participate in Project SMART (eight schools), negative effects were observed for the affective program after 24 months, whereas the social influence program was found to delay the onset of tobacco and marijuana use for at least a year (Hansen et al., 1988). Although the results for alcohol showed similar trends, they may have been attributable to preexisting differences in the social milieu surrounding drinking in the treatment schools. Within two years, most differences favoring the social influence program had disappeared.

The Midwestern Prevention Project (Project STAR) is a school-based program with several community components. Also developed at USC, the program was implemented in 50 schools in Kansas City (Kansas and Missouri) beginning in 1984–1985, and in 57 schools in Indianapolis, Indiana, three years later. Elements of the intervention include a 10-session school curriculum, which incorporates a social-skills, assertiveness-training model; parent programs (involving, for example, homework assignments with their children); training for community leaders; changing community health policies; and media campaigns.

Results of Project STAR have been reported for various Kansas City subsamples. To compensate for the lack of random assignment, the first analysis (of students from eight schools) tested several statistical models, concluding that the program produced reductions in cigarette use after one year but had no effect on drinking and ambiguous results for marijuana use (Dwyer et al., 1989). Another study yielded different results after one year: Reporting school-level findings for 42 schools (not randomly assigned), it found reductions of 30% in current (last month) use of alcohol, cigarettes, and marijuana (Pentz et al., 1989). A more recent analysis covered three years and individuals from eight schools; it reported modest reductions in recent cigarette and marijuana use, but not in recent alcohol use (Johnson et al., 1990).[9]

Another major research project testing the social influence model is Project ALERT (Adolescent Learning Experiences in Resistance Training), a longitudinal multisite experiment conducted in 30 California and Oregon schools. The curriculum, developed by Phyllis Ellickson and her colleagues at the Rand Corporation, is targeted to seventh and eighth graders. It extends the social influence approach by incorporating aspects of the health belief model (Becker, 1974) and the self-efficacy theory of behavior change (Bandura, 1977a). To motivate young people to resist, the program (eight lessons in grade seven, three boosters in grade eight) addresses their beliefs about the consequences of drug use and their own susceptibility to those consequences, builds confidence in their ability to resist prodrug pressures, helps students recognize that most teenagers do not use drugs, and clarifies the benefits of resistance. To develop resistance skills, the curriculum offers a repertoire of ways to say no and provides repeated practice in how to identify and resist internal as well as external pressures (Ellickson et al., 1988).

Specifically designed to overcome methodological limitations of earlier drug prevention research, this study randomly assigned schools to three treatment conditions (with teen leaders, without teen leaders, and control), tested the curriculum in a variety of school environments, used extensive statistical controls to rule out alternative explanations of the findings, and adjusted for within-school correlation of outcomes when reporting levels of significance. Results after 3, 12, and 15 months showed that Project ALERT reduced both marijuana and cigarette use. It was effective for both low- and high-risk students and with minorities as well as whites (Ellickson & Bell, 1990a, 1990b). The program delayed marijuana initiation among nonusers of marijuana and cigarettes (a reduction of about one-third) and held down regular (weekly) marijuana use among prior users. It also curbed frequent, heavy smoking among students who had previously experimented with cigarettes and induced a significant number to quit.

However, it was less successful against alcohol—early effects disappeared by grade eight—and it had a boomerang effect on students who were confirmed smokers by grade seven. The authors suggest that the short-lived results for alcohol reflect the favorable social climate surrounding drinking, and that the negative effect on confirmed smokers indicates that those students need earlier, more comprehensive, and more intensive interventions. Follow-up analyses showed that the program's impact on drug use eroded after students made the transition into high school, although its effect on cognitive risk factors lasted considerably longer. The authors conclude that adolescents need continued reinforcement for resisting drugs during the high school years (Ellickson, Bell, & McGuigan, 1993; Bell, Ellickson, & Harrison, 1993).

In Michigan, T. E. Dielman and associates have developed a social influence program aimed at preventing alcohol misuse. The Alcohol Misuse Prevention Study (AMPS) favors intervention in elementary school; it defines alcohol misuse as overindulgence (getting drunk, getting sick), trouble with friends (of the same or the opposite sex), or trouble with adults (parents, teachers, or police). An early evaluation of the AMPS on fifth and sixth graders who had received the intervention in 1984 found no effects on alcohol use, although subjects' awareness of the curriculum content had increased (Dielman, Shope, Butchart, & Campanelli, 1986). Evaluation after two years (213 classrooms from 49 randomly assigned schools) found that the treatment reduced the rate of increase in alcohol misuse among eighth graders who had received the program in grade six and had already used alcohol in unsupervised settings (as well as supervised settings). These results were significant after the authors controlled for within-school correlation of outcomes (school effects). There was no impact, however, on the amount or frequency of their drinking. Also, there were no effects for children who received the program in fifth grade or for children who either had no previous alcohol experience or had used alcohol only in supervised settings (Dielman, Shope, Leech, & Butchart, 1989). Later analyses suggest that the impact on alcohol misuse lasted as long as grade ten for unsupervised drinkers who had the initial lessons in grade six, about one sixth of the targeted group (Shope et al., 1992; Dielman, in press). The authors conclude that the social influence approach can curb alcohol misuse among a high-risk subgroup, but may be less appropriate when delivered to younger (grade five and below) elementary school students.

Another program targeted solely at alcohol was conducted under the auspices of the World Health Organization in 25 schools in Australia, Chile, Norway, and Swaziland. The five-session program, taught largely by peer leaders in some schools and by teachers in others, proved more efficacious with the first delivery method. For both abstainers and drinkers, the peer-led program produced lower alcohol use scores at the one-month follow-up than the teacher-led or control conditions across the four countries. Within countries, however, the results were less positive. In Australia and Swaziland, there were no significant outcomes. In Norway and Chile, modest effects showed up for nondrinkers but not for previous drinkers. Overall, the teacher-led program yielded a boomerang effect (higher use scores) for both nondrinkers and drinkers (Perry et al., 1989).

In 1983, the Los Angeles Police Department and the Los Angeles Unified School District jointly developed Project DARE (Drug Abuse Resistance Education), a program that has since been implemented in many other areas of the country. Specially trained police officers, assigned full-time to DARE, teach students about the consequences of using drugs and how the media promotes drug use. Other curriculum components include information about techniques for enhancing their self-esteem and resisting peer pressures to use drugs, as well as making responsible decisions and managing stress. The curriculum, adapted from the one used in Project SMART, is typically taught in fifth- or sixth-grade classrooms, although versions for older adolescents have also been developed.

A key, but untested, assumption underlying the DARE program (and others using police officers in program delivery) is that the officers' experience and expertise in drugs give them greater credibility than regular teachers. Indeed, anecdotal evidence indicates that the officers are well-received by students, and evaluators (Clayton, Cattarello, Day, & Walden, 1991) have judged them to be highly qualified for delivering the curriculum (they received 80 hours of training) and dedicated to teaching it as written. However, DARE officers appear to place less stress on participatory learning and student–teacher interaction than providers of other social influence programs do (Tobler, 1992).

Evidence on DARE's effectiveness against drug use has not been very encouraging. An early study found that DARE produced small but significant reductions in use of cigarettes and hard liquor (DeJong, 1987), but it had serious methodological limitations (ad hoc comparison schools and no pretest data). More rigorous evaluations of

DARE have shown little impact on drug use. For example, first- and second-year results from a longitudinal evaluation of DARE in Kentucky indicate the program has had some effect on attitudes, but little on drug use. Indeed, DARE actually increased marijuana use among the treatment school students after one year, an effect that disappeared by the second-year follow-up (Clayton, Cattarello, Day, & Walden, 1991; Clayton, Cattarello, and Walden, 1991). Reports from two sophisticated evaluations in North Carolina (20 schools) and Illinois (36 schools) were not much more positive. The first showed no effects on drug use at the immediate posttest, but positive effects on attitudes toward using (Ringwalt, Ennett, & Holt, 1991). The second showed no impact on drug use one or two years after the program (Ennett et al., 1994). A recent meta-analysis that compared eight DARE evaluations with the results from an earlier meta-analysis of 25 drug prevention studies showed that DARE's effect on drug use is slight. Moreover, DARE does considerably worse than other drug prevention programs, particularly those that use the interactive style of delivery associated with the social influence approach (Ennett, Tobler, Ringwalt, & Flewelling, 1994).[10] Thus, DARE appears to function more like the earlier didactic or affective models of prevention than like the highly participatory social influence model.[11]

Botvin (1987) completed a multiyear test of the Life Skills Training program on the use of tobacco, alcohol, and marijuana, following an initial sample of 1,200 seventh graders in greater New York schools until the end of grade 10. The ten schools were randomly assigned to five conditions: teacher-led, teen-led, teen-led plus grade eight and nine boosters, teacher-led plus grade eight and nine boosters, and controls. In the booster schools, students received 10 booster lessons during grade eight and five more during grade nine.

Analyses controlling for baseline use but not for school effects indicated that LST produced substantial results in the teen-led condition with boosters. Those results were strongest after one year, when students had received twenty seventh-grade lessons and ten booster lessons. By eighth grade, students in the teen booster schools smoked significantly less compared with those in the control schools, used less marijuana, and consumed smaller amounts of alcohol.[12] However, the comparable teacher-led program with boosters produced boomerang results for both cigarette and alcohol use. After two years, some smoking reductions persisted in the teen plus booster schools, but the effects on marijuana were no longer significant, and a boomerang effect showed up for alcohol. After three years, negative effects showed up for all three substances in the teacher booster schools.

These results suggest that booster lessons help extend program effects while students are still in junior high. After they entered high school, however, the LST booster lessons appeared less efficacious: they helped curb smoking among ninth graders, but not marijuana or alcohol use. By grade ten, when students had received no maintenance sessions for a year, program effects were no longer present. The data also suggest that older teens are more effective than teachers as program deliverers. However, Botvin attributes this result to poor implementation by some teachers; additional analyses showed that teachers with high implementation ratings did as well as the teen leaders.

Conclusions

This review has shown that information alone is not enough to reduce adolescent drug use, that affective education programs have not, by themselves, demonstrated results, and that the social influence model shows the most promise of all drug education approaches. Social influence–affective hybrids also show promise, but it is not clear what the affective components contribute. To determine whether the addition of general skills components provides an extra preventive effect requires a comparison of the pure and the hybrid models in an experimental test.

The results clearly demonstrate that school programs can work, a conclusion bolstered by recent meta-analyses (Tobler, 1986; Rundall &

Bruvold, 1988). Social influence programs have been particularly effective in curbing use of cigarettes and marijuana, the substances that are most closely linked with progression to hard drugs. They have produced results for both high- and low-risk children, have worked across a variety of school environments, and have curbed regular as well as occasional use. Thus the model's potential is not confined to keeping nonusers from the onset of drug use, but also includes helping curb frequent use among those who already use drugs. Moreover, social influence programs appear to work in both high-minority, urban settings and predominantly white, middle-class, suburban environments. In the RAND field trial, program results were similar across low- and high-minority schools; where they differed, they tended to favor the high-minority schools.

However, as we noted for the smoking-only curricula, the net effects of drug prevention programs are likely to be modest and, in the absence of a continued maintenance program, to last for only one to two years. Booster lessons appear essential for long-term prevention, but we have little evidence about whether continued program inputs during high school actually make a difference. Botvin's data suggest that they may prolong effects for tobacco use. What we know for sure is that one-shot inoculations are unlikely to guarantee long-term immunity.

The available research yields little basis for choosing among different program deliverers— teachers, peers, or older teens. As we noted earlier, some studies support including peers or older teens in classroom delivery; others conclude that teachers are equally effective with or without the assistance of same-age or older peers. However, unmotivated teachers are highly likely to produce null or negative results. Evaluations of DARE cast doubt on the efficacy of police officers as prevention teachers, but DARE's comparatively poor results may reflect differences in curriculum substance as well as in who delivers the program and how they do it.

It is also true that social influence programs are not a panacea. They do not help all children, nor do they work equally well for all substances.

Because classrooms and schools have diverse student populations, programs offered to an entire cohort do not necessarily meet the needs of all children within that cohort. Michigan's alcohol misuse curriculum, which emphasized high-risk behavior, did not work for abstainers or for children whose prior drinking experience was supervised. Project ALERT, which focused on preventing initiation and the transition to regular use, triggered a rebellious reaction among more confirmed smokers (but not among confirmed marijuana users). These variations in who benefits and who does not underscore the need for ascertaining how the unaffected or negatively affected children can be helped.

Curbing alcohol use presents a complex problem. Several studies have had no effect on drinking behavior or produced early results that eroded within a year (Ellickson & Bell, 1990b; Dwyer et al., 1989; Hansen, Malotte, & Fielding, 1988; Hansen et al., 1988). The AMP curriculum curbed problems associated with drinking for some children, but not how much or how often children drank (Dielman, Shope, Leech, & Butchart, 1989). Another program that focused on developing conservative norms about the prevalence and acceptability of alcohol use curbed drunkenness after one year but had no effect when combined with resistance training (Hansen & Graham, 1991). Botvin's LST curriculum yielded mixed results at the one year follow-up and a negative impact after two years.

Drinking is an integral part of social life for many Americans, whereas smoking and marijuana use are considerably less common and less accepted. Although less than 10% of the adult population are heavy drinkers, about two-thirds drink occasionally. Among high school seniors, more than half report current drinking, but less than 30% report smoking and only 12% report using marijuana. Similarly, 70% disapprove of trying marijuana once or twice, whereas only 33% disapprove of trying one or two drinks (Johnston, O'Malley, & Bachman, 1993). Expecting a short-term prevention program to counter such prevailing norms and attitudes is

clearly unrealistic. As long as the signals from the media and most adults directly contradict program messages, social influence programs are unlikely to realize their potential for curbing adolescent drinking.

In the absence of substantial changes in society's attitudes toward alcohol use, more limited goals for alcohol prevention may produce better results. Dielman's work suggests that efforts aimed at reducing problems associated with alcohol misuse yields payoffs for children who have already engaged in unsupervised drinking. Societal messages about alcohol *misuse,* which are more consistently disapproving, may provide the broader reinforcement needed for alcohol prevention to work. The difficult task, however, is to develop programs that take advantage of such social reinforcement while avoiding a message that promotes experimental drinking by children.

Our analysis also suggests that an underlying base of societal disapproval is a precondition for effective prevention. Thus, the media could play an important role in altering the current climate surrounding alcohol use. Cigarette ads are banned from television; alcohol ads are not. Between 1950 and 1975, major changes in public attitudes about smoking and significant reductions in consumption occurred in the wake of prolonged publicity about the hazards of smoking (Warner, 1977). Studies in both the United States and Britain suggest that antismoking campaigns played an important role in reducing cigarette consumption (Warner, 1979; Russell, 1973). Similar efforts targeted at alcohol might help reduce adolescent drinking.

The importance of the prevailing social context for prevention also has implications for the issue of legalizing marijuana and other drugs. Today's social climate puts enormous pressures on young adolescents to drink. In contrast, the social climate surrounding marijuana use is considerably more disapproving. To shrink that base of disapproval by legalizing marijuana might very well remove an essential precondition for effective prevention efforts in the schools. Changing the legal classification of marijuana, cocaine, or other drugs could convey the message that these substances are now acceptable, thereby weakening current social norms against their use.[13]

FUTURE DIRECTIONS

This review suggests that schools should give priority to social influence programs that are designed for students in grades six to eight. However, drug prevention is a difficult and challenging undertaking and we still have much to learn about it. No single approach carries a guarantee of success. Although the results to date indicate that social influence programs can yield positive results, those results are modest and typically hold up for only one to two years. They must be supplemented by maintenance sessions in high school and ground-building efforts in elementary school. Still other approaches are needed for high-risk children.

In this section, we discuss possible strategies for each of these groups—high school students, elementary school children, and high-risk youth. The discussion largely rests on an assessment of which drug use antecedents should be addressed when, and what approaches are appropriate for different ages. Where available, evidence about programs that appear to be effective with younger, older, or high-risk children is included.

High School Programs

Only a few programs designed specifically for high school students have been evaluated, and still fewer have shown positive results in preventing substance use. Programs for older adolescents based on the informational or general skills approach have fared no better with them than with younger students, and social-influence programs have usually proved less effective with high school students than with younger adolescents (Johnson, Hansen, Collins, & Graham, 1986; Perry et al., 1983).

During high school, prodrug influences increase and intensify while links between psycho-logical stress and problem use become more apparent. Hence, an appropriate focus for high school students would seem to be a combination of elements from the social influence model (adapted to accommodate the greater sophistication of older teenagers) together with elements that deal with the relationship between emotional distress and problem use.

This strategy would address risk factors associated with social influences, normative beliefs, and psychological vulnerabilities. If offered following a program for junior high students, these components might reinforce earlier resistance training, help older adolescents learn ways of coping with emotional and family problems, and help prevent erosion of earlier prevention results. Within this overall approach, high school programs should also take into account the older teenager's vulnerability to alcohol-related accidents, helping students to understand the dangers of drinking and driving (or riding with an intoxicated driver) and teaching them how to avoid such situations.[14]

Finally, school drug policy has an important role to play at both the junior and senior high levels (Moskowitz & Jones, 1988). Drug education efforts can be enhanced by fostering a school climate in which drug use is viewed as socially inappropriate. Encouraging clear and consistent rules about drug use on school campuses and fostering parent–school interactions that encourage drug resistance (such as contracts for alcohol- and drug-free parties) can help make drugs an unpopular choice.

Programs for Young Children

For younger children, social influence programs do not appear to be appropriate. Children in kindergarten through grade three lack the cognitive and experiential prerequisites for understanding what social influence means, particularly the subtle ways in which people can be pressured without being offered drugs directly. Those in grades four and five may have similar limitations.[15]

Kindergarten through Grade Three

Unfortunately, there is little evidence about what might constitute effective prevention for young children. We do know that we should choose programs that avoid harm and are tailored to the target group's developmental capacities, limitations, and experiential background (Ellickson & Robyn, 1987). Between kindergarten and grade three, it seems appropriate to concentrate on helping young children learn how to stay healthy (eat nutritiously, stay physically fit, avoid unsafe activities, and avoid putting unhealthy substances in their bodies). Examples include the American Lung Association's Growing Healthy Curriculum (for grades K–3) and Minnesota's nutrition program for third graders. Aimed at changing unhealthy eating patterns, the latter proved more effective when delivered via a correspondence format that involved both parents and children in activities (Perry et al., 1988). The results thus underscore the crucial role parents play in promoting healthy behavior and the efficacy of a novel approach for obtaining parental participation.

Grades Four and Five

By grade four or five, it is possible to lay the groundwork for successful resistance by fostering positive peer relationships and academic achievement. Activities enhancing cooperative learning, assertiveness skills, and the ability to communicate more effectively can be targeted to this group, along with introductory drug information. Although such programs have shown little effect on actual drug use in the past, they might increase the effectiveness of programs for older children by providing a behavioral base for learning specific resistance skills.

Programs for High-Risk Children and Adolescents

The Rand study pointed out that some high-risk children need much more than drug prevention alone. By grade seven, children who had already said "yes" to cigarettes had also developed strong prosmoking attitudes and a network of friends who smoke, drink, and use marijuana. In addition, they also exhibited several other signs of being on the fast track to trouble—they were more likely to have stolen something from a store, to be doing poorly in school, and to have impaired or disrupted family relations (Ellickson & Bell, 1990a). Although smoking cessation lessons might reduce their cigarette use, they clearly need earlier and more intensive interventions aimed at their multiple problems.

Since 1987, the Center for Substance Abuse Prevention (CSAP) has funded dozens of high-risk youth demonstration projects, but evaluation of these activities has been limited. Among school-based programs for high-risk youth, two approaches stand out: counseling services for junior high and high school students (secondary prevention) and whole-school programs for younger children in high-risk communities.

The former, typified by Student Assistance Programs, generally serve students who already have problems (dysfunctional drug use, poor school performance, truancy). Hence, they mitigate the stigma dilemma—labeling youngsters as troubled before problem behavior appears and possibly creating the problem.[16] In addition to individual and group counseling at school or elsewhere, they may offer treatment services as appropriate. Originally designed to use mental health professionals from outside the school system, many programs now use school counseling staff. One such effort reported reductions in alcohol and marijuana use, quantity of alcohol consumed, and days "drunk or very high" among assisted students (Moberg, 1988).

Two programs targeted at changing institutions, one developed by J. David Hawkins in Seattle and the other created by James P. Comer in New Haven, also avoid the stigma problem noted above. Both are whole-school efforts designed for all children and families in high-risk communities. They do not single out particular youngsters as potential problems. Because they focus on strengthening the child's bonds with the family and school, they are particularly appropriate for elementary school children, whose links to these institutions are still being formed.

Hawkins focuses on the risk factors that tend to precede exposure to prodrug social influences and heighten susceptibility to those influences, such as early antisocial behavior, poor family relationships, poor school performance, low degree of commitment to education, alienation, and rebelliousness. Based largely on Hirschi's (1969) social control theory, his "social development" model posits that adolescents who exhibit deviant behavior are poorly integrated into traditional social institutions (Hawkins & Weis, 1985). Through improved social bonding to parents and schools, these early risk factors can be reduced. Other risk factors (such as parental drug use, association with drug-using peers, and early drug use) are addressed by techniques that parallel the social influence model: fostering social norms that are antithetical to drug use and teaching children the skills they need to live according to those norms. Thus the unique aspect of Hawkins's approach is its focus on changing families and schools.

In 1981, an experimental test of the social development model was launched in Seattle. Aimed at preventing juvenile delinquency and drug abuse, the test involves several components: parent and teacher training, conflict-resolution services for high-risk children, and home–school liaison services. The program is targeted to public elementary schools located in racially mixed urban areas and serving children from high-crime neighborhoods. The parent-training program teaches effective family management practices, and the teacher-training component is designed to improve academic performance, reduce antisocial behavior, and increase children's bonds of attachment and commitment to school.[17]

A recent analysis of short-term effects (Hawkins, Von Cleve, & Catalano, 1991) indicates that the program has had significant effects on one of the risk factors for adolescent drug abuse—early antisocial behavior. At the end of second grade (i.e., after two years in the program), white boys in an experimental group from eight participating elementary schools were significantly less aggressive than those in the control group, and white girls were significantly less self-destructive. However, no effects were found for black children. Analyses for later grades will examine whether the program curbed initial drug use and delinquent behavior.

A systems approach to improving schools has been tested by Comer in Connecticut and Maryland. Comer describes his intervention as a process rather than a curriculum or set of teaching techniques. The program, which is based on mental health principles, aims to create a social environment in high-risk schools (serving poor, usually minority, children) that promotes a child's psychological development and supports learning. Though not designed with substance use in mind, it does address risk factors (poor school performance, weak attachment to school) associated with drug use. Bonding to the teacher is considered essential. The theory is that children who suffer a mismatch between mainstream values and those learned at home, which Comer calls "sociocultural misalignment," will not form such bonds because the teacher will not react positively to them. Such children are likely to have trouble learning and to seek self-affirmation in nonmainstream groups, which may put them at risk for dropping out, teenage pregnancy, drug abuse, crime, or other problem behaviors.

First implemented in two New Haven public schools in 1968, Comer's program includes four school management elements (details of the program vary for each school): a governance and management group composed of teachers and parents; parent participation in classroom and school activities; mental health staff who provide services to children, staff, and parents; and overall academic goals and strategies established for the entire school, with education programs tailored to the individual needs of at-risk students.

Data on program outcomes are confined to school-related behaviors and the initial analyses lacked a control or comparison group. The intervention, tracked from 1969 to 1984, resulted in improved attendance, improved reading and math skills, and improved parent participation within the test schools. A follow-up study comparing seventh graders who had participated in the program in elementary school with a matched control group showed the former to score significantly better on achievement tests, to meet their grade level in mathematics and reading, and to have better grades (Comer, 1985). When implemented in 10 largely black schools in Maryland, the program yielded average percentile gains on California Achievement Test scores that exceeded those for the district as a whole (Comer, 1988).

Evidence that a school management approach may curb both drug use and delinquency comes from a study conducted by Denise Gottfredson in four middle and three high schools (Gottfredson, 1986). Designed to promote achievement, attachment to school, and improved self-concept by changing the general school climate, this program facilitated shared decision making among school and community members, implemented specific academic and career innovations (cooperative learning; reading, studying, and test-taking programs; job-seeking skills) and enhanced school climate through peer counseling and special activities. One year later, the comparison high school showed small but measurably higher increases in overall scores for serious delinquency and drug involvement, whereas the treatment schools showed decreases.

All of these approaches must be carefully and rigorously evaluated to establish their effectiveness and portability across different environments. Without such information, we lose the chance to learn how to improve programs for future generations. Features that have detracted from earlier evaluations include lack of random assignment, failure to assess attrition or the validity of self-reports, inadequate statistical controls for preexisting differences that may explain program effects, and overly liberal statistical tests.[18] Because boomerang effects are not uncommon in prevention research, studies that report one-tailed tests of significance give the evaluated program an unwarranted advantage.

Future evaluations also must provide information on how programs affect different risk groups and, if they are successful, how they work. By accumulating information about who is helped, who is not, and why, we can fine-tune successful approaches, adding supplementary or compensating features for those who were not helped by the original version and increasing the likelihood that prevention effects will endure. Developing a balanced approach to prevention means choosing promising prevention models, assessing their results, and learning from that assessment.

NOTES

1. That susceptibility is underscored by the developmental changes typical of this age: the transition out of the more sheltered environment of the elementary school and into one with new faces and routines, an increasing orientation toward peers rather than adults, and the shift toward greater independence and nonconformity (Ellickson & Robyn, 1987).

2. Nevertheless, because most seventh graders had not tried alcohol more than once or twice, curbing the transition to regular drinking was still possible for most students.

3. A person may also continue to use addicting substances in order to avoid withdrawal symptoms.

4. See, for example, Chassin and Presson, 1984; Fredericks and Dossett, 1983; Kandel, Kessler, and Margulies, 1978; Ellickson and Hays, 1991b.

5. See, for example, Blum, Blum, & Garfield (1976); Branca, D'Augelli, & Evans (1975); Carney (1971).

6. The strategy derives from both social learning and communications theory. Social learning theory posits that adolescents learn from significant others in two ways: direct modeling of the behavior of peers or adults, and reinforcement of beliefs, attitudes, and behavior through social approval or disapproval (Bandura, 1977b). Peer role models who do not use drugs and who disapprove of doing so are relevant to both ways of learning. Communications theory stresses the greater persuasiveness of credible communicators (McGuire, 1964; Hovland, Janis, & Kelley, 1953; Kiesler, Collins, & Miller, 1969). Factors that increase credibility include familiarity (perceived similarity to the audience), which the use of peers provides.

7. However, most of them failed to correct for within-school correlation of outcomes (school effects) when analyzing individual-level data, and thus typically reported overly liberal tests of significance.

8. Known as the "bogus pipeline" technique, the saliva collection strategy is thought to motivate more honest reports of smoking behavior by convincing students that smoking can be detected by analyzing their saliva (Evans, Hansen, & Mittelmark, 1977; Luepker et al., 1981).

9. However, this report failed to adjust for school effects (within-school correlation of outcomes) and relied on one-tailed tests of significance rather than the standard, more stringent two-tailed test.

10. DARE had an average effect size of close to zero for drug use; by contrast, social influence programs had an average effect size of 0.40.

11. Indeed, in a later analysis of 56 programs, Tobler (1992) omitted DARE from the category of interactive programs (which included social influence programs and social influence plus general skills programs).

12. Significant reductions showed up for the smoking index and recent smoking (month, week, day); for marijuana, the reductions occurred for use in the past month and the index measure.

13. This argument does not necessarily apply to decriminalization, which involves lowering or eliminating the penalties for marijuana possession without changing its legal classification. Such changes have already occurred in several states, with little or no subsequent impact on use levels or adolescent beliefs and attitudes about marijuana (Johnston, O'Malley, & Bachman, 1981). Decriminalization is likely to have a more limited impact on social norms against use than is legalization because it does not alter the link between written law and informal social controls (MacCoun, 1993) and because it tends to have lower salience than legalization, to generate less publicity, and to be geographically circumscribed (implemented in individual states).

14. Evidence about whether such an approach might work is sparse. One evaluation found no effects on actual riding behavior but greater ability to refute pro-drinking and driving arguments (Duryea, Mohr, Newman, & Martin, 1984).

15. Dielman notes that the alcohol abuse curriculum, when delivered to fifth graders, had no effect, despite the fact that fifth graders also received booster lessons a year later (Dielman, Shope, Leech, & Butchart, 1989).

16. Targeting children who already exhibit problem behavior diminishes the likelihood of creating the problem, but it does not remove the possibility that grouping troubled youngsters together may reinforce both the "troubled" label and the undesired behavior.

17. Parents of children in grades one through three are taught to monitor, reward, and discipline their children, to improve family interaction and communication, and to help their children succeed in school. The parent curriculum for grades five and six addresses attitudes and rules about drug use as well as decision-making and coping skills. Teachers are trained in proactive classroom management (providing clear instructions, maintaining order without disrupting the class, praising and encouraging students), social skills (such as conflict resolution), and interactive teaching (measuring students by their mastery of specific learning objectives rather than against other students).

18. Inadequate statistical controls and inappropriate tests of significance can contribute to overstated estimates of program effects. The Rand researchers found a 45% reduction in marijuana initiation before controlling for multiple baseline variables; that reduction was reduced to one-third after the appropriate controls were implemented (Ellickson & Bell, 1990b). In the same study, 24% of the differences that were significant at the .05 level were dropped after adjusting the *t*-statistics downward to account for school effects (an important caution when analyzing data from many individuals clustered within comparatively few schools).

REFERENCES

Akers, R., Krohn, M., Lanza-Kaduce, L., & Radosevich, M. (1979). Social learning and deviant behavior: A specific test of general theory. *American Sociological Review, 44* (4), 636–655.

Bachman, J., Johnston, L., & O'Malley, P. (1981). Smoking, drinking and drug use among American high school students: Correlates and trends, 1975–1979. *American Journal of Public Health, 71*, 59–69.

Bachman, J., O'Malley, P., & Johnston, L. (1984). Drug use among young adults: The impacts of role status and social environment. *Journal of Personality and Social Psychology, 47* (3), 629–645.

Bachman, J., Wallace, J., O'Malley, P., Johnston, L., Kurth, C., & Neighbors, H. (1991). Racial/ethnic differences in smoking, drinking, and illicit drug use among American high school seniors, 1976-89. *American Journal of Public Health, 81,* 372–377.

Bandura, A. (1977a). Self-efficacy: Toward a unifying theory of behavioral change. *Psychology Review, 84,* 191–215.

Bandura, A. (1977b). *Social learning theory.* Englewood Cliffs, NJ: Prentice Hall.

Becker, M. H. (Ed.) (1974). The health belief model and personal health behavior. *Health Education Monographs, 1,* 324–473.

Bell, R., Ellickson, P., & Harrison, E. (1993). Do drug prevention effects persist into high school? How Project ALERT did with ninth graders. *Preventive Medicine, 22,* 463–483.

Berndt, T. (1979). Developmental changes in conformity to peers and parents. *Developmental Psychology, 15,* 608–616.

Best, J., Thomson, S., Santi, S., Smith, E., & Brown, K. (1988). Preventing cigarette smoking among school children. *Annual Review of Public Health, 9,* 161–201.

Bettes, B. A., Dusenbury, J., Kerner, J., James-Ortiz, S., & Botvin, G. J. (1990). Ethnicity and psychosocial factors in alcohol and tobacco use in adolescence. *Child Development, 61,* 557–565.

Biglan, A., Severson, H., Ary, D., Faller, C., Gallison, C., Thompson, R. Glasgow, R., & Lichtenstein, E. (1987). Do smoking prevention programs really work? Attrition and the internal and external validity of an evaluation of a refusal skills training program. *Journal of Behavioral Medicine, 10,* 159–171.

Blum, R, Blum, E., & Garfield, E. (1976). *Drug education: Results and recommendations.* Lexington, MA: Lexington Books.

Botvin, G. J. (1987). *Factors inhibiting drug use: Teacher and peer effects.* Rockville, MD: National Institute on Drug Abuse.

Botvin, G. J., Batson, J. W., Witts-Vitale, S., Bess, V., Baker, E., & Dusenbury, L. (1989a). A psychosocial approach to smoking prevention for urban black youth. *Public Health Reports, 104,* 573–582.

Botvin, G. J., Dusenbury, L., Baker, E., James-Ortiz, S., & Kerner, J. (1989b). A skills training approach to smoking prevention among Hispanic youth. *Journal of Behavioral Medicine, 12,* 279–296.

Botvin G. J., Eng, A., & Williams, C. (1980). Preventing the onset of cigarette smoking through life skills training. *Preventive Medicine, 11,* 199–211.

Botvin, G. J., Renick, N. L., & Baker, E. (1983). The effects of scheduling format and booster sessions on a broad-spectrum psychosocial smoking prevention program. *Journal of Behavioral Medicine, 6,* 135–379.

Branca, M. D., D'Augelli, J. F., & Evans, K. L. (1975). *Development of a decision-making skills education program, Study 1.* Addictions Prevention Laboratory, Pennsylvania State University, State College, Pennsylvania.

Brook, J., Whiteman, M., Brook, D., & Gordon, A. (1981). Paternal determinants of male adolescent marijuana use. *Developmental Psychology, 17,* 841–847.

Brunswick, A., & Messeri, P. (1985). *Causal factors in onset of adolescents' cigarette smoking.* New York: Haworth Press.

Carney, R. E. (1971). *An evaluation of the effect of a values-oriented drug abuse education program using the risk taking attitude questionnaire.* Coronado, CA: Coronado Unified School District.

Carney, R. E. (1972). *An evaluation of the Tempe, Arizona 1970–71 drug abuse prevention education program using the RTAQ and B-VI: Final report.* Tempe, AZ: Tempe School District.

Carney, R. E. (1975). *An evaluation of the effects of a program to enhance responsible behavior (especially drug abuse prevention) in grades 4 through 6 in representative schools in five Orange County, California, school districts: 1973–75.* Santa Ana: California School of Professional Psychology.

Chassin, L. (1984). Adolescent substance use and abuse. In P. Karoly & J. J. Steffen (Eds.), *Advances in child behavioral analysis and therapy,* vol. 3. Lexington, MA: Lexington Books, pp. 99–153.

Chassin, L., & Presson, C. (1984). Predicting the onset of cigarette smoking in adolescents: A longitudinal study. *Journal of Applied Social Psychology, 14,* 224–243.

Clayton, R. R., Cattarello, A., Day, L. E., & Walden, K. P. (1991). Persuasive communication and drug prevention: An evaluation of the D.A.R.E. program. In L. Donoher, H. Sypher, & W. Bukoski (Eds.), *Persuasive communication and drug abuse prevention.* Hillsdale, NJ: Lawrence Erlbaum Assoc., pp. 295-313.

Clayton, R. R., Cattarello, A., & Walden, P. (1991). Sensation seeking as a potential mediating variable for school-based prevention intervention: A two-year follow up of DARE. *Health Communication, 3,* 229–239.

Cleary, P. D., Hitchcock, J. L., Semmer, N., Flinchbaugh, L. J., & Pinney, J. M. (1988). Adolescent smoking: Research and health policy. *Milbank Quarterly, 66* (1), 137–171.

Comer, J. P. (1985). The Yale–New Haven primary prevention project: A follow-up study. *Journal of the American Academy of Child Psychiatry, 24,* 154–160.

Comer, J. P. (1988). Educating poor minority children. *Scientific American, 259,* 42–48.

D'Augelli, J. F. (1975). *Brief report: Initial evaluation of a televised effective education program as a primary prevention strategy.* State College: Pennsylvania State University, Addictions Prevention Laboratory.

DeJong, W. (1987). A short-term evaluation of Project DARE (Drug Abuse Resistance Education): Preliminary indications of effectiveness. *Journal of Drug Education, 17,* 279–294.

Dembo, R., Farrow, D., Jarlais, D.C.D., Burgos, W., & Schneidler, J. (1981). Examining a causal model of early drug involvement among inner-city junior high school youths. *Human Relations, 34,* 169–193.

Dielman, T. E. (in press). Research on the prevention of adolescent alcohol use and misuse. *Journal of Research on Adolescence.*

Dielman, T. E., Shope, J. T., Butchart, A. T., & Campanelli, P. C. (1986). Prevention of adolescent alcohol misuse: An elementary school program. *Journal of Pediatric Psychology, 11,* 259–282.

Dielman, T. E., Shope, J. T., Leech, S. L., & Butchart, A. T. (1989). Differential effectiveness of an elementary school-based alcohol misuse prevention program. *Journal of School Health, 59,* 255–263.

Donovan, J. E., & Jessor, R. (1983). Problem drinking and the dimension of involvement with drugs: A Guttman scalogram analysis of adolescent drug use. *American Journal of Public Health, 73,* 543–552.

Duryea, E., Mohr, P. L., Newman, I., & Martin, G. (1984). Six-month follow-up results of a preventive alcohol education intervention. *Journal of Drug Education, 14* (2), 97–105.

Dwyer, J. H., MacKinnon, D. P., Pentz, M. A., Flay, B. R., Hansen, W. B., Wang, E.Y.I., & Johnson, C. A. (1989). Estimating intervention effects in longitudinal studies. *American Journal of Epidemiology, 130* (4), 781–795.

Ellickson, P. L. (1984). *Project ALERT: A smoking and drug prevention experiment, first year progress report.* Santa Monica, CA: The RAND Corporation, N-2184-CHF.

Ellickson, P. L., & Bell, R. M. (1990a). Drug prevention in junior high: A multi-site longitudinal test. *Science, 247,* 1299–1305.

Ellickson, P. L., & Bell, R. M. (1990b). *Prospects for preventing drug use among young adolescents,* R-3896-CHF. Santa Monica, CA: The RAND Corporation.

Ellickson, P. L., Bell, R. M., & Harrison, E. R. (1993). Changing adolescent propensities to use drugs: Results from Project ALERT. *Health Education Quarterly, 20* (2), 227–242.

Ellickson, P. L., Bell, R. M., & McGuigan, K. (1993). Preventing adolescent drug use: Long term results of a junior high program. *American Journal of Public Health, 83* (6), 856–861.

Ellickson, P. L., Bell, R. M., Thomas, M. A., Robyn, A. E., & Zellman, G. L. (Dec. 1988). *Designing and implementing Project ALERT: A smoking and drug prevention experiment.* Santa Monica, CA: The RAND Corporation, R-3754-CHF.

Ellickson, P. L., & Hays, R. D. (1991a). Antecedents of drinking among young adolescents with different alcohol use histories. *Journal of Studies on Alcohol, 52* (5), 398–408.

Ellickson, P. L., & Hays, R. D. (1991b). Beliefs about resistance self-efficacy and drug prevalence: Do they really affect drug use? *International Journal of the Addictions, 25* (11A), 1353–1378.

Ellickson, P. L., & Hays, R. D. (1992). On becoming involved with drugs: Modeling adolescent drug use over time. *Health Psychology, 11* (6), 377–385.

Ellickson, P. L., Hays, R. D., & Bell, R. M. (1992). Stepping through the drug use sequence: Longitudinal and scalogram analysis of initiation and regular use. *Journal of Abnormal Psychology, 101* (3), 441–451.

Ellickson, P., McGuigan, K., Adams, V., Bell, R. M., & Hays, R. D. (submitted for publication). Teenagers and alcohol misuse: By any definition, it's a big problem.

Ellickson, P., & Robyn, A. (1987). Goal: Effective drug prevention programs. *California School Boards, 45* (4), 24–27.

Elliott, D., Huizinga, D., & Ageton, S. (1985). *Explaining delinquency and drug use.* Beverly Hills, CA: Sage.

Elliott, D. S., & Morse, B. J. (1989). Delinquency and drug use as risk factors in teenage sexual activity. *Youth & Society, 21* (1), 32–60.

Ennett, S. T., Rosenbaum, D. P., Flewelling, R. L., Bieler, G. S., Ringwalt, C. L., & Bailey, S. L. (1994). Long-term evaluation of drug abuse resistance education. *Addictive Behaviors, 19,* 113–125.

Ennett, S. T., Tobler, N. S., Ringwalt, C. L., & Flewelling, R. L. (1994). How effective is drug abuse resistance education? A meta-analysis of project DARE outcome evaluations. *American Journal of Public Health, 84* (9), 1394–1401.

Evans, R. I., Hansen, W. B., & Mittelmark, M. B. (1977). Increasing the validity of self-reports of behavior in a smoking in children investigation. *Journal of Applied Psychology, 62,* 521–523.

Evans, R. I., Rozelle, R. M., Mittelmark, M., Hansen, W. B., Bane, A., & Havis, J. (1978). Deterring the onset of smoking in children: Knowledge of immediate psychological effects and coping with peer pressure, media pressure, and parent modeling. *Journal of Applied Social Psychology, 8,* 126–135.

Fisher, D. A., Armstrong, B. K., & De Klerk, N. H. (1983). *A randomized trial of education for prevention of smoking in 12-year-old children.* Paper read at Fifth World Congress on Smoking and Health, Winnipeg, Canada.

Flay, B., Koepke, D., Thomson, S. J., Santi, S., Best, J. A., & Brown, K. S. (1989). Six-year follow-up of the first Waterloo School Smoking Prevention Trial. *American Journal of Public Health, 79,* 1371–1376.

Fredricks, A. J., & Dossett, D. L. (1983). Attitude–behavior relations: A comparison of the Fishbein–Ajzen and the Bentler–Speckart models. *Journal of Personality and Social Psychology, 45,* 501–502.

Friedman, L., Lichtenstein, E., & Biglan, A. (1985). Smoking onset among teens: An empirical analysis of initial situations. *Addictive Behavior, 10,* 1–13.

Gersick, K. E., Grady, K., Sexton, E., & Lyons, M. (1981). Personality and sociodemographic factors in adolescent drug use. In D. J. Lettieri & J. P Ludford (Eds.), *Drug abuse and the American adolescent,* Research Monograph 38. Rockville, MD: National Institute on Drug Abuse.

Glynn, T. J. (1981). From family to peer: Transitions of influence among drug-using youth. In D. J. Lettieri & J. P. Ludford (Eds.), *Drug abuse and the American adolescent.* Rockville, MD: National Institute on Drug Abuse.

Glynn, T. J. (1989). Essential elements of school-based smoking prevention programs. *Journal of School Health, 59* (5), 181–188.

Goodstadt, M. S. (1978). Alcohol and drug education: Models and outcomes. *Health Education Monographs, 6,* 263–279.

Gottfredson, D. C. (1986). An empirical test of school-based environmental and individual interventions to reduce the risk of delinquent behavior. *Criminology, 24,* 705–731.

Hansen, W. B., & Graham, J. W. (1991). Preventing alcohol, marijuana, and cigarette use among adolescents: Peer pressure resistance training versus establishing conservative norms. *Preventive Medicine, 20,* 414–430.

Hansen, W. B., Johnson, C. A., Flay, B. R., Graham, J. W., & Sobel, J. (1988). Affective and social influences approaches to the prevention of multiple substance abuse among seventh grade students: Results from Project SMART. *Preventive Medicine, 17* (2), 135–152.

Hansen, W. B., Malotte, C. K., & Fielding, J. E. (1988). Evaluation of a tobacco and alcohol abuse prevention curriculum for adolescents. *Health Education Quarterly, 15,* 93–114.

Hawkins, J. D., Von Cleve, E., & Catalano, Jr., R. F. (1991). Reducing early childhood aggression: Results of a primary prevention program. *Journal of American Academy of Child and Adolescent Psychiatry, 30,* 208–217.

Hawkins, J. D., & Weis, J. G. (1985). The social development model: An integrated approach to delinquency prevention. *Journal of Primary Prevention, 6,* 73–97.

Hays, R. D., & Ellickson, P. L. (1990). How generalizable are adolescents' beliefs about pro-drug pressures and resistance self-efficacy? *Journal of Applied Social Psychology, 20* (4), 321–340.

Hirschi, J. (1969). *Causes of delinquency.* Berkeley: University of California Press.

Hovland, C. I., Janis, I. L., & Kelley, H. H. (1953). *Communication and persuasion.* New Haven, CT: Yale University Press.

Huba, G. J., & Bentler, P. M. (1984). Casual models of personality, peer culture characteristics, drug use and crucial behavior over a five-year span. In D. Goodwin, K. Van Dusen, & S. Mednick (Eds.), *Longitudinal research in alcoholism.* Boston: Kluwer-Nijhof.

Huba, G. J., Wingard, J. A., & Bentler, P. M. (1981). A comparison of two latent variable causal models for adolescent drug use. *Journal of Personality and Social Psychology, 40,* 180–193.

Hurd, P., Johnson, C., Pechacek, T., Bast, L., Jacobs, D., & Luepker, R. (1980). Prevention of cigarette smoking in seventh grade students. *Journal of Behavioral Medicine, 3,* 15–28.

Jessor, R., & Jessor, S. L. (1977). *Problem behavior and psychosocial development: A longitudinal study of youth.* New York: Academic Press.

Johnson, C., Hansen, W., Collins, L., & Graham, J (1986). High-school smoking prevention: Results of a three-year longitudinal study. *Journal of Behavioral Medicine, 9,* 439–453.

Johnson, C. A., Pentz, M. A., Weber, M. D., Dwyer, J. H., Baer, N., MacKinnon, D. P., & Hansen, W. B. (1990). Relative effectiveness of comprehensive community programming for drug abuse prevention with high-risk and low-risk adolescents. *Journal of Consulting and Clinical Psychology, 58* (4), 1–10.

Johnston, L. D., O'Malley, P. M., & Bachman, J. G. (1978). Drugs and delinquency: A search for causal connections. Washington, DC: Hemisphere-Wiley.

Johnston, L. D., O'Malley, P. M, & Bachman, J. G. (1981). *Marijuana decriminalization: The impact on youth, 1975–1980,* (Monitoring the Future Occasional Paper No. 13). Ann Arbor, MI: Institute for Social Research.

Johnston, L. D., O'Malley, P. M., & Bachman, J. G. (1993). *National survey results on drug use from the Monitoring the Future Study, 1975–1992.* Rockville, MD: National Institute on Drug Abuse.

Kandel, D, B, (Ed) (1978). *Longitudinal research on drug use: Empirical findings and methodological issues.* Washington, DC: Hemisphere-Wiley.

Kandel, D. (1985). On processes of peer influences in adolescent drug use: A developmental perspective. In J. S. Brook, Lettieri, D. J., & Brock, D. W. (Eds.), *Alcohol and substance abuse in adolescence.* New York: Haworth Press.

Kandel, D. B., & Adler, I. (1982). Socialization into marijuana use among French adolescents: A cross-cultural comparison with the United States. *Journal of Health and Social Behavior, 23,* 295–309.

Kandel, D. B., Davies, M., Karus, D., & Yamaguchi, K. (1986). The consequences in young adulthood of adolescent drug involvement. *Archives of General Psychiatry, 43,* 746–754.

Kandel, D. B., & Faust, R. (1975). Sequence and stages in patterns of adolescent drug use. *Archives of General Psychiatry, 32,* 923–932.

Kandel, D. B., Kessler, R., & Margulies, R. (1978). Antecedents of adolescent initiation into stages of drug use: A developmental analysis. *Journal of Youth and Adolescence, 7,* 13–40.

Kandel, D., & Logan, J. (1984). Patterns of drug use from adolescence to young adulthood: I. Periods of risk for initiation, continued use, and discontinuation. *American Journal of Public Health, 74,* 660–666.

Kaplan, H. (1980). Self-esteem and self-derogation theory of drug abuse. In D. Lettieri, *Theories on drug abuse.* Rockville, MD: NIDA.

Kellam, S. G., & Brown, H. (1982). *Social adaptational and psychological antecedents of adolescent psychopathology ten years later.* Baltimore: Johns Hopkins University.

Kiesler, C. A., Collins, B. E., & Miller, N. (1969). *Attitude change: A critical analysis of theoretical approaches.* New York: John Wiley and Sons.

Kim, S. (1981). An evaluation of ombudsman primary prevention program on student drug abuse. *Journal of Drug Education, 11,* 27–36.

Kinder, B., Pape, N., & Walfish, S. (1980). Drug and alcohol education programs: A review of outcome studies. *International Journal of Addictions, 7,* 1035–1054.

Krosnick, J., & Judd, C. (1982). Transitions in social influence at adolescence: Who induces cigarette smoking? *Developmental Psychology, 18,* 359–368.

Leventhal, H., & Cleary, P. D. (1980). The smoking problem: A review of the research and theory in behavioral risk modification. *Psychology Bulletin, 88,* 370–405.

Luepker, R. V., Pechacek, T., Murray, D., Johnson, C., Hund, F., & Jacobs, D. (1981). Saliva thiocyanate: A chemical indicator of smoking in adolescents. *American Journal of Public Health, 71,* 1320–1324.

Maccoby, N., & Farquhar, J. (1975). Communication for health: Unselling heart disease. *Journal of Communication, 25,* 114–126.

MacCoun, R. J. (1993). Drugs and the law: A psychological analysis of drug prohibition. *Psychological Bulletin, 113* (3), 497–512.

Maddahian, E., Newcomb, M. D., & Bentler, P. M. (1985). Single and multiple patterns of adolescent substance use: Longitudinal comparisons of four ethnic groups. *Journal of Drug Education, 15* (4), 311–326.

Maddahian, E., Newcomb, M. D., & Bentler, P. M. (1986). Adolescents' substance use: Impact of ethnicity, income, and availability. *Advances in Alcohol and Substance Abuse, 5,* 63–78.

McAlister, A., Perry, C., & Maccoby, N. (1979). Adolescent smoking: Onset and prevention. *Pediatrics, 63,* 650–658.

McGuire, W. (1964). Inducing resistance to persuasion. In L. Berkowitz (Ed.), *Advances in experimental social psychology.* New York: Academic Press, 191–229.

Mensch, B. S., & Kandel, D. B. (1988). Dropping out of high school and drug involvement. *Sociology of Education, 61,* 95–113.

Mills, C., & Noyes, H. (1984). Patterns and correlates of initial and subsequent drug use among adolescents. *Journal of Consulting and Clinical Psychology, 52,* 231–243.

Moberg, D. (1988). *Evaluation results for a student assistance program.* Paper presented at the Annual Meeting of the American Public Health Association, Boston, Nov. 14.

Morgan, M. C., Wingard, D. L., & Felice, M. E. (1984). Subcultural differences in alcohol use among youth. *Journal of Adolescent Health Care, 5* (3), 191–195.

Moskowitz, J. M., & Jones, R. (1988). Alcohol and drug problems in the schools: Results of a national survey of school administrators. *Journal of Studies on Alcohol, 9* (4), 299–305.

Murray, D. M., Davis-Hearn, M., Goldman, A. I., Pirie, P., & Luepker, R. V. (1988). Four- and five-year follow-up results from four seventh-grade smoking prevention strategies. *Journal of Behavioral Medicine, 11,* 395–405.

Murray, D., Johnson, C. A., Luepker, R. V., & Mittelmark, M. B. (1984). The prevention of cigarette smoking in children: A comparison of four strategies. *Journal of Applied Social Psychology, 14,* 274–289.

Murray, D. M., Pirie, P., Luepker, R. V., & Pallonen, U. P. (1989). Five- and six-year follow-up results from four seventh-grade smoking prevention strategies. *Journal of Behavioral Medicine, 12,* 207–218.

Newcomb, M. D., & Bentler, P. M. (1986). Frequency and sequence of drug use: A longitudinal study from early adolescence to young adulthood. *Journal of Drug Education, 16,* 101–120.

Newcomb, M. D., & Bentler, P. M. (1987). Impact of adolescent drug use and social support on problems of young adults: A longitudinal study. *Journal of Abnormal Psychology, 97,* 64–75.

Newcomb, M. D., & Bentler, P. M. (1988). *Consequences of adolescent drug use: Impact on psychosocial development and young adult role responsibility.* Beverly Hills, CA: Sage.

Newcomb, M. D., & Bentler, P. M. (1989). Substance use and abuse among children and teenagers. *American Psychologist, 44* (2), 242–248.

Newcomb, M. D., Maddahian, E., & Bentler, P. M. (1986). Risk factors for drug use among adolescents: Concurrent and longitudinal analyses. *American Journal of Public Health, 76,* 525–531.

Newcomb, M. D., Maddahian, E., Skager, R., & Bentler, P. M. (1987). Substance abuse and psychosocial risk factors among teenagers: Associations with sex, age, ethnicity, and type of school. *American Journal of Drug and Alcohol Abuse, 13,* 413–433.

NIDA (1991). *National household survey on drug abuse: Main findings, 1990.* Rockville MD: U.S. Department of Health and Human Services.

Oetting, E., & Beauvais, F. (1987). Peer cluster theory, socialization characteristics, and adolescent drug use: A path analysis. *Journal of Counseling Psychology, 34,* 205–213.

Oetting, E. R., Edwards, R., Goldstein, G. S., & Garcia-Mason, V. (1980). Drug use among adolescents of five Southwestern Native American tribes. *International Journal of Addictions, 15,* 439–445.

Office on Smoking and Health (1987). *Smoking and health: A national status report. A report to Congress.* U.S. Department of Health and Human Services, Public Health Service, DHHS Publication no. (PHS) 87-8396.

Office on Smoking and Health (1990). *Executive summary, smoking and health: A national status report. A report to Congress,* 2nd Edition. U.S. Department of Health and Human Services, Public Health Service, DHHS Publication no. (CDC)87-8396.

Orive, R., & Gerard, H. B. (1980). Personality, attitudinal, and social correlates of drug use. *International Journal of Addictions, 15,* 869–881.

Paton, S., Kessler, R., & Kandel, D. (1977). Depressive mood and adolescent illegal drug use: A longitudinal analysis. *Journal of Genetics and Psychology, 131,* 267–289.

Pentz, M. A., Dwyer, J., MacKinnon, D., Flay, B., Hansen, W., Yang, E., & Johnson, C. (1989). A multi-community trial for primary prevention of adolescent drug abuse: Effects on drug use prevalence. *Journal of American Medical Association, 261* 3259–3266.

Perry, C. L., & Grant, M. (1988). Comparing peer-led to teacher-led youth alcohol education in four countries. *Alcohol Health & Research World, 12,* 322–326.

Perry, C. L., Grant, M., Ernberg, G., Florenzano, R. U., Langdon, M. C., Myeni, A. D., Waalhberg, R., Berg, S., Andersson, K., Fisher, K. J., Blaze-Temple, D., Cross, D., Saunders, B., Jacobs, Jr., D. R., & Schmid, T. (1989). WHO collaborative study on alcohol education and young people: Outcomes of a four-country pilot study. *International Journal of the Addictions, 24* (12), 1145–1172.

Perry, C., Luepker, R., Murray, D., Kurth, C., Mullis, R., Crockett, S., & Jacobs, D. (1988). Parent involvement with children's health promotion: The Minnesota Home Team. *American Journal of Public Health, 78* (9), 1156–1160.

Perry, C. L., Telch, M., Killen, J., Burke, A., & Maccoby, N. (1983). High school smoking prevention: The relative efficacy of varied treatments and instructors. *Adolescence, 18,* 561–566.

Reuter, P., Haaga, J., Murphy, P., & Praskac, A. (July 1988). *Drug use and drug programs in the Washington metropolitan area.* Santa Monica, CA: The RAND Corporation, R-3655-GWRC.

Ringwalt, C., Ennett, S. T., & Holt, K. D. (1991). An outcome evaluation of project DARE (Drug Abuse Resistance Education). *Health Education Research, 6,* 327–337.

Robins, L., & Przybeck, T. (1985). Age of onset of drug use as a factor in drug and other disorders. In C. Jones & R. Battjes, *Etiology of drug abuse: Implications for prevention.* Rockville, MD: National Institute on Drug Abuse.

Rundall, T., & Bruvold, W. (1988). A meta-analysis of school-based smoking and alcohol use prevention. *Health Education Quarterly, 15* (3), 317–334.

Russell, M.A.H. (1973). Changes in cigarette price and consumption by men in Britain, 1946–71: A preliminary analysis. *British Journal of Preventive Social Medicine, 27,* 1–7.

Schaps, E., Moskowitz, J., Malvin, J., & Schaeffer, G. (1986). Evaluation of seven school-based prevention projects: A final report on the Napa Project. *International Journal of the Addictions, 21,* 1081–1112.

Schinke, S. P., Gilchrist, L. D., & Snow, W. H. (1985). Skills intervention to prevent cigarette smoking among adolescents. *American Journal of Public Health, 75,* 665–667.

Shedler, J., & Block, J. (1990). Adolescent drug use and psychological health: A longitudinal inquiry. *American Psychologist, 45* (5), 612–630.

Shope, J. T., Dielman, T. E., Butchart, A. T., Campanelli, P. C., & Kloska, D. (1992). An elementary school-based alcohol misuse prevention program: A follow-up evaluation. *Journal of Studies on Alcohol, 53* (2), 106–121.

Simcha-Fagan, O., Gersten, J., & Langner, T. (1986). Early precursors and concurrent correlates of patterns of illicit drug use in adolescence. *Journal of Drug Issues, 16,* 1–28.

Skager, R., & Austin, G. A. (1993). Fourth biennial statewide survey of drug and alcohol use among California students in grades 7, 9, and 11. Winter 1991–92 Report to the Attorney General. Sacramento, CA: Office of the Attorney General.

Skager, R., Austin, G., & Frith, S. L. (1991). *Biennial survey of drug and alcohol use among California students in grades 7, 9, and 11. Winter 1989–1990 report to the Attorney General.* Sacramento, CA: Office of the Attorney General.

Skager, R., Frith, S. L., & Maddahian, E. (1988). *A statewide survey of drug and alcohol use among California students in grades 7, 9, and 11. Winter 1987–1988 report to the Attorney General.* Sacramento, CA: Office of the Attorney General.

Skinner, W., Massey, J., Krohn, M., & Lauer, R. M. (1985). Social influences and constraints on the initiation and cessation of adolescent tobacco use. *Journal of Behavioral Medicine, 8,* 353–375.

Smith, G. M., & Fogg, C. P. (1978). Psychological predictors of early use, late use, and non-use of marihuana among teenage students. In D. Kandel (Ed.), *Longitudinal research on drug use: Empirical findings and methodological issues.* Washington, DC: Hemisphere-Wiley.

Statistical Abstracts of the United States, 1986. Washington, DC: U.S. Bureau of the Census, December 1985, Tables 115 and 1050.

Stuart, J. (1974). Teaching facts about drugs: Pushing or preventing? *Journal of Educational Psychology, 66,* 189–201.

Swisher, J. D. (1974). The effectiveness of drug education: Conclusions based on experimental evaluation. In M. Goodstadt (Ed.), *Research on methods and programs of drug education.* Toronto: Addiction Research Foundation.

Tobler, N. (1986). Meta-analysis of 143 adolescent drug prevention programs: Quantitative outcome results of program participants compared to a control or comparison group. *Journal of Drug Issues, 16,* 537–567.

Tobler, N. (1992). Drug prevention programs can work: Research findings. *Journal of Addictive Diseases, 11* (3), 1–28.

U.S. Department of Health and Human Services (1989). *Reducing the health consequences of smoking: 25 years of progress. A report of the Surgeon General.* Public Health Service, Centers for Disease Control, Center for Chronic Disease Prevention and Health Promotion, Office on Smoking and Health. DHHS Publication No. (CDC)89-8411.

U.S. General Accounting Office (1993). *Drug education: Limited progress in program evaluation, statement of Eleanor Chelimsky/testimony before the subcommittee on select education and civil rights, committee on education and labor, House of Representatives.* GAO/T-PEMD-93-2, March 31.

Vicary, J., & Lerner, J. (1983). Longitudinal perspectives on drug use: Analyses from the New York longitudinal study. *Journal of Drug Education, 13* (3), 275–285.

Warner, K. (1977). The effects of the anti-smoking campaign on cigarette consumption. *American Journal of Public Health, 67,* 645–650.

Warner, K. (1979). Clearing the airwaves: The cigarette ad ban revisited. *Policy Analysis, 5,* 435–450.

Welte, J. W., & Barnes, G. M. (1985). Alcohol: The gateway to other drug use among secondary school students. *Journal of Youth and Adolescence, 14,* 487–498.

Welte, J. W., & Barnes, G. M. (1987). Youthful smoking: Patterns and relationships to alcohol and other drug use. *Journal of Adolescence, 10,* 327–340.

Winfree, L. (1985). Peers, parents, and adolescent drug use in a rural community: A two-wave panel study. *Journal of Youth and Adolescence, 14* (6), 499–512.

Wingard, J., Huba, G., & Bentler, P. (1979). The relationship of personality structure to patterns of adolescent substance use. *Multivariate Behavioral Research, 14,* 131–143.

Yamaguchi, K., & Kandel, D. (1984). Patterns of drug use from adolescence to young adulthood: II. Sequences of progression. *American Journal of Public Health, 74,* 668–672.

Zucker, R. (1976). Parental influences on the drinking patterns of their children. In M. Greenblatt & M. Schuckit (Eds.), *Alcoholism problems in women and children.* New York: Grune & Stratton, 22–23.

CHAPTER 6

HEALTH CARE PROVIDERS

J. THOMAS UNGERLEIDER
NAOMI J. SIEGEL
BERNARD B. VIRSHUP

INTRODUCTION: THE CHALLENGE OF PREVENTION FOR THE HEALTH CARE PROFESSIONAL

The projected cost to the nation for alcohol abuse alone for 1990 is estimated to be approximately $130 billion, with $70 billion in lost worker productivity and unemployment. In 1983, $13 billion was spent on treatment of complications of alcohol; it is estimated that half the hospital beds in this country are occupied by people who have abused alcohol, cigarettes, or other drugs. Our justice system is clogged. The costs in terms of personal, family, and social anguish are huge. What can the health care professional do to help alleviate this national tragedy?

Medicine does not have a good history of prevention. Semmelweis, who espoused hand washing to prevent the spread of puerperal fever, was the object of scorn and ridicule and lost his medical career. William Dock, who proved conclusively by 1948 that coronary artery disease could be prevented by a low-fat diet and exercise, died in 1990 learning that the medical profession was grudgingly accepting this "new" finding. America, with the best medical care in the world, has one of the highest infant mortality rates among industrialized nations; according to some, a third of all underweight births could be prevented if the country addressed the medical, social, and economic conditions underlying the disproportionately high U.S. rates of low birth weight and infant death. As a society, we are more willing to pay massive amounts for curing the afflicted or imprisoning the guilty than to pay the smaller cost of dealing with primary causes by emphasizing prevention. Treatment is much more costly, both in direct outlay of funds and in lost productivity because we have just that many fewer people who are functioning at their best. In drug addiction prevention, this flawed tradition continues.

PROBLEMS AND OBSTACLES

The Health Care System

From a health care provider's prevention viewpoint, there are many problems with our health care system. The primary problem is that it is almost exclusively treatment-reimbursed; prevention efforts are not financially rewarded.

The health care system in the United States is complex, with multiple components; these include physicians, nurses, social workers, psychotherapists (psychologists, psychiatrists, social workers, counselors), researchers, pharmacists and the pharmaceutical industry, health maintenance organizations, hospitals, emergency rooms, clinics, public health officers, dieticians, and wellness communities. In addition, there are a sizeable number of people selling and promoting fads and unproven "cures."

Thus, although most people perceive a visit to the family doctor as their contact with the health care system, the practicing physician is but one link in a chain of interrelated organizations, attitudes, and policies. In addition to the common goal of maintaining and delivering good health care to our population, these components often have adopted values and set policies that have created obstacles to the development of effective substance abuse prevention strategies.

Lack of Federal Leadership

On the federal level, governmental health care and legislative agencies help define our national policies. The Surgeon General is a major spokesperson who articulates these policies. More than 200 years ago, Benjamin Rush, M.D., our first Surgeon General, labeled "intemperance" a disease (Lewis, Niven, Czechowicz, & Trumble, 1987). No Surgeon General, however, played any major role in alerting the public, even during the mid-1960s, when national concern regarding substance abuse reached epidemic proportions. It was not until the 1970s that the Surgeon General required that tobacco cigarette packages carry warning labels.

Various governmental bodies have made drug abuse policy statements, issued health research and prevention reports, appointed national and presidential commissions, passed legislation, and provided funds for research and treatment (U.S. Secretary of Health, Education, and Welfare, 1991a, 1991b; U.S. Department of Education, 1988). This has been particularly true since President Nixon first "declared war" on drugs in 1970 and established the Special Action Office of Drug Abuse Prevention (SAODAP), headed by Jerry Jaffe, M.D. This agency advised the president on matters of drug abuse, with special emphasis on treatment. The National Commission on Marijuana and Drug Abuse, created by Congress and appointed by the president, recommended in 1973 that schools of medicine, nursing, pharmacy, and public health include in their curricula a block of instruction dealing with the social and medical aspects of drug use (National Commission on Marijuana and Drug Abuse, 1973).

Presidents Carter and Reagan also had special advisors in the White House. Both were physicians: Peter Bourne, M.D. (Carter), and Donald Ian Macdonald, M.D. (Reagan), with primary advisory roles. Although more emphasis was placed on prevention issues, no major policy positions were taken in this area. Neither the Alcohol nor Psychoactive Drug Liaison Task Panels to President Carter's Commission on Mental Health in 1978 addressed the education of the Health Care Professional (Report of the President's Commission on Mental Health, 1978). Likewise, the Second Triennial Report to the Congress (1987) from the Secretary of Health and Human Services neglected to address this issue.

Under President Bush, stimulated by the perceived "crack" crisis, a major new post was established. The Office of National Drug Control Policy and the establishment of a "Drug Czar" (William J. Bennett) saw the first commitment of funding to attempt a major attack on all aspects of the drug problem.

However, federal policy, as developed by this office, has placed major emphasis on funding enforcement aspects of the drug problem (70%); treatment, research, and prevention efforts receive only 30%. The National Drug Control Strategy, prepared by this office in September 1989, reflected this focus on supply reduction. No mention was made of the need for any efforts directed toward physicians or other health care professionals (*National Drug Control Strategy,* 1989). Paradoxically, this followed by one year the publication of a manual by the World Health Organization, with majority input from American health professionals, on teaching about substance abuse in medical and other health settings (Arif & Westermeyer, 1988).

Toward the end of 1990, Drug Czar Bennett resigned and both he and President Bush, citing the statistics that showed casual use (not abuse) declining, declared our nation well on the road to winning the war on drugs.

Inadequate Federal and State Funding for Preventive Efforts

A major problem for the health care provider is inadequate federal funding for preventive efforts.

For political and conceptual reasons, federal funds and effort are diverted from preventive efforts to largely ineffective attempts to interdict the flow of a few drugs, largely ignoring the much greater health costs of alcohol and cigarettes. Punishment of offenders who turn to crime to fund their habits is a high priority. There has been little emphasis on, or funding for, studying and implementing measures aimed at substance abuse prevention.

It might appear that the problem of prevention of addiction is basically a public health problem. After all, drug addiction is a communicable disease that is threatening the health of our nation, and surely deserves the full attention and services of the Public Health Service. However, the public health service, chronically crippled by lack of funds, has been as effectively bypassed in this effort as have local public health services.

State policies that drastically curtail general health care and care for mental illness (including dually diagnosed drug abusers) and substance abuse have also dealt a major blow to prevention efforts. In addition, state programs, like their federal counterparts, now allocate 70% of their substance abuse budget for enforcement versus 30% for treatment and prevention. This budgetary ratio persists despite growing evidence that prevention is an effective deterrent to substance abuse.

The state of California published a report in December 1990, called "Families and Substance Abuse: The Case for a Comprehensive Approach," which was based on testimony and studies during the preceding three years. The report emphasized the special need to include families in all treatment and prevention efforts, rather than continuing with policies that criminalize the family. Despite such reports, budget constraints continue to destroy outstanding programs. One such program in California targeted families with children in which parents, grandparents, or other relatives had been identified as substance abusers or alcoholics and were living in the home. The program, which provided comprehensive services to the children and adults, was discontinued because the Office of Substance Abuse Prevention had to

eliminate funding beyond the top 7% of their programs, and this one was in the top 10% (Smith, 1990).

The Health Care Professional

Surely the health care professional sees the need for addiction prevention and is prepared to implement it. However, the health care provider faces formidable obstacles in this arena:

— The health care provider is usually uneducated in the nature of addiction, its detection, and its treatment. For example, despite the myriad physical effects of alcoholism, many physicians just do not routinely consider alcohol problems in their differential diagnosis with patients.

— Medical schools have been slow to train physicians in the prevention, diagnosis, and treatment of substance abuse. No major efforts have been made to include addiction in the education of the health care provider at medical school and postgraduate professional levels. Health care education in general usually doesn't emphasize the concept of prevention, and education about addiction is no exception. Educational efforts in prevention will be only partially successful until they focus on the prevention of addiction.

— The psychological aspects of addiction make many health care providers uncomfortable, so they tend either to deny these problems or to immediately refer these patients to a psychiatrist. This attitude is counterproductive in both the treatment and the prevention of addiction.

— Considerable moral stigma is attached to addiction. Many now accept that it is an illness, rather than willful misconduct, and a treatable one; nevertheless, old habits die hard, and many health care providers are critical of the addict, reflecting society's tendency to punish rather than help.

— The professional often has some of the same psychological processes at work as does the addict. Indeed, many health care providers have their own addictions. It is difficult for them to face in the addict what they will not face in themselves.

— Many health care professionals entered their profession in order to help people as a way of feeling good about themselves. However, the addicted patient can be very difficult to treat, often being hostile, manipulative, and in denial about his or her problem. Understandably, the caregiver reserves care for those more likely to show improvement quickly and gratefully.

— Little financial remuneration for the health care professional who practices prevention is available. No social mechanism rewards such services. Remuneration is almost exclusively reserved for the actions involved in reversing the effects of addiction.

— Prevention requires a degree of involvement in the personal lives of their patients that many health care workers feel is intrusive, unless there is a clear indication such as child abuse (and even there, many hesitate). One would like to perceive health care professionals as deeply compassionate and intimately involved in the lives of their patients. For too many professionals, this is just not true. Although compassion and caring do exist, they are often severely compromised by the training of the professional, by limitations of time, and by financial constraints.

The Prescribing of Pharmaceuticals

A widespread perception is that physicians have contributed to a national desire for a chemical solution to problems of daily living by prescribing admittedly useful and therapeutic drugs as an alternative to helping their patients cope with emotional distress. Pharmaceutical companies have been included in this perception. By 1970, 200 million prescriptions were being written annually for psychoactive substances, comprising about 20% of all prescriptions and refills. Advertising efforts to promote this chemical solution have been directed at the general public and physicians alike.

Special Interest Groups

Many policies are influenced by special interest groups such as the tobacco and alcohol industries. Major television and radio advertising campaigns by the alcohol industry recently led to the defeat, at the California polls, of the popular "nickel a drink" tax initiative, with its estimated nearly $1 billion annually earmarked for treatment of the direct and indirect health casualties from substance abuse.

Health Insurers

The insurance industry plays a major role in the provision of health care in this country. Until recently, it has been reluctant to reimburse for substance abuse and alcohol treatment services (Luckey, 1987). This policy has been based on the inaccurate and disproved notion that alcohol and drug treatment are largely ineffective.

The Dysfunctional Family

Drug addiction thrives in dysfunctional families, and a large number of American families are dysfunctional. Parenting practices are uncritically passed along from generation to generation. Abused children abuse their children. A child who has experienced bad parenting has little knowledge of good parenting. Most children today, even if they have not been previously abused, have little knowledge of good parenting skills. For parents to learn good parenting skills, they must learn good living skills for themselves. A parent so stressed by life pressures and behavioral maladjustments that he or she lives with constant or recurrent episodes of anxiety, anger, or depression is less able to learn empathic and caring communication and other good parenting skills.

If we are to teach parenting skills, who is to teach them? Health care workers are presently more trained to treat than to teach, and teachers are reluctant and not well-trained to address the psychological needs of their students. Typically, neither is psychologically attuned to teach good parenting.

WHAT IS THE HEALTH CARE PROVIDER ACCOMPLISHING?

Federal Leadership

In the mid-1980s, C. Everett Koop, M.D., used his position as Surgeon General as a bully pulpit to warn citizens more fully about the dangers of tobacco smoking. Koop is largely credited with the recent major change in public attitudes about cigarette smoking; more than 40 million Americans have given up smoking in the past decade. This dramatic statistic clearly illustrates how a strong government policy can serve as an effective prevention strategy. Cessation of cigarette smoking and the change in attitudes is an important primary prevention tool for young people not only in relationship to nicotine use, but for other drug use as well; cigarettes and alcohol are gateway drugs to illicit drug use. Those who never smoke cigarettes or drink alcohol rarely abuse other substances (Yamaguchi & Kandel, 1984). Before his retirement, Koop had also begun to target drunk drivers for public scrutiny and outrage.

Koop's action with regard to cigarette addiction prevention provides an example of what strong government leadership can and should do. His banishment, just after he announced that the alcohol industry's advertising practices and drunk driving were his next targets, attest to the political and economic power of the addiction industry.

Federal Funding

Another major component of the federal governmental role in the health care system is found in the national institutes that fund research, education, and treatment projects.

The National Institute of Health (NIH) was the parent organization. In the 1970s, the Alcohol, Drug Abuse, and Mental Health Administration (ADAHMA) was formed to oversee the National Institute of Mental Health (NIMH), the National Institute on Alcohol Abuse and Alcoholism (NIAAA), and the National Institute on Drug Abuse (NIDA).

NIAAA and NIDA were established to oversee and fund research, treatment, prevention, and education in alcohol and drug abuse. As one example of the latter effort, NIDA and NIAAA have set up a Health Educations Program to fund the design of a better curriculum for training medical and nursing students in early diagnosis and treatment of substance abuse.

A career teacher program in Alcohol and Drug Abuse was initiated by the federal govern-

ment in 1971 at approximately 60 medical schools. These career teachers began to develop substance abuse curriculum objectives in each medical school. When even the minimal funding for this program was discontinued after 10 years, by Ronald Reagan, the organization moved to the private sector, and persists to this day as the Association for Medical Education and Research in Substance Abuse (AMERSA).

A newer agency under ADAHMA, the Office of Substance Abuse Prevention (OSAP), formed in 1986 and now called CSAP (Center for Substance Abuse Prevention), has recently funded demonstration projects in medical schools for the development of curricula and faculty in substance abuse education. It has also funded events for medical school faculty such as the California Area Health Education Center (AHEC) conferences on "Educating Physicians, Residents and (Medical) Students on Substance Abuse Prevention" in 1988 and again in 1990. These conferences are attended by delegations of medical students, house officers, faculty, deans, and members of the school's curriculum committee representing, among others, each of the University of California Medical Schools (Ways, 1990).

CSAP also supports the National Clearinghouse for Alcohol and Drug Information (NCADI), which publishes and distributes free health information about the substances of abuse to the public (NCADI Publication #EN 8400, 1990).

Physician Organizations

Physicians have formed new societies at the state level, including the California Society for the Treatment of Alcoholism and other Drug Dependencies and the Southern California Physicians Association on Drug Dependence.

On the national level, new societies include the American Society for Addiction Medicine (ASAM). ASAM has enrolled several thousand physicians, given a certifying exam, and addressed the educational needs of its members and of physicians in general. This group now cosponsors educational activities with the American Medical Association (AMA).

The American Academy of Psychiatrists on Alcoholism and Addictions (AAPAA) is the most recent addition to the professional groups. It has more than 900 members to date, and has requested subspecialty recognition from the American Boards of Psychiatry and Neurology, a position endorsed by the American Psychiatric Association's Council on Addiction Psychiatry and its Assembly (*Psychiatric News,* 1990).

The American College of Physicians, the American Academy of Pediatrics, and the American Board of Family Practice have all been active in addressing special aspects of alcohol and other drug dependence (National Clearinghouse for Alcohol and Drug Information, 1989).

The AMA puts on educational symposia and publishes booklets for physicians such as "The Busy Physician's 5 Minute Guide to the Management of Alcohol Problems" and the "AMA Handbook on Alcoholism and Drug Abuse" (National Clearinghouse for Alcohol and Drug Information, 1989).

The California Medical Association (CMA) also has extensive education and prevention programs for physicians and the public. The CMA's Committee on Chemical Dependency is charged with developing a comprehensive program with the following goals:

— To analyze and make recommendations on proposed legislation and regulations affecting physicians, patients, and prevention
— To continue to design and present continuing medical education on chemical dependency issues
— To provide liaison between the CMA and the Department of Alcohol and Drug programs, the California Society of Addiction Medicine, and other state departments and organizations

The CMA has taken a particularly strong public policy position regarding chemical dependency, stating that the organization believes that chemical dependency must be recognized and treated as a disease and encouraging insurance coverage of the treatment of alcoholism and other drug dependencies. The organization's primary prevention efforts for the public are educational and include the publication of *Health Tips,* a newsletter appropriate for display in physicians' offices (California Medical Education, 1985). The CMA works in collaboration with the Medical Board of California, publishes guidelines for prescribing controlled substances for chronic conditions, and provides programs for impaired physicians.

The Washington State Medical Association has joined with nonmedical groups in sponsoring a proposal to control liquor advertising (Balzar, 1991). Noting that alcohol-related traffic accidents are the number-one killer of 16- to 24-year-olds in the state, the Medical Association has asked the Liquor Control Board to ban liquor industry advertisements that specifically target the young, especially beer ads.

A partnership between the American Bar Association and the AMA is a particularly exciting new collaborative effort that should be an effective primary prevention program in that its goals are to affect policy, encourage the involvement of influential community members, provide authoritative and practical information, promote a healthy lifestyle, strengthen social competencies and peer resistance skills, and involve members who will act as positive role models.

Pharmaceutical Companies

Pharmaceutical company advertisements are controlled by the Food and Drug Administration (FDA) with AMA guidelines (Coombs, 1976). The National Commission on Marijuana and Drug Abuse, in its Second Report to the Congress, recommended that manufacturers of psychoactive substances undertake a major campaign to educate both health professionals and the public about the appropriate role of psychoactive compounds for various stress-related and depressive conditions (National Commission on Marijuana and Drug Abuse, 1973).

Also in the 1970s, some pharmaceutical companies began to fund medical conferences and other educational efforts directed at physicians and various aspects of substance abuse. Smith, Kline, and French led the way, funding the Haight Ashbury Free Clinic's Amphetamine Research Project, followed by their PCP Project. Other examples include Roche Laboratories' sponsorship of the Benzodiazepine Project, Pfizer's Free Clinic Council Conference, Upjohn's emphasis on proper prescribing practices, and Mead Johnson's look at issues of dual diagnosis.

It should be noted that the pharmaceutical industry consists not only of manufacturing firms, but of drug wholesalers and community, hospital, and mail-order pharmacies.

Dwaine Lawrence of the University of Southern California School of Pharmacy has played a crucial role in an effort to involve pharmacists in a national grass-roots effort to inform people of options they have in the fight against addictions and other public health illnesses. Like physicians' offices, community pharmacists are an integral part of every neighborhood, and ideally suited to serve as agents of change. Unfortunately, as in medicine, present-day economics have seen the gradual replacement of the individual pharmacist by large, "efficient" chain operations in which the pharmacist is kept behind a glass wall filling prescriptions, and thus is only minimally able to interact with his or her clients. There is, however, considerable pressure on the part of pharmacists to resist this change and to reestablish communication with their clients. This is an important struggle for the community, and one to be followed with interest.

Direct Service Providers

Direct service providers, in the form of the substance abuse treatment industry, have raised the national consciousness regarding the health needs of the population of substance abusers, primarily by advertising the services they offer. Drug treatment has become big business, an important component of what the National Commission on Marijuana and Drug Abuse called the drug abuse industrial complex (National Com-

mission on Marijuana and Drug Abuse, 1973). Some medical corporations that provide chemical dependency treatment sponsor conferences for health care providers and the public, educating them on recent advances and issues in chemical dependency treatment. In addition, they offer free telephone consultations and interventions for individuals concerned about a family member. The treatment industry is now looking at the development of effective outpatient treatment because statistics indicate that this is a valuable and cost-effective method (Peluso, 1990). If chemical dependency experts do not take the lead in this area, insurance companies will be designing programs by default by deciding independently the type of services they will reimburse.

Health Insurers

New techniques for assessing treatment efficacy indicate that if costs are measured against benefits, mandated treatment is worthwhile. An exhaustive study in the state of Oregon, which has mandated treatment, shows that the total cost for delivering treatment and all associated services is 1.1% of the total for all health care costs. These statistics are similar to a report that shows that chemical dependency treatment comprises 1.23% of total HMO costs (O'Neill, 1990).

Because the projected cost to the nation for alcohol abuse alone for 1990 is estimated to be approximately $130 billion, with $70 billion in lost worker productivity and unemployment, the benefits of treatment appear to warrant the costs. In addition, studies show that after treatment, chemically dependent plan members use fewer medical services than untreated individuals (Holder & Blose, 1986). Another aspect of this problem indicates the importance of properly diagnosing chemical dependency early in the disease process. Of the $13 billion spent in 1983 on alcoholism treatment, $12 billion was spent on treatment of complications, such as alcohol-related liver disease, versus $1 billion on treatment administered by specialists in alcoholism (Holden, 1987).

Medical School Education

This is a critical component in prevention efforts. Some special efforts from the private sector in this area are noteworthy.

After AMERSA was established, the Kroc Foundation funded Project CORK, the Dartmouth version of a model undergraduate medical curriculum in substance abuse, and a similar project in the University of Washington's Department of Family Medicine (Lewis, 1989). Other major training projects were started at Harvard, Virginia, Louisiana State University, Brown, Johns Hopkins, and several other medical schools (The Pediatric Substance Abuse Curriculum Project, 1986; Dube et al., 1989). Schools of nursing, particularly at the University of Connecticut, New York University, and Ohio State, also emphasized teaching about substance abuse.

The J.M. Foundation and the Pew Charitable Trusts have both funded medical student educational programs in substance abuse. The Pacific Institute for Research and Evaluation has initiated projects that target health professionals who work with children for special training (National Clearinghouse for Alcohol and Drug Information, 1989). Pediatricians have also received information addressing special prevention strategies (MacDonald, 1986).

There is a need for an integrated approach to drug and health prevention policies, on all levels, that takes into account current knowledge regarding substance abuse. Upgrading medical education at the university level is crucial.

Model educational programs on substance abuse are beginning to be developed in medical schools, targeting medical students, residents, and faculty (The Pediatric Substance Abuse Curriculum Project, 1986; Dube et al., 1989). Aims and objectives, methods for achieving them, and evaluation of effectiveness are included in these ambitious projects, funded by NIDA and NIAAA (Coggin, 1989; "The AIMS Program . . .," 1989). Workshops are held, audio–visual materials have been developed, and special programs for intervening with impaired faculty have been created. Special government publications attempt to coor-

dinate and disseminate this information (National Clearinghouse for Alcohol and Drug Information, 1989).

Some innovative programs designed not only to provide information but to change attitudes of health workers early in their professional training have been developed. We will describe one such program, UCLA Medical School's Interactive Teaching (IAT) Seminar on Substance Abuse, in detail (Ziedonis, Ungerleider, & Noble, 1989).

All first- and second-year medical students at UCLA choose several "selectives" to sharpen their ability to think critically and to help develop tools for lifelong self-learning. The basic concept of the IAT is to provide students with an opportunity to self-direct their learning and teach one another relevant information, with instructors acting as expert consultants.

More than half of the first- and second-year students now take an IAT seminar in substance abuse. It has been offered five times yearly for the past three years (more than 200 students have completed the course), with a waiting list remaining at the end of each year. Students meet in groups of 14 for two hours weekly, over an eight-week period (some beginning as early as the first week of their first year) to explore issues and topics pertaining to aspects of the four major areas of substance abuse: treatment, research, prevention and education, and law enforcement.

Another innovative feature of this course is that it helps students understand the impact between health problems and societal problems, so social policy issues involving these four areas are emphasized. To obtain the information for their presentations in the seminar, teams of two students make three site visits to various university and community facilities; these teams then present their assigned topics and lead the group in a discussion of the issues.

The primary goals for the IAT are simple: to let the students know that substance abuse is treatable; to show that their attitudes are vital to effective diagnosis, intervention, and treatment; and to show that they must critically examine and challenge any teaching to the contrary.

In pairs, students visit a 12-step program such as Alcoholics Anonymous, Cocaine Anonymous, Narcotics Anonymous, Alanon, Adult Children of Alcoholics, or Overeaters Anonymous for one of their three site visits. (There are more than 2,000 such meetings in Los Angeles each week.) One factor in the underdiagnosis of substance abuse is the physician's own reluctance to examine his own and his colleagues' drug use behaviors. Physicians often believe that only "skid-row" people really have a substance abuse problem. To change this belief, all students attend these 12-step meetings with a "recovery teacher," a physician or professional who has been in recovery from substance abuse for at least two years. The recovery teacher briefs the students before the meeting, accompanies them to the meeting, and then discusses with them what they have all experienced together. Impressions are shared, and the different 12-step programs are compared and contrasted during the IAT session titled "Twelve Step Day."

Sites for the student's second visit include the Los Angeles Police Department's prevention and education program in the city schools (DARE) and their Drug Detection Unit (working at the city jail), a walk-along with a street outreach team, or visits with a detoxification center, an adolescent residential facility, a methadone maintenance program, or a drug diversion program. The students prepare reports on what they have learned about prevention, education, and treatment from the resource professionals they meet and from the substance abusers they interview at each site.

For their third presentation, students are involved in a debate, a report, or a role play. Students select issues to debate, such as the disease concept of alcoholism, the ethics of random urine testing among medical students and house staff (the Johns Hopkins Model), or social policies of zero tolerance or drug legalization, including needle-exchange programs.

Other students select topics for reports such as an overview of treatment modalities, the psychological dynamics of 12-step programs, drug abuse as a family disease, the impaired physi-

cian, and theories of prevention and education. Additional reports have included Fetal Alcohol Syndrome, the addicted newborn, genetic implications of alcoholism, AIDS and drug abuse, and the biological and psychological effects of the different classes of psychotropic drugs, including nicotine.

Students have also created their own topics for reports; for example, some have contacted the state medical board, the hospital's medical ethicist, or the hospital attorney. Others have appeared before the hospital credentials committee. One group of students surveyed their entire class about their drug attitudes, by ethnic background. Each year, after the course, several students participate in the Betty Ford Center's Professional in Residence (PIR) week-long experiential teaching program for physicians and medical students.

Some nontraditional teaching techniques are used in an attempt to bring affect into the learning situation and to influence students' attitudes. Role playing has been used when topics of early diagnosis and intervention are presented. For the section on early diagnosis, a "programmed patient" (actor) who has studied a case history of a drug abuse patient is interviewed by each student. An internist facilitator is present, who "freezes" the patient, explores new avenues of inquiry, and gives feedback to the students.

In the intervention segment, students play the roles of family members and friends of the "programmed patient" while a professional interventionist leads them in an intervention; the classroom serves as the patient's living room.

Material for all debates, reports, and role plays comes primarily from team meetings with a resource professional who has special expertise in the student's chosen area of interest. More than 60 resource professionals and recovery teachers from a variety of departments on the UCLA campus, in the UCLA Medical Center, and from throughout the community have enthusiastically participated.

The students also explore their attitudes toward substance abusers through the use of audio–visual materials such as the Project CORK Tapes. Videotapes are used extensively, including many on current events. Each session begins with a general discussion called "This Week in Drug Abuse"; here the students present what they have learned that week from the mass media. Particularly lively discussions follow events such as John Tower's physician telling the media that his patient did not have a drinking problem because his liver function tests were normal or Pete Rose's use of his gambling "addiction" as a defense against his ban from baseball.

THE FUTURE: WHAT CAN AND SHOULD HEALTH PROVIDERS DO TO PREVENT ADDICTION?

Federal and State Leadership and Funding

With adequate funding and direction, governmental agencies could help address this problem in a variety of ways:

— The Surgeon General must continue speaking out about the health care problems involved in cigarettes and alcohol, despite pressures from the tobacco and alcohol industry.

— The Office of National Drug Control should reverse the major emphasis of funding so that a majority is allocated to prevention and treatment rather than to enforcement, with closer involvement of and cooperation with addictionologists and the support of prevention programs and treatment facilities.

— The government funding agencies should better support academic programs that emphasize teaching of prevention and the health providers who attempt to implement it.

— States should recognize that prevention and treatment programs are more cost-effective than treatment programs alone, and should fully support them. Especially worthy of such intervention effort are those targeting families in which parents, grandparents, or other relatives have been identified as substance abusers.

— A revitalized Public Health Service should become involved in implementing and testing the effectiveness of programs to care for the children of alcoholics and drug addicts and other dysfunctional families. It could establish test programs in camps and day-care centers for children of the disadvantaged, where they could receive intervention by child-care workers. It could support adolescent centers, run by social workers and paraprofessionals, who could help these children learn how to cope with the stresses in their families and lives, and to experience some success. Such success enhances self-respect and builds self-esteem. With such activities adequately funded, the Public Health Service could play a major part in our prevention efforts against addiction.

Many of these functions can be assumed by private and nonprofit agencies. Peggy Amante of the University of Texas School of Public Health describes the efforts of the Greater Southeast Community Hospital in Washington, D.C., a hospital that has developed a program to address the health and economic needs of the community residents—a program that, in words of the hospital president, has been "aggressive and aimed at preventive care to ensure that we use our resources as wisely as we can." They work with community groups to better coordinate services directed at drug and alcohol abusers, but in addition have sponsored an impressive program of public health services that, in the long run, may be even more effective in combatting drug and alcohol abuse.

It begins with an adolescent pregnancy program that, going beyond traditional obstetrics classes, helps young mothers obtain prenatal care, develop parenting skills, and improve their lives after they deliver. It continues with a high-risk infant care program that, combatting one of the highest infant mortality rates in the country, emphasizes health education for all family members. It has a volunteer nursing assistant certification program aimed at undereducated, unemployed, or underemployed single women; this program provides the patient-care experiences these women need to find jobs in the health field. The community development program, run through the hospital's parent corporation, has renovated more than 500 housing units that provide clean, affordable accommodations for more than 1,700 community residents (Amante, 1991).

The Health Care Provider Network

Physicians in their offices and other health care workers comprise a widespread network that interacts with the general public as an important source of information. Prevention, however, requires a much closer interaction between the physician's office and the public it serves than now exists. Prevention requires the involvement of health care providers in many aspects of the family lives of their patients. Health care providers must learn to inquire into family psychological health. They must know what to do for dysfunctional families. They must break down the wall of professional distance that too often separates them from their patients.

The physician's office must provide services similar to a local mental health center by participating in the mental health of the community, becoming involved with local community groups in promoting the essentials of good mental health, by training mothers in good child care and good self-care.

Role models for this type of interaction do exist. Bruno Cortis, a cardiologist in Chicago, holds weekly meetings in his waiting room for his patients, where they discuss the implications of their illness on their personal lives, the effects of their personal lives on their illness, and ways of coping with both (Cortis, 1988).

William Manahan of Mankato, Minnesota, describes a family practice that includes society-oriented efforts at interaction with the community, including counseling services. He writes, "I slowly began to really learn about battered women, incest, codependency, food addictions, alcoholism, and many other topics about which I thought I already knew. I was amazed to learn how many of my own patients had these types of problems, without my having been aware of them." He adds, "I firmly believe that physicians can not only survive but can thrive, personally and financially, in a wellness-oriented, preventive-medicine practice" (Manahan, 1990, pp. 1–6).

Shouldn't family physicians learn that such wellness-oriented, preventive-medicine practice can be personally and financially rewarding? Shouldn't training in the special skills required for this type of practice be available in medical school and residency?

Make no mistake: Special attitudes and skills are required. They include attitudes of caring, compassion, and community involvement. They include skills of active listening, interpersonal relating, psychological understanding, and therapeutic support. They include the willingness to interact emotionally with people, to listen without needing to cure, and to feel, without needing to avoid one's own feelings.

The Prescribing of Pharmaceuticals

Effective as present-day psychoactive drugs are in the treatment of mental illness, they do not prevent drug addiction, and are inappropriate when used as a quick fix for situational problems. Advertising of the quick cure must be checked so that at least it is balanced by the understanding of the need to learn skills for better coping with psychological difficulties. Furthermore, the pharmacist stands in an ideal position as counselor for those seeking such drug relief for emotional distress; he or she should be used more widely for this purpose by the community.

Health Insurers

Financial incentives for nonsmoking, nondrinking members might prove to be a creative and effective form of prevention. Because many believe that the economic incentives to market health insurance at reduced costs are low, reduced premiums are unlikely unless mandated by Congress or state legislatures (Hurt 1990). It seems certain that the tobacco and alcohol industries will object.

Insurance companies could cut costs further by becoming involved in primary prevention efforts, such as prevention programs aimed at families covered in their plans. In addition, secondary prevention efforts, such as providing a thorough screening of all members for substance abuse during physical examinations and during hospital admissions, could easily be done. With appropriate chemical dependency treatment provided when indicated, it could decrease the need for more costly treatment of the major medical complications resulting from untreated chemical dependency.

Upgrading Substance Abuse Education in Medical Schools

The medical profession, as the primary representative of the health care system, must take the lead in developing effective prevention programs, and must begin by upgrading substance abuse education in medical schools. Model courses, such as the one at UCLA, must be present in every medical school in the country, and they must be expanded to include the psychosocial causes of addiction.

Thus physicians can perform primary, secondary, and tertiary prevention in their offices with each patient (and patient's family) they encounter. However, a single course is only the beginning. Each medical school should develop a division of addiction medicine, with faculty from each department providing courses illustrating the relationship between substance abuse and other medical conditions. Faculty members trained specifically in addiction medicine should be on the full-time staff of every medical school. The Center for Fellowship Studies has data on 38 full-time fellowship programs in addiction medicine. There are 41 physicians who began such fellowship programs in 1990, and 107 physicians currently in these fellowship programs (Fleming, 1990). Even if all of these physicians choose academic careers, which is unlikely due to the continuing lack of strong support within medical schools for addiction studies, the numbers are insufficient to meet the real need.

Michael Fleming has proposed a seven-point program for the improvement of medical education in substance abuse that would create the environment necessary to meet the challenges of this disease (Fleming, 1990). His strategies are as follows:

1. Develop a comprehensive plan to train 100 physicians per year for academic careers in addiction medicine.
2. Establish politically active working groups in specialties of family medicine, internal medicine, pediatrics, sports medicine, emergency medicine, and obstetrics (psychiatry already has such a group).
3. Develop and fund additional full-time fellowship programs within family medicine, internal medicine, pediatrics, and psychiatry.
4. Develop, fund, and test alternative part-time faculty development models to enhance the skills and expertise in addiction medicine.
5. Work within medical schools and universities to create faculty positions for physicians with expertise in addiction medicine.
6. Encourage medical students to choose addiction medicine as a special area of interest.
7. Develop comprehensive evaluation studies to assess the effectiveness of training models.

We suggest the following additions to this excellent list:

8. Medical schools must pay special attention to the well-being of their own students.
9. Schools must provide groups and workshops in which students can learn how to share their feelings with their peers.
10. Students must learn the social skills of listening, reflecting, affirming, and empathizing, not only with patients, but with each other.
11. They must learn how to listen to the feelings of others without being overwhelmed (empathy, not sympathy).
12. They must learn how to accept their own feelings of concern, sadness, anxiety, regret, and even shame and inadequacy in the face of failure.
13. They must learn how to hear criticism without becoming unduly defensive or aggressive. All this improves their coping skills and ultimately their sense of self-worth. This is primary prevention at its best.

Within the general medical community, continuing medical education upgrading for physicians is crucial. In addition, many advocate the establishment of a certified subspecialty in substance abuse.

At present, most physicians recognize the disease of alcohol addiction only when it presents at the terminal stage of cirrhosis of the liver with its secondary manifestations of ascites, hypoalbuminemic edema, and bleeding esophageal varices. Although 10% of the population suffers from alcoholism, fewer than 1% of patients going through the primary physician's office are so diagnosed. It is incumbent on the practicing physician to become more skilled at recognizing the disease at an earlier stage, when the functioning alcoholic in denial comes in with the following symptoms:

- Insomnia, depression, nightmares, poor memory, nervousness
- Nonspecific abdominal pain, morning vomiting, diarrhea, GI bleeding
- Polyuria, impotence, decreased libido, menstrual disorders
- Palpitations, hypertension
- Repeated trauma
- Behavioral problems such as increased absenteeism at work and repeated legal problems

At this point, the skilled health care provider has a chance to intervene, reframe the life experience of the individual, present supportive treatment options, and possibly prevent the progression of this disease.

To achieve this, the physician and other health care providers must become more skillful in introducing the topic of using alcohol as a destructive way of coping with stress. The history should include nonthreatening invitations to discuss family problems (including a family history of alcoholism), social difficulties, difficulties at work or with the law (such as DUIs), and a supportive and empathic investigation into personal emotional problems centered around feelings of diminished self-worth and possible suicidal feelings. The CAGE questions (Have you ever felt the need to *Cut* down on your drinking?, Have you ever been *Annoyed* by criticism of your drinking?, Have you ever felt *Guilty* about your drinking?, and Have you ever had a drink first thing in the morning to settle the "shakes" or get rid of a hangover [*Eye* opener]?) are useful for developing a high index of suspicion for alcoholism. They can be followed up with more specific questions about drinking to get high, drinking alone, looking forward to drinking, increased tolerance, blackouts, losing control, drinking as relief from painful feelings, and maintaining an excessively large supply of alcohol (Clark, 1981, 1985).

Programs to Improve Parenting Skills

One point at which intervention would be especially effective in preventing alcohol and other drug abuse is early in the parent–child relationship. Programs that improve parenting skills would greatly reduce the child's need for drugs to quiet the tumultuous distress of adolescence.

How do we know this? "Among the family variables directly related to drug use among adolescents, the most important are the affective relationships between the parents and between parents and child. It is generally and consistently observed that the likelihood of the adolescent's becoming involved in drug use increases with the degree of discord in the affective relationships in the home. Drug consumption by parents is the other main factor. . . . Consumption by offspring increases with the consumption of legal or illegal drugs by parents" (Lopez, Redondo, & Martin, 1989, pp. 1067–1079).

Furthermore, "[t]he predisposition to heavy, chronic use of a specific drug or class of drugs originates early in life. Persons who become committed to heavy, chronic use of a specific substance do so because their drug of choice . . . either allows temporary escape from currently experienced problems or creates the illusion that these problems have been solved by pharmacological means" (Shontz & Spotts 1989, p. 1097).

Using this type of information about modifiable aspects of the parent–child relationship, a Drug Risk Scale has been created that predicts the risk for drug use in high school students (Climent, de Aragon, & Plutchik, 1989). The scale includes data on the sharing of affection and communication with children, parental interest in the children's activities, and the degree of parental approval of drug use. Students are asked the following questions about their parents:

— Do they show affection?
— Do they do pleasant things with you?
— Do they talk to you about your life (plans, friends, play)?
— Do they talk to you about your problems?
— Do they show interest in helping you?
— Do they show that they care about you?
— Do they try to give you whatever you need?
— Are they fair with you?
— Do they express love for you?
— Do they know where you are when you are out?
— Do they know whom you are with when you are out?
— Do they enjoy talking to you about the things you do?
— Do they enforce curfews in a consistent way?
— Do they talk to you about your sexual interests?

These are, of course, students' perceptions of their parents. The questionnaire also asks about the students' perceptions of parental attitudes toward soft drinks, alcohol, aspirin, cigarettes, coffee, tranquilizers, and marijuana, as well as cocaine, crack, and other "hard" drugs. It asks several questions related to impulsivity and impulsivity control. This scale was cross-validated against non-drug-using high school students, against drug-using high school students, and against true drug addicts.

The major work of the prevention addictionologist, then, will be to educate parents to build relationships with their children through affection and communication, based on students' responses to the questionnaire.

The field work, of major importance in training parents, will most likely have to be done by another new professional, one trained and closely supervised by the prevention addictionologist. These addiction paraprofessionals will require special training that will cross existing professional lines. Furthermore, these must be professionals whose own well-being is well-tended so that they are psychologically able to teach empathic, caring parenting.

The nature of the parental training, and training of the professional to train the parent, will undoubtedly differ from institution to institution, and from area to area, probably creating turf and theoretical wars. Many social and economic factors are important, and must be considered in each program. We believe, however, that certain aspects of the training must be universal in order for the program to be successful. These include the following:

— The development of evaluation instruments, so that methods can be tested, changed, and improved
— Attention to the emotional health, well-being, and personal development of the professional
— Helping the parents accept and respect the personality and needs of their child as a separately evolving human being
— Attention to communication skills, including active listening, attention to nonverbal cues, empathic listening skills, and effective feedback skills
— Attention to individual personal and psychological characteristics, needs and traits, and the need to personalize instruction appropriately
— Improving interpersonal skills and empathy training
— Improving handling of stressful situations and painful emotions
— Improving self-esteem, reducing shame and guilt, developing assertiveness skills, and otherwise promoting the psychological growth of the parent (and, thus the child), without formal psychotherapy
— The use of nonpunishing methods of setting behavior limits (such as time outs)
— Active interaction with the parent, with a minimum of didactic instruction, using person-to-person and group interaction, videotapes, art, and other nonverbal therapy techniques, and whatever auxiliary teaching aids can be developed by the institution

The most efficient point at which to teach good parenting skills is when the mother is pregnant. At that point, motivation is highest, old habit patterns are most easily modified, and new skills are most applicable. Such programs have been in place in several areas, most notably for pregnant women who are themselves disadvantaged. Some believe that they should be mandatory for all parents (Anastasiow, 1988). Los Angeles County requires recipients of welfare to attend programs conducted by teachers to improve their coping skills, and the State of California has given official recognition of the value of programs that improve self-esteem in all walks of life.

Peer pressure, another important factor in drug experimentation and continued use, must not be neglected either.

Prevention Addictionology

Addictionology is now a recognized medical specialty. So far, however, it is largely limited in its scope to diagnosis and treatment, albeit early diagnosis and treatment. An inescapable conclusion is that prevention addictionology is a psychologically oriented specialty that differs from diagnostic and therapeutic addictionology, and needs special skills, not necessarily medical. The prevention addictionologist primarily needs the skills and talents of the teacher, social worker, and psychologist, as well as a basic medical understanding of the physiology, pathology, and symptomatology of drug addiction.

SUMMARY

The disease concept of addiction is becoming more accepted. This change thrusts health care providers into a central role in the prevention of and education about substance abuse.

What has been a fragmented and often neglected effort now, more than ever before, needs a coordination of planning on the part of that disparate and variegated entity known as health care providers.

Many problems concerned with the prevention of alcohol and other addictions face the health care provider; among them is the lack of leadership or support at the federal level, so that funds are diverted to paramilitary operations to interdict the supply of drugs and to incarcerate the abuser for a variety of criminal offenses, rather than to education and treatment. The health care provider is shackled by inadequate education in the prevention, diagnosis, and treatment of substance abuse; this shortcoming is often coupled with a defensive denial of his or her own vulnerability.

Pharmaceuticals are widely used and prescribed as a way of coping with personal problems, encouraging the use of more widely available and effective antianxiety drugs such as alcohol, a use aided and abetted by alcohol industry advertising. Health insurers have been reluctant to pay for preventive measures thus far. The dysfunctional and alcoholic family is largely ignored by our therapeutic community, allowing the emergence of dysfunctional and alcoholic offspring.

There are some encouraging and useful activities. The Surgeon General has demonstrated the power of effective federal preventive strategies. The National Institutes of Health and other agencies give limited support to research and to efforts to establish curricula in medical schools relating to drug and alcohol addiction. Physician organizations are developing education and prevention programs for physicians and the public, and are beginning to line up against alcohol industry advertising. Direct service providers, advertising their services, have made the public more aware of treatment options for the abuser. Studies have demonstrated that prevention and treatment *are* cost-effective for health insurers. Educators are (however slowly) moving alcohol and drug abuse programs into some medical school curricula.

Much remains to be done. The federal and state governments should redirect their efforts to prevention and treatment. Physicians must integrate themselves into the mental health of their communities and to learn to recognize and treat early signs of abuse. Pharmaceuticals must be integrated with programs for coping with stress. Health insurers must move in the direction of better support for preventive measures. Medical schools must upgrade substance abuse education. The problem of dysfunctional families is a major one; parents-to-be need increased educational opportunities to learn good parenting skills. Preventive addictionology should be established as a new and important specialty.

In this chapter, we have attempted to look at the major components of the health care provider complex in terms of what they have and have not done in the prevention of substance abuse, why they act as they do, and what they might do in the future. The obstacles are formidable, but they are not insuperable. People in general, and the medical profession in particular, are usually able to unite in the face of crisis. Drug addiction is a crisis of unprecedented proportions. With careful planning and adequate funding, we have the opportunity to change the drug ambience of our country. The alternative will not be pleasant.

REFERENCES

The AIMS Program: Aid for impaired medical students. Memphis: University of Tennessee Medical Center, 1989.

Amante, P. (Feb. 1991). The field of public health. Address to the Texas Association of Allied Health Professionals.

Anastasiow, N. (1988). Should parenting education be mandatory? *Topics in Early Childhood Special Education, 8* (1), 60–72.

Arif, A., & Westermeyer, J. (1988). *Manual of drug and alcohol abuse: Guidelines for teaching in medical and health institutions.* New York: Plenum Books.

Balzar, J. (1991). Doctors offer a cure for bad taste liquor ads. *Los Angeles Times,* Jan. 16.

California Medical Association (1985). *Health tips.* San Francisco: California Medical Education and Research Foundation.

Clark, W. D. (1981). Alcoholism: Blocks to diagnosis and treatment. *The American Journal of Medicine, 71,* 275–286.

Clark, W. D. (1985). The medical interview: Focus on alcohol problems. *Hospital Practice,* Nov 30, 59–68.

Climent, C. E., de Aragon, L. V., & Plutchik, R. (1989). Prediction of risk for drug use in high school students. *International Journal of the Addictions, 24* (11), 1053–1064.

Coggin, P. (1989). *Resource manual for alcohol and other drug abuse education in family medicine medical school and residency programs.*

NIDA/NIAAA Contract #ADM 281-85-0002 and 281-85-0012.

Coombs, R. H., Fry, L. J., & Lewis, P. G. (Eds.) (1976). Preconditions in drug abuse. In *Socialization in drug abuse.* Cambridge, MA: Schenkman.

Cortis, B. (1988). Finding your support group. *Bulletin of the Society for Professional Well-Being, 1* (2), 3.

Dube, C. E., Goldstein, M. G., Lewis, D. C., Cyr, M. G., & Zwitch, W. (1989). Project Adept: The development process for a competency-based alcohol and drug curriculum for primary care physicians. *Substance Abuse, 10* (1), 5–15.

Fleming, M. (1990). I have a dream. *Substance Abuse, 11* (3) 123–124.

Holden, C. (1987). Alcoholism and the medical cost crunch. *Science, 235,* 1132–1133.

Holder, H., & Blose, J. (1990). Alcoholism treatment and total health care utilization and costs. *Journal of the American Medical Association, 256* (11), 1456–1460.

Hurt, R. (1990). Beyond Koop. *Professional Counselor, 4* (4), 34–41.

Lewis, D. C. (1989). Putting training about alcohol and other drugs into the mainstream of medical education. *Alcohol Health and Research World, 13* (1), 8–14.

Lewis, D., Niven, R. G., Czechowicz, D., & Trumble, J. G. (1987). A review of medical education in alcohol and other drug abuse. *Journal of the American Medical Association, 257,* 2945–2948.

Lopez, J. M., Redondo, L. M., & Martin, A. L. (1989). Influence of family and peer group on the use of drugs by adolescents. *International Journal of the Addictions, 24* (11), 1065–1082.

Luckey, J. (1987). Justifying alcohol treatment on the basis of cost savings: The 'Offset' literature. *Alcohol, Health and Research World, 12* (1), 8–15.

MacDonald, D. I. (1986). Prevention of adolescent smoking and drug use. *Pediatric Clinics of North America, 3,* 995–1005.

Manahan, W. (1990). Can a physician survive financially in a wellness-oriented medical practice? *Bulletin of the Society for Professional Well-Being, 2* (3), 1–6.

National Clearinghouse for Alcohol and Drug Information (1989). *Alcohol Health and Research World, 13* (1).

National Commission on Marijuana and Drug Abuse (March 1973). *Drug use in America: Problem in perspective.* Washington, DC: USGPO, pp. 377–82.

National Drug Control Strategy (Sept. 1989). Washington, DC: U.S. Government Printing Office.

NCADI Publications (1990). Catalog #EN 8400. Rockville, MD: OSAP.

O'Neill, C. (1990). The cost savings of mandated alcohol drug treatment. *Professional Counselor, 4* (4), 42–43.

The Pediatric Substance Abuse Curriculum Project, Johns Hopkins University (1986). NIDA/NIAAA Contract #281-86-0009.

The Pediatric Substance Abuse Curriculum Project, Johns Hopkins University (1987). Department of Medicine Contract #ADM 281-86-0020.

Peluso, E. (1990). Why out is in. *Professional Counselor, 4* (4), 45–47.

Psychiatric News, November 2, 1990, p. 6.

Report of President's Commission on Mental Health, vol. 4 (1978). Appendix.

Shontz, F. C., & Spotts, J. V. (1989). From theory to practice: The planned treatment of drug users. *The International Journal of the Addictions, 24* (11), 1091–1136.

Smith, L. (1990). Treatment: It's all in the family. *L.A. Times,* Dec. 7, pp. E1–E3.

U.S. Department of Education (1988). *Drug Prevention Curricula.* Washington, DC: U.S. Government Printing Office.

U.S. Secretary of Health, Education, and Welfare (1991a). *Drug abuse and drug abuse research,* Triennial reports to Congress. Washington, DC: USGPO.

U.S. Secretary of Health, Education, and Welfare (1991b). *Marijuana and health; Annual reports (biannual) to the U.S. Congress.* Rockville, MD: NIDA.

U.S. Secretary of Health and Human Services (1987). Summary of research into prevention of drug abuse; Drug abuse and drug abuse research, Second triennial report to Congress. Washington, DC: USGPO.

Ways, P. (1990). AHEC Conference Coordinator, personal communication.

Yamaguchi, K., & Kandel, D. (1984). Patterns of drug use from adolescence to young adulthood: II. Sequences of progression. *American Journal of Public Health, 74,* 668–672.

Ziedonis, D. M., Ungerleider, J. T., & Noble, E. P. (1989). Teaching substance abuse using an interactive teaching model. *Substance Abuse, 10* (2), 97–102.

CHAPTER 7

EMPLOYERS

PAUL M. ROMAN
TERRY C. BLUM

THE DRUG–WORK CONNECTION: WHAT IS THE PROBLEM?

Some years back, it was rare to find either re-search or theory that established a clear linkage between drugs and work (Trice & Roman, 1972). Indeed, as recently as 20 years ago, there was little evidence of a societal consensus that America had a significant alcohol problem. However, a multitude of social changes have brought both drugs and alcohol to the forefront of public concerns in the interim. Most evident is the continuing "war on drugs," initiated by the federal government, but now supported by all levels of government as well as through nongovernmental resources.

This "war" consists mainly of drug interdiction efforts, but includes drug problem treatment and a variety of educational and preventive efforts. Despite many of its questionable emphases and tactics, the "war on drugs" has made citizens aware of multiple dimensions of drug problems, including the drug–work connection. Evidence abounds through the media and through highly visible government-sponsored activities that American employers should combat the workplace drug problem, prevent the use or misuse of drugs by workers, and ultimately produce a drug-free American workforce. Although these responsibilities fall on employers, American citizens, as employees, are expected to support these efforts, much as the citizenry is mobilized in any war.

More recently, the departure of the Republican strategists of the "war on drugs" has marked the downplay of drugs as the problem and at least partially turned the focus toward drug abuse as the problem. The treatment of drug problems and rehabilitation of the drug abuser have moved onstage as important elements in dealing with all drug problems among both the employed and the unemployed. This has not supplanted, but rather supplements, the interdiction emphases.

Given this level of attention and the centrality of work as an American social institution, one would expect abundant research literature on the drug–work connection. This is not the case however, for at least four different reasons.

First, federal drug policy was developed and implemented without the perceived need for a base of research evidence or guidance. In the atmosphere of a "war," the technology of screening urine samples for evidence of drug metabolites was quickly adopted and diffused. The "emergency" allowed little time to examine possible adverse side effects or other long-term consequences of using this technology.

Second, even under the best of circumstances, and when research funding is at its highest levels, money for psychosocial research is very scarce relative to the research dollars available to

The authors acknowledge partial support from Research Grant no. R01-DA-07417 from the National Institute on Drug Abuse and Research Grants R01-AA-07250 and R01-AA-07192 from the National Institute on Alcohol Abuse and Alcoholism.

pursue the biomedical causes and cures of drug dependence. Thus, within the National Institute on Drug Abuse (NIDA), a massive amount of research resources are centered on the biodynamics of psychoactive chemicals within the human organism, but a much lower priority is assigned to studying the patterns of drug problem identification, or the consequences of a variety of interventions directed at those who are directly or indirectly affected by drug abuse. This has recently been exacerbated by the organizational relocation of the NIDA within the National Institutes of Health, an organizational setting that nearly guarantees an overwhelming emphasis on biological considerations, with relegation of psychosocial science to case counting and evaluation studies. Despite the administration's promises that no research programs would be disrupted by the move of NIDA to NIH, a fledgling research unit dedicated to supporting studies of workplace drug problems and policies was essentially abolished in the transfer process.

Third is a problem of research methodology. Researchers must go into the workplace to understand the dynamics of drug use, abuse, its tolerance, its identification, and the range of solutions that can be undertaken without disrupting the flow of work activities or undermining the basic goals of work organizations. But in contrast to the public schools or to the streets and neighborhoods of this land, the workplace is not an easy place within which to mount sound research. Workplaces are closed systems with increasingly tight concerns with efficiency, typically without the slack to devote workers' or managers' time to participate in research. Further, obtaining access to conduct serious research within a single worksite is very difficult, to say nothing of the challenges associated with studies that should be grounded in a representative sample of worksites.

Finally, at least part of the neglect of the drug–work connection by researchers can be traced to the assumption by federal policymakers (taking their lead from former president Reagan) that the drug–work connection presented the simplest of issues, namely that the connection had to

be broken and the workplace made drug-free. Such a conclusion does not seem to demand extensive research. It is an exemplar of pragmatism and common sense. The stated policy position of the Reagan administration, enunciated by the president himself in a speech at Duke University, was that people without jobs who used drugs should be excluded from employment and people with jobs who use drugs should have those jobs taken away. Surely to suggest that such clear ideas should be researched before they are implemented would have attracted massive derision.

Despite this apparent practicality and simplicity, since the early 1980s webs of complexity have grown around the "war on drugs." Just Say No has become an increasingly hollow and sometimes laughable slogan. The other seemingly straightforward policy approaches to the American drug problem have become increasingly problematic. The "get rid of 'em" strategy directed toward the workplace was not feasible, and quickly became altered through court decisions based on the Bill of Rights, followed by a stream of related litigation that remains prominent across all levels of the judicial system.

Thus, it is not mere ideology to argue that the organization of work in American society provides a poor fit with Reagan's double-pronged "exclusion solution," despite the popular attraction of a Supreme Commander's pragmatic simplicity in the early stages of war. Today's drug–work connection involves not only questions about testing and identification, but also concerns about equity and fairness, as well as attention to conserving human resources that have become stigmatized or debilitated by drug use.

CAFFEINE AND HEROIN IN THE WORKPLACE: A COMPARISON

Meaningful discussions about drugs and work can quickly run aground when people operate with incompatible definitions. This is a common occurrence, because psychoactive drugs surround us in great variety and abundance. Furthermore, our culture places scientific knowledge on a sacred pedestal, the practical face of which is technology. Quite beyond and apart from the lurid scenes of young people toking and snorting or addicts sharing needles, we Americans use drugs to make ourselves feel better, to improve our performance, to lubricate our social events, and to save our lives.

When we consider the relationship between drugs and the workplace, definition is thus a natural first question. "Drugs" range from caffeine, readily available to children in soft drinks and to adults in coffee, tea, and pills, as well as soft drinks. These potions are seen as common, useful, and safe, falling more or less in the category of foods.

A sharp contrast can be made to heroin, a substance viewed as without redeeming value, dangerous, poisonous, and enslaving. Heroin is typically envisioned as emanating from some dark nefarious corner of the earth, used by people who unwittingly take a single dose and become addicted for life. The elaboration of this stereotype has the heroin addict driven to crime and deprivation in order to maintain the high-cost habit. Without the drug, the addict is believed to go into a hellacious withdrawal, the fear of which drives the addiction.

It is notable that these two examples both have relevance in the workplace. A comparison of reactions to these two drugs in the workplace provides an important sociological context for much of the material that follows.

Caffeine is practically ubiquitous, readily and easily available at most worksites. It is regularly consumed by the majority of adult Americans, conservatively 125,000,000 in number. It is not uncommon for employers to provide unlimited amounts of caffeine to their employees. Although there are employees who find for a variety of health-related reasons or personal discomforts that they have to give up caffeine and switch to decaf, there is little evidence of the social costs of widespread caffeine dependence or addiction.

Perhaps of greater significance, there is no anticaffeine lobby or association. Despite the technical existence of a caffeine dependence syndrome in medical classification, there are essentially no social resources directed toward the identification, treatment, and rehabilitation of caffeine addicts. Although the NIDA supports some biomedical research to consider some of the basic psychopharmacology of caffeine, federally funded research on caffeine related problems is practically nonexistent.

Heroin is the opposite in essentially all respects. Probably more than any other drug, heroin is feared by both nonusers of drugs and by those who have experimented with illegal drugs or who are recreational users. For many, it seems that the notion of addiction is exemplified by the heroin addict, an individual believed to organize a life of stealth and theft around a constant craving and a need for a steady supply of the drug (Trice & Roman, 1972; Chambers & Heckman, 1972). In many respects, the antidrug lobbies and voluntary organizations have been centered on heroin addiction and use it as the model for describing more recently discovered dependencies on cocaine and marijuana.

Workplace managers go to great lengths and expense to ensure that both heroin and heroin users are not present in the workplace. The reactions of employers to cases of employee heroin use are varied. Whether most heroin users can be successfully targeted by interventions and returned to "normal" work performance is a question that cannot be answered from our current base of research data. The level of effort seems driven much more by the cultural image of this drug than by its actual socioeconomic impact, for curiously, even the most inflated estimates of the population of regular heroin users in the United States do not exceed 500,000.

Thus it is clear that caffeine and heroin, two very different drugs, have different impacts and elicit different responses in the workplace. Why? It seems simple to say that caffeine is weak and heroin is strong, yet there is little doubt that one can become significantly strung out on several rapidly successive cups of coffee or cola drinks. The idea that caffeine is not importantly addictive while heroin is very importantly addictive is defied by the numbers cited above. It may be equally defied by the obvious drug-dependent behavior one can observe among the American adult population in the hours immediately following their awakening on a typical weekday (Ray, 1978). One can only imagine the results of a contrived experiment in which caffeine in all forms was removed from a community for a single day.

The more direct answer to why caffeine seems to be cherished in the workplace while heroin is abhorred lies in the perception of these drugs' effects on work and the expected behaviors of both types of drug users within the workplace. Caffeine is perceived as enhancing energy and work performance whereas heroin is seen as creating an intense set of sensory experiences in which work would have no relevance and during which any attempt at job performance would be foolhardy.

Beyond direct effects on performance, we need to look further at the cultural imagery surrounding the drugs and the users of different drugs. Although there may be a physiological addiction to caffeine that develops over a pattern of long-term regular use, caffeine users in the workplace are typically viewed as those who are committed to and involved in their work, employees who use this substance to stay alert and do better.

The heroin user, by contrast, is seen as an extreme deviant engaging in the use of an illegal substance about which substantial warnings have been communicated to all members of society. This is not perceived as accidental straying but behavior that has evolved into deliberate deviance, reflecting an attitude of defiance and rejection of society's cherished beliefs and values about conformity and participation. In many ways, the heroin user is a rebel. Finally, by being in the workplace, many if not most heroin users are seen as doubly deviant. They not only spoil their social identities by engaging in acts of substance use judged to be distinctively wrong by society, but are believed to steal from the employer or attempt to sell heroin and other drugs to co-workers in order to raise enough money to support their habits.

The workplace is in many ways a microcosm of society. In a crucial sense, workplace behaviors supposedly capture the implementation of core values about individual conformity, commitment, and achievement. In this context, the broader historical imagery associated with different psychoactive substances becomes relevant. This imagery is not necessarily based on the public's exposure to scientific data. The public is heavily educated by the mass media, but the mass media are distinctively outside the business of education, instead competing for segments of the audience most satisfactory to the commercial sponsors that pay for the media's existence. The horrors of addiction and the many dreadful consequences of drug abuse make good copy.

What the public learns about drugs also reflects careful selection of scientific data by image-makers and policy proponents to effectively bolster a particular construction of "truth." This need not be deliberate distortion, but reflects the fact that researchers and policymakers must engage in certain amounts of marketing in their competition for scarce research and program dollars, because these dollars are sought with equal fervor by the constituencies surrounding other problems believed to undermine the strength and fiber of American society. Often, the target of marketing efforts is Congress and the various state legislatures. It is clear that these groups will not sustain their bases of power by encouraging or accepting visions of drug problems or drug problem solutions that are at odds with what they perceive to be the beliefs of the voters who put them in office.

Thus, one of the key notions about caffeine pervasive in our culture is that it is harmless, a perspective doubtlessly disputed by scientific data describing the risks caffeine consumption may present in the presence of other conditions (Ray, 1978). As has been mentioned, little is made of the addictive nature of caffeine, despite scientific evidence.

Heroin, on the other hand, is seen as extremely harmful to the human organism, despite evidence that much of the harm associated with heroin use stems from the lifestyles associated with distribution and use of this highly illegal substance. Heroin is seen as instantly addictive, with a respected psychiatrist at one time titling a book about its dangers *It's So Good Don't Even Try It Once* (Smith, 1973). By contrast, scientific data (systematically neglected or ignored) describe patterns of recreational and controlled heroin use in some settings ("chipping"), with addictive use suggested to be a function of socially induced expectations rather than inevitable physiological processes (Zinberg, 1984). The present authors (as well as fellow researchers) can testify to the adamant and even furious reactions and rejections that descriptions of this research can generate among otherwise calm and well-educated citizens.

These observations suggest that the drug–work connection is a combination of realities and perceptions as well as a combination of value-based beliefs and scientific evidence. We stress that such combinations are typical of approaches to any social problem in American society. As a society, we like to believe that we rationally deal only in facts and evidence, but emotional perceptions and beliefs are always present and often very influential. Whatever their association with truth, perceptions and beliefs provide definitions of the situation, and these definitions can produce very real consequences.

While we tend in this chapter to use the term *drugs* in a rather generic fashion, our implicit focus is on the drugs that are viewed as having the most adverse impacts on the workplace in terms of the combination of their effects and the prevalence of their use. These are alcohol, a legal drug, and cocaine and marijuana, both illegal drugs. To a lesser extent, our considerations encompass heroin, the use of which is much less common than these other drugs.

BASES FOR EMPLOYER ACTION

Working from a broad perspective, the following can be listed as adverse impacts of drug use on work. Each of these impacts can be challenged, and we do not include here a critical review of the methodologies of studies from which these observations are drawn:

- Drug use reduces workers' productivity in terms of both quality and quantity of performance.
- Drug use creates unpredictable and disruptive behavior in the workplace, affecting the behavior and productivity of co-workers.
- Drug use is a threat to safety in the workplace.
- The presence of illicit drug use is typically an indicator of illicit drug dealing. Not only does this imply the presence of serious criminal behavior in the workplace, but also suggests the increased likelihood that pushing will occur, which may induce nonusing employees to use drugs.
- Drug-using habits are expensive and encourage theft from both the employer and fellow employees.

Two further, related impacts have been suggested:

- Employees' performance and attendance may be affected by the drug-using behaviors of their dependents and family members.
- Drug-using behavior is not only illegal but "wrong"; the presence of drug use in the workplace or tolerance of it undermine respect for other workplace rules.

Thus, there is no shortage of reasons for employers' concern about employees' use of drugs. Assessing the validity of each of the above generalizations offers a complicated set of issues, some of which are explored in the other chapters in this book. For present purposes, it is important to stress that many employers believe that these generalizations are valid, and they act on these beliefs. In line with the principle set forth by sociologist W. I. Thomas, these beliefs are real "stuff" because they produce real consequences. Regardless of their accuracy, these generalizations are powerful because they are the bases for action.

THE SOURCES OF EMPLOYEE DRUG ABUSE

One rather obvious issue that deserves comment is employers' perception of the causes of drug use among employees. It would seem that the conditions of work might be a major source of stress, which would lead some employees to adopt drug use as a relief or escape, a notion sometimes conceptualized as self-medication. There is a direct connection between such an idea and the employer undertaking steps to eliminate the causes of stress and thus reduce drug use in the workforce.

As obvious as such approaches seem to be, they are rarely adopted. First, a variety of regulations associated with Worker's Compensation place liability on employers for working conditions that lead to employee disease or injuries. Although there is a large literature on employer liability for diseases and physical injuries, the issue of such responsibility for employees' behavioral problems has long been ambiguous (Trice & Belasco, 1966).

Second, although a great deal of research has attempted to link working conditions with employees' psychiatric problems as well as their use of psychoactive substances, the conclusions of such research are vague and equivocal (Newcomb, 1988). Thus, assuming that an employer was motivated to find the work-based sources of employees' drug use, there is little available guidance from the research literature. Furthermore, it would be very difficult to mount a study that would conclusively provide evidence of the causal linkage between work stress and drug use, drinking, or psychiatric conditions. It is perhaps ironic that some researchers have noted that the association between work and drinking may be grounded in the cultures of occupations or work groups (Sonnenstuhl & Trice, 1987). These findings indicate that it is not unusual that the culture that promotes or facilitates the behavior is essentially a "play" or solidarity culture, rather than one based on escapism or rebellion against the employer.

Thus, for the most part, employee drug problems are perceived and defined as rooted in the employees' lives and behaviors outside work. Although the problem of establishing causality is as problematic here as within the workplace, it is surmised that these external causes reside in employees' personal physiologies or lifestyle choices that may be linked to drug use.

Reflecting one well-known approach to the study of organizations, it is both convenient and consistent with much organizational research to view employee drug use as an intrusion from the external environment surrounding the organization (Thompson, 1967). In such a framework, employee drug use represents a potential cost and disruption against which the organization should be prepared to buffer itself.

PAST AND CURRENT PREVENTION PROGRAMS AND STRATEGIES

In response to the belief that there is drug abuse among employees that requires action, two types of organizational interventions have been widely adopted. These are drug screening programs (DSPs) and employee assistance programs (EAPs). Before considering these strategies in detail, we examine their evolution.

The early history of work in the United States was marked by the integration of alcohol consumption with work (Rorabaugh, 1979; Ames, 1989). This was in part a cultural transfer from the European backgrounds of those who inhabited the country, both during the colonial period and for nearly 50 years after the American Revolution. Historians have shown that alcohol abuse was not a major social problem. This can be at least partially explained by the level of technology guiding most work. There was relatively little interaction between workers and complex machines, and the modern clock-conscious and limb-grinding workplace was yet to emerge.

In large part, the Industrial Revolution made the consumption of mind-altering drugs into a social problem and a workplace problem. The entry of machine-based technologies and the factory as a principal mode of work organization made the impairment of the worker an evident problem. Not only could alcohol consumption affect job performance and productivity, but it could also create risks and hazards for others, particularly in the presence of large and potentially dangerous machinery.

EMERGENCE OF THE "UNIVERSAL" WORKPLACE POLICY

This transformation has been the subject of considerably detailed analyses, and it is germane here to describe the role of workplaces in responding to the emergent problems of alcohol in the workplace. The initial and enduring response originated as the suggestion of temperance, the notion that drinkers should moderate their use of alcohol to minimize its impact on their own and others' well-being. In part due to the ambiguity of defining *temperance,* a norm of moderation became quickly transformed into advocacy for total abstinence for individuals, to be facilitated or required for the entire population by national Prohibition (Clark, 1976).

Recent analyses offer compelling evidence that the potency of the movement for Prohibition during the nineteenth century was based on strong support from the emerging class of industrial capitalists (Rumbarger, 1989). It is obvious that alcohol consumption by workers offered little if anything of value to the successful sweep of the Industrial Revolution and the accompanying emergence of the construction, transportation, communication, and services industries. Thus the good and desirable worker was an abstemious individual, regular in his habits and behavior, and a dedicated employee whose other basic life commitment was to the support of his wife and children.

The combined political forces of these industrialists, religious leaders, and large numbers of the middle class supportive of the temperance movement led to the passage of Prohibition in the form of a constitutional amendment, effective in 1920. The societal support for such means of maximizing social order in an increasingly large and heterogenous society was reflected several years earlier in the 1914 passage of the Harrison Act, which effectively constituted societywide prohibition of manufacture and distribution of a range of nonalcoholic drugs (Morgan, 1981; Roman & Blum, 1992).

If we remove historical blinders and define *prohibition* as laws forbidding the manufacture and distribution of certain substances, it is evident that beliefs in the utility of the concept have not faded with time. Rather than viewing Prohibition as a historical relic of antiquated ideas of social control, we must recognize that such a concept is the highly supported and valued centerpiece of the contemporary "war on drugs." There is little argument that indeed, the American public of the late twentieth century is strongly supportive of this particular version of prohibition.

Furthermore, the concept of prohibition (at the local or organizational level) is the longest-surviving strategy for dealing with problems of drugs and alcohol in the workplace (Staudenmeier, 1989). Although we know of no survey data that specify the actual prevalence of workplace rules of conduct that prohibit the use or distribution of alcohol or drugs by employees during work hours, it is obvious that it is a high proportion. Even in sites where such rules may not be visible or widely diffused, it is typically understood that such rules apply.

This is a classic example of an attempt at primary prevention. Here we define primary prevention as measures intended to curb the incidence of new problem events. Although there are no controlled studies comparing worksites that do and do not prohibit the use or distribution of alcohol, it is clear that the relative absence of alcohol and drugs from the workplace affects the occurrence of a whole series of potential problems that might occur if workers were allowed to drink on the job in a fashion paralleling the norms of colonial America. Thus, few if any employers question the utility of a prohibition policy; they simply adopt and typically enforce such policies. Worksite-level prohibition of the use of drugs and alcohol can be reasonably described as an institutionalized policy in the United States.

Such policies are not, however, without their deficiencies. Commonly cited examples of inconsistencies in such policies include the following:

- Providing alcohol to employees under company auspices at office parties, picnics, and ceremonial events such as retirement parties.
- Allowing certain classes of workers, such as field sales personnel or upper-level executives, to consume alcohol at lunch or business dinners and as part of business activities, sometimes on company premises.
- Having no clear rules for employee drinking during lunch hours, especially when lunch breaks are allowed off-premises.
- Whereas some rules prohibit drinking on the job, others prohibit only intoxication or some other level of use that might be established through a blood or breath test. These latter rules imply that a certain level of alcohol intake does not impair acceptable job performance, although it would be rare for any such policy to implicitly accept any level of use of nonalcoholic drugs.
- Unclear implications of the acceptability of drinking before coming to work. Although it is clear that drinking immediately before coming to work would probably be viewed as a breach of rules of conduct, research evidence has determined the impact on job performance of hangover effects resulting from drinking during the previous evening (Yesavage, Leirer, Denari, and Hollister, 1985). This becomes more ambiguous when there are unusual hours of work, such as in the transportation industry. Given the nature of drug testing described below, it is clear that alcohol and drugs are on different regulatory planes in this regard.

Whereas the first four of these concerns apply primarily to alcohol in the workplace, it is clear that the last two center on concerns affecting both alcohol and drugs.

Thus, prohibition is very widespread as a primary prevention strategy for dealing with alcohol and drugs in the workplace. There are no precise measures of this policy's effectiveness across a variety of types and sizes of settings, but unlike total prohibition of alcohol or drug availability in society, partial prohibition in the workplace has not been a costly or cumbersome policy to implement or maintain. The exceptions to this generalization are incidents in which employers have searched workers, their lockers, and their cars or used drug-sniffing dogs.

For many workplaces, prohibition is not enough. As mentioned, the two main categories of interventions used to deal with drug and alcohol problems in the workplace are DSPs and EAPs. We look first at the evolution of DSPs.

THE FIRST CAMPAIGN FOR A "DRUG-FREE WORKPLACE"

The past decade has been marked by much attention to efforts to create "drug-free workplaces" in the United States, but this is the "second round" in the battle against employee drug abuse (Roman & Blum, 1992). It is important to note that the two drugs that became of central concern as problems, opiates and cocaine, were widely used and generally viewed as nonproblematic in American culture until the last quarter of the nineteenth century, when concerns began to escalate, culminating in the Harrison Act.

The submergence of specific concern about drugs in the workplace from 1900 until the 1970s tends to support an assumption that drug abuse tended to be concentrated among those in marginal social categories; other than occasional commentary about drug use and addiction among medical professionals (Winick, 1961; Simon & Lumry, 1969; Smith & Blachly, 1966) and those in the performing arts (Winick, 1960; Becker, 1953), there is no literature in the ensuing period that describes any general pattern of nonalcohol drug problems in the workplace.

It is well-known that the cohort entering young adulthood during the early 1970s became extensively involved with illegal drugs, with marijuana and the hallucinogens gaining the most attention. The interest and concern about drugs and the workplace arose in concert with the movement of this cohort toward full-time employment. This brief movement included the following elements (Roman & Blum, 1992):

- The drug abuser was viewed as a menace who threatened order and profitability in the workplace.
- The drug problem was seen as new and therefore difficult for companies to understand and combat.

- Although objective detection of heroin use was possible through urine screening, use of other drugs could not be easily detected.
- Companies could expect theft and other dishonesty among employees who use illegal drugs.
- The effectiveness of treatment intervention for drug abusers was regarded as very poor.
- In part due to greater hiring of minorities, drug problems were moving from the ghetto to the workplace (Wilcke, 1970).

For a series of complex reasons that are described elsewhere (Roman & Blum, 1992), this fledgling interest played itself out until reemerging in a different form in the mid-1980s. We briefly describe the events that occurred in the interim.

EMERGENCE OF THE SECOND "DRUG-FREE WORKPLACE"

The history of current efforts to deal with drugs in the workplace is relatively complex (Roman & Blum, 1992), but a brief synopsis is useful here.

A pivotal effort to address employee drug problems was a policy statement by the U.S. Civil Service Commission (now the Office of Personnel Management) in 1973. This policy included methods for handling both drug users and drug distributors and thus was a mixture of treatment and criminal concerns. Of importance was its orientation toward treating the employed drug abuser in a constructive fashion, following a prototype of an EAP policy. Because accompanying financial support was minimal, this policy produced what were essentially "paper programs" throughout the federal establishment.

Another important development in the early 1970s was the establishment of the National Institute on Drug Abuse (NIDA). Its mandate was centered on a medical model of drug-related problems. It was given authority to award and administer demonstration, treatment, prevention, and research grants. During the 1970s and into the early 1980s, however, there was little evidence of either NIDA-supported demonstration projects or research activity focused on drug abuse in the workplace.

This situation changed dramatically in the early 1980s with the emergence of the "war on drugs" and its inclusion of the goal of a drug-free workplace in the United States. The 1985 establishment of the Office of Worksite Initiatives (OWI) within NIDA was one means of implementing the administration's interest, and concern with employee drug abuse and the subgoal of a drug-free workplace was part of the goal of a drug-free America.

The initial position of the OWI was centered on the implementation of drug screening in the workplace. OWI was the base for several initiatives that were originally focused on drug testing, including standards and certification for laboratories that process the body fluids taken in the drug screening process, studies of the effectiveness of both pre- and post-employment drug screening, and support for an informational hotline for employers desiring to address drug problems in their workplaces.

The federal drug free workplace initiative has been a major stimulus for the rapid growth of a drug-testing industry. These businesses function to promote the development of screening of all types in the workplace, in many instances ensuring workplaces' conformity with federal regulations.

At the same time, for-profit alcoholism treatment programs have broadened their coverage to include the treatment of drug abuse. This availability taps employed clients who have access to third-party health insurance reimbursement for drug abuse treatment.

Although OWI was initially positioned to offer drug screening as practically the sole mechanism for dealing with workplace drug abuse, it subsequently moved toward a position that has been vital in the integration of DSPs and EAPs. This new position envisions the complementarity of DSPs and EAPs, suggesting that offers of assistance to drug abusing employees through EAP mechanisms follow the identification of employed drug abusers through DSP mechanisms.

In 1990, OWI was transformed into the Workplace Research Branch within NIDA. This organization essentially vanished when NIDA was merged into the NIH in 1992.

EMERGENCE OF EAPS

In the decades following the repeal of Prohibition, gradual changes in institutional responses to alcohol problems became evident. From its founding in 1935, Alcoholics Anonymous demonstrated that explicit "steps" taken within an environment of acceptance could produce recovery from alcoholism. Eventually, the National Council on Alcoholism, a public policy organization emanating largely from the activities of AA members, began promoting the workplace as a setting for alcoholism rehabilitation (Trice & Schonbrunn, 1981), an approach that proved attractive to a handful of major corporations during the 1950s and 1960s.

A huge leap forward for alcoholism interests came with the establishment of the National Institute on Alcohol Abuse and Alcoholism (NIAAA) in 1970. It adopted as its goal mainstreaming alcoholism into the health care delivery system (Roman & Blum, 1987). Under this strategy, the workplace offered a potentially reliable source of clients covered by health insurance who could be treated in a newly emerging system of alcoholism treatment centers. This combination was seen to legitimize alcoholism as a disease like any other.

The EAP model emerged as NIAAA's transformation of the early AA-based industrial alcoholism program (Blum & Roman, 1989). The centerpiece of this new model was that it did not require the supervisor to identify the employee's problem, but instead emphasized that supervisory monitoring of employee behavior should be limited to job performance issues. Self-referral of employees for personal problems that they perceived to affect their jobs was also encouraged. Thus, the new approach afforded identification and referral of a broad range of employee problems, including but not limited to alcohol problems. This change proved to be critical for the eventual integration of employee drug abuse problems under this programmatic umbrella. The change also proved effective in tapping employer receptivity to EAPs, as is discussed later in this chapter.

CURRENT FORMS OF DSPS

Having reviewed their evolution, we now examine aspects of DSPs and EAPs in the contemporary American workplace. We first consider the several different kinds of DSPs (Blum, 1989).

— The most prevalent form is pre-employment screening. The technology here is straightforward and well-known. Job applicants are required to provide a urine sample (produced under varying degrees of surveillance) that is tested at a contracting laboratory for the presence of residues or metabolites of a variety of substances. These tests do not provide information as to the time of drug ingestion or the pattern of drug use. Unless blood or breath tests are used during pre-employment screening, the employer typically has no information as to the alcohol use by prospective employees.

— Random testing of all or some preselected segments of the workforce is a rarely used type, but is the subject of the most controversy.

— Closely related is universal drug testing of all employees, sometimes as part of a preannounced medical check-up.

— Drug testing "for cause" has been recently incorporated into long-standing fitness-for-duty policies. A supervisor with evidence that a subordinate is impaired, but without evidence of the cause of the impairment, asks to have the employee's fitness for work verified by a medical functionary, who may use a drug test. Subsequent procedures or referrals are contingent on the policies of a particular workplace, but increasingly involve a suggested referral to an EAP.

— Related to this type of screening is post-accident testing. Employers are often anxious to discover whether employees' personal behaviors can be imputed as a cause of an accident that may involve employer liability.

— DSPs may test current employees before they are promoted, after they return to work from extended absences, or when they are transferred into job categories regarded as particularly sensitive to drug abuse impact.

— Drug testing is also used as a follow-up technique with employees who have been through treatment (fully or partially paid for by the employer's health insurance plan) to confirm these employees' compliance with the abstinence goals of treatment.

CURRENT FORMS OF EAPS

The structure of EAPs often varies by the size of the organization. In large organizations, they tend to be in-house programs staffed by company employees who are usually based in the human resources management function. In some large companies and in most medium-sized and smaller settings, EAP services are provided under contract by an external provider. These arrangements vary from employees having telephone access only to the contractor to situations in which the contractor has on-site staff whose activities resemble in every way the operation of an in-house program.

EAPs are usually based on a written policy statement. They provide access for supervisors to appropriate professional consultation in dealing with subordinates whose performance is affected by any of a range of personal problems, nearly all of which are encompassed by substance abuse, psychiatric, or marital and family problems. EAPs also provide for employee self-referral. The basic functions of EAP services include clinical assessment of employee problems, referral to appropriate community resources, follow-up of the employee at the workplace following service use, and training and consultation available to supervisors and managers about appropriate EAP use.

CORE TECHNOLOGY OF EAPS

On the basis of our own research and observations, as well as the experience of others, we believe that EAPs offer substantial potential in resolving drug abuse problems in the workplace (Roman, 1989). In order to further understand their dynamics, we first consider the key techniques that define the uniqueness of EAP strategy (its core technology), a matter considered in more detail elsewhere (Blum & Roman, 1989; Roman, 1990).

First, EAPs provide for the identification of drug-abusing employees via documented evidence of impaired job performance. Performance-based identification is more complex than it may appear. It is a crucial substitute for the natural tendency to directly address a suspected substance abuser with evidence of the apparent symptoms of his or her drug use behavior. In contrast to the denial that such accusations encourage, the supervisors' addressing job performance issues represents both a firm basis for confronting a problem employee and a legitimate role for supervision. Performance problems should be much less equivocal than the ambiguity inherent in the signs and symptoms of drug use. Direct accusations raise the further problem of potential slander.

Second, as a way of implementing serious attempts at job performance management, EAPs provide consultative assistance to supervisors and managers in how to appropriately implement EAP policy with suspected drug abusers. Thus, supervisors or shop stewards who believe that they are dealing with an employee who has a drug abuse problem are strongly encouraged to immediately consult with the EAP about what to do next. This ensures that policy guidelines will be followed, that potential problems with the employee will be sidestepped, and that the supervisor will proceed in a context of organizational support.

The third element of the core technology is constructive confrontation (Trice & Beyer, 1984). This is a specific method of motivating employees with drug abuse problems to use the EAP. Constructive confrontation uses evidence of job problems to precipitate a crisis and as the basis for insisting that steps be taken to shape up if one desires to avoid discipline or maintain employment. This demand is counterbalanced by the opportunities for assistance offered through the EAP in an atmosphere of confidentiality.

The fourth technique is creating linkages between employees and community resources most appropriate to assisting with their drug abuse problems. Without an EAP, the employee either does not seek services or does so with haphazard guidance about which resources to use. Thus, the program can provide the "microlinkage" that affords the employee the best quality service matched to employee's problems, work situation, insurance coverage, and geographic location.

Closely related is EAPs' ability to create long-term linkages between workplaces and the service provider systems in the community. These linkages place the employer in a position to negotiate with providers for the treatment services most appropriate for employed populations. Such negotiations are especially important as treatment services for drug abuse are in a stage of emergence.

The sixth and final element of the core technology is institutionalization of the concept that the workplace can provide constructive assistance for dealing with employees' substance abuse problems. The outcome is that organizational culture comes to tolerate, accept, or even encourage recovery from drug dependency. At the same time, this culture does not reward supervisors who support a pattern of cover-up for an employee with an alcohol or drug abuse problem.

EAPs emerged from industrial alcoholism programs, and have had as their goals the treatment and rehabilitation of employees with personal problems that affect their work. Thus, EAPs are positioned to receive referrals of employees with performance problems that may turn out to be based in drug abuse. Likewise, EAPs may receive self-referrals of employee drug abusers who are seeking assistance in controlling their behavior. Neither of these types of referrals need involve drug screening.

In reviewing the different types of drug screening, it is clear that in many instances current employees who test positive for drugs may be referred to the EAP to be offered a chance at rehabilitative assistance. Thus, in some ways we may view the three types of programs as complementary and synergistic.

These three strategies exhaust the alternatives that are used in the workplace to deal with employee drug abuse. Although there are smatterings of efforts to educate employees about the dangers of drug misuse, such efforts are not widely used and are rarely evaluated. Proponents of wellness and health promotion efforts sometimes suggest that regimens of exercise and healthy lifestyles offer alternatives to substance abuse, but again such emphases are minimal.

It is observed that rates of positive drug screens have declined since workplace screening programs were originated several years ago. This suggests the possibility of primary prevention through deterrent effects, but there is no empirical evidence to support such a claim. Thus, primary prevention is limited to the prohibition strategy. DSPs and EAPs are appropriately classified as secondary prevention because they are oriented to the identification of existing behaviors and problems.

PROBLEMS WITH PRESENT AND FUTURE PREVENTION PROGRAMS IN THE WORKPLACE

To what extent do DSPs and EAPs constitute reasonable intervention-solutions for dealing with drug abuse in the workplace?

Pre-employment screening has spread very rapidly and is quickly moving toward being the norm in the American workplace. These practices may seem to protect employers from the entry of active drug users, but there is no evidence to show that employers who use such screening experience lower rates of employee drug problems over the long run (Blum, 1989). In other words, individuals who do not produce a positive screen on entry into employment cannot be certified as drug-free for the life of their employment.

Pre-employment screening may protect a given employer from hiring those with positive screens, but what happens to these individuals in the larger labor market? At the minimum, socially responsible employers might inform applicants who produce positive screens that this is the reason they are not being hired. This might encourage prospective employees to request a second testing, but given the problems in test reliability relative to actual drug usage, this would be a reasonable demand. Alternatively, those with positive screens might be given guidance toward treatment or counseling, with the offering of an opportunity for another employment interview and rescreening at a later date. It does not appear reasonable that employers turn drug users back into the community without a sense that the employers are part of the community and may eventually share the consequences of these persons' failure to become integrated into work life and productivity.

Further, although pre-employment tests may be reliable in their indication of the presence of a certain amount of substances that indicate prior drug use, there is some question as to whether the drug use that is detected has any bearing on projected patterns of future job performance, in either the short or the long term. To a considerable extent, the tests reveal marijuana use during the previous days or weeks, but there is little evidence that would support the conclusion that drug-positives who have been casual users of marijuana will be substandard performers (Normand, Salyard, & Mahoney, 1990).

Beyond pre-employment screening, DSPs may serve some useful functions in that they identify current employees in need of assistance. We do not suggest that all current employees who test positive for drugs are in need of treatment, nor do we suggest that all such individuals should be willing to accept a diagnosis or possible referral to treatment. But for drug-abusing employees who do receive services through an EAP, a number of important functions are served for the employer that deserve further discussion here.

FUNCTIONS SERVED BY EAPS

EAPs can serve five critical functions for employers' attempts to manage employee drug abuse problems. First, EAPs allow for retaining employees who may have developed drug abuse problems but in whom the workplace has a substantial training investment. This function is like-

wise important in recognizing the employee's commitment to the workplace, independent of personal problems that have developed. This recognition is important for the morale of other employees. Fundamental is the point that EAPs offer employees opportunities to accept treatment and rehabilitation and thus may prevent costly turnover.

Second, EAPs reduce or eliminate supervisory, managerial, and union shop stewards' costly, disruptive, and inefficient efforts at "counseling" or otherwise attempting to "straighten out" the drug-abusing employee. In the absence of an EAP, supervisors and managers are implicitly assigned responsibility to deal with the suspected drug abuser according to their best instincts. In some instances, they may be effective in bringing about a successful outcome by leading the employee either to rehabilitation or to legitimate discipline. However, long-term experience has demonstrated that such amateur (and unsupported) counseling efforts are inefficient.

Third, as a key to minimizing conflict, grievances, and future litigation, EAPs provide a standardized means for dealing with employed drug abusers that specifically includes the offer of assistance if employees choose to pursue it. Thus, the EAP policy provides due process for drug-abusing employees whose personal behaviors have broken organizational rules. This also describes how equitable implementation of the EAP policy can foster an atmosphere in which unions work supportively with management in dealing with the drug abuser who may be a union member. Experience has indicated strong union support for EAPs as a reasonable resolution for dealing with such problems (Sonnenstuhl & Trice, 1986).

Fourth, EAPs provide a gatekeeping function in employees' use of health care services for substance abuse, psychiatric problems, and family problems. Most employees do not have the information needed to select effective providers for substance abuse treatment services. Direction about appropriate resources from EAP staff sharply reduces the likelihood of the employee using an overly expensive or ineffective treatment resource.

A related but distinctively different benefit is that EAPs control employers' cost of health care insurance by drug-abusing employees. Employees with alcohol problems are heavy users of health care services; this heavy use extends to abusers' families as well (Fein, 1984; Holder, 1987; Holder & Hallan, 1986). Data indicate further that these levels of usage decline markedly following successful interventions to deal with alcohol problems. Parallel data support the impact of intervention in reducing health care use among employees with psychiatric problems (Jones & Vischi, 1979). It follows that these dynamics extend to employees who abuse drugs other than alcohol.

Experience has shown that there are substantial opportunities for the integration of DSPs and EAPs in providing constructive opportunities to employees with drug abuse problems. It is our firm position that employers will benefit substantially by linking all drug testing of current employees to opportunities for referral to the EAP.

One can become overly sanguine about the extent to which these linkages exist. We must take care not to exaggerate the extent of this integration, for there are a great many instances in which a positive drug test of a current employee will lead to immediate dismissal, or in some instances, discipline. There is marked inconsistency in such policies across different workplaces. Such inconsistency in the DSP–EAP linkage is also found among the federal agencies that require the use of drug testing by organizations under their regulatory control or by contractors that provide services to the agencies.

In light of the numerous functions EAPs can serve for an organization, it would be maximally beneficial if drug screening policy statements provided that any employee who tests positive on a drug screening test is given the opportunity to undergo an appropriate diagnosis and, if necessary, has the opportunity for counseling or treatment assistance. Those who do not accept such opportunities would be governed by the workplace rules applicable to their subsequent job performance, whereas those who undergo treatment would be treated in a manner similar to other employees with health problems.

Any policy that offers no second chances is quite foolhardy. Examination of these systems of drug use detection and identification indicates numerous opportunities for error or misunderstanding. No-second-chance policies preclude any kind of flexibility to consider extenuating circumstances. If policies include opportunities for second chances, then it seems reasonable that the EAP be included in the loop of potential opportunities for behavioral correction and return to acceptable job performance.

Although drug screening programs are specifically and exclusively focused on drug abuse in the workplace, they are generally limited in their attention to illegal drugs, may or may not involve screening for prescription drug use, and very rarely deal with alcohol use or abuse. This definitely reveals a degree of "moral concern" embedded in these tests, independent of rational and equitable concerns limited to safety risks and job performance decrements.

It should be stressed that EAPs' target population differs from that of DSPs. Whereas DSPs seek objective physiological evidence of drug use, independent of behavior, performance, or self-report, EAPs' design limits their drug-related service usage to instances of impaired job performance, peer or self-motivated initiation of requests for personal assistance by drug using employees, or self-motivated initiation of requests for assistance in dealing with a drug-using family member. Nearly all of these modes of identification involve subjective indices or perceptions. This difference in target employee populations sets the stage for considerable confusion about the relative utility and importance of the two strategies.

This highlights a critical point for future consideration. By their design, neither DSPs or EAPs are equipped to deal with the entire range of drug use and abuse events in a workforce or in a workplace. It is also not reasonable to conclude that the combined efforts of both programs would accomplish such a comprehensive goal. Both programs have problems in the reliability and validity of their identification strategies. Furthermore, neither program has the wherewithal to detect what is probably the most common and perhaps even the most costly drug-related issue in the workplace, the use of alcohol during off-work hours that creates risks for job performance problems and accidents, but cannot be reliably detected through either performance monitoring or tests of body fluids.

Drug screening mandated by law or public regulation is only in its infancy, and this is even more distinctively the case with EAPs. The fact that so much activity has developed in a context of voluntary adoption by employers is notable, indicative of the facts that substantial numbers of employers have perceived significant problems in terms of employee drug and alcohol abuse, but have also seen enough merit in DSPs and EAPs to make voluntary investments in various levels of implementation.

As we move toward the future, much more research and evaluation focused on both DSPs and EAPs is needed. It is important that each program type be considered in the context of broader labor force considerations. Of great importance is the development of standards for the definition and evaluation of these programs in specific worksites. At present, the term *EAP* can be applied to practically any type of workplace-based good intention or program sold by an unlicensed and unregulated external vendor. An EAP is of little value in protecting the rights of employees with positive drug screens unless all of the elements of the core technology are present. In addition to comprehensive research about program structure and process, data should also be collected on the long-term work-related outcomes associated with different patterns of program-related experience of drug abusing employees who are identified, dismissed, disciplined, or offered constructive assistance through these mechanisms.

THE STRUCTURE OF SOCIAL SUPPORT FOR WORKPLACE EFFORTS

Despite apparent logic, strong research evidence, and policymakers' passions in favor of certain strategies, such interventions generally have little prospect of long-term impact without a firm base of social support from the affected community. This is well-illustrated in the case of drug problems in the workplace. It is not uncommon for there to be a substantial policy–practice gap between the attitudes of the affected public and the favored strategies of government leaders and academic researchers.

The present authors' research program has involved a substantial amount of data collection centered on the attitudes of employees and the general public toward drug abuse issues, with special concerns about what the public sees as the most appropriate ways to manage drug use and abuse in the workplace. In this section, we describe some of these findings, which generally show a firm base of support for workplace drug testing as well as for workplace EAPs.

In 1991, we collected data on a variety of issues related to workplace alcohol problems from a nationally representative sample of 3,001 full-time employed adults, using random-digit dial telephone survey techniques. In 1992, we conducted a follow-up survey of this sample, and were able to complete interviews with 61.4% of this panel, or 1,842 respondents. This follow-up survey included a substantial range of questions about drug abuse issues. In reviewing these findings, it is important to keep in mind that many of the estimates may be conservative because we are studying a substantially stable group of workers. Not only does our sampling frame exclude part-time and unemployed people, but our follow-up strategy also eliminated those whose job changes and other problems made them unavailable for the second interview.

The vast majority of the respondents, 66%, reported that they perceived no problem with illegal drug use in their workplaces. Of all respondents, 27% reported a minor problem, 7% indicated a moderate problem, and less than 1% indicated that their workplace had a major problem with employees using illegal drugs. On one hand, this might appear to minimize the extent of workplace drug problems, but a somewhat different perspective emerges when these data are seen as finding a third of American full-time workers perceiving some level of drug abuse problem in their workplace.

In a somewhat similar vein, several interpretations are possible for the finding that 10.4% of the respondents report that at least one close co-worker is a drug user. Although it might be said that nearly 90% of the full-time workforce is not affected by drug users in their work surroundings, the potential costs and impacts of having a tenth of the workforce exposed in this fashion should not be underestimated or minimized. Exposure to drug use on the job is considerably more likely at work than at home. Only 2.3% of the respondents reported that someone in their household was currently a drug user.

Looking at the types of drug screening programs reported by respondents, 30.9% reported that their employers use pre-employment drug screening, 25.6% report that their employers use drug screening of current employees when there is probable cause that drug use may explain employee behavior, and 16.8% indicate that their employers routinely conduct random drug screening of employees.

Contrary to the impressions that might be garnered from the scholarly literature that is critical of drug screening, this survey revealed a very high level of support for drug screening among full-time employees in the United States. When asked their opinion about these methods of dealing with drug use in the workplace, 80% indicated they strongly or mildly approved of pre-employment drug screening, 85.6% indicated that they strongly or mildly approved of for-cause drug screening, and 67.9% indicated that they strongly or mildly approved of random drug screening.

Personal experience with drug testing, however, is less extensive than might be expected. Only 14% of the respondents reported that they had undergone a drug screening test as part of the requirements for obtaining their current job. When asked to indicate their reactions to the drug screening experience, only 4% reported it to be very distressing, 13% said it was somewhat distressing, and 83% reported that it was not at all distressing. Although these are low levels of reported distress, it should of course be noted that these persons successfully passed the drug screen and obtained the desired employment.

For those in workplaces that use random screening, only 36.3% indicated that they had been selected to submit to such a test. Of these individuals, only 4% described the testing experience as very distressing, 11% indicated that it was somewhat distressing, and 85% reported that it was not at all distressing. Thus, we again find a discrepancy between employees' reported experiences and the concerns in scholarly papers about the humiliation, degradation, and invasion of privacy involved in workplace drug testing.

This data collection also involved a range of attitudinal questions regarding drug testing and drug use. Here we generally find a mixture of ideas that seem to question some aspects of drug screening, albeit indirectly. There was strong agreement (88%) with the statement that drug testing provides for safer workplaces. However, when asked whether job applicants who have a positive drug test should be refused employment by the employer requesting the test, 66% agreed, making it somewhat surprising that one-third of the respondents apparently believe that drug-positive individuals should not be necessarily barred from employment.

In a somewhat similar vein, 61% of respondents agreed that pre-employment drug testing keeps undesirable individuals out of the workplace, again indicating that more than one-third did not agree that drug testing was effective in this manner.

Some insights into this apparent ambivalence are revealed by responses to several other items. First, a surprisingly high proportion, 77% of the respondents, agreed that it was possible that persons who are not drug users could produce a positive result on a drug test. It is perhaps curious that the overall high level of confidence in drug testing as a valuable policy alternative and strategy is coupled with a remarkably high level of skepticism about the accuracy of the technology. Second, only 24% of the respondents agreed that current employees who test positive on a drug screen should be fired, with 76% disagreeing with the appropriateness of this outcome. Indeed, 85% of the full-time employees indicated that a current employee who produces a positive drug test should be subjected to further testing before any action is taken. Thus, there is evidence of a high degree of concern about the technical validity of workplace drug testing, but once again it is important to emphasize the context of broad support within which these doubts exist.

Contrary to the notion of many policy leaders that drug testing is primarily an exclusionary device to create a drug-free workplace, the data reveal that 86% of the respondents believe that drug testing is a means of ultimately providing help to employees. There is practically universal agreement in the sample (95.2%) that a current employee with a positive drug test should be offered help, a finding that must be taken as a strong challenge to the assumption that the popular opinion supports drug testing as a means of ridding the workplace of undesirables.

In order to gain a more complete picture of structural support for drug-related strategies, it is important to examine some more general attitudes toward drug abuse within this sample of employed Americans.

When asked whether drug dependency should be treated as an illness, 88.2% of the respondents agreed. Furthermore, and perhaps in contrast to political decision makers, employed people in this sample showed a very high level of agreement (90.2%) with the statement that most drug dependency could be successfully treated.

Some consistency in these attitudes is indicated by the parallel finding of a low level of agreement (8.7%) with the statement that people who are dependent on drugs should be viewed and treated as criminals. A considerably higher proportion (26.9%) agreed that drug users should be punished. This is definitely an attitude of a minority, but it appears to indicate that many make a clear distinction between drug-using and drug-dependent individuals.

A similar proportion (28.5%) agreed with the statement that weak moral character is a primary cause of drug dependency. Of great importance for those desiring to develop support for intervention efforts is the finding of 88.2% of the respondents agreeing that people should be held responsible for becoming dependent on drugs. Thus, the medicalization of drug dependence has some unique features if that trend is seen as establishing the view that drug dependence is a disease like any other. It may also be observed that the public has rarely been queried about the extent to which they would hold individuals responsible for the development of "real diseases" such as heart disease, diabetes, cirrhosis of the liver, or lung cancer.

A context for these findings is offered by comparison of parallel attitudes toward alcoholism. Impressions garnered from both research and the mass media tend to support the position that alcohol abuse and alcoholism are far more medicalized within public attitudes than are other types of drug dependence (Mulford & Miller, 1961; Reis, 1977; Orcutt, Cairl, and Miller, 1980; Peele, 1989). Such a generalization is not fully supported by data from this national sample of employed persons.

When asked whether alcoholism should be viewed and treated as an illness, 90.2% agreed, a nonsignificant difference from the 88.2% endorsing this attitude toward drug dependence. Similarly, 92.4% agreed that most alcoholics could be successfully treated, as compared to 90.2% agreeing about the potential of treatment for drug-dependent people.

Although not a strong difference, significantly fewer respondents agree that weak moral character is a primary cause of alcoholism (23%) as compared to 28.5% agreement on this item for drug dependency. Finally, a fairly strong difference is found in the extent of agreement with the statement that people should be held responsible for becoming alcoholics. Although a majority of 70.2% agreed, the 88.2% agreeing with this statement for drug dependent persons is significantly higher.

These data suggest that within the workplace, there are somewhat parallel attitudes toward drug and alcohol problems. Certainly the relative stigma placed on drug problems is much less than might be expected from some generalizations that have been made. On the other hand, the medicalization of both problems is far from complete, and on a number of items it is clear that employed people hold stringent attitudes toward drug dependency and drug use, somewhat more stringent than parallel attitudes toward alcohol problems.

In terms of the alternative strategies that have been discussed in this chapter, some perspective may be gained from reports of experiences and attitudes toward EAPs that were revealed in this national survey of full-time employees. EAPs are reported present in 59% of the respondents' workplaces, offering an approximate estimate of their nationwide workplace presence. The institutionalization of EAPs as a workplace human resource management practice is indexed not only by this scope of program presence but also by the fact that the first survey of this panel found EAPs present in 49% of the respondents' workplaces, indicating steady growth in EAP implementation over a one-year period.

The respondents are favorable toward the program, with 73% indicating that it is very likely or somewhat likely that they would seek help from the EAP for a personal problem. Interestingly, there is even a higher level of confidence in the EAP when respondents were asked whether they would seek help from it if they had a drug problem: 76% indicated it was very likely or somewhat likely that they would do so.

Actual EAP use is remarkably high. In the first survey of this panel, respondents in workplaces with EAPs were asked whether they had used the EAP for a problem of their own, to which 8.4% responded affirmatively. Another 5.5% indicated that they had used the program for a problem affecting a family member, and 15.5% of respondents who are supervisors indicated that they had used the program to get help

for someone whom they supervised. Furthermore, 47.5% of the respondents in workplaces with EAPs indicated that someone with whom they work closely has used the EAP.

Looking only at those in the initial interview who were users of EAP services, 43% found the program to have been very helpful and 42% found it somewhat helpful, indicating that only 15% were not satisfied with the help they received through the EAP.

Respondents also reported that support for the EAP from their own supervisor was strong. Two-thirds (67.1%) of the respondents in workplaces with EAPs reported that their supervisors strongly supported the EAP, and 31.4% indicated mild support by their immediate supervisor. Opposition to the EAP by one's superior was reported by only 1.6% of the respondents.

We have examined three sets of data: attitudes toward drug testing, attitudes and experiences related to drug use (with comparisons of parallel attitudes toward alcohol problems), and attitudes and experiences related to EAPs. These data offer a somewhat complex picture of the profile of social support for different interventions related to drug problems in the workplace.

There is support for both drug testing and EAP strategies. The attitudes indicate, however, that full-time employed Americans tend to see the two strategies as complementary rather than as alternative strategies. There is clearly a desire to provide opportunities for treatment and help to current employees who are found to have drug problems (or who may refer themselves to an EAP for help with a drug problem). Exclusionary strategies are seen as much less appropriate for those who are already employed than for those who may be seeking employment. This linkage between reduced social distance and greater desire to provide help is a common finding in studies of attitudes toward substance abusers (Roman, 1982; Blum, Roman, & Bennett, 1989).

There is a remarkably high degree of confidence, support, and positive experiences in workplace settings where EAPs are present. On the other hand, it would be a definite mistake to assume that the full-time American workforce has adopted a fully medicalized view of drug abusers, an image that they have little or no responsibility for their problem, or the notion that substance abuse should be regarded as a disease like any other. However, there is far more compassion, acceptance of the value of treatment, and lower social rejection of the drug user than might be expected from widely diffused societal stereotypes.

SUMMARY

There is a somewhat different way in which to frame these conclusions. The drug–work connection seems to be firmly established. To use sociological language, it is a linkage that has become institutionalized. This means that a set of norms have become routinized and accepted and are no longer the basis for controversy or the object of calls for major change. In this instance, the norms of interest are those that on one hand support exclusion of drug users from employment but on the other hand are sympathetic toward providing treatment for employees who develop drug problems. There is no doubt a substantial degree of ambivalence in the minds and actions of many Americans toward the proper role of their workplaces in dealing with drug problems. We do not know the extent to which this ambivalence is an impediment to constructive actions toward peers or subordinates with drug problems, for doubts and confusion are indeed the foundations for indecision and denial.

It is clear that more research is needed to better understand the attitudes and behavioral predispositions across all levels of employed people. One would be foolhardy to suggest that current norms will soon be swept away from the legalization of most or many of the drugs that are currently the objects of major concerns and actions. Thus, it is imperative to know more about the vast number of interventions that have been put into place in worksites over the past decade in terms of how they affect those who do and do not use illegal drugs.

REFERENCES

Ames, G. (1989). Alcohol-related movements and their effects on drinking policies in the American workplace. *Journal of Drug Issues, 19,* 489–510.

Becker, H. S. (1953). Becoming a marihuana user. *American Journal of Sociology, 59,* 236–242.

Blum, T. C. (1989). The presence and integration of drug abuse intervention in human resource management. In S. Guste (Ed.), *Drugs in the workplace: Research and evaluation data,* National Institute on Drug Abuse research monograph no. 91. Washington, DC: U.S. Government Printing Office, pp. 271–286.

Blum, T. C., & Roman, P. M. (1989). Employee assistance and human resources management. In K. Rowland & G. Ferris (Eds.), *Research in personnel and human resources management,* vol. 7, Greenwich, CT: JAI Press, 258–312.

Blum, T. C., Roman, P. M., & Bennett, N. (1989). Public attitudes toward alcoholism: Data from a Georgia survey. *Journal of Studies on Alcohol, 50,* 5–14.

Chambers, C., and Heckman, R. (1972). *Employee drug abuse: A manager's guide to action.* Boston: Cahners Books.

Clark, N. S. (1976). *Deliver us from evil: An interpretation of American prohibition.* New York: Norton.

Fein, R. (1984). *Alcohol in America: The price we pay.* Minneapolis: Care Institute.

Holder, H. D. (1987). Alcoholism treatment and potential health care cost savings. *Medical Care, 25,* 52–71.

Holder, H. D., & Hallan, J. B. (1986). Impact of alcoholism treatment on total health care costs: A six-year study. *Advances in Alcohol and Substance Abuse, 6,* 1–15.

Jones, K. R., & Vischi, T. R. (1979). Impact of alcohol, drug abuse and mental health treatment on care utilization. *Medical Care, 17,* Supplement 12.

Morgan, H. W. (1981). *Drugs in America: A social history, 1800–1980.* Syracuse, NY: Syracuse University Press.

Mulford, H. A., & Miller, D. E. (1961). Public definitions of the alcoholic. *Quarterly Journal of Studies on Alcohol, 22,* 312–320.

Newcomb, M. D. (1988). *Drug use in the workplace: Risk factors for disruptive substance abuse among young adults.* Dover, MA: Auburn House.

Normand, J., Salyards, S. D., & Mahoney, J. J. (1990). An evaluation of pre-employment drug testing. *Journal of Applied Psychology, 75,* 629–639.

Orcutt, J. D., Cairl, R. E., & Miller, E. T. (1980). Professional and public conceptions of alcoholism. *Journal of Studies on Alcohol, 41,* 652–660.

Peele, S. (1989). *The diseasing of America.* Lexington, MA: D.C. Heath.

Ray, O. (1978). *Drugs, society, and human behavior* (2nd edition). St. Louis: C.V. Mosby, 186–199.

Reis, J. K. (1977). Public acceptance of the disease concept of alcoholism. *Journal of Health and Social Behavior, 18,* 338–344.

Roman, P. M. (1982). Barriers to the use of constructive coercion with employed alcoholics. *Journal of Drug Issues, 12,* 369–382.

Roman, P. M. (1989). The use of employee assistance programs to deal with drug abuse in the workplace. In S. Guste (Ed.), *Drugs in the workplace: Research and evaluation data,* National Institute on Drug Abuse monograph no. 91, 245–270. Washington, DC: U.S. Government Printing Office.

Roman, P. M. (1990). Strategic considerations in designing interventions to deal with alcohol problems in the workplace. In P. M. Roman (Ed.), *Alcohol problem intervention in the workplace: Employee assistance programs and strategic alternatives.* Westport, CT: Quorum Press, 371–406.

Roman, P. M., & Blum, T. C. (1987). Notes on the new epidemiology of alcoholism in the USA. *Journal of Drug Issues, 11,* 321–332.

Roman, P. M., & Blum, T. C. (1992). Employee assistance and drug screening programs. In D. Gerstein (Ed.), *Treating drug problems,* vol 2. Washington, DC: National Academy of Sciences Press.

Roman, P. M., Blum, T. C., & Martin, J. K. (1992). Distribution of employee assistance programs across American workplaces: Results from a national survey, University of Georgia, unpublished manuscript.

Rorabaugh, W. J. (1979). *The alcoholic republic: An American tradition.* New York: Oxford University Press.

Rumbarger, J. (1989). *Power, profits and prohibition.* Albany: State University of New York Press.

Simon, W., & Lumry, G. K. (1969). Alcoholism and drug addiction among physicians: Chronic self destruction? *Drug Dependence, 1,* 11–14.

Smith, D. (1973). *It's so good don't even try it once.* Englewood Cliffs, NJ: Prentice Hall.

Smith, S. M., & Blachly, P. H. (1966). Amphetamine usage by medical students. *Journal of Medical Education, 41,* 167–170.

Sonnenstuhl, W., & Trice, H. (1986). *Strategies for employee assistance programs: The crucial balance,* Key issues no. 30. Ithaca, NY: ILR Press.

Sonnenstuhl, W., & Trice, H. (1987). The social construction of alcohol problems in a union's peer counseling program. *Journal of Drug Issues, 17* (3), 223–254.

Staudenmeier, W. J. (1989). Contrasting organizational responses to alcohol and illegal drug abuse among employees. *Journal of Drug Issues, 19,* 451–472.

Thompson, J. D. (1967). *Organizations in action.* New York: McGraw Hill.

Trice, H. M., & Belasco, J. A. (1966). *Emotional health and employer responsibility,* bulletin no. 47. Ithaca: Publications Division of the New York State School of Industrial and Labor Relations at Cornell University.

Trice, H., & Beyer, J. (1984). Work-related outcomes of constructive confrontation strategies in a job-based alcoholism program. *Journal of Studies on Alcohol, 45,* 393–404.

Trice, H. M., & Roman, P. M. (1972). *Spirits and demons at work: Alcohol and other drugs on the job.* Ithaca: Publications Divisions of the New York State School of Industrial and Labor Relations at Cornell University.

Trice, H. M., & Schonbrunn, M. (1981). A history of job-based alcoholism programs, 1900–1955. *Journal of Drug Issues, 11,* 171–198.

Wilcke, G. (1990). Growing use of narcotics saps industry. *New York Times,* April 6.

Winick, C. (1960). The use of drugs by jazz musicians. *Social Problems, 7,* 240–248.

Winick, C. (1961). Physician narcotic addicts. *Social Problems, 9,* 174–186.

Yesavage, J. A., Leirer, V. O., Denari, M., and Hollister, L. (1985). Carry-over effects of marihuana intoxication on aircraft pilot performance. *American Journal of Psychiatry, 142,* 1325–1329.

Zinberg, N. (1984). *Drug, set and setting: The basis for controlled intoxicant use.* New Haven, Yale University Press.

CHAPTER 8

RELIGIOUS ORGANIZATIONS

STEPHEN J. BAHR
RICKY D. HAWKS

INTRODUCTION

There is considerable evidence that religious involvement tends to retard drug abuse. Individuals affiliated with a religion have lower rates of drug use than those not affiliated with a religion. Regardless of denomination, people who attend church regularly are less likely to use drugs than those who do not attend regularly. Individuals who belong to religions that teach abstinence have a lower prevalence of drug use than persons whose religion does not proscribe the use of alcohol and tobacco (Amoateng & Bahr, 1986; Bahr, 1991; Kandel, 1980).

The purpose of this chapter is to explore the influence of religious involvement on drug use and the role of religious organizations in drug abuse prevention and treatment.

There are three different aspects of religious involvement that may influence drug use: affiliation, attendance, and beliefs. These three dimensions do not necessarily vary together. For example, one may be affiliated with a religious organization but rarely attend. Some who regularly attend religious services do not believe in core religious tenets. Others may be very religious in their individual beliefs but may not attend nor be affiliated with a religious organization.

Religious organizations may influence individual drug use at three different levels: primary, secondary, and tertiary. Primary influence includes prevention activities designed to deter initiation to drug use. It may involve direct teachings against drug use as well as providing purpose to life so that substance abuse is not attractive.

Secondary influence is intervention to keep experimental or occasional drug use from escalating. Tertiary influence includes programs to help those who regularly abuse drugs avoid relapse. The impact of religious organizations on drug use may include one of these elements without including another. For example, abstinent teachings of a religious organization may deter nonusers from experimenting but may have little effect on those who are experimenting or who are already heavy users of a drug.

RELIGION AND DRUG USE

Research on religion and drug use is not as extensive as research on how other social characteristics are related to drug use. Nevertheless, a growing body of research has found that religious affiliation and attendance are associated with drug use. We begin this section with a brief review of existing research on the association between religion and drug use.

Previous Research

In a review of existing research on adolescent drug use, Kandel (1980) found that involvement in religion had a negative association with alcohol and marijuana use. Burkett (1980) observed that antidrinking beliefs learned from religious groups tended to deter drinking among adolescents. In a study of more than 3,000 adolescents, Cochran (1991) reported that religiosity was negatively associated with the frequency of use of several different types of drugs. Hadaway, Elifson, and Petersen (1984) discovered that even after controlling for other important influences, religion still had a significant effect on alcohol and drug use. Several other scholars have found that religiosity is inversely associated with alcohol and drug use (Beeghley, Bock, & Cochran, 1990; Gorsuch & Butler, 1976; Newcomb, Maddahian, & Bentler, 1986; Rohrbaugh & Jessor, 1975).

The negative association between religious involvement and drug use appears to be particularly strong among members of religious groups that teach abstinence. For example, Crowley (1985) observed that there were more nondrinkers and fewer heavy drinkers among fundamentalist Protestants than among other Protestants, Catholics, or those with no religion. Dudley, Mutch, and Cruise (1987) found that religious commitment was important in preventing or limiting drug use among Seventh-Day Adventists. In a comparison of several different religions denominations, Amoateng and Bahr (1986) observed that the association between religious involvement and drug use was stronger among members of religions that taught abstinence than among members of religious groups that did not teach abstinence.

Current Data on Religion and Drug Use

There is a need for more extensive and current information regarding the association between religion and drug use (Cochran, 1991). In this section, we analyze data from two recent national surveys to determine rates of drug use among major religious organizations in the United States.

Adults

We analyzed data from the General Social Survey (Davis & Smith, 1991) to estimate drug use among adults. Each year, the National Opinion Research Center conducts the General Social Survey (GSS) among a random sample of about 1,500 adults in the United States. We combined

the GSS for the years 1972–1990, for a total sample of more than 27,000. GSS does not have extensive information on drug use, but asks whether the respondents currently drink alcohol, whether they sometimes drink more than they should, whether they smoke cigarettes, and whether they approve of the legalization of marijuana. The respondents were grouped into five major religious categories: Protestant, Catholic, Jew, Other, and None.

In the GSS, the percentage of adults who drink alcohol was 85 among Catholics and Jews and 86 among those with no religion. The proportion who drink was significantly lower among Protestants and Others, the percentages being 64% and 67%, respectively.

The Jews were the least likely to report that they sometimes drink more than they should. Only one-fourth (26%) of the Jews admitted that they sometimes drink too much, compared to about one-third of the Protestants, Catholics, and Others, and almost half (48%) of those with no religion.

The percentage of adults who favor legalization of marijuana was 52% among those with no religious preference and 42% among Jews. It was lowest among Catholics (22%) and Protestants (18%), as shown in Table 8.1.

Adolescents

To estimate adolescent drug use, we examined data from the 1984–1987 Monitoring the Future surveys. Monitoring the Future (MTF) is an annual survey of high school seniors conducted by the Survey Research Center at the University of Michigan (Johnston, O'Malley, & Bachman, 1992). Data collection took place in approximately 125 public and private schools selected to provide an accurate cross-section of high school seniors throughout the United States. In each school, questionnaires were administered in classrooms during normal school hours.

A multistage sampling procedure was used to secure a representative sample of high school seniors in the United States. More than 15,000 seniors were sampled each year, making the total

TABLE 8.1 Drug and Alcohol Behavior and Attitudes Among U.S. Adults, by Religion, 1972–1990

	PROTESTANT	CATHOLIC	JEWISH	OTHER	NONE	TOTAL
Drink alcohol	64.1%	84.5%	84.5%	67.4%	85.6%	71.2%
Sometimes drink too much	37.1	36.9	25.9	33.1	47.8	37.6
Smoke	34.5	37.1	28.0	34.1	48.7	36.1
Approve legalization of marijuana	17.4	21.9	41.8	29.3	51.6	21.9
Sample Size	10,361	4,002	323	290	1,172	16,148

Source: General Social Survey, 1972–1990.

sample in the pooled 1984–87 surveys approximately 62,000.

The respondents were asked detailed questions about drug use. In this section, we report data on alcohol, cigarettes, marijuana, and cocaine. The questions on religious preference were collapsed into seven major categories: Mainline Protestant (Episcopal, Lutheran, Methodist, Presbyterian), Fundamentalist Protestant (Baptist, Churches of Christ, Disciples of Christ, United Church of Christ, Other Protestant), Roman Catholic, Jewish, Mormon (LDS), Other, and None.

Table 8.2 shows alcohol use by religious affiliation. Seventy-nine percent of the Jews and 75% of the Catholics reported alcohol use during the past month. For both Mainline Protestants and "None," the results were 70%. Only 58% of Fundamentalist Protestants consumed alcohol during the past month. About half of those belonging to "Other" religions reported alcohol use. The lowest proportion of alcohol users was among Mormons at 33%.

As an indicator of excessive alcohol use, the respondents were asked whether they had five or more drinks in a row during the past two weeks (See Table 8.2, column 2). Catholics, Jews, None, and Mainline Protestants were similar, ranging

from 37% among Jews to 44% among Catholics. Fundamentalist Protestants were noticeably lower at 31%. Only one in four of seniors who belonged to "Other" religions had consumed five or more drinks in a row during the past two weeks, and Mormons were the lowest at 18%.

Marijuana is the most commonly used illicit drug. The proportion of seniors who have used marijuana during the past month is shown in Table 8.3. Almost one in four high school seniors in the United States said that they have used marijuana during the past month. This percentage was highest among those with no religious affiliation (32%), followed by Jews (28%) and Catholics (25%). It was lowest among "Other" (19%) and Mormons (14%).

The percentage of high school seniors who have used cocaine is shown in Table 8.4. Sixteen percent used cocaine sometime in their lives and 6% did so within the past month. The highest percentage of users was among those with no religion. Almost one in four of the seniors with no religion had tried cocaine and almost 10% said they used cocaine during the past month. Of those who were affiliated with a religious organization, Jewish seniors had the highest proportion of cocaine users; 22% had tried cocaine sometime in their lives and 8% used it within the past

TABLE 8.2 Percentage of U.S. High School Seniors Who Have Used Alcohol During the Past Month, by Religion, 1984–1987

RELIGION	ALCOHOL PAST MONTH	5+ DRINKS IN A ROW PAST 2 WEEKS
Mainline Protestants	70.3	38.8
Episcopalian	73.9	39.6
Lutheran	76.2	44.6
Methodist	66.1	35.0
Presbyterian	68.6	37.7
Fundamentalist Protestant	57.7	31.0
Baptist	55.4	28.5
Churches of Christ	62.7	37.7
Other	59.0	32.5
Roman Catholic	75.2	44.1
Jewish	79.0	37.0
Mormon	33.0	17.9
Other	50.5	25.4
None	70.1	40.1
Total	66.3	37.0

Source: National High School Senior Survey, 1984–1987 (Johnston, O'Malley, and Bachman, 1989).

TABLE 8.3 Percentage of U.S. High School Seniors Who Have Used Marijuana in the Past Month, by Religion, 1984–1987

RELIGION	MARIJUANA USE PAST MONTH
Mainline Protestants	22.8
Episcopalian	27.9
Lutheran	24.3
Methodist	20.3
Presbyterian	23.1
Fundamentalist Protestant	21.3
Baptist	20.5
Churches of Christ	24.8
Other	20.4
Roman Catholic	25.4
Jewish	28.0
Mormon	13.5
Other	18.7
None	31.7
Total	23.8

Source: National High School Senior Survey, 1984–1987 (Johnston, O'Malley, and Bachman, 1989).

TABLE 8.4   Percentage of U.S. High School Seniors Who Have Used Cocaine, by Religion, 1984–1987

RELIGION	LIFETIME	PAST YEAR	PAST MONTH
Mainline Protestants	14.0	10.0	4.6
Episcopalian	19.0	14.6	6.9
Lutheran	15.3	11.0	5.1
Methodist	11.2	7.6	3.5
Presbyterian	15.6	11.3	5.2
Fundamentalist Protestant	13.3	9.2	4.4
Baptist	11.5	7.6	3.8
Churches of Christ	19.0	14.0	6.7
Other	13.9	10.2	4.8
Roman Catholic	18.0	13.8	6.7
Jewish	22.4	16.6	8.0
Mormon	10.6	8.3	4.5
Other	14.7	10.5	4.8
None	23.8	17.9	9.0
Total	16.2	11.9	5.7

Source: National High School Senior Survey, 1984–1987 (Johnston, O'Malley, and Bachman, 1989).

month. Methodists, Baptists, and Mormons had the lowest percentage of seniors who had ever used cocaine, which was about 11% among all three groups. Use during the past month was lowest among Methodists and Baptists; less than 4% of them said they used cocaine during the past month.

Overall, drug use tended to be highest among those with no religion, followed by Jews and Catholics. Mainline Protestants tended to be in the middle compared to other religions. Methodists were consistently lower than the other Mainline Protestant religions. Fundamentalist Protestants had rates of drug use that were somewhat lower than Mainline Protestants. Baptists were consistently lowest among the Fundamentalists. The "Other" religious group (which included non-Christian denominations) had the lowest percentage of drug users except for Mormons.

Paradoxical Alcohol Use

Skolnick (1958) and Cahalan, Cisin, and Crossley (1969) suggested that when members of absti-nence-teaching religions use alcohol, they often show a paradoxical drinking pattern. That is, although most members of abstinence-teaching religious groups were found not to consume alcohol, the small percentage who did tended to be involved with heavier and more frequent drinking than members of religious groups that did not teach abstinence. The paradoxical alcohol use pattern is theorized to exist among religious groups that teach abstinence from alcohol, including Muslims, Buddhists, Baptists, Mormons, and Seventh-Day Adventists.

A number of scholars have observed evidence consistent with a paradoxical pattern of alcohol use. In a study of adult Jews, Cahalan, Cisin, and Crossley (1969) found that 10% of all Jews in the United States were classified as heavy drinkers, compared with the 12% among the general population. Cahalan and his colleagues concluded that, compared with other religious groups, more Jewish men drank but fewer drank heavily or were problem drinkers.

Using a college population, Gusfield (1970) found that Protestant students who drank had a

TABLE 8.5   Review of Research Studies in which Mormons were Included in the Research Sample and Paradoxical Drinking Was Discussed as Part of the Research

STUDY	DESCRIPTION	SUPPORT FOR PARADOXICAL DRINKING
Straus and Bacon (1953)	16,747 college students 778 Mormon drinkers	yes
Snyder (1958)	secondary analysis Straus and Bacon's data	yes
Skolnick (1958)	secondary analysis Straus and Bacon's data	yes
Smith (1969)	5,000 college sociology students— 2,500 Mormon	yes
Preston (1969)	516 junior and high school students— Mormon collapsed with other religions	yes
Moss and Janzen (1980)	1,811 Native American family heads—90 Mormon	yes
Albrecht (1985)	per-capita alcohol and estimate of alcoholics—50 states	yes
Hawks and Bahr (1992)	secondary analysis 5,000 Utah adults	no

higher consumption rate than Jewish students. Cahalan and Room (1974) also found the paradoxical tendency among drinkers from conservative Protestant sects or from "dry" regions. In a national survey of treated alcoholics, it was discovered that alcoholism was more common in the South and among Protestants, demographic characteristics that tend to be associated with abstinence (Armor, Polich, & Stambul, 1978). A number of other researchers have reported results consistent with paradoxical drinking (Skolnick, 1958; Smith, 1969; Moss & Janzen, 1980; Albrecht, 1985).

However, not all research has supported the paradoxical drinking phenomenon. For example, Krohn, Akers, Radosevich, and Lanza-Kaduce (1982) found no evidence of paradoxical drinking or marijuana use among adolescents. In an analysis using measures of alcohol frequency and quantity from 5,200 Utah adults, Hawks and Bahr (1992) observed no evidence of paradoxical drinking among Mormons. A listing of the research studies on paradoxical drinking is shown in Table 8.5.

THEORETICAL EXPLANATIONS

The above data show that religion is a powerful influence on drug use and abuse. Regardless of the denomination, individuals who are affiliated with a religion are less likely to abuse most drugs than individuals not affiliated with a religion.

Among church members, individuals who attend church services regularly have substantially lower rates of drug use than individuals who are not actively involved in their religion. Members of religions that teach abstinence have the lowest rates of drug use, particularly for alcohol, tobacco, and marijuana.

Although we know that religion influences drug use, we are just beginning to explore the nature of that influence. What are the mechanisms by which religious involvement influences drug use? The answer to that question will help us understand drug use and be more effective in prevention and treatment. In this section, we explore two theories that seem helpful in understanding how religion influences drug use: social control theory and social learning theory. Then we discuss how they relate to a values approach to addiction.

Social Control Theory

Social control theorists assume that humans are inherently antisocial and naturally capable of committing criminal acts. Because deviant behavior is a natural response to rules and scarce resources, conformity rather than deviance must be explained (Hirschi, 1969). In the context of drug use, it is assumed that drugs are readily available in our society and that it is natural for people to experiment with and use drugs. Rather than asking why people use drugs, the question is, Why don't people use drugs? Hirschi argued that conformity is based on a bond that is developed between individuals and society that keeps them from violating the rules.

Hirschi's (1969) social bond consists of four elements: attachment, commitment, involvement, and belief. For youths, attachment consists of affective ties to parents, school, and friends. Commitment refers to a youth's aspirations for attending college and obtaining a prestigious occupation. Involvement is participation in traditional activities such as spending time on schoolwork and obtaining good grades. Belief is respect for the rules of society. Hirschi's theory predicts that individuals who are high on attachment, commit-

ment, involvement, and belief are less prone to deviate from the norms of society, including norms regarding drug use. Although Hirschi's theory is broad and lacks conceptual clarity, research has generally supported social control theory as an explanation of drug use (Marcos & Bahr, 1988; Marcos, Bahr, & Johnson, 1986).

An important social institution not included by most social control theorists is religion. Bonds to religious organizations may deter drug use in several ways. First, individuals may become attached to a church and the people they associate with at church. Because of that attachment and negative sanctions that may follow drug use, people who attend a church may be less likely to use drugs than those who do not attend a church. Second, involvement in religious activities may leave less time available for drug experimentation. Involvement may also provide a network of support that may insulate people from opportunities to use drugs. Third, commitment to a religious organization and its goals may provide meaning to life that makes drug use less attractive. Fourth, the belief system of most religious groups is against drug use and those teachings may reinforce personal beliefs against drug use. In short, religious organizations tend to involve people in conventional activities and a social network that does not approve of illicit drug use.

Social Learning Theory

Another theory that is useful in explaining drug use is social learning theory. There are many varieties of social learning theory, but many are based on Sutherland's differential association theory (Sutherland & Cressey, 1978). Some versions are couched in operant conditioning language, but their central theme is that deviant or criminal behavior is primarily influenced by the associations one has with definitions or behavior patterns that either promote (reinforce) or proscribe (punish) such behavior. An important corollary is that those definitions or behavior patterns are primarily derived from one's close acquaintances.

Social learning theorists assume that conformity is natural, and ask, Why do people violate normative rules? The answer, according to differential association theory, is that one learns to be deviant as one learns anything else, through intimate associations in primary groups. Thus, those who use drugs tend to have friends who use drugs. From their friends, they acquire attitudes favorable to drug use, learn techniques necessary to use drugs, and receive support for their attitudes and behavior (Jacquith, 1981; Matsueda, 1982).

Sutherland and Cressey (1978) said that the ratio of prodeviance to antideviance definitions was the primary cause of deviance, and not just the level of prodeviance definitions. Therefore, people with drug-using friends might refrain from drug use if they receive high levels of counterbalancing definitions. They might receive those antidrug definitions from religion as well as from parents and friends.

Most social learning theorists have said little about religion, but it may play an important part in learning attitudes about drug use. Religious organizations often teach against drug use and provide an interpersonal network in which drug use may be considered inappropriate, harmful, or evil. If through church activity individuals develop a network of friends who do not use drugs and whose attitudes are not tolerant of drug use, religions may be an important place to learn and reinforce attitudes against drug use.

Although these two theories have somewhat different assumptions, there is some overlap in the concepts of belief and definitions. Furthermore, processes of control and learning appear to be operating in drug use and an integration of the two theories seems fruitful. Marcos, Bahr, and Johnson (1986) have developed a model of drug use in which the two theories are integrated; their data provide support for such an integration.

Both theories provide insights into how religion may influence drug use. Social learning theory focuses on the learning of antidrug definitions through direct teachings and a network of non–drug-using peers. Social control theory assumes that drug use is deterred by bonds to a religious organization and other people involved in the religion. Religious organizations may also supplement and reinforce bonds to other conventional groups, including family and educational institutions.

Values and Addiction

Peele (1988, 1990) maintains that the current "war on drugs" will not succeed because it ignores personal values and assumes that addiction is a medical problem that can be solved by reducing the drug supply and by providing medical treatment. As an alternative, Peele offers a values approach to addiction that takes into account the actor and the setting. He contends that to reduce addiction, people must be taught constructive values and become involved in family and community. Important values include learning, achievement, work, empathy, responsibility, and community. Peele says we need clearer messages about right and wrong along with an increase in positive alternatives.

Peele's (1990) focus on inculcating values and increasing community involvement integrates two key ideas from social learning and social control theories. Religious organizations are an important social structure for performing all of the elements suggested by Peele. A key aspect of religious organizations is teaching right from wrong and punishing misbehavior.

Peele (1990) maintains that addiction occurs because people lack purpose. Religious organizations play an important role in helping people gain purpose by reaching out to unproductive groups, teaching constructive values, providing constructive alternatives, and involving people in the community. The need for this type of involvement may be particularly important in inner cities and high-addiction areas. In the spring of 1992, there were riots in Los Angeles after the acquittal of the four police officers who beat Rodney King. Following the riots, religious organizations played a key role in reaching out and helping individuals and communities rebuild. This type of involvement by religious organizations may be vital in reducing addiction by giving people purpose, inculcating values, creating a sense of community involvement, and helping to provide better choices. It is also consistent with the theoretical orientations of social control and social learning theories.

RELIGIOUS POSITIONS TOWARD ALCOHOL AND DRUG ABUSE

The influence of various religious groups on drug use may depend on their official positions toward the use of various substances. Although most religious groups do not encourage drug abuse, their specific positions vary considerably. Some religious groups have strong positions against the use of any drug, including alcohol and tobacco, and consider the use of drugs a sin. Others say relatively little about drug use and consider abuse a medical rather than moral problem. Many religions accept the moderate use of substances such as alcohol and tobacco. In this section, we review some of the specific positions of major religious groups toward drug use and abuse.

For many years, various religious groups have been concerned about the harmful effects of alcohol and other substances. Religious groups often have specific rules relating to health and conduct. For example, traditional Jewish prohibitions against certain foods are among the most well-known religious dietary codes and some date from the time of Moses. Orthodox Jews avoid food products from animals that have a cloven hoof but do not chew cud, such as pigs. Drunkenness is condemned by most religious groups, although many accept the use of alcohol in moderation.

Jews and Catholics

Jews and Catholics do not forbid the use of alcohol but are opposed to drunkenness (De Ropp, 1987). In 1972, the U.S. Catholic Conference established the Catholic Office of Drug Education (CODE) and rehabilitation centers have been established in many dioceses in the United States

(Broderick, 1987). Catholic Charities USA makes available a guide titled *Substance Abuse Agency Resources Guide* (1990). The booklet contains a list of substance abuse resources that have been used by Catholic parishes across the United States. In addition, the official Catholic Church's position on chemical dependency can be found in the document titled *New Slavery New Freedom; A Pastoral Message on Substance Abuse* (U.S. Catholic Conference, 1990).

Protestants

The position of Protestants is similar to that of Jews and Catholics. They are opposed to the abuse of alcohol and drugs but tolerate drinking in moderation. Fundamentalist Protestants such as Southern Baptists, Seventh-Day Adventists, and Pentecostal religions are opposed to the consumption of alcohol or drugs.

Lutherans are opposed to alcoholism. They supported the temperance movement and consider excessive drinking to be sinful (Lueker, 1975).

The Southern Baptist Council has opposed alcohol consumption for many years and regularly passed resolutions condemning alcohol use and abuse. During the sixties and seventies, other types of drugs were included in their proscriptive resolutions (Wood, 1982).

Several of these religions have organized themselves to fight drugs use. For example, the Episcopal Church created the National Episcopal Coalition on Alcohol and Drugs (NECAD). The NECAD is an independent, nationwide network of Episcopal laity, clergy, dioceses, parishes, schools, agencies, and other institutions, all with a shared commitment to address the issues associated with the use and misuse of alcohol and other drugs. The NECAD emerged from the efforts of Diocesan Commissions in Province III to implement the 1979 General Convention resolution on alcohol. In a similar fashion, the Presbyterian Church has made available an *Alcohol and Drug Abuse Ministry Planning Package,* which includes written documents plus a video titled "Is There an Elephant in the Sanctuary?"

Other Religious Groups

Pentecostal religions are opposed to the sale, distribution, and consumption of alcohol. Seventh-Day Adventists abstain from liquor, tobacco, tea, and coffee. The Mormon Church has a health code that forbids the use of alcohol, tobacco, tea, and coffee (Backman, 1983). Many religious people have a common understanding that the body is a sacred temple and should be treated as such. These beliefs greatly influence one's use of alcohol and drugs. In some religions, such as Mormons, full participation in church activities is refused to church members who violate this code of health.

Moral or Medical Problem?

Perhaps one of the most challenging issues facing various religious groups is whether drug use is a sin or a sickness. As early as 1956, the American Medial Association (AMA) accepted alcoholism as a disease. However, among some contemporary religious leaders, there is still no agreement. Should drug users be referred to their clergy to facilitate repentance or should they be referred to a hospital for treatment?

Lorch and Hughes (1988) conducted a survey of all church pastors in a western city of about 250,000 people. Twenty-four religious groups were represented in their study. They found considerable differences among the churches in their attitudes toward addicts. The researchers arranged the various religious groups along a fundamentalism–liberalism continuum. The more liberal groups were more likely to view the problems of alcoholism and drug addiction as illnesses rather than as sins, immorality, or lack of willpower. Well over half of the Methodist, Lutheran, Episcopal, Presbyterian, Catholic, and Jewish religious groups considered both alcoholism and other types of drug addiction as illnesses. At the other end of the scale, the fundamentalist religious groups were more likely to consider both alcoholism and drug addiction as sins. More than 50% of the clergy from Baptist, Mormon, and "Other" religions considered both alcoholism and drug addiction as sins. Mormons were more likely than any other group to view drug abuse as a sin; all of the Mormon clergy considered drug abuse to be "a sin" or "morally wrong," and 86% said alcohol use was "a sin" or "morally wrong."

In churches in which addiction is a moral issue, shame and guilt are often used to motivate members to abstain. The aim is to label drug use as sin and cause avoidance of substances by encouraging avoidance of sin (Royce, 1985). However, most specialists in drug prevention and treatment maintain that using shame and guilt is ineffective in preventing alcohol and drug problems.

RELIGION, MENTAL HEALTH, AND DRUG USE

One of the ways in which religion may reduce drug use is by fostering good mental health. Religious involvement may foster good mental health by providing meaning to life, support during various stresses, friendship networks, recreational activities, and a set of standards that provide structure and meaning. Good mental health may help insulate individuals from pressures to experiment with illicit drugs and abuse them. On the other hand, indicators of poor mental health, such as depression, alienation, and low self-esteem, may predispose some individuals to experiment with illicit drugs.

There are conflicting views regarding the impact of religion on mental health. Some clinicians have suggested that religiosity is associated with a variety of mental disorders. After reviewing the empirical literature on this topic, Bergin (1983) concluded that religion was not related to mental illness. More recently, Bergin (1991) portrayed religion as multifactorial in nature and suggested that there are healthy and unhealthy ways of being religious. He observed that religious involvement tends to be negatively correlated with problems of social conduct such as sexual permissiveness, teenage pregnancy, suicide, drug abuse, alcohol use, and delinquency.

There is evidence that religiously devout people have a frame of reference that may help them cope with deprivation, trauma, and other kinds of adversity. Their belief in God, trust in God, religious convictions, and religious habits and attitudes may be a great strength.

Regardless of denomination, religion has been and continues to be an important influence on what people think of themselves and how they take care of their bodies. Because religious organizations influence people's health beliefs and practices, churches, synagogues, and other religious institutions may be strong allies in efforts to improve both physical and mental health.

RELIGION AND THE PREVENTION AND TREATMENT OF DRUG ABUSE

Religious organizations have a long history of involvement in prevention and treatment of drug abuse. The temperance and prohibition movements of the late 1800s and early 1900s were led by religious groups. By the early 1900s, the leader of the temperance movement was the Anti-Saloon League of America, which often referred to itself as "the church in action." The Anti-Saloon League organized the mainstream Protestant leaders of America, particularly the Methodist and Baptist denominations, to achieve the passage of the Eighteenth Amendment. At its height, the league had more than 50% of the churches in the country in active affiliation (Conley & Sorensen, 1971)

Although religious groups and their clergy have contributed significantly to the prevention and treatment of substance abuse, there is not always a close working relationship between the clergy and professional substance abuse workers. The Florida Drug-Free Communities Project is an example of religious organizations working cooperatively with substance abuse professionals. The Florida project is a primary prevention effort sponsored by the governor. The mobilization of religious communities has been identified as a top priority. The project links religious leaders from a variety of faiths and assists them in developing community-based coordination and information sharing. Several resources, including a clergy training guide and video, have been created to assist in achieving their goals. The Florida program is exemplary because it has successfully networked government, alcohol and drug professionals, and a variety of religious leaders in drug abuse prevention.

We now turn to a discussion of some of the specific types of prevention and treatment programs available from various religious organizations. Numerous study guides, manuals, support groups, and pilot projects are available from a variety of different religious groups, private corporations, and religious individuals. These substance abuse education, prevention, and treatment services have been merged with religious tenets in various ways. They have been made available to specific church populations and in some cases to the general population. In the following discussion, the various programs and resources are categorized into primary, secondary, and tertiary prevention. The following listing is not meant to include all programs available but is rather a representative list of the many services.

Primary Prevention

Primary prevention interventions focus on school-based education programs such as K–12 and general population awareness and information programs. These services are designed to preclude the onset of alcohol and other drug use. *Drugs, God and Me* (Eschner & Nelson, 1988) and *An Ounce of Prevention* (Christian Civic Foundation, 1986) are examples of curriculums for primary prevention.

The Archdiocese of New York Drug Abuse Prevention Program (ADAPP) is an example of a school-based prevention program providing substance abuse intervention, prevention, and education services to students, teachers, and parents in the parochial schools of the Archdiocese of New York. The education component includes general seminars and workshops on drug and alcohol information, including children of alcoholics, issues of adolescent development, parenting, and communication skills. Crisis consultation and referral are also available. The ADAPP program is funded by the New York State Division of Substance Abuse Services.

Right Start is a primary prevention program provided by a private corporation named Rapha. It contains a video and book series that includes up-to-date facts, statistics, sermon material, and Sunday school lessons on a variety of drug-related issues.

Secondary Prevention

Secondary prevention, or targeted prevention, is a type of prevention that includes school, church, and community-based education to meet the needs of specific high-risk populations. High-risk groups are those that exhibit factors that have been found to be related with substance use, such as children of alcoholics. Within a targeted prevention program, the typical pattern is to include a variety of exercises to educate and build interpersonal skills. In addition, in first-offender and diversionary programs, first-time alcohol and drug offenders are given specialized services. The goal of secondary prevention is to identify persons exhibiting risk factors toward addiction and reduce the likelihood that problematic alcohol and drug use will develop. Here we identify two examples of secondary prevention programs, *The Church and Alcohol—A Resource Manual* and The Creating Lasting Connections Program.

The Church and Alcohol—A Resource Manual is the product of a pilot project funded by the Alamo Area Council of Governments in Texas. It is an attempt to put some alcohol abuse prevention programs in local congregations. The project staff (an Episcopal priest and a Methodist lay person) conducted alcohol awareness education within normative religious education experiences, consulted and trained clergy and other church members to become in-house alcohol awareness providers, and assisted children and families already affected by alcohol problems. The manual provides a guide to help church

members duplicate the pilot project within their own congregations. The manual includes hymns, scriptures, suggestions, and agendas for retreats.

The Creating Lasting Connections Program is a project offered by The Council On Prevention and Education: Substances, Inc. (COPES). This project is an application of a model ecumenical community-based project and focuses on reducing community, family, and personal risk factors. The project is done in collaboration with the Catholic Archdiocese of Louisville and the West Louisville Community Ministries. This program is designed to work with church communities and families in acquiring information to strengthen healthy attitudes and skills necessary to increase the whole family's ability to resist unhealthy influences. This program serves youths between the ages of 12 and 14 and their families and is a demonstration project for the Center for Substance Abuse Prevention (CSAP). The project includes 10–20 weeks of skill-building sessions and each family is assigned a staff member who stays in touch with them for one year and assists them in finding recreational and social activities, after-school programs, support services, or social services in the community.

Tertiary Prevention

The goal of tertiary prevention is to help people with serious substance abuse habits recover from their addiction and avoid relapse. There are a number of religion-oriented programs designed to help people recover from alcohol and drug abuse. These programs can be divided into support groups patterned after Alcoholics Anonymous (AA) and programs that provide an inpatient or residential treatment program. We turn now to a discussion of some of these programs.

12-Step Support Groups

One of the most well-known tertiary programs is AA, which is a spiritual movement with roots in religion. The theological formula of confession, repentance, reconciliation, and redemption is the basis of the 12 steps of AA.

In 1935, Bill W., the founder of AA, was attending the Calvary Church in New York searching for answers to his personal alcohol problems. Through a church directory in a hotel lobby, Bill W. eventually met and held the first AA meeting with Bob S. in Akron, Ohio. Feeling lonely and at risk of drinking, Bill W. made a phone call to a local clergyman (Apthorp, 1990). Conley and Sorensen (1971) suggested that the founders based AA on the principles of the Oxford Group movement, a religious movement inspired by a Lutheran minister named Reverend Frank Buchman. Many believe that the therapeutic function of AA is similar to that of conversion to a religious movement.

AA, Cocaine Anonymous, Alanon, and similar Christian 12-step groups can be immeasurably helpful to people recovering from addiction. Religiously tailored 12-step support groups are able to serve people who already have a spiritual or religious concept. There are no fees or dues to join a 12-step support group. Several Christian-tailored support groups have been patterned after AA, including Overcomers Outreach, SAVE, and Alcoholics for Christ. In addition, many faiths support 12-step meetings by allowing the groups to meet in their church facilities. Reverend Richard Bulwith of Catholic Charities of the Archdiocese of Chicago goes one step further and provides special Catholic masses for members of 12-step recovery groups.

Overcomers Outreach was organized to provide a support system for individuals and families within evangelical Christian churches who suffer from chemical addiction by providing a Christian 12-step support group. Overcomers Outreach Inc. includes more than 800 groups in 48 states.

Alcoholics for Christ (AC) is an incorporated nondenominational, nonprofit lay-Christian fellowship for substance abusers and their families. Members come from a variety of Christian denominations. This group has adapted the 12 steps of AA and includes Bible study as part of their program. AC also has support groups for adult children of alcoholics, parents, and teen

substance abusers. A 12-step recovery workbook using scriptural examples is also available. Both AC and Overcomers support groups are tailored for Christians in general.

Substance Abuse Volunteer Efforts (SAVE) was organized in 1983 to accommodate members of the Church of Jesus Christ of Latter-day Saints (Little, 1985; Hawks & Buckner, 1985). SAVE was patterned after the AA's 12 steps but was tailored to meet the needs of Mormons.

Inpatient and Residential

Perhaps the oldest and most popular religious residential program for alcoholics is the rescue missions. The rescue mission approach to alcoholism and drug addiction usually requires the recipient of the services to attend religious meetings. These meetings typically are a gospel or prayer meeting. In addition, the recipient receives a place to stay and food. If the convert decides to stay at the mission, he or she may be assigned to do work around the mission. When recovery has been sufficient, the convert might become involved with the mission's employment service. Some rescue missions maintain fellowship groups for ex-alcoholics. Alcoholics Victorious is one such group. The Salvation Army is an example of a rescue mission. Many homeless alcoholics and drug addicts have been helped by rescue missions throughout the world. Both New Life and Minirth-Meier clinics are examples of private corporations that provide substance abuse counseling using Christian concepts and the 12 steps of AA.

The Victory Outreach Ministries International is another example of a private incorporation of Christians organized to provide substance abuse services. Victory Outreach is located in many metropolitan cities in the U.S. It became known as The Addict Church because of its large membership of recovering alcoholics and drug addicts. Victory Outreach offers the substance abuser a new way of life through Christianity. This corporation provides "victory homes" for alcohol and drug rehabilitation, drug and gang prevention rallies, and a weekly television program.

Perhaps one of the better-known Christian programs is the National Teen Challenge Inc. The Teen Challenge program has more than 100 centers in major metropolitan areas in the United States and Puerto Rico, and many more centers in countries around the world. It provides a variety of services including education, evangelism, crisis intervention and referral, and residential treatment facilities. The Teen Challenge facilities depend on the "changing power of Jesus Christ" to provide the incentive for change.

National Organizations

There are several national organizations that attempt to network and invite religious groups to deal with alcohol and drug problems. The American Council on Alcohol Problems (ACAP) and the North Conway Institute are two of the best known. ACAP is a nonprofit organization whose roots were in the formation of the American Anti-Saloon League in Washington, D.C., in 1895. The name was changed to the National Temperance League in the 1930s and to the American Council on Alcohol Problems in 1964. Although the name has changed several times, the primary purpose of the organization has remained essentially the same: to provide a channel of cooperation through which state temperance organizations, national religious bodies, and similar concerned groups and individuals can unite to deal with the problems caused by alcohol and other drugs.

The North Conway Institute is an ecumenical, interfaith national association organized in 1954. Its goal is to act as a catalyst to facilitate cooperative action by churches and synagogues to reduce alcohol and other drug-related harm and to promote personal and social development.

Another national religious organization designed to train and establish community networks is Wings of Hope, an anti–substance abuse project started by the Southern Christian Leadership Conference. It currently has operations in Atlanta, Cleveland, Chicago, and Los Angeles. Wings of Hope was begun with the belief that the police response to drug abuse is inadequate, ineffective, and detrimental to communities. It is mobilizing churches, mosques, temples, synagogues, and other religion-based community groups to effectively address the issue of substance abuse. It provides a six-week training program and supervises the establishment of Wings of Hope church committees in congregations and communities. The committees help to establish educational programs, develop Afrocentric 12-step substance abuse treatment programs, and promote church "adoption" of families at risk. Wings of Hope is an example of a religious organization consistent with the values approach discussed by Peele (1990). It is an organization that operates primarily in inner-city and urban areas that have relatively high rates of drug abuse.

A relatively new religious organization involved in the prevention and treatment of drug abuse is the Interfaith Coalition. It was begun because of a need for various religious groups to share ideas and cooperate in the fight against drug abuse. The Office of National Drug Control Policy has been instrumental in forming the Interfaith Coalition, a national organization based in Washington, D.C. The goal of the Interfaith Coalition is to gain representation from national religious leaders and unite their efforts in combating alcohol and drug abuse. Missouri and Florida have state organizations that function to network religious denominations in the fight against substance abuse. It is hoped that the Interfaith Coalition can do a similar thing on the national level.

Literature and Media

In recent years, individual clergy have made significant contributions to the literature on the treatment of alcoholism and drug abuse. Because of his work with substance abuse, Vernon E. Johnson, an Episcopal minister, wrote *I'll Quit Tomorrow* (1980), one of the most useful books on the practical aspects of treating addiction.

Father Martin, dressed in preacher attire, lectured in the movie series *Chalk Talk*, which was produced by the General Services Administration (1972). Father Martin discussed many aspects of alcoholism in the film series. *Chalk Talk* has been shown to thousands of educational classes across the nation for many years.

Guide for the Family of the Alcoholic and *Alcoholism a Merry-Go-Round Named Denial* are pamphlets distributed by Alanon. They were written by Joseph Kellerman, who worked for 23 years as a pastor before entering the field of alcoholism in 1958.

Literature for Clergy

Literature helpful to clergy in dealing with substance abuse includes *Good News for the Chemically Dependent* (VanVonderen, 1985) and *Alcohol and Substance Abuse: A Handbook for Clergy and Congregations* (Apthorp, 1990).

Government Publications

The National Council on Alcoholism has provided written literature concerning clergy's involvement with substance abuse. These documents include *How to Produce a Clergy Workshop on Alcoholism* (Schmidt, 1983); *Pastoral Counseling and the Alcoholic* (Verdery, 1983); and *Stumbling Blocks or Stepping Stones: Overcoming Clergy Inhibiting Attitudes* (Schneider, 1977).

Two national guides to alcohol and drug prevention programs are available: The *Citizen's Alcohol and Other Drug Prevention Directory* (U.S. Department of Health and Human Services, 1990) and the *National Directory of Drug Abuse and Alcoholism Treatment and Prevention Programs* (U.S. Department of Health and Human Services, 1989). The *Citizen's Alcohol and Other Drug Prevention Directory* reviews hundreds of state and national prevention organizations. Each organization is listed with a brief written description of services provided, contact information, and suggestion on how the public can get involved. However, no religiously tailored prevention programs are listed.

The *National Directory of Drug Abuse and Alcoholism Treatment and Prevention Programs* lists prevention and treatment programs by state. Contact information and a coding line is shown for each service listed in the directory. The coding line provides additional information concerning the program. Some religiously tailored programs are listed in this directory.

PREVENTION POSSIBILITIES

There is extensive involvement by religious organizations in the prevention and treatment of drug abuse and their involvement appears to have increased in recent years. In this section, we explore some of the ways religious organizations might improve their efforts at drug prevention.

Networking

Religious organizations could do much more to form networks to share information and resources. As noted earlier, The American Council on Alcohol Problems, the North Conway Institute, and the Interfaith Coalition were organized to encourage networking. Wings of Hope is another organization that is attempting to develop networks and encourage cooperation among religious organizations. More must be done to enable various religious groups to share experiences and evaluative data. This type of sharing will not occur unless some type of communication network is established. This could be done among religious organizations or more directly among various prevention programs. Because it is expensive to gather evaluative data, evaluation resources and expertise could be shared. Regular meetings and some type of newsletter or journal may facilitate communication of this type. If it operates as planned, the Interfaith Coalition could do much to facilitate this type of networking.

Direct Involvement

Religious leaders should take advantage of the numerous opportunities to include messages about drug abuse in programs taking place within their respective religious communities. The most obvious of these is to use the pulpit to give messages. There are many passages in scripture that can focus on substance abuse and coping with day-by-day stress. A religious community may make space in its pamphlet racks and on its bulletin boards for alcohol and other drug abuse literature and program information.

In addition, religious leaders must prepare themselves to deal with alcohol and other drug abuse problems in a counseling and referral setting. Their effectiveness as gatekeepers is increased as they become aware of how to recognize substance abuse problems and where to refer people for help. It is useful for each religious leader to have at least two resources for information and referral.

Religious organizations should continue lending their facilities for aftercare and support groups. Many churches allow 12-step meetings to be held in their facilities. In addition, religious organizations could hold regularly scheduled retreats for recovering persons and their families.

Promote Evaluation Research

One of the glaring weaknesses of almost all religiously sponsored prevention and treatment programs is the absence of evaluation. Programs have been developed and implemented without any plan to systematically evaluate their effectiveness. Without such evaluative data, money and time may be allocated to programs with limited effectiveness. Furthermore, promising prevention strategies may not be identified and expanded if their effectiveness is not documented. More programs such as those sponsored by the Center for Substance Abuse Prevention (CSAP) are encouraged. For example, The Creating Lasting Connections Program has research built into the project.

Preliminary evaluative data could be obtained inexpensively if administrators gathered simple observational and questionnaire data from people involved in their programs. Prevention workers should be required to systematically record their observations. The individuals who attend various prevention programs could be given short questionnaires to obtain their evaluations. The administrators should analyze and report such data in books and other written material about their programs.

In addition, more complete data could be obtained by allocating a fixed percentage of operating funds to evaluation research. Independent scholars could be hired to systematically evaluate the organization and outcomes of programs. Funds for evaluation might be obtained from both government and private sources. Without such evaluative data, there is no way to determine which types of programs are effective. Good empirical data would save money because resources could be put into the most effective programs.

Organize Family-Centered Activities

Because religious participation is often family-centered, religious organizations may have a unique opportunity to influence drug prevention through families. Local church organizations could prepare lessons and written materials for individuals at various age levels. Classes, discussion groups, and activities could be organized that include parents and their children. State and national organizations could identify activities at local levels, help evaluate those activities, and disseminate information about successful programs.

There is some evidence that adolescents in highly cohesive families are less likely to abuse drugs than individuals from families low in cohesion (Barnes, 1984; Barnes, Farrel, & Cairns, 1986; Glynn, 1984; Hundleby & Mercer, 1987). This finding suggests that religious organizations may influence drug abuse indirectly by encouraging family togetherness.

One example of this type of policy is the Family Home Evening program established by the Mormon Church. No formal religious meetings or activities of any kind are ever scheduled by the Mormon Church on Monday evenings and all families are encouraged to spend the evening together. The purpose is to promote family togetherness and encourage parents to teach their children. Many families give a short spiritual message and participate in an enjoyable activity. To the extent that this type of policy builds cohesion among families, it may reduce the chance of drug abuse.

Another example of this type of activity is the church "adoption" of families at risk promoted by Wings of Hope. This provides a supportive network that could be invaluable for families with special stresses and needs.

Raise Money for Drug Prevention

At the state and national level, religious organizations could organize drug prevention activities. For example, some religious groups have held special fast days in which members go without food for one or two meals and contribute the amount of money they would have spent on the food to the church. The church collects the money and uses it to purchase food and other necessities for the needy. Drug abuse is a serious problem that also could benefit from such a policy. A religious group could ask its members to fast for two meals and send that money to the church to be used for drug prevention and treatment programs. Those programs could be organized within a given church organization or the money could be contributed to an independent prevention program.

Establish Organizations Separate from Religions

Some religious organizations are large bureaucracies that have a multitude of interests and competing demands for resources. They are hierarchical organizations and it is often time-consuming and difficult to get new programs approved, let alone money allocated to them. Although drug prevention is important to most religious groups, they have many other priorities that may supersede drug prevention. This may restrict the amount of money and attention that a religious organization may devote directly to drug prevention.

One way to circumvent this problem is to establish a private, nonprofit organization that is legally separate from a religious organization. Such an organization could raise money specifically for drug prevention, prepare prevention resources such as pamphlets, books, and videos, and organize evaluation of programs. It could focus on drug prevention that is consistent with the principles of a church, yet would not need formal church sanction for all of its policies and procedures.

Organize and Evaluate Population-Specific Programs

There may be unique problems associated with a specific religious group. For example, some religions advocate complete abstinence from alcohol. If people who are members of such a group develop a problem with alcohol, they may face guilt and rejection not faced by other problem drinkers. Family and friends may view them as sinners who have violated a commandment of God and the drinker may feel ostracized and unworthy. Prevention and treatment in such a population may require different approaches than among people where moderate drinking is the norm. Children of alcoholics and members of different ethnic groups are other populations that may have special characteristics that influence prevention and treatment. Wings of Hope is attempting to deal with the special problems faced by black, urban families by developing Afrocentric 12-step substance abuse treatment programs.

In addition, prevention should be tailored to the level of drug use, as noted earlier. Prevention of initial use may be very different from prevention of abuse among occasional users, which is different from treatment of regular users of a drug. Strategies that are adequate for preventing experimentation may be wholly inadequate for encouraging appropriate social use and preventing abuse.

The findings of Hawks (1989; 1990) confirm that strategies that are effective for one religious group may not be effective for another. Using data from a national sample of high school seniors, Hawks (1989) compared Mormons, those with no religion, and members of other religious groups. The cumulative effects of national and local anti-alcohol campaigns appeared to be less influential on Mormon seniors than on others, as evidenced by a lack of decline in alcohol use frequency among Mormons.

Religious prevention programs must identify some of the unique characteristics of their populations and determine how these characteristics might affect treatment. This will require research that explores the effectiveness of various prevention and treatment strategies among various religious and ethnic groups at different levels of use.

Encourage Political Activity

Each church and synagogue should take a clear, responsible, and visible position regarding the misuse of alcohol and the abuse of illicit drugs. The most significant response any faith or religious community can make is to establish, publish, and adhere to a policy statement on the use of alcohol and mood-altering drugs for all events.

At times, religious groups might explicitly take a stand for or against an existing or proposed law, such as against legalization of marijuana or for a law giving stricter penalties to drunk drivers. They could encourage their members to write their political representatives to express their views regarding drug issues. This could include requests to allocate more funds to drug education and prevention and less to interdiction. Often religious organizations are reluctant to take formal political positions, but there are drug-related issues where religious groups could take a political stand that is consistent with their professed beliefs. Such a stand could focus attention on drug issues and help obtain needed political and monetary support for drug prevention efforts.

Emphasize Secondary Prevention

Much religious involvement has focused on primary and tertiary prevention but not secondary prevention. The aim of primary prevention is to divert nonusers from initial drug involvement. Tertiary prevention focuses on treating individuals who have serious drug problems. Although both of these types of prevention are important, many individuals experiment with and use substances regularly but are not classified as addicts. Religious organizations have not given these experimental and modest users the same attention they have given to nonusers or addicts. Religious organizations could do more to prepare prevention activities for these experimental and non-addicted users. This type of prevention could keep many users from becoming addicted.

SUMMARY

People affiliated with a religion have lower rates of drug use than those not affiliated with a religion. Those who belong to religions that teach abstinence tend to have lower rates of drug use than people whose religions do not proscribe the use of alcohol and tobacco. Regardless of religious affiliation, people who attend church regularly have lower rates of drug use than those who do not attend regularly.

A variety of prevention and treatment programs have been implemented by religious organizations. Some of the ways in which religious organizations could improve drug prevention are by networking among religious organizations to help disseminate and evaluate drug prevention information, becoming directly involved in drug prevention efforts, promoting systematic evaluation of religiously oriented drug programs, encouraging family-centered activities, raising money for drug prevention, establishing supplemental organizations that focus on drug prevention, organizing and evaluating population-specific programs, encouraging political activity, and placing more emphasis on secondary prevention.

Peele (1990) argues that drug policy in the United States is based on misconceptions about drug abuse. He maintains that drug abuse is the result of a personal orientation that often includes an inability or an unwillingness to become involved in productive work, a lack of concern for and commitment to families and communities, and an acceptance of excess and unconsciousness. To reduce drug abuse, he recommends that we inculcate constructive values and involve people in work and social institutions. He identifies values such as hard work, honesty, commitment to family and community, and sobriety.

Peele's position is consistent with social control and social learning theories of drug abuse, and both theories have received substantial empirical support. If Peele (1990) is correct, religious organizations have a vital role in reducing drug abuse, not only through religion-based prevention programs, but by teaching constructive values and reaching out to those who feel discouraged and alienated. In the long run, Peele suggests that teaching constructive values and helping to integrate unproductive individuals may do more to reduce drug addiction than specific drug prevention programs.

REFERENCES

Albrecht, S. L. (1985). *Alcohol consumption and abuse.* Paper presented at Utah Academy of Arts and Sciences, Brigham Young University, Provo.

Amoateng, A. Y., & Bahr, S. J. (1986). Religion, family, and adolescent drug use. *Sociological Perspectives, 29*, 53–76.

Apthorp, S. (1990). *Alcohol and substance abuse: A handbook for clergy and congregations* (2nd ed.). Harrisburg, PA: Morehouse.

Armor, D. J., Polich, J. M., & Stambul, H. B. (1978). *Alcoholism and treatment.* New York: Wiley.

Backman, M. V., Jr. (1983). *Christian churches of America: Origins and beliefs* (Revised edition). New York: Scribner.

Bahr, S. J. (1991). *Religion and adolescent drug use.* Paper presented at the Sunstone Symposium XIII, Salt Lake City, Utah, August 8.

Barnes, G. M. (1984). Adolescent alcohol abuse and other problem behaviors: Their relationships and common parental influences. *Journal of Youth and Adolescence, 13*, 329–348.

Barnes, G. M., Farrel, M. P., & Cairns, A. (1986). Parental socialization factors and adolescent drinking behaviors. *Journal of Marriage and the Family, 48*, 27–36.

Beeghley, L., Bock, E. W., & Cochran, J. K. (1990). Religious change and alcohol use: An application of reference groups and socialization theory. *Sociological Forum, 5*, 261–278.

Bergin, A. (1983). Religiosity and mental health: A critical reevaluation and meta-analysis. *Professional Psychology: Research and Practice, 14*, 170–184.

Bergin, A. (1991). Values and religious issues in psychotherapy and mental health. *American Psychologist, 46*, 394–403.

Broderick, R. C. (Ed.) (1987). *The Catholic encyclopedia* (Revised and updated edition). Nashville: Thomas Nelson.

Burkett, S. R. (1980). Religiosity, beliefs, normative standards and adolescent drinking. *Journal of Studies on Alcohol, 41*, 662–671.

Cahalan, D., Cisin, I. H., & Crossley, H. M. (1969). American drinking practices: A national study of drinking behavior and attitude. *Monographs of the Rutgers Center of Alcoholism Studies, 6*.

Cahalan, D., & Room, R. (1974). *Problem drinking among American men.* New Brunswick, NJ: Rutgers Center of Alcohol Studies.

Catholic Charities USA (1990). *Substance abuse agency resources guide.* Alexandria, VA: Catholic Charities USA.

Christian Civic Foundation (1986). *An ounce of prevention.* Bridgeton, MO: Christian Civic Foundation.

Church of Jesus Christ of Latter-day Saints (1984). *Resource manual for helping families with alcohol problems.* Salt Lake City, UT: Church of Jesus Christ of Latter-day Saints.

Cochran, J. K. (1991). The effects of religiosity on adolescent self-reported frequency of drug and alcohol use. *Journal of Drug Issues, 22*, 91–104.

Conley, P. C., & Sorenson, A. A. (1971). *The staggering steeple.* Philadelphia: Pilgrim Press.

Crowley, J. E. (1985). The demographics of alcohol use among young Americans: Results from the 1983 national longitudinal survey of labor market experience of youth. Columbus: Center for Human Resource Research, The Ohio State University.

Davis, J. A., & Smith, T. W. (1991). *General social surveys, 1972–1991: Cumulative codebook.* Chicago: National Opinion Research Center.

De Ropp, R. S. (1987). Psychedelic drugs. In M. Eliade (Ed.), *The encyclopedia of religion,* vol. 12. New York: Macmillan.

Dudley, R. L., Mutch, P. B., & Cruise, R. J. (1987). Religious factors and drug usage among Seventh-Day Adventist youth in North America. *Journal for the Scientific Study of Religion, 26,* 218–233.

Eschner, K. H., & Nelson, N. G. (1988). *Drugs, God and me.* Loveland: Lutheran Social Services of Colorado.

General Services Administration (1972). *Chalk talk* (Film, two reels). Washington, DC: National Audiovisual Center.

Glynn, T. J. (1984). Adolescent drug use and the family environment: A Review. *Journal of Drug Issues, 14,* 271–295.

Gorsuch, R. L., & Butler, M. (1976). Initial drug abuse: A review of predisposing social psychological factors. *Psychological Bulletin, 83,* 120–137.

Gusfield, J. (1970). The structural context of college drinking. In *G.L. Collegians.* New Haven: Yale University Press.

Hadaway, C. K., Elifson, K. W., & Petersen, D. M. (1984). Religious involvement and drug use among urban adolescents. *Journal for the Scientific Study of Religion, 23,* 109–128.

Hawks, R. D. (1989). Alcohol use trends among LDS high school seniors in America from 1982–1986. *Journal of Association of Mormon Counselors and Psychotherapists, 15,* 43–51.

Hawks, R. D. (1990). Alcohol use among LDS and other groups teaching abstinence. In R. R. Watson (Ed.), *Drug and alcohol abuse prevention.* Clifton, NJ: Humana Press, pp. 133–149.

Hawks, R. D., & Bahr, S. J. (1992). Religion and drug use. *Journal of Drug Education, 22,* 1–8.

Hawks, R. D., & Buckner, E. (1985). S.A.V.E. . . . More than just a four-letter word. *Journal of Association of Mormon Counselors and Psychotherapists, 11,* 69–73.

Hirschi, T. (1969). *Causes of delinquency.* Berkeley: University of California Press.

Hundleby, J. D., & Mercer, G. W. (1987). Family and friends as social environments and their relationship to young adolescents' use of alcohol, tobacco, and marijuana. *Journal of Marriage and the Family, 49,* 151–164.

Jacquith, S. M. (1981). Adolescent marijuana and alcohol use: An empirical test of differential association theory. *Criminology, 19,* 271–280.

Johnson, V. E. (1980). *I'll quit tomorrow.* New York: Harper & Row.

Johnston, L. D., O'Malley, P. M., & Bachman, J. G. (1989). *Drug use, drinking, and smoking: National survey results from high school, college, and young adult populations, 1975–1988.* Rockville, MD: National Institute on Drug Abuse.

Johnston, L. D., O'Malley, P. M., & Bachman, J. G. (1992). *Smoking, drinking, and illicit drug use among American secondary school students, college students, and young adults, 1975–1991.* Rockville, MD: National Institute on Drug Abuse.

Kandel, D. B. (1980). Drug and drinking behavior among youth. *Annual Review of Sociology, 6,* 235–285.

Krohn, M. D., Akers, R. L., Radosevich, M. J., & Lanza-Kaduce, L. (1982). Norm qualities and adolescent drinking and drug behavior. *Journal of Drug Issues, 12,* 343–359.

Little, R. A. (1985). Mormons face alcoholism. *Alcoholism, 5,* 24–25.

Lorch, B. R., & Hughes, R. H. (1988). Church, youth, alcohol and drug education programs, and youth substance use. *Journal of Alcohol and Drug Education, 33,* 14–26.

Lueker, E. L. (Ed.) (1975). *Lutheran encyclopedia* (revised edition). St. Louis: Concordia Publishing House.

Marcos, A. C., & Bahr, S. J. (1988). Control theory and adolescent drug use. *Youth and Society, 19,* 395–425.

Marcos, A. C., Bahr, S. J., & Johnson, R. E. (1986). Test of a bonding/association theory of adolescent drug use. *Social Forces, 65,* 135–161.

Matsueda, R. L. (1982). Testing control theory and differential association: A causal modeling approach. *American Sociological Review, 47,* 489–504.

Moss, F. E., & Janzen, F. V. (1980). *Types of drinkers in Indian communities.* Salt Lake City: University of Utah, Western Region Alcoholism Training Center.

Newcomb, M. D., Maddahian, E., & Bentler, P. M. (1986). Risk factors for drug use among adolescents: Concurrent and longitudinal analyses. *American Journal of Public Health, 76,* 525–531.

Peele, S. (1988). A moral vision of addiction: How people's values determine whether they become and remain addicts. In S. Peele (Ed.), *Visions of Addiction: Major Contemporary Perspectives on*

Addiction and Alcoholism. Lexington, MA: Lexington Books, pp. 201–233.

Peele, S. (1990). A values approach to addiction: Drug policy that is moral rather than moralistic. *Journal of Drug Issues, 20,* 639–646.

Preston, J. D. (1969). Religiosity and adolescent drinking behavior. *The Sociological Quarterly, 10,* 372-383.

Rohrbaugh, J., & Jessor, R. (1975). Religiosity in youth: A control against deviant behavior. *Journal of Personality, 43,* 136–155.

Royce, J. E. (1985). Sin or solace? Religious views on alcohol and alcoholism. *Journal of Drug Issues, 15,* 51–62.

Schmidt, M. L. (1983). *How to produce a clergy workshop on alcoholism.* New York: National Council on Alcoholism.

Schneider, K. A. (1977). *Stumbling blocks or stepping stones: Overcoming clergy inhibiting attitudes.* New York: National Council on Alcoholism.

Skolnick, J. H. (1958). Religious affiliation and drinking behavior. *Quarterly Journal of Studies on Alcohol, 19,* 452-470.

Smith, W. E. (1969). *The word of wisdom. A test of the predictability of human behavior.* Provo, UT: Brigham Young University.

Snyder, C. R. (1958). *Alcohol and the Jews.* New Haven: Yale University Press.

Straus, R., & Bacon, S. D. (1953). *Drinking in college.* New Haven: Yale University Press.

Sutherland, E. H., & Cressey, D. R. (1978). *Criminology* (10th ed.). Philadelphia: Lippincott.

U.S. Catholic Conference (1990). *New slavery new freedom: A pastoral message on substance abuse.* Washington, DC: U.S. Catholic Conference.

U.S. Department of Health and Human Services (1989). *National directory of drug abuse and alcoholism treatment and prevention programs,* DHHS publication no. (ADM) 89-1603. Rockville, MD: U.S. Department of Health and Human Services.

U.S. Department of Health and Human Services (1990). *Citizen's alcohol and other drug prevention directory,* DHHS publication no. (ADM) 90-1657. Rockville, MD: Office of Substance Abuse Prevention, U.S. Department of Health and Human Services.

VanVonderen, J. (1985). *Good news for the chemically dependent.* Nashville, TN: Thomas Nelson, Inc.

Verdery, E. A. (1985). *Pastoral counseling and the alcoholic.* New York: National Council on Alcoholism.

Wood, J. A. (1982). Alcohol and other drugs. In *Encyclopedia of Southern Baptists* (vol. IV). Nashville, TN: Broadman Press, pp. 2078–2079.

CHAPTER 9

VOLUNTARY ORGANIZATIONS

SUE RUSCHE

For a variety of reasons, it is difficult for science to measure broad social movements led by grassroots citizens' groups. Such movements tend to erupt spontaneously. They spread in nonscientific ways from one community to the next as people share strategies that have worked for them with others who want to achieve similar results. Nor do such movements lend themselves to experimental and control groups. They are up and running and spreading across communities and states before funding mechanisms can be established to allow investigators to measure them. Although financing for grass-roots organizations would accelerate changes citizens are trying to make, and financing for research would establish whether their efforts actually bring about such changes, social movements nonetheless proceed without funding as people respond to problems that affect their communities and come together to try to resolve them.

Such may be the case with a grass-roots, community-based substance abuse prevention movement that began in the United States in the mid-1970s. The use of nearly all illicit drugs peaked in the nation a few years after this movement began. In 1979, 24 million Americans were current users of illicit drugs (meaning they had used an illicit drug at least once during the month preceding the survey). By 1992, that number had been cut to 11 million. Cocaine use peaked in 1985, when 5.8 million Americans were current users, more than four times the number who use cocaine today: 1.3 million (see Figure 9.1). The Department of Transportation announced that minimum-drinking-age laws saved more that 13,000 lives between 1975 and 1992. Tables 9.1 and 9.2 illustrate how these declines in drug use occurred among youth (ages 12–17) and young adults (ages 18–25) between 1979 and 1992 (National Institute on Drug Abuse, 1991; Substance Abuse and Mental Health Services Administration, 1993).

Since the mid-1970s, citizens from many different communities have been banding together to identify problems that contribute to substance abuse and to resolve those problems through education and political action at the local, state, and federal level. Initially, as illicit drug use spread downward in the '70s from Vietnam veterans and college students to adolescents in middle- and upper-income communities, parents formed groups across the country to stop this trend. Leading the parent movement were at least three national organizations, the National Federation of Parents for Drug-Free Youth, Parents Resource Institute for Drug Education (PRIDE), and National Families in Action. Paralleling the parent drug prevention movement was an anti-drunk driving movement led by Mothers Against Drunk Driving (MADD) and other groups whose goal was to reduce alcohol-related deaths on the highway, particularly among young people, for whom drunk driving was the leading cause of death. Both of these movements also organized youth groups to engage young people in prevention efforts.

As the prevention movement expanded into the late '70s and early '80s, other groups organized, as various interests realized they had roles

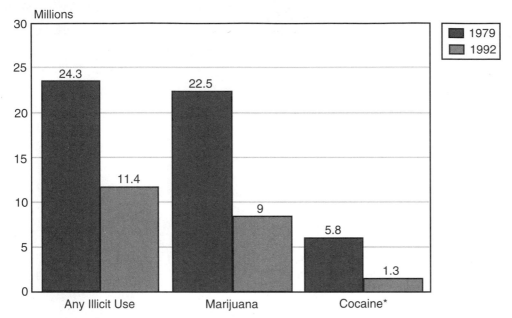

FIGURE 9.1.   Past Month Drug Use, 1979–1992
*Peak of 5.8 million users occurred in 1985.

to play in reversing attitudes or dealing with specific aspects of substance abuse. Organizations such as the Scott Newman Center, the Entertainment Industries Council, and the Academy of Television Arts and Sciences formed to address overt drug references in television and films. The Partnership for a Drug-Free America mounted a billion-dollar effort to use the power of the advertising media to educate Americans about the harmful effects of illicit drugs, particularly cocaine. The Partnership later broadened its reach to include other drugs and to target specific at-risk populations.

Still other groups include the American Council on Drug Education, the U.S. Chambers of Commerce, and countless employers who have initiated drug-free workplace policies, employee assistance programs, and other workplace programs. In addition, led by the umbrella group, United Way of America, many United Way agencies across the nation created special drug task forces and partnerships to assist voluntary prevention efforts. Specific professions, such as the

American Medical Association and the American Bar Association, formed voluntary organizations to involve their members in the drug prevention effort. With the explosion of crack cocaine, these movements were soon joined by specific ethnic and cultural groups concerned about the overall impact of substance abuse in their communities, as well as the overabundance of alcohol and tobacco advertising targeting African-Americans, Hispanics and Latinos, Native Americans, and Asian-Americans.

More recent variations of voluntary organizations are community partnerships, where all interests in a community, private and public, come together to resolve every aspect of the drug problem facing their community. This effort was stimulated by the Robert Wood Johnson Foundation's "Fighting Back" program and later expanded by the Center for Substance Abuse Prevention, which, through the efforts of the Office of National Drug Control Policy, was able to provide a considerable boost in funding for community partnership grants from assets seized

TABLE 9.1 Lifetime Prevalence of Drug Use

DRUG	AGE GROUP	1979	1992
Any illicit drug	Young adults	69.9%	51.7%
	Youth	34.3	16.5
Marijuana	Young adults	68.2	48.1
	Youth	30.9	10.6
Cocaine	Young adults	27.5	15.8
	Youth	5.4	1.7
Alcohol	Young adults	95.3	86.3
	Youth	70.3	39.3
Cigarettes	Young adults	82.8	68.7
	Youth	54.1	33.7

by the federal government in drug-smuggling operations. In addition, the President's Drug Advisory Council created a national umbrella group for community partnerships, funded or not, called Community Anti-Drug Coalitions of America, Inc. Finally, as the nation's understanding evolves about the relationships between substance abuse and HIV/AIDS, violence, teen pregnancy, and child abuse, the substance abuse prevention movement continues to broaden and expand with the formation of additional prevention groups.

Two common themes prevail throughout the efforts of most voluntary organizations. One is the understanding that drugs of abuse are addictive and gradually lead people to behave in ways that are destructive to themselves, their families, and their communities. The other is the belief that citizens in a democratic society must take responsibility for widespread social problems and find ways to solve them.

For nearly two decades, citizens have been doing precisely this. Since their efforts began, experimental and regular use of illicit drugs in the United States has declined significantly. Experimental and regular use of alcohol and tobacco has declined somewhat, and deaths from alcohol-related automobile crashes have dropped to their lowest level since 1980 (from 26,000 to 17,700 in 1992). Because no one has measured the community-based, grass-roots prevention movement or any of the other factors that might have brought about these declines, no one can say for sure what caused them. Because citizens'

TABLE 9.2 Current (Past Month) Drug Use

DRUG	AGE GROUP	1979	1992
Any illicit drug	Young adults	37.1%	13.0%
	Youth	17.6	6.1
Marijuana	Young adults	35.4	11.0
	Youth	16.7	4.0
Cocaine	Young adults	9.3	1.8
	Youth	1.4	0.3
Alcohol	Young adults	75.9	59.2
	Youth	37.2	15.7
Cigarettes	Young adults	42.6	31.9
	Youth	12.1	9.6

prevention efforts are probably contributing to the decline in substance abuse, this chapter will examine in more detail the first wave of that effort, the parent drug-prevention movement, in an attempt to elucidate how drug abuse escalated throughout the '60s and '70s and what these groups did to try to reverse the trend.

BACKGROUND

In the early '70s, research convinced many drug-abuse experts that drug education alone did not change behavior. This belief was so widespread that in 1972 Congress placed a moratorium on all publicly funded drug-education materials for students in elementary and high school.

Congress' moratorium created a vacuum that was soon filled by social, political, and commercial pressures and concerns. As marijuana and other recreational drugs, once limited to the counterculture of the '60s, became socially acceptable in the '70s, drug use escalated. How much it escalated, and how rapidly, can be seen when one realizes that in 1962 less than 2% of the entire population of the United States had had any experience with any illicit drug (Cissin, Miller, & Harrell, 1977). By 1979, 68% of the nation's young adults, 60% of its high school seniors, and 31% of its teenagers had tried marijuana, and large numbers of people were using other illicit drugs as well.

Before this escalation, in response to an earlier heroin epidemic, Congress established the National Commission on Marijuana and Drug Abuse as part of the Comprehensive Drug Abuse Prevention and Control Act of 1970. Congress charged the commission with studying the problem and making recommendations to solve it. The commission issued two reports, one on marijuana and one on other drugs. In the first report, the commission said that it found little scientific or medical evidence to suggest that marijuana was harmful and recommended that the United States decriminalize and eventually legalize the drug. Of the two, the marijuana report is the better remembered, perhaps because many who served on the commission soon founded the Na-

tional Organization for the Reform of Marijuana Laws (NORML) to advocate the implementation of the commission's recommendation. (Some 15 years later, NORML underwent a metamorphosis with the creation of the Drug Policy Foundation, which advocates the legalization of all drugs. Although NORML still exists, many of its former staff and board members now serve on the staff or board of the Drug Policy Foundation.)

At about the time the Marijuana Commission's work was beginning, the Ford Foundation conducted a national survey to determine what Americans' most pressing concerns might be. The survey found that citizens' number-one concern, even in 1970, was drug abuse. In response, the foundation established the Drug Abuse Council, a Washington think tank whose mandate was to analyze public drug-abuse policy. The Council drew on both the Marijuana Commission and NORML for much of its leadership, and not surprisingly, echoed the recommendations of both in its final report (Drug Abuse Council, 1980), namely that the United States should decriminalize and eventually legalize all drugs, beginning with marijuana.

Throughout the '70s, some states acted on at least one of these recommendations. From 1972 to 1978, 11 state legislatures decriminalized marijuana and there was a great deal of talk by advocates in the press about extending decriminalization to cocaine and other drugs.

These laws, along with an increasing social acceptance of marijuana and, to a lesser extent, other drugs, stimulated the creation of the drug paraphernalia industry. By 1978, there were an estimated 30,000 "head shops" (places where "heads"—"pot heads," "acid heads," etc.—could buy drug accoutrements). Drug paraphernalia toys and gadgets to enhance or conceal drug use, along with a host of magazines, books, pamphlets, and comic books that glorified drug use, provided a significant amount of commercial pressure to engage young people in the drug culture. And engage them it did. By 1978, daily marijuana use was nearly double that of daily alcohol use among high school seniors (10.7% versus 5.7%, respectively).

ACCURATE INFORMATION

As an increasing number of young people be-came involved with marijuana and other drugs, an increasing number of parents were learning that, contrary to popular belief, marijuana had many harmful effects on the health, learning ability, and social functioning of their children. What they were seeing in their own children was substantiated in the medical and scientific litera-ture, which they obtained and read and in which they found ample, solid evidence that contra-dicted the public perception that pot and other illicit drugs were harmless. Parents mounted an intense effort to share that information. They ed-ucated other parents, their own children, and those who worked with children about the harm-ful effects of drugs. This effort gave birth to the prevention movement and to the first of three fundamental principles on which it is based: One can change young people's behavior by teaching them, and all who influence them, that drugs can hurt them.

As Figures 9.2, 9.3, 9.4, and 9.5 show, the year that use of a particular drug peaked among high school seniors was the same year that the fewest seniors believed that the drug could hurt them. In contrast, the more seniors who believe that a specific drug can hurt them, the fewer se-niors use that drug (National Institute on Drug Abuse, 1991; Substance Abuse and Mental Health Services Administration, 1993).

PREVENTION RATHER THAN INTERVENTION GOALS

The second principle of the prevention move-ment involves clarifying the difference between intervention strategies and prevention strategies. Traditional intervention strategies seek to reduce the problems associated with drug use, rather than to prevent it from occurring at all, and by definition, target people who already use drugs.[1] But despite the escalation of drug use among American adolescents in the '70s, not all teen-agers used drugs. Parents developed strategies that target nonusers to prevent them from initiat-ing drug use and that target users to help them quit, rather than tolerating use and trying to re-duce problems associated with it.

In contrast with prevention strategies, inter-vention strategies often condone behavior that conflicts with the law. When the prevention movement began, the majority of drug-education materials available to young people contained in-tervention messages with stated goals of reduc-ing drug use rather than preventing it. These ma-terials sought to reduce problems associated with drug use by teaching young people how to use drugs "responsibly." A textbook for high school and college students titled *Responsible Drug and Alcohol Use,* by Ruth C. Eng (1979), lists the following hints for the responsible use of mari-juana: (1) Smoke with friends, (2) use a bong, and (3) don't drop ashes or you'll burn holes in your clothes.

In *Chocolate to Morphine: Understanding Mind-Active Drugs* (1983), coauthors Andrew Weil and Winifred Rosen explain that there is no such thing as a bad drug, just "bad relationships" with drugs. The authors state that the goal of drug education should be to teach young people how to have "good relationships" with drugs such as marijuana, cocaine, PCP, LSD, and many others.

LEGISLATIVE ACTION

Nowhere in these materials and others like them is there any acknowledgement that possessing, using, or selling drugs is against the law. The prevention movement not only clarified this issue, but reversed the logic imbedded in the be-lief that accompanied it, from "drugs don't hurt people and should be legal" to "drugs are illegal because they hurt people." With this reversal, the prevention movement based its strategy on the twin precepts of the health and legal conse-quences of drug use, and gave rise to the third principle underlying that strategy, that of teach-ing children to obey the law.

Parents set out to protect children from be-coming involved with drugs by teaching them about the harmful effects of those drugs. They

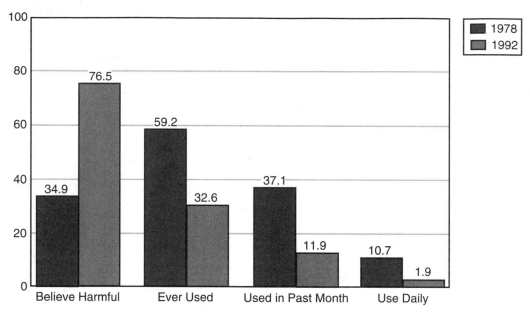

FIGURE 9.2. Percentage of High School Seniors Who Believe Marijuana Is Harmful Versus Percentage Who Use, 1978–1992

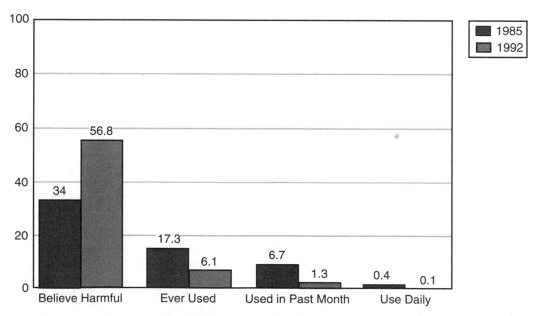

FIGURE 9.3. Percentage of High School Seniors Who Believe Cocaine Is Harmful Versus Percentage Who Use, 1985–1992

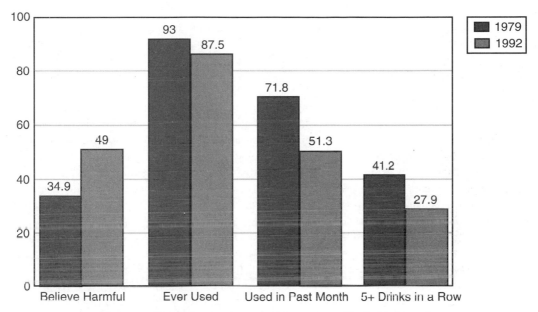

FIGURE 9.4. Percentage of High School Seniors Who Believe Alcohol Is Harmful Versus Percentage Who Use, 1979–1992

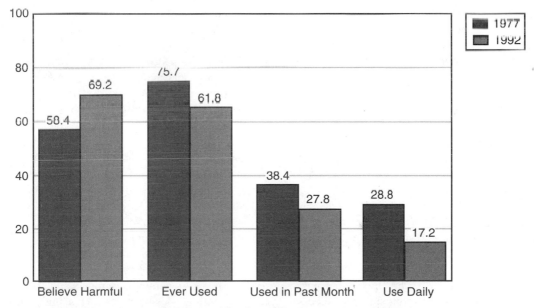

FIGURE 9.5. Percentage of High School Seniors Who Believe Cigarettes Are Harmful Versus Percentage Who Use, 1977–1992

soon recognized that they would also have to protect families and communities from drug abuse. To do this requires an ongoing process that brings people together to identify a problem and then find a solution for it. That solution often is centered in a legal framework.

In some cases, parents focused on existing laws and stressed the importance of obeying them. Such discussions might point out the legal risks teenagers took when they gave or sold drugs to friends. They might examine the legal liabilities to which parents exposed themselves when they allowed teenage parties to take place in their homes where drugs or alcohol (illegal for teenagers) were present. Such discussions helped parents recognize the responsibility they had to obey the law themselves in order to model appropriate behavior for their children.

In other cases, parents pressured authorities to enforce laws and assured officials that they would support them for doing so. Parents lobbied school officials to set and enforce limits about drugs and alcohol that complied with society's laws. Others worked with police, prosecutors, and judges to strengthen the enforcement of laws that young people were breaking while authorities looked the other way. Many parents established drug watches in Neighborhood Watch programs to assist police in apprehending drug dealers, and then worked with judicial officials to mandate those who were addicted into treatment.

In still other cases, parents worked to pass new laws. They shared an almost universal revulsion toward head shops, which served as learning centers for fledgling drug abusers. If drugs were illegal, how could implements that enhance their use be legal? In state after state, parents lobbied local and state officials to pass laws banning the sale of drug paraphernalia. By the early 1980s, nearly all states had passed some kind of paraphernalia law, and, after a long struggle in federal district and appellate courts, the United States Supreme Court upheld the paraphernalia statutes as constitutional. The success parents achieved in this effort acquainted them with the legislative process and encouraged them

to advocate other laws to constrain the exploitation of children for commercial gain.

The parent movement, for example, worked hard to stop further efforts to decriminalize marijuana. As noted above, 11 states decriminalized marijuana between 1972 and 1978. During this time, marijuana use and the use of other drugs escalated to unprecedented levels: from 14 to 31% among adolescents and from 48 to 68% among young adults. Parents worked to stop additional states from taking similar action; in 1980, when a federal bill to decriminalize marijuana nationwide was introduced in Congress, parents mounted an intense effort to defeat the bill. They also succeeded in ending decriminalization at the state level. No state has decriminalized marijuana since 1978. Some, again at the instigation of parent groups, have actually recriminalized the drug. Oregon, one of the first states to decriminalize, recently increased the penalty for possessing an ounce or less of marijuana to a maximum fine of $1,000 and a mandatory minimum fine of $500. Alaska, where it was legal to possess up to four ounces of marijuana (enough to make about 160 joints), and where marijuana use among teenagers was double that of their mainland counterparts (Segal, 1988), recriminalized the drug after parents mounted a statewide petition drive to get the issue on the ballot. Moreover, parents' efforts have ended most serious discussion about legalization as the answer to the nation's drug problem, at least for the time being. Public opposition to legalization has risen significantly over the past decade, as measured by Gallup polls. This reflects the understanding that keeping drugs illegal holds use down. Once an addictive drug is legal, legitimate industries are created to produce and sell that drug. Some of the profits generated from sales are used to advertise and market the drug to increase consumption. As more people purchase and use the drug, more taxes are generated for local, state, and federal governments and controlling or limiting sales becomes increasingly difficult.[2] Just how difficult can be seen by comparing current use of illegal drugs with current use

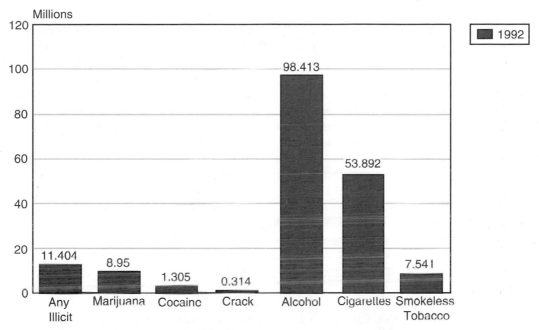

FIGURE 9.6.   Number of Americans Who Used Drugs in the Past Month, 1992

of society's most popular legal drugs, alcohol and tobacco, as measured by the 1992 National Household Survey (see Figure 9.6).

Parent prevention groups have lobbied for thousands of other local, state, and federal laws, including laws to raise the drinking age to 21, to suspend young peoples' drivers licenses until they reach age 18 if they are convicted of a drug or alcohol offense, to increase funding for the prevention and treatment of alcoholism and drug addiction, and to ban smoking areas from public schools. The list of new laws sought by parents is endless, as is the unceasing effort of parent-group leaders to educate fellow citizens about the need to obey existing laws and to pressure officials to enforce them.

As serious as the nation's illicit drug problem is, because they are legal and because far more people use them, alcohol and tobacco kill more Americans than all illegal drugs combined: nearly 500,000 tobacco-related deaths and 100,000 alcohol-related deaths each year compared to an estimated 6,000–30,000 annual

deaths related to illicit drug use. Alcohol alone has been the leading cause of death of American teenagers and was responsible for so many premature deaths among them that theirs was the only age group (15–24) whose life span decreased while the life spans of all other age groups increased (*Health, United States,* 1987). Alcohol-related automobile crashes topped the list, but many teenagers suffered alcohol-related deaths that did not occur in cars as well, such as deaths from alcohol overdoses, drownings, and falls from high places.

Voluntary organizations such as Mothers Against Drunk Drivers (MADD) and Remove Intoxicated Drivers (RID) have done a good job of raising awareness about drunk driving deaths, which constitute about one-fourth of the total number of alcohol-related deaths. However, the nation has virtually ignored the other three-fourths of alcohol-related deaths, those that don't take place in cars. A major reason may be that, as with the drug-education materials of the '70s and early '80s, many of today's alcohol-education materials are based on intervention rather than prevention strategies and contain a preponderance of "responsible use" messages. Such messages are appropriate for adults, but inappropriate for adolescents, who cannot legally purchase or possess alcohol.

One of the clearest examples of this was seen with Students Against Drunk Driving (SADD) and the SADD Contract, a source of controversy throughout the '80s until SADD's leadership changed, triggering a change in the contract. The drinking age in every state is 21, making it against the law for anyone younger to purchase or possess alcohol. In Georgia, for example, purchase or possession is a misdemeanor punishable by up to one year in jail and up to $1,000 in fines. The original SADD Contract required teenagers to promise their parents not that they wouldn't drink, as the law requires, but that they wouldn't drive if they had had too much to drink. This promise offered no protection to young people who die alcohol-related deaths that do not take place in cars and little protection to teenagers who drank and had to determine precisely when they'd drunk "too much." Teenagers interpreted the SADD message to mean that it was okay to drink, as long as they didn't drink "too much." (The same criticism has been leveled at designated driver programs for the same reasons.)

Over the years, parent prevention groups pressured SADD's leadership to modify the SADD contract in order to bring it in compliance with the law. The organization's leaders eventually agreed to change the contract pending approval of its board of directors, but the board refused to change it. At the time, SADD's board of directors consisted primarily of representatives of the alcohol industry (such as Anheuser-Busch, the Wine Institute, DISCUS, and the Beer Institute), some of whom also funded SADD. That SADD consistently refused to clarify the distinction between underage young people and adults is not surprising because the alcohol industry, in its advertising, marketing, and educational efforts, also consistently refused to do so. The industry has traditionally emphasized responsible drinking, but said little about the fact that this message is totally inappropriate for underage young people for whom drinking itself (except in the home in the presence of parents) is unlawful. (The single exception at this writing is a current campaign by Anheuser-Busch that states quite clearly that it wants to stop underage drinking before it starts, signaling a significant shift in strategy by one of the nation's largest brewers. This marks a peculiar irony because SADD finally acquiesced to public pressure and changed its contract to reflect the legal drinking age at the same time it rejected further funding from Anheuser-Busch. However, this may change once again because SADD is experiencing considerable financial problems and announced that it may be forced to accept money from the alcohol industry.)

Just how committed the alcohol industry is to bringing the responsible-use message to people under the legal drinking age is illustrated in testimony before Congress June 15, 1989, by the president of the Beer Institute:

> *Brewers continue to be heavily involved in public education campaigns to promote* responsible consumption, *such as "Know When to Say When," sponsored by Anheuser-Busch; "Alcohol Information from Miller"; "Alcohol, Drugs and You," sponsored by Adolph Coors Company; and "Friends Don't Let Friends Drive Drunk," sponsored by the Licensed Beverage Information Council.* Stroh Brewing Company and the National Beer Wholesalers Association have developed curricula for primary and secondary schools. *(Emphasis added.)*

The alcohol industry's public education effort, including curricula it designs for school children, fails to distinguish between underage and legal drinkers and promotes responsible consumption to an age group that is not only too young to legally consume the industry's product, but is suffering an excessive amount of premature and unnecessary death as a result of consuming it.

The parent prevention movement has devoted a considerable amount of energy to making that distinction. In fact, it is a cornerstone of all prevention efforts. Parents and communities object whenever this distinction is missing from alcohol (and tobacco) prevention and education programs. As with the ongoing effort to clarify and reinforce their expectation that all concerned will obey and enforce the drug laws, so too are parent leaders bringing pressure on communities to obey and enforce the alcohol laws, particularly with respect to alcohol sales to minors.

STATE NETWORKS

When the parent drug prevention movement began, the first parent groups to form usually did so in capitals of states where they could influence legislators, work to ban drug paraphernalia sales, and lobby for other statewide legislation. Because this initial activity gave each group a great deal of visibility, people in other parts of their states contacted the originating group for help in forming similar family and community action groups locally. In helping others organize, in sharing information, and in lobbying for prevention with state legislators and state agencies, these early parent groups generally assumed the role of networking concerned parents, families, and communities throughout each state. The state networks are the heart of the parent movement and constitute much of its vitality.

Most state networking groups share common goals and objectives and provide similar services. These include the following:

— Educate young people, families and communities about the harmful effects of drugs of abuse.
— Emphasize that alcohol is an addictive drug and is illegal for those under age 21.
— Stress that tobacco is an addictive drug and is illegal for those under 18 in most states.
— Establish a no-use message for every illegal drug.
— Equip families and communities with technical skills to prevent illegal drug use in their homes, communities, and schools.
— Network with political, business, and religious leaders; social and professional organizations; educators; law enforcement officials; the judicial system; and all others who play a role in children's lives.

— Refer family members for support, counseling, and treatment as needed.
— Train parents and families to teach them how to form parent and community groups throughout the state.
— Conduct annual statewide conferences to share ideas through workshops and networking.
— Stimulate the formation of youth groups and coordinate their efforts statewide.
— Publish statewide newsletter.
— Generate and monitor legislation within the state.
— Monitor activities of state agencies to ensure that they are responsive to the needs of citizens.
— Encourage coalition building.
— Sponsor throughout the state programs and projects generated by local, state, and national parent and youth prevention leaders and groups, such as Project Graduation, Red Ribbon Week, and Safe Homes.
— Serve as statewide resources for information and referral, operating a toll-free statewide telephone referral service, if possible.
— Network local, state, and national legislative issues between and within state networks. Advocate prevention policies to strengthen the prevention field.
— Generate, support, and coordinate formulation of policy issues with national prevention organizations.

ETHNIC AND CULTURAL GROUPS

With the introduction of crack in the mid-80s, drug abuse spread to inner city communities made vulnerable by high rates of poverty, teen pregnancy, absent fathers, and violence. The prevention movement broadened and expanded as countless more citizen organizations formed to fight back against overwhelming odds to restore their communities to lives free of drug use, drug dealing, and drug addiction. The following provides a few examples of the energy, determination, and dedication citizens who live in the inner city bring to fighting drug abuse in their communities.

Hispanos en Minnesota is a nonprofit agency that helps Hispanic families living in St. Paul organize prevention groups. The Atlanta Religious Mobilization Against Crime, a group of multidenominational clergy, encourages drug users to seek spiritual enlightenment instead of crime. The Lone Pine Parents Prevention Forum was organized in Inyo County, California, by Native American parents who were concerned about alcohol and drug abuse among youth.

Community of Hope offers support to Washington, D.C., grandmothers who are caring for grandchildren their daughters neglect because of drugs. Take Back the Neighborhood: Milwaukee Mobilizes Against Drug and Alcohol Abuse forums led to citizens' decision to organize a neighborhood group to force drug dealers out by keeping daily logs of events occurring at suspected drug houses. Stop the Madness Foundation was organized by a Washington, D.C., mother whose son was gunned down in a drug-related incident. The Foundation is an antidrug, antiviolence, antigun organization of parents determined to prevent further tragedies by reaching out and guiding youth through troubled times and troubled streets.

Project 2000, led by the group Concerned Black Men in the Washington, D.C., area, offers weekly mentoring sessions to young black boys. We The People Reclaiming Our Streets is an organization of senior citizens in Detroit who, carrying pots and pans as their weapons marched on a crack house. Emboldened by the success of moving dealers out of the crack house, they now move through neighborhoods block by block, establishing drug-free beachheads as they go.

SOSAD, Save Our Sons and Daughters, is another parents' organization in Detroit, this one made up of families who have lost a child to drug-related violence. These parents are determined to prevent further needless deaths by drawing youth away from drugs and gangs. Stop the Violence is a group of inner-city Milwaukee parents dedicated to ridding their communities of drug dealers by recording their license-plate numbers and turning that information over to police. They also work to stop the sale of crack paraphernalia and have been assisted in their efforts by Reverend George Clements, a Roman Catholic African-American priest who started the inner-city antiparaphernalia effort in his hometown of Chicago.

The Advisory Neighborhood Commission is a group of Washington, D.C., citizens and clergy who are ridding their neighborhoods of public phones used by drug dealers to conduct their illicit business. In Atlanta, Brothers Against Drugs is a coalition of former drug addicts and drug dealers who patrol the streets of public-housing communities urging addicts to get help and dealers to move on.

The Fairlawn Coalition in Washington, D.C.'s Anacosta section, where drug-related violence was out of control, is patrolled every night by a group of residents organized by a phone-company employee. Residents wear bright orange caps, carry video cameras, and confront drug dealers by videotaping their activities.

Mad Dads is a group of angry, primarily black fathers who patrol drug-infested streets in Omaha, Nebraska. Chapters of their organization have sprung up in Denver and interest in organizing similar groups has come from Boston, Seattle, San Francisco, Miami, Albuquerque, Des Moines, Providence, and Washington.

Residents of inner-city neighborhoods in Detroit and Harlem have targeted the proliferation of billboards in their neighborhoods that advertise high-alcohol beverages and cigarettes designed to appeal exclusively to African Americans and Hispanics. Groups in Philadelphia forced manufacturers to withdraw Uptown, a new cigarette designed exclusively for African Americans.

These efforts represent the originality, activism, and civic responsibility citizens of every race are making to reclaim their communities from alcohol, tobacco, and other drug abuse.

COMMUNITY PARTNERSHIPS

The most recent wave of activity in the multifaceted effort to prevent substance abuse emanates from the community-partnership movement. Information about three partnerships is presented to give the reader some idea of the kinds of things partnerships do to fight drugs. All are based on the understanding, backed by fairly extensive research, that it takes all parts of a community to come together and jointly address the problem.

In Kansas City, Alvin Brooks and friends formed the Ad Hoc Group Against Crime in 1977 in response to the murders of nine black women. The group set four goals: Raise the level of awareness about the impact crime and violence were having on the black community, improve community–police relations, establish a 24-hour crime-reporting hotline, and establish a fund to pay rewards to witnesses and to assist victims. The Ad Hoc Group has many partners, including community groups, police, U.S. Attorneys, county prosecutors, juvenile court officials, school officials, FBI agents, detention centers, and the mayor's office. Together they have raised and given out more than $150,000 in rewards to anonymous witnesses and to victims of crimes. A strong court watch program combines facets of the partnership. The Ad Hoc Group monitors all homicide, rape, and drug cases where the defendant is black. It takes large groups of young students to these trials and the young people deliberate in a separate room just as the jury does. Prosecutors, judges, and defending attorneys come in to talk with the young people to acquaint them with the law and the particulars of cases as each sees them. The Ad Hoc Group also accompanies rape victims to the trials of their assailants and provides assistance to witnesses to hold down intimidation of the victim by family members and friends of the accused.

Initially, the Ad Hoc Group did not concern itself with drug abuse, but that changed when crack infiltrated black neighborhoods. The group has conducted more than 300 marches on crack houses and shut down more than 200 of them. By working closely together, this partnership of citizens and law enforcement officials ensures a high rate of problem-solving to reduce crime and violence, much of it associated with drugs.

In Fort Worth, Texas, Challenge ACE (Activated, Committed and Empowered) involves an even larger cast of players. Challenge began in 1984 when a coalition of volunteer groups put together a blue-ribbon committee of business and civic interests to study problems in the community and to make an inventory of services available to cope with those problems. The study revealed that one in five citizens in Fort Worth over age 12 was a substance abuser. For the next 18 months, small groups, committees, and task forces met to analyze the findings of the study and make recommendations as to how things could be done differently and more effectively. This led to a publication (*Forth Worth Accepts the Challenge*) and Fort Worth Challenge was created to implement some 35 recommendations from the report. In essence, the group served as a catalyst to help existing agencies reform and shape new services needed to resolve identified problems.

Throughout this period, crack was invading inner-city communities. Residents hard-hit by the crack epidemic called Fort Worth Challenge for help in organizing ways to resist the influx of crack and the devastation it was bringing to families. Residents wanted to create and provide services of their own, but didn't know where to turn for help. Fort Worth Challenge responded to their calls by obtaining a grant that puts impoverished neighborhoods in the driver's seat and builds from the grass roots up rather than the more traditional other way around. This community partnership, funded by a grant from the Center for Substance Abuse Prevention, allows Challenge to act as an institutional partnership in service to neighborhoods. Fort Worth Challenge is serving as a community mobilization manager, bringing the power of its institutional members to assist its neighborhood partners. Now that the first year of the grant is behind them, Fort Worth Challenge feels that significant recruitment and trust-building issues have been addressed and that year two will see much progress as disparate segments of the community learn how to work with each other to resolve entrenched problems.

The Miami Coalition is one of the oldest and most widely emulated community coalitions in the nation. More than 85 representatives from other parts of the United States and other nations have traveled to Miami to learn how its coalition works. The coalition has more than 1,500 volunteers, operates nine different task forces, has a board of directors that consists of 115 people and an executive committee of 30, and has set itself 22 major goals, all directed to reducing drug abuse in Dade County. Drug use in Dade County is substantially below national usage rates, according to 67 of 70 criteria established in an evaluation process that began when the coalition first formed. The Coalition assembled a scientific advisory committee of academics from universities in the area and took a benchmark survey at its initiation. Each year, subsequent surveys point to further reductions over the previous year in Dade County and over national rates.

The Miami Coalition set out to bring diverse groups together to learn how to respect each others' needs and to work together to solve problems. Determined not to reinvent anyone's wheel, the coalition has taken pains to help programs already started become even more effective. It got commitments from the *Miami Herald, El Nuevo Herald,* and *Diaro Los Americus* to give two pages every week to promote coalition-sponsored efforts. It is working with the state legislature to obtain a tax to support drug treatment. It has raised funds to support the Dade County drug court program, which diverts drug users from jails, places them in treatment, and provides them with education and job training. The recidivism rate from this effort is 10%. Even more astonishing, it costs the same amount of money to keep a person in the drug court program for a year as it costs to keep that person in jail for just 14 days.

The Miami Coalition is represented on the President's Drug Advisory Council through one of its founders, who spearheaded the effort to create the Community Anti-Drug Coalition of America to carry on the Council's work when its charter ended. The Council convened two national conferences, Leadership Forums One and Two, which brought together 456 people from 176 cities the first year, and 740 people from 266 cities the second, to take part in defining and expanding the role of community partnerships to bring America's drug problem to an end. Community Anti-Drug Coalitions of America, Inc., is now operating and encouraging other community coalitions to join the effort.

SUMMARY

The United States has an unprecedented opportunity to continue to reduce substance abuse and its related problems. Many of the mechanisms needed are in place to achieve this goal. Wave after wave of ordinary people from every community—rich, poor, black, white, mothers, fathers, children, grandparents, aunts, uncles, sisters, brothers, as well as local business, political, and religious leaders—are working to reclaim their communities. They are taking ownership of the problem. They are taking responsibility for solving it. In the process, without consciously understanding that they are doing so, they are exercising the responsibilities of citizenship in the best and truest sense of the word.

One hopes that Congress will provide funding to investigate whether their efforts are contributing to the decline in substance abuse the nation is experiencing. If it is shown that they are, one also hopes that Congress will provide funding to help local organizations continue and expand the important work they are doing.

NOTES

1. This is not to be confused with the treatment intervention goal that seeks to teach families how to intervene in a family member's addiction and restore that person to a life free of addiction through treatment.
2. For a fascinating account of the growth of the tobacco industry in the United States, see Chapters 9 (Tobacco, United States, 1850–1945) and 10 (Tobacco, United States, 1945–1973), Gregory A. Austin, *Perspectives on the History of Psychoactive Substance Use: Research Issues.* Rockville, MD: National Institute on Drug Abuse, 1978.

REFERENCES

Cissin, I., Miller, J. D., & Harrell, A. V. (1977). *Highlights from the national survey on drug abuse.* Rockville, MD: National Institute on Drug Abuse, p. 15.

Drug Abuse Council (1980). *The facts about "drug abuse."* New York: Free Press, Macmillan.

Eng, R. C. (1979). *Responsible drug and alcohol use.* New York: Macmillan.

Health, United States (1987). National Council for Health Statistics.

National Institute on Drug Abuse (1991). *Preliminary estimates from the 1991 National Household Survey on Drug Abuse.* Rockville, MD: National Institute on Drug Abuse.

Segal, B. (1988). *Drug-taking behavior among Alaskan youth—1988: A follow-up study.* Anchorage: Center for Alcohol and Addiction Studies, University of Alaska.

Substance Abuse and Mental Health Services Administration (1993). *Preliminary estimates from the 1992 National Household Survey on Drug Abuse.* Rockville, MD: Substance Abuse and Mental Health Services Administration.

Weil, A., & Rosen, W. (1983). *Chocolate to morphine: Understanding mind-active drugs.* Boston: Houghton Mifflin.

CHAPTER 10

SPORTS ORGANIZATIONS

GARY I. WADLER
ERIC D. ZEMPER

Sport is the "play of the spirit, the challenge of the mind, and the perfection of the body" (Wadler & Hainline, 1989, p. ix). Ironically, for many, sport has become the field of play for the abuse of drugs.

During the 1980s, it seemed that hardly a day would pass when there was not one elite athlete or another, in one sport or another, in the news because of drug abuse. Organized sports has been playing catch-up as it has attempted to come to grips with the dimensions of drug abuse in sports, as well as its root causes. Detection and remediation have been the principal foci of attention, and efforts aimed at prevention have seemingly lagged behind.

Other chapters in this book address drugs of abuse such as marijuana, alcohol, and heroin, which might be dubbed recreational, social, or pleasure drugs. Sports organizations must also address the abuse of so-called performance-enhancing or ergogenic drugs, such as anabolic–androgenic steroids, amphetamines, human growth hormone, and erythropoietin (EPO). Another factor further complicates the issue of drug use and abuse in sports—the drug testing protocols of many sports organizations have made "illegal" the use of legitimate therapeutic drugs because of the belief that they are performance-enhancing, even when used in pharmacological doses. Drugs in this category include diuretics (often used by athletes to mask the presence of performance-enhancing drugs), over-the-counter decongestants containing sympathomimetic amines (central nervous system stimulants), and even beta blockers (used to slow down the heart rate, which is an advantage in sports such as shooting and archery).

To better understand the role of sports organizations in drug abuse prevention, it is essential to put the athlete, particularly the elite athlete, into proper perspective.

THE YOUTH ATHLETE

It has been estimated that more than twenty million North Americans participate in organized sports (Vallerand, Deci, & Ryan, 1987), and more than five million youngsters participate in high school sports at the varsity and junior varsity levels (National Federation of State High School Associations, 1990). It has been shown that children first enter sports as a way to have fun, to relate to their peers, to test their skills, and to enhance their sense of well-being and fitness. Surprisingly little has been written about the psychological profile of the young athlete who rises to the elite level, and even less has been written about the elite athlete's motives for participating in competitive athletics. For some, competitive athletics represents an opportunity to demonstrate skills or to please themselves and others. For others, it represents a passport to higher education, as evidenced by a 1990 survey in which it was noted that more high school students think that their best chance for a college scholarship will come from athletics (16.2%) than from academics (13.9%) or other skill areas (Kelly, 1990). For some, the lure of a career in professional athletics is the driving force for participation in competitive athletics. As Vallerand has noted: "The instant fame and enormous wealth that accrue to athletes who make a great play in front of millions of television viewers lead participants, parents, and coaches alike to covet making the big time" (Vallerand, Deci, & Ryan, 1987). However, of the more than five million high school athletes participating at the varsity or junior varsity levels, only 1 in 50 makes a college team and only 1 in 1,000 makes it to the pros (*USA Today,* 1990).

A 1990 NBC/*USA Today* survey of 645 families provides some statistical insights into the perceptions of athletes between the ages of 10 and 17 (*USA Today,* 1990):

- 88% participate in sports to have fun.
- 83% participate in sports to get fit.
- 69% prefer a coach who puts a higher priority on having fun than on learning the sport.
- 37% prefer not to have parents watching them play their sport.
- 74% feel hard work is required to be an athlete.
- 13% feel natural ability is required to be an athlete.
- 33% state that they have played when injured.
- 41% have awakened in the middle of the night worrying about a game or athletic competition.
- 14% list football as their favorite sport.
- 7% list soccer as their favorite sport, yet 45% of those polled played organized soccer.
- 3% of parents rate their child's coaches as poor, 22% as fair, 55% as good, and 19% as excellent.

The trip along the athletic road is not without its obstacles and pitfalls. As Kirshenbaum (1984) has noted: "The attempt to perform effectively in any sport, even the most intricate of team sports, can be a very solitary endeavor" (p. 159). Particularly for those with collegiate or professional aspirations, other interests may be blunted or never developed, and socialization may be limited to fellow athletes. At all levels, the athlete will be subjected to many of the same peer pressures as the nonathlete with regard to use of recreational drugs, but as they rise through the performance levels, they also may be subjected to additional pressures regarding the use of performance-enhancing drugs.

THE COLLEGE ATHLETE

The studies discussed below shed light on the many issues in college sports that have either direct or indirect bearing on any programmatic efforts of prevention or early intervention of drug abuse by the college athlete.

Summary Results from the 1987–88 National Study of Intercollegiate Athletics

This study, conducted by the American Institutes for Research (AIR) for the Presidents Commission of the National Collegiate Athletic Association (NCAA), provides important insights into the college student athlete (American Institutes for Research, 1988). The study involved 4,083 student athletes and comparison students at 42 Division I campuses. The student athletes included football players, male and female basketball players, men and women who had athletic scholarships in sports other than football and basketball, and students athletes without athletic scholarships who participated in sports other than football and basketball. For the purpose of comparison with the athlete group, students extensively involved in extracurricular activities such as orchestra, drama, and campus work-study programs also were selected for study, and are referred to here as extracurricular students. As expected, the picture of the college student athlete is a complex one, and only a few of the many subjects covered are summarized here.

At the time of enrollment in college, 23% of football and basketball players and 30% of scholarship recipients in other sports reported that they expected to become professional athletes, and by the senior year this expectation remained high at 21% and 25%, respectively. This seems to be an unrealistic expectation given that, in 1990, only 331 college football players were drafted by the NFL, and only 140 actually became active players in the league. With much smaller squad sizes, the numbers for professional basketball are significantly smaller.

Football and basketball players spent approximately 30 hours per week involved with their sports during the season, which was more time than they spent preparing for and attending classes. Even in the off-season, the time spent in their sports was substantial. Although extracurricular students spent less time on their activities than student athletes did on their sports, the extracurricular students also spent more time on their activities than on preparing for and attending classes. Student athletes had, on average, lower grades than students in extracurricular activities, with football and basketball players having the lowest grade point averages, 2.46 versus 2.79 for the extracurricular students. In terms of course performance, student athletes and extracurricular students were equally likely to repeat courses, receive incompletes, or be placed on academic probation.

However, when the players in the more successful competitive football and basketball programs were compared with players in the less successful competitive programs, it was noted that student athletes in the more successful programs were more likely to struggle academically. The AIR report also stated that "Football and basketball players in more successfully competitive programs report more often having experienced physical and mental abuse and feelings of isolation than do football and basketball players in less successfully competitive programs" (American Institutes for Research, 1988, p. 14).

Approximately 50% of student athletes reported having sustained an injury as a result of participating in their sport. Approximately 25% of football and basketball players and 12% of other athletes had felt intense or extremely intense pressure to ignore their injuries. No distinction was made as to whether these pressures were externally applied or internally derived as a result of the athlete's competitiveness.

In addressing the subject of drug abuse, 39% of football and basketball players, 46% of other athletes, and 36% of extracurricular students reported that being an athlete or extracurricular student made it easier for them to avoid drugs, although neither specific drugs nor categories of drugs were specified. On the other hand, 12% of the football and basketball players,

6% of the other student athletes, and 7% of the extracurricular students felt that being an athlete or an extracurricular student made it harder to avoid drugs. With respect to alcohol, football and basketball players and extracurricular students provided comparable ratings as to the ease or difficulty of avoiding alcohol, whereas student athletes in other sports reported that it was slightly easier to avoid alcohol as a function of being an athlete.

The study attempted to identify profiles of student athletes who had experienced multiple problems in college. These "problem profiles" were based on 16 indicators of problems grouped into five areas: psychological stress, physical distress, difficulty in avoiding drugs or alcohol, mental and physical abuse, and unsatisfactory academic performance. Twelve percent of football and basketball players had problems in at least two areas, and 4% of the other athletes and 7% of the extracurricular students were identified as having problems in at least two areas. Further analysis suggested that student athletes with multiple problems were found more often in colleges that had more successful football and basketball programs. For example, about 14% of the football and basketball players in the more successful programs fell into the problem group, as contrasted with only 7% in the less successful programs. Similar correlations existed for students who were more intensively recruited than for those not so recruited. There also was a correlation, though to a lesser extent, between those football and basketball players who had problems in at least two of the areas and who had coaches perceived as being ineffective in nonathletic areas. It should be noted that these results cannot be interpreted in a causative manner. As emphasized by the authors, "our findings are preliminary and merely suggest certain relationships. They do not prove that more successfully competitive programs or unsupportive coaches cause problems for student athletes. Rather, these findings show only that football and basketball players with multiple problems are more likely to be found at institutions with these characteristics" (American Institutes for Research, 1988, p. 71).

Although the AIR study was not able to examine graduation rates, a separate study by the NCAA provides some insight into the performance of athletes and nonathletes on this ultimate measure of academic performance. A 1989 NCAA report of academic performance of student athletes at Division I schools (the largest schools with the largest athletic programs) showed five-year graduation rates for all students (47.8%) and for student athletes (48.0%) to be essentially the same (National Collegiate Athletic Association, 1989). Graduation rate was defined as the number of students graduating in a given year divided by the total number of students enrolled in that class five years earlier.

Study of the Substance Use and Abuse Habits of College Student Athletes

An initial study of the substance abuse habits of college athletes was contracted by the NCAA and was conducted by the College of Human Medicine at Michigan State University during the fall of 1984 (Anderson & McKeag, 1985). In this first major study of the drug use habits of college student athletes, 2,039 participants in five men's and five women's sports from six Division I, three Division II, and two Division III schools completed a carefully administered, anonymous questionnaire. The questionnaire was similar to the *Monitoring the Future* questionnaire used by the National Institute on Drug Abuse. In 1989 and again in 1993, the study was replicated, using 2,205 student athletes in 1989 and 2,505 in 1993, in the same 10 men's and women's sports and each time at 11 different randomly selected NCAA member institutions (Anderson & McKeag, 1989; Anderson, Albrecht, & McKeag, 1993). These replications provided data regarding the trend of drug use and opinion changes during the intervening years, the reaction of student athletes to drug education and drug testing programs administered at their institutions, and the effectiveness of drug education and drug testing programs administered by the NCAA during these years. For the purposes of these studies, the drugs studied were categorized either as ergogenic (performance-enhancing) or as social/recreational. Ergogenic drugs included amphetamines, anabolic–androgenic steroids, barbiturates/tranquilizers, and major pain medications; social/recreational drugs included alcohol, cocaine/crack, psychedelics, marijuana/hashish, and smokeless tobacco.

An extensive list of research questions were addressed concerning factors such as the type, frequency, and amount of drugs used, where they are obtained, why and with whom drugs are used, when athletes began using drugs, and reasons for stopping or never starting the use of specific drugs. Research questions also addressed athletes' opinions about alcohol, drugs, and drug testing, and attempted to identify important demographic characteristics related to drug use. Finally, the study attempted to identify what variables predicted athlete drug and alcohol use. Although addressing all of these provocative questions is clearly beyond the scope of this chapter, certain observations and conclusions from these studies are noteworthy when considering drug abuse prevention strategies.

Ergogenic Drugs

The overall use rate for anabolic–androgenic steroids remained stable at 4.4% and 4.9% in 1985 and 1989, but dropped to 2.5% in 1993. The greatest use of steroids occurred in football, between 8% and 10% in 1985 and 1989 but dropping to 5% in 1993. The use of amphetamines was reported at 8.1% in 1985, but declined to 2.8% and 2.1% in 1989 and 1993, respectively. Barbiturate and tranquilizer use was low across all three replications of this study, dropping from 2.1% in 1985 to 1.4% in 1993. Major pain medications were widely used, with 27.7% (1985), 34.3% (1989), and 30.1% (1993) of the student athletes saying they had used them in the previous year.

The reasons put forth by the student athletes for having used ergogenic drugs varied for the different drugs studied. As might be expected, for major pain medications, more than 75% of these uses were for sports-related injuries, and in approximately 80% of the cases were obtained directly from physicians. For anabolic–androgenic steroids, the great majority stated that the main reason was to improve athletic performance. By contrast, only about one-third of amphetamine users said performance enhancement was the main reason for their use of these drugs, while about one-quarter stated that their principal motivation was to give them more energy, although such use might be construed as a component of performance enhancement.

In addressing the issues of prevention and early intervention of performance enhancing drug use, knowledge of when these drugs are initially used by the athlete is especially important. With the exception of anabolic–androgenic steroids, the majority of ergogenic drug use began at the high school or junior high school level, although by 1993 nearly 43% of steroid users started before reaching college. By 1993, 52% of amphetamine users had started in high school or junior high school, which was down from approximately 70% in previous years. The proportion of barbiturate and tranquilizer users who start in high school or junior high school has remained relatively stable at approximately two-thirds over the course of this study.

It has been reported that eating disorders have been problematic in a variety of sports (Wadler & Hainline, 1989; Warren, Stanton, & Blessing, 1990; Clark, Nelson, & Evans, 1988). This is particularly evident in individual sports in which a low body weight or low body fat percentage may be an important physical characteristic (such as gymnastics, wrestling, and distance running). Accordingly, the 1989 Michigan State study included nonprescription weight control products in the list of drugs studied and included these drugs in the "perceived ergogenic" category. These products generally include laxatives, diuretics, and diet pills containing phenylpropanolamine. Five percent of all the student athletes studied had reported usage of nonprescription weight control products in the preceding 12 months.

When asked why these nonprescription weight control products had been taken, 53.1% indicated the principal reason was to "improve my appearance," 36.7% indicated "improve athletic performance," 4.1% to "make me feel good," and 6.1% for other reasons. As many as 13% initially used these products in junior high school or in elementary school and 46% started using them in high school, 20% during the first year of college, and 20% after the first year. Eighty-one percent of all the student athletes using weight loss products had bought the products themselves, and only 4% obtained them from a physician.

With respect to racial and ethnic differences in reported ergogenic drug use, the data revealed that Caucasian athletes reported as much or more use than athletes who described themselves as being in other racial or ethnic categories.

Social/Recreational Drugs

By far the most commonly used drug in this category was alcohol, with between 88% and 89% having reported usage during the previous 12 months in all three replications of this study. In contrast, the use of cocaine/crack fell dramatically, from 17.0% (1985) to 5.4% (1989) to 1.1% (1993). Marijuana and hashish use fell from 35.9% to 21.4% during this period. However, the use of smokeless tobacco rose from 19.8% in 1985 to 27.6% in 1989 and 26.9% in 1993.

Of those who had used any of the four categories of social/recreational drugs, approximately 75% for each category had first used them in high school or junior high school. Throughout the period of this study, by far the predominant source of cocaine/crack and marijuana/hashish for these athletes was a friend or relative. Throughout the study, the vast majority of student athletes reported using alcohol (more than 80%), cocaine/crack, marijuana/hashish, and smokeless tobacco (each more than 60%) for recreational or social reasons, with the second most common reason being "it makes me feel good."

This survey of college athletes also attempted to get a sense of why they had chosen not to use a specific drug, or why use of a specific drug was discontinued. Across all four drug categories in the 1993 replication, the two predominant responses were "concerns about my health" and "no desire for the effect," with "I don't like it" also receiving frequent mention for alcohol and smokeless tobacco.

THE PROFESSIONAL ATHLETE

An analysis of the professional athlete is difficult because their numbers pale when contrasted with the numbers of high school and college athletes and because there are no in-depth studies of professional athletes comparable to the NCAA study discussed above. Moreover, great variations exist in the sociology, psychology, and physical demands of each professional sport. Nonetheless, some factors, specifically fame, fortune, free time, and a feeling of invincibility, at least to some extent, appear to be common to many professional athletes. It is these very elements that may well enhance their vulnerability to drug abuse during their professional careers. As noted by Arnold M. Nicholl, Jr., consulting psychiatrist for the New England Patriots professional football team, "because of their outstanding talent, some of the players have been indulged for most of their lives. Parents and teachers have bent the rules and moved boundaries to accommodate them. Consequently, a few players have failed to internalize the controls that most people acquire before reaching late adolescence and early adulthood. In one sense, athletic development has proceeded at the expense of emotional development." He further noted, "many players come out of college in limited financial circumstances, and then, at a very young age, begin to earn huge sums of money. They also find themselves with a great deal of public recognition. . . . This sudden access to money, recognition and an excess of free time imposes considerable stress on a person just out of college" (Nicholl, 1987, p. 1096). Like others in the public eye—politicians, musicians, or actors—some athletes have come to believe that they are exempt from the everyday obligations society imposes (Rosecan, Spitz, &

Gross, 1987). This sense of entitlement too often extends to drug abuse.

Professional athletes in sports such as football in many cases feel a great deal of pressure to use anabolic–androgenic steroids, whether to win or maintain a place on a team or to recover from injuries or strenuous training, especially if they feel others are using the drugs. With huge salaries at stake, they do not feel they can afford to be placed at any disadvantage in the competition to earn or hold their place on the team.

The primary focus of the four major professional sports leagues has been on recreational drugs such as alcohol and cocaine, although professional football has made efforts to eliminate the use of anabolic–androgenic steroids as well. Specific policies among the other major professional sports leagues regarding secondary prevention (drug testing) and tertiary prevention (required participation in rehabilitation programs after the second or third positive drug test) are aimed principally at recreational drugs. Some sports do mention performance-enhancing drugs in their primary prevention efforts for their athletes, but it is very seldom that a positive test for anything but recreational drugs has become public knowledge. However, this may be partly explained by confidentiality requirements with regard to drug testing. It often is the case that an athlete testing positive for recreational drugs also has had some contact with law enforcement officials on public record (such as DUI), leading to revelations by the media, whereas those testing positive for performance-enhancing drugs are better able to keep the results confidential.

At the moment, football is the only professional sport that releases data on the results of its testing program. However, because of confidentiality issues raised by team management and by players' unions in all professional sports, and a general reluctance by both to cooperate in any type of well-designed study of the actual rate of drug use by athletes, we are left with only the purely anecdotal evidence provided by media coverage. As any researcher can attest, conclusions based only on anecdotal evidence usually are very distorted. Whatever the causes, whatever the numbers, it is clear that drug abuse by professional athletes has, too often, become a regular feature of sports headlines and stories.

SOCIAL/RECREATIONAL DRUGS IN SPORTS

This chapter does not permit a review of the array of drugs that fall into this general category, such as alcohol, marijuana and cocaine, which have received the most public attention and are covered elsewhere in this book. However, smokeless tobacco is one drug in this category that has not received as much public attention and tends to be often associated with athletes, and therefore will be covered here.

Smokeless Tobacco

While headlines have focused on cocaine, alcohol, and anabolic–androgenic steroids, smokeless tobacco has insidiously become an ever-increasing and alarming problem in sports. However, the problem is not limited to sports. The use of smokeless tobacco is widespread among young persons in the United States, especially in rural areas, as well as in select groups such as baseball players (Benowitz, Jacob, & Yu, 1989). As noted previously, the Michigan State study of college athletes indicated that between 1984 and 1989, the use of smokeless tobacco increased from 20% to 28%. In that study, 57% of the baseball players, 40% of the football players, 29% of the male tennis players, 20% of the male track athletes, and 9% of the female softball players had used smokeless tobacco. Forty percent of these athletes used it from one to five times a day and 14% used it six or more times per day.

The study indicated that 21% of the smokeless tobacco users initiated their use in junior high school or before and 54% did so while in high school. Despite the common belief that the use of smokeless tobacco is more common in certain parts of the country, the use was evenly spread across all regions. However, in the East the use of these products increased from 15% to 25% between 1984 and 1989, and in the Midwest it increased from 19 to 33%.

The Michigan State study provides some insight into the athlete's motivations for the use of smokeless tobacco. Sixty-two percent used it for recreational reasons, 28% because it made them feel good, and only 1.3% use it to improve performance. Whether nicotine is, in fact, ergogenic is not completely understood. Research tends to suggest that it may potentially enhance performance by means of its calming effects, although this may represent relief from craving associated with nicotine withdrawal and an enhancement of information-processing tasks (Wadler & Hainline, 1989). However, Edwards, Glover, and Schroeder (1987) found no beneficial effects of smokeless tobacco on three perceptual tasks (reaction time, movement time, total response time), and another study noted that smokers had a substantial deficit in performing complex tasks involving both cognitive and reflex responses (Spillich, 1987).

With the increasing use of smokeless tobacco, initiated at increasingly younger ages, the adverse health effects of this form of tobacco use are of increasing concern. Particularly disturbing are the findings of Ernster and colleagues (1990) of a 46% incidence of precancerous lesions (leukoplakia) of the mucous membranes of the athletes' mouths in those currently using smokeless tobacco. The presence of oral leukoplakia was greater in those whose use exceeded three years. It also increased with hours used per day and amount of tobacco used. This study did not reveal any oral cancers per se, but this is not surprising because the subjects of this study were relatively young and had used smokeless tobacco for less than a decade. Previous studies (Winn et al., 1981) have indicated that the development of these cancers is generally associated with decades of smokeless tobacco use. Overall, although the Ernster et al. study did not reveal an increase in dental caries, gingivitis, or plaque formation in the users of smokeless tobacco, there were significant increases in gum recession and attachment loss at the locations where the tobacco was held.

There has been a misperception that smokeless tobacco is a safe alternative to smoking.

However, there is no question that it shares the addiction potential of cigarettes. As noted by Goldstein and Kalant (1990), on a relative addiction risk scale of 1 to 5, with 1 representing maximum addictive potential (cocaine), nicotine is scored as a 2 along with the opiates. In a study of professional baseball players, 19% of all users and 26% of snuff users described themselves as "hooked" or "unable to stop," despite the widespread knowledge among users that smokeless tobacco is potentially harmful to their health (Connolly, Orleans, & Kogan, 1988).

DRUGS OF ABUSE UNIQUE TO SPORTS

An overview of representative or particularly problematic drugs unique to organized sports is a prerequisite to a discussion of prevention efforts by sports organizations. The performance-enhancing drugs are a major concern to sports organizations in their efforts to ensure that all athletes are playing on a level playing field, and until the past decade were the historic focus of athletic drug testing efforts. In recent years, the use of recreational drugs such as alcohol or cocaine has become a more public concern in relation to athletes, but these drugs are covered elsewhere in this book. With the exception of the possibly exacerbating effects of the unusual social situation of the elite or professional athlete mentioned in the last section (fame, fortune, free time, and a feeling of invincibility), the problems of the athlete with regard to recreational drugs are not too different from those of the general population. This section highlights some of the problems with two types of performance-enhancing drugs of particular concern to the athletic community: anabolic–androgenic steroids and erythropoietin.

Anabolic–Androgenic Steroids

In what has become a silent epidemic, anabolic–androgenic steroid abuse has spilled over from the world of competitive athletics into the nation's high schools to an alarming degree. From being a drug whose principal illicit use was limited to increasing an athlete's body mass and strength, it has become the drug of choice for the teenager who seeks to contour muscles or to lower the percentage of body fat. In 1989, it was estimated that $500 million was spent for illicit anabolic–androgenic steroids. Studies have estimated the incidence of steroid use by male senior high school students between 6% and 7% (Buckley et al., 1988). It has even been reported that as many as 11% of eleventh grade boys have used these drugs (United States General Accounting Office, 1989). In absolute terms, various reports suggest that between 250,000 and 500,000 high school students have used anabolic–androgenic steroids (United States General Accounting Office, 1989). At least as disturbing is the fact that approximately 40% of these students have used five or more cycles of these drugs, a cycle ranging between six and eight weeks, and approximately 40% began using these steroids before the age of 16 (Wright & Cowart, 1990). Females have not been immune to the problem. A 1990 report released by the Inspector General of the Department of Health and Human Services estimated that between 0.5% and 2.5% of girls in grades 7 through 12 also are involved (Cowart, 1990).

Anabolic–androgenic steroids, the synthetic derivatives of the male hormone testosterone, as well as testosterone itself, have been used by athletes principally to increase their lean body mass and strength. Thus, it is not surprising that these drugs are used primarily in sports in which these physical characteristics are important attributes, such as weightlifting and football. However, as the Michigan State study (Anderson, Albrecht, & McKeag, 1993) and others have shown, these drugs also are used in sports in which strength and an increased lean body mass are not of paramount importance. In some sports, for instance, steroids are used more to decrease recovery time from workouts or injuries than for their muscle-building qualities. Still others take steroids to increase their aggressiveness. In addition, the controversy surrounding the disqualification of sprinter Ben Johnson for a positive drug test during the 1988

Olympic Games has certainly suggested the possibility that anabolic–androgenic steroids may be of benefit to athletes who depend on acceleration, as contrasted with speed, in their sport.

The use of anabolic–androgenic steroids by men far exceeds that by women, as noted in the Michigan State study (Anderson, Albrecht, & McKeag, 1993). In addition, the 1986 Hazeldon-Cork/Women's Sports Foundation's Elite Women Athletes Survey found that 3% and 5% of Olympic and professional athletes, respectively, admitted to anabolic–androgenic steroid use during their lifetime (Elite Women's Athlete Survey, 1987). Although many reasons for the low prevalence of steroid use by women may be advanced, there can be little doubt that the virilizing effect of these drugs—hirsutism, acne, deep voice, and loss of breast tissue—has been a major factor.

Information on the adverse side effects of anabolic–androgenic steroid use are derived primarily from reports on patients with underlying medical conditions and taking normally prescribed doses, rather than healthy athletes who take vastly greater doses than used when these drugs are prescribed by physicians. Despite these limitations, there is no doubt that the adverse effects of these drugs include alterations of liver chemistries and liver structure (peliosis hepatitis) and breast enlargement in males (gynecomastia). Reversible effects include testicular atrophy and azoospermia. Profound changes in cholesterol metabolism have been noted, but as yet there is no definite evidence of accelerated atherosclerosis in steroid-abusing athletes. Occasional reports have appeared of malignant neoplasms (kidney, liver, prostate) occurring in individuals using anabolic–androgenic steroids, but these data are scant at best. In adolescents, the premature closure of the epiphyses in those using these steroids will result in failure to reach full growth potential. In recent years, a further problem is the danger of the spread of AIDS through shared needles, which has been reported in association with the use of injectable steroids (Sklarek et al., 1984).

In addition to the physical side effects, there have been reports of behavioral and psychological effects of taking anabolic–androgenic steroids. These include depression, suicidal ideation, euphoria, irritability, and, on occasion, extreme aggressiveness, a behavior pattern referred to as "Roid Rage." Various psychotic states, including homicide and near homicide, have been reported in the medical literature (Pope & Katz, 1988). Although it remains speculative as to whether or not steroid use produces an actual addiction, there appears to be mounting evidence that chronic usage does produce a state of dependency. According to Kashkin and Kleber (1989), evidence includes the following: the use of these hormones continues over a longer period of time than was desired or originally planned; attempts to stop are often not successful; use of these drugs continues despite information regarding the problems associated with them; characteristic drug withdrawal symptoms can occur, such as joint pain, depression, apathy; and the drug may be reinstituted to relieve these symptoms.

The use of anabolic–androgenic steroids has had a major impact on one of the primary means used by sports organizations to prevent the use of performance-enhancing drugs by athletes: drug testing. When drug testing was initially used in sports during the late 1960s, it was aimed at detecting central nervous system stimulants such as amphetamines, which is a relatively straightforward process. Because these stimulants act over only a brief span of time before they are cleared from the body, testing immediately at the completion of competition was an effective deterrent against the use of stimulants. This approach to drug testing was quickly found to be ineffective against the use of anabolic–androgenic steroids. Depending on the specific anabolic–androgenic steroid used, the steroid or its metabolites may be present in the body for weeks to as long as nine months after use. The sought-after effects are not transient like those of the psychomotor stimulants; they can persist long after the steroid or its metabolites are cleared by the body. Thus, to avoid detection, the athlete typically stops using the steroid before competition, in time for it or its metabolites to clear the body before drug testing.

Recognizing this, sports organizations have resorted to year-round, out-of-competition, random, unannounced drug testing.

Testing for anabolic–androgenic steroids is a complicated process. Testing may be done for the parent compound or for its unique metabolites, or metabolic breakdown products excreted in the urine. Some synthetic steroids can have as many as a dozen or more metabolites, and there are numerous anabolic–androgenic steroids available. Further complicating the issue is the fact that athletes often use more than one type of steroid simultaneously. It is an extremely complex process to sort out and identify all of the varied metabolites of an anabolic–androgenic steroid from among all the normal metabolites produced by the body. Proper analysis of the athlete's urine samples requires specific equipment, including a mass spectrometer, which operates at the molecular level to identify extremely small amounts of compounds, and a laboratory staff with a great deal of experience identifying the myriad combinations of metabolites. For this reason, testing for anabolic–androgenic steroids is expensive and cannot be adequately done by most drug testing laboratories, even if they have a mass spectrometer. Not only is the process complex and costly, but when done for forensic reasons, it also requires adherence to precise quality control standards. Accordingly, the International Olympic Committee maintains a rigorous certification and recertification program for drug testing laboratories. At the time of this writing, the only laboratories in North America that have received IOC certification are located in Montreal, Los Angeles, and Indianapolis, and they are regularly used by national sports governing bodies for their drug testing programs.

The complexity of testing for anabolic–androgenic steroids has led to a continuous cycle of competition between athletes trying to find new ways to beat the drug tests and the drug testers trying to stay ahead of these attempts. In recent years, these attempts have most often taken the form of using other drugs, such as diuretics, to dilute the urine and help mask the presence of steroid metabolites; probenecid, to

inhibit urine secretion; or the new anabolic–androgenic steroids that have not yet had their metabolites characterized and are thus invisible to the testing procedure. The responses have included adding drugs that can be used as urine manipulators to the list of banned drugs, and a vigorous research program to quickly characterize the metabolites of new steroids.

The pressures to use anabolic–androgenic steroids can take many forms. At the high school level, the use of steroids can be seen as the path to a college athletic scholarship, with the pressure coming from parents, coaches, or from within the athlete. At the collegiate and international level, it becomes pressure to be successful in national or international competition, with the desire not to have to compete at a disadvantage against other athletes who are believed to be using steroids. These pressures can be extremely coercive to a competitive athlete, inducing him or her to use the drugs despite the dangers. At the professional level, as mentioned previously, it can become a monetary issue for the athlete. Over all levels hangs the pervasive social penchant for glorifying only the winners; winning at any cost gradually has become the accepted and even expected norm.

Erythropoietin

Endurance athletes have long known that they can improve athletic performance by increasing the transport of oxygen to working muscles. To accomplish this, they have used a variety of techniques to increase the number of oxygen-carrying red blood cells in the circulatory system. These techniques have included physiological methods such as training at high altitudes to physiologically stimulate the production of an increased number of red blood cells, as well as illegal and dangerous methods such as blood doping (the intravenous infusion of homologous red blood cells) and, most recently, the use of erythropoietin.

Erythropoietin (EPO) is a naturally occurring hormone, produced by the kidney, that helps govern the rate of formation of new red blood cells. When the kidney senses a decrease in the number of circulating red blood cells (via a drop in oxygen tension), it releases EPO into the circulatory system, which in turn stimulates the bone marrow to produce more red blood cells. EPO is produced in such small quantities in the body that it is impossible to harvest enough of the natural product from healthy people to be of therapeutic value for patients who require it for medical reasons. Because of its enormous potential as a therapeutic agent for the treatment of certain anemias, research was successfully undertaken to produce the hormone by means of recombinant DNA techniques (genetic engineering). Although the drug was approved in 1989 for treatment of the marked anemia of patients with advanced kidney failure, its use has been extended to the management of other anemias. It is not at all surprising that EPO has now found its way into the athletic community as an alternative to blood doping.

The primary danger to the athlete using EPO lies in the combination of increased red blood cell volume and dehydration during endurance activities. As the number of red blood cells increases, and therefore the proportion of RBC's in the total blood volume increases, the blood begins to thicken and becomes more difficult to move through vital organs; the increased numbers of red blood cells literally begin to clog the capillaries. This situation is exacerbated in endurance athletes because dehydration reduces the volume of plasma in the blood, thereby intensifying the effects of the increased numbers of red blood cells from use of EPO. The indiscriminate use of EPO may substantially increase the risks of hypertension, stroke, heart attack, and even sudden death (Cowart, 1989; Wadler, 1994).

With respect to drug testing, EPO poses a real dilemma because the hormone is rather rapidly metabolized in the liver. Shortly after its administration, it is no longer detectable in the blood, even though the increase in red blood cells continues for several days. Because it is negligibly eliminated in the urine, currently there is no available urine drug testing technique to detect the use of EPO by athletes. Undoubtedly this is one of the primary reasons the International Olympic Committee is now considering the use of blood testing as an indirect marker of EPO abuse as part of its doping control program in the future. Perhaps more than any other drug, erythropoietin highlights the complex issues attendant to the use of performance-enhancing drugs by athletes: EPO does artificially enhance performance and therefore can be considered a means of cheating in sports, it is not detectable by current urine drug testing methods, and it is dangerous.

DRUG TESTING

One of the predominant means of preventing drug abuse in athletes at the college level and beyond, particularly the use of performance-enhancing drugs, is the use of drug testing as a deterrent. Although in many other settings it often is used as a means of secondary prevention (detection of those at an early stage of drug abuse), drug testing in sports also may be considered a means of primary prevention because of the often strict consequences of a positive test (loss of one or more years of eligibility or lifetime banishment from participation in a sport) designed to deter use of drugs. Drug testing in athletics has been, and continues to be, a highly complex and controversial subject. This section is intended only to highlight some of the issues that are completely or substantially unique to sports. For more detailed discussions, the reader is directed to the publications by Wadler and Hainline (1989) and Zemper (1991).

It is imperative that any sports organization that plans to conduct a drug testing program must first explicitly define the philosophical objectives of the program. For example, is it the sole intent of the program to eliminate the use of performance enhancing drugs in order to level the playing field for all competitors? Is it to eliminate the use of all illicit drugs from the sport, whether they are recreational or performance-enhancing? Is it the intent of the sports organization to completely eliminate or to limit the association of its athletes with the use of alcohol and tobacco on the grounds that the organization believes its athletes should be perceived as positive role models ·for young people? The answers to these and similar questions serve as the blueprints for the development of a drug testing program that will fulfill the philosophical objectives of the sports organization.

Sports, as noted in the introduction to this chapter, start in early childhood at the local recreational level and span the athletic spectrum to the international and professional levels. This heterogeneity confounds the already complex subject of drug testing by introducing countless variables—amateur versus professional athletes, type of drug being tested for (performance enhancing, recreational, therapeutic), adult versus minor, drug detectability, rights of privacy and related legal issues, national versus international considerations, the economics of amateur and professional sports, sponsorships, costs, and collective bargaining issues, to name but a few.

To illustrate the complexity of some of these issues and their attendant impact on programs of prevention, two examples will be cited.

Sympathomimetic Amines

Phenylpropanolamine (PPA), ephedrine, and pseudoephedrine are members of a class of drugs referred to as sympathomimetic amines. They are central nervous system stimulants that are readily available as over-the-counter medications. PPA is a common ingredient of diet pills and decongestants. Ephedrine and pseudoephedrine are commonly used in the treatment of asthma, hay fever, sinusitis, allergy rhinitis, and other allergy disorders. When PPA and ephedrine are combined with caffeine, they may simulate amphetamines, and when so combined they have been referred to as the "look-alikes" (Wadler & Hainline, 1989).

Anecdotal evidence suggests that the sympathomimetic amines have been abused in organized sports as a stimulant to improve performance. Thus, it is not surprising that the International Olympic Committee and the U.S. Olympic Committee, as well as the NCAA, have banned these drugs. On the face of it, testing for these drugs appears to make sense. However, according the USOC's *1988 Drug Education and Control Policy* (in Wadler & Hainline, 1989), doping is defined as "the administration of or use by a competing athlete of any substance taken in *abnormal quantity* or taken by an abnormal route of entry into the body with the *sole intention* of increasing in an artificial and unfair manner his/her performance in competition" (p. 257; emphasis ours). Given this definition of doping, the categorical banning of sympathomimetic amines presents a number of very real problems:

— The scientific evidence that therapeutic doses of sympathomimetic amines are in fact performance enhancing is at best scant.
— The urinary excretion patterns of these drugs are not well enough understood to clearly discriminate between therapeutic and ergogenic doses.
— The sympathomimetic amines are legal drugs, usually available as over-the-counter drugs, and are among the most widely used drugs in the United States.

Recent NCAA drug testing data underscore the magnitude of the problem of testing for this category of drugs (F. Uryasz, personal communication, 1991). Between 1986 and 1989, of 12,950 tests administered by the NCAA, there were 392 positive tests. Of these 392 positives, 292 were for sympathomimetic amines and only 100 for other categories of banned drugs. No distinctions were reported between therapeutic doses and abnormally high levels of sympathomimetic amines. Recognizing the aforementioned problems, the NCAA dealt with these findings by not revoking eligibility for positive tests for sympathomimetic amines, and finally removed this category from its list of banned drugs. However, the IOC and the USOC continue to include sympathomimetic amines on their banned lists, as do a number of national sports governing bodies, such as USA Track and Field.

From a practical point of view, there is no question that an athlete may abuse these drugs to obtain an unfair athletic advantage or, more to the point, to cheat. However, the NCAA data strongly suggest that it is more likely that athletes innocently using over-the-counter medications for the symptomatic relief of allergies or an upper respiratory infection might find themselves being banned from a sport, stripped of a championship, and possibly losing their well-earned reputation. Thus, it is entirely reasonable to suggest that the imposition of penalties for athletes testing positive for sympathomimetic amines should be eliminated unless it can be demonstrated that the levels in the urine clearly discriminate between therapeutic use and ergogenic abuse, and that these drugs are in fact performance-enhancing.

Erythropoietin

EPO is not detectable in the urine by currently available drug testing methods. However, it unquestionably is a performance-enhancer. Because EPO is not eliminated in the urine, and more invasive testing techniques such as blood testing have not yet been approved by sports organizations, thought has been given to using tracer amounts of a radioisotope as a marker in all manufactured EPO. Although this would make the use of EPO relatively easy to detect in a sports drug testing situation, because large numbers of patients with chronic anemia receive regular doses of EPO, it is unreasonable to continuously subject these patients to radioactive isotopes in order to prevent the unscrupulous behavior of a relatively few endurance athletes. Because it enhances performance and because it cannot be detected, EPO presents and will continue to present a special and very difficult challenge to the sports community and to its efforts to prevent ergogenic drug abuse.

PREVENTION: WHOSE RESPONSIBILITY?

As indicated at the beginning of this chapter, an individual's exposure to sports begins early in childhood. Along the athletic road, from the child's first participation in sports until the end of

his or her career in high school, college, or professional sports, there are countless individuals, teams, and organizations who are in a position to act as agents of drug abuse prevention and early intervention.

It is essential to reflect on a child's initial motivation for engaging in sports—to have fun, to develop skills, to relate to one's peers. Winning is not a priority! Parents and amateur coaches must be ever-mindful of this. During these early years, attitudinal foundations as well as skill foundations are put into place. Virtually every parent with a child who has participated in sports can recount stories of the local coach who lost sight of these principles.

Similarly, parents must be cautious not to act out their own frustrations, desires, and ambitions through their child. How often has the story been told of the overinvolved parent berating his or her child because of a perceived failure on the part of the child, or of a parent berating a coach, referee or, even worse, someone else's child?

As skills improve and athletic talent is identified, other influences come into play. Although fun is still at the forefront, winning and excelling begin to move to center stage. Making the team and starting take on added significance. However, being a bench jockey and learning to lose graciously also become important elements in the athletic development process. With increasing successes, local fame, together with a developing sense of invincibility, takes on added significance. Formalization of the athletic process—league play and the publication of individual results and team standings—moves the athletic experience to a new level. At the same time, coaches become more skilled, but they also become more invested. It is during these dynamic processes that one must be particularly attentive to the possibility of drug abuse and to the opportunities for prevention and intervention strategies.

The athlete, particularly at the high school level, can be subjected to a great deal of pressure, seeming to live in a fishbowl environment. Whereas a student who does poorly on an exam usually has to deal with such a failure only through a teacher and maybe parents, an athlete who drops a pass or misses a free throw does it in front of teammates, peers, and a major segment of the community, and it may even show up in the local newspaper or on television. Student athletes may have the opportunity for some moments of glory on the athletic field, but they also must face the real risk of criticism from friends and strangers. Young athletes often are ill-equipped to handle such attention, and this provides a setting for easy gravitation toward the use of alcohol and other drugs to help cope. This is where coaches, parents, and peers can provide the support needed to prevent drug use as a means of escape from these pressures.

As noted in the Michigan State study, the majority of athletes who use drugs begin doing so in high school or earlier. This fact alone is a strong indication that the focus for primary prevention efforts must be on the young athlete at the beginning stages of his or her participation in sports. Primary prevention efforts tend to be much less expensive than secondary prevention (such as drug testing) and tertiary prevention (such as mandatory rehabilitation after failing drug tests), which are more appropriately left to the college and professional levels of sport with the money to support them. Primary prevention of the use of performance-enhancing and recreational drugs must begin with the youth sports programs and junior and senior high school sports programs. At these levels, the burden of responsibility will fall on program administrators, and particularly the coaches who interact with the athletes on a regular basis. Beyond the high school level, there are opportunities for primary and secondary prevention for not only the coaches, but also the athletic trainer and the team physician, who become regular members of the sports team at these levels. If a high school has an athletic trainer or a regular team physician (which is seldom the case), obviously they should also be resources for prevention and intervention at this level.

In developing specific prevention and intervention approaches, it must be emphasized that,

as with drug testing, the philosophy of the sports organization must be explicitly defined, whether the organization is a local youth sports group, a high school league, a college or professional sports organization, or a national or international sports governing body. This philosophy must be unquestionably understood by all individuals involved in the chain of command—university presidents, team owners, administrators, athletic directors, coaches, athletic trainers, and team physicians.

It would be naïve to ignore the realities of elite college and professional sports. There are enormous pressures to win and vast amounts of money are at stake. Therefore, it often takes extreme situations before changes in the status quo are initiated. At the international level, it took the amphetamine-related deaths of Danish cyclist Kurt Enemar Knud Jensen during the 1960 Olympics and English cyclist Tommy Simpson during the 1967 Tour de France to get the Medical Commission of the IOC to publish a list of banned drugs for the 1968 Olympics (Wadler & Hainline, 1989). At the national level, the 1986 cocaine-related deaths of University of Maryland basketball star Len Bias and Cleveland Brown football star Don Rogers awakened the United States to the problem of athlete drug abuse. The disqualification of gold medalist Ben Johnson in the 1988 Olympic Games forced major attention to the pervasiveness of anabolic–androgenic steroid abuse. Wadler and Hainline (1989) list more than 200 athletes whose names were prominent in the news during the 1980s for problems related to drug abuse.

The coach, the athletic trainer, and the team physician are professionals with important roles to play in the prevention and early intervention of athlete drug abuse.

The Coach

The coach, at all skill levels, from youth sports to the professional level, sets the tone for the team. In years past, drug abuse (performance-enhancing or recreational drugs) was rarely a subject the coach had to address. This is no longer the case. In addition to establishing the game plan, the coach must set a moral and an ethical standard consistent with the philosophy of the team and the governing body of the sport. Inherent in these standards must be an unambiguous policy, preferably written, concerning drug use by athletes. When that policy is violated, previously defined courses of action must be implemented in a consistent, predictable, and evenhanded manner.

The Athletic Trainer

In college and professional sports, the athletic trainer is in a unique position with respect to drug abuse prevention, detection, and early intervention. The trainer relates to the athlete in a manner distinctly different from others in the team's administrative hierarchy, having the primary day-to-day responsibility of keeping the athlete fit and tending to his or her injuries. There usually is a close bond and a sense of trust between the athletic trainer and the athlete. So entrusted, the trainer has a responsibility to keep abreast of issues regarding the athlete's health and well-being. Included in these issues is the subject of athlete drug use. This subject must be an integral part of the athletic trainer's formal education at the undergraduate, graduate, and continuing education levels. By virtue of his or her relationship with the athlete, the trainer is in a unique position to influence the athlete's decision-making regarding the use and abuse of drugs. In essence, the athletic trainer can be a very significant primary source for drug abuse prevention.

Additionally, it is likely that the athletic trainer will be one of the first members of the team to detect drug abuse by the athlete. In the case of anabolic–androgenic steroids, for example, the trainer may note unusually rapid gains in weight and strength and increased irritability. In the case of cocaine abuse, the trainer may become aware of increased episodes of tardiness, weight loss, and changes in behavior. The ath-

letic trainer is in a special position to facilitate early intervention when such problems are encountered.

The Team Physician

The team physician or sports medicine physician should be a major resource on the subject of drug use for the entire sports organization. However, for the team physician to be effective in this capacity, he or she must have a comprehensive understanding of the subject. As Beresford has noted in Wadler and Hainline (1989, p. 244):

> One might argue that it would be unreasonable to expect a team physician whose specialty is orthopedics to meet the standards that apply to a psychiatrist specializing in the treatment of drug abuse and dependency. However, epidemiologic data suggest considerable drug use and abuse among athletes. This information, coupled with the detailed discussion in this text on the psychophysiologic makeup of the athlete, the drugs used by athletes and the therapeutic, ergogenic, and adverse effects of these drugs, and the principles of recognition and management of drug-related problems, present a compelling argument that team/sports medicine physicians should accept responsibility for recognizing and ensuring proper treatment of athletic drug-related problems.

Without doubt, this concept must be extended to that of drug abuse prevention.

REPRESENTATIVE ORGANIZATIONAL APPROACHES TO PREVENTION

As noted in the previous discussion of the Michigan State studies of the drug use patterns of college athletes, the majority of athletes involved in drug use begin their use in high school or even junior high school. The obvious implication is that any successful drug prevention program for athletes must include a primary component aimed at these younger age groups. This section briefly outlines the drug education programs of two sports organizations, the National Federation of State High School Associations and the National

Collegiate Athletic Association, both of which involve a focus on the young athlete at the high school and junior high school level.

National Federation of State High School Associations

In 1984, the National Federation of State High School Associations (NFSHSA) established a nonprofit organization named TARGET as a service to assist schools develop and implement drug education programs. Information on TARGET programs is distributed by the NFSHSA to all local schools through each state high school activities association. The TARGET approach is to foster a coalition of school staff, parents, community leaders, and student leaders in each school to address the problems of tobacco, alcohol, and other drugs. A primary focus is to train and encourage student leaders, including athletes, to take advantage of opportunities to lead and demonstrate positive role-modeling skills among their peers with regard to drug use and other health and well-being issues. A basic assumption is that student leaders are a major peer influence in any school, and that most often these leaders are involved in athletics, music, and other activities. It is a flexible approach that can be used to help implement new programs or to complement and strengthen existing programs.

TARGET provides a number of support resources, including a student leadership training program, free and low-cost printed materials, videotapes, monthly publications, and, for athletes, a program emphasizing the dangers of anabolic–androgenic steroids and other performance-enhancing drugs. Technical assistance is offered through a National Resource Center at the NFSHSA national office.

A primary TARGET tool to reach school athletes, parents, and staff is the preseason meeting. Before the start of each athletic season, a meeting is held for athletes, parents, school administrators, and coaches. During this meeting, information is provided to athletes and parents regarding a number of important issues, including insurance, physicals, district policies, program philosophy, eligibility, team policies, and schedules. There also is discussion of concerns unique to athletes, such as eating disorders, drug use (performance-enhancing and recreational), and the potential for physical injury while participating in sports. Specific guidelines, rules, and consequences of rule violations are discussed and, before participation is allowed, all athletes and their parents must sign a statement affirming that they understand the policies regarding team rules and drug use and that they understand the physical risks of sports participation. These meetings also present the opportunity to get parents more directly involved in the school program, opening lines of communication and establishing shared responsibility for school programs. These preseason meetings have proven so successful that many schools now have them for other school programs besides athletics.

National Collegiate Athletic Association

The NCAA Drug Education Committee was formed in 1973 and has developed programs that reach out to the grade school, junior high, high school, and college athlete. A brief overview of the scope of these activities is presented to illustrate the types of programs this sports organization is implementing.

Publications and Educational Materials

Educational materials available from the NCAA include *Drugs and the Athlete . . . a Losing Combination,* a nine-page booklet presenting facts, myths, and possible side effects of frequently abused drugs; and *Alcohol Choices and Guidelines for College Students,* a publication included in a packet distributed each year to more than 500,000 first-year students—athletes and nonathletes—at colleges and universities throughout the nation. Also available are posters dealing with anabolic–androgenic steroids and other performance enhancing drugs; and *The Sports Sciences Education Newsletter,* a quarterly newsletter mailed to all athletic directors, senior administrators, head athletic trainers, and counseling centers at all NCAA member institutions, containing up-to-date information on drug abuse prevention, drug testing, and other health and wellness issues.

In addition to a bibliography of drug education videotapes available for purchase or rent from a variety of sources, the NCAA has its own videotapes available describing the policies and procedures of the NCAA drug testing program, and a four-part videotape series, *Drugs and the Collegiate Athlete*, with an instructional manual, combining classroom instruction with video support. Drug education research by the NCAA includes the Michigan State studies *Substance Use and Abuse Habits of College Student Athletes,* described earlier in this chapter, and the *NCAA Annual Drug Education Survey,* begun in 1984, which includes a list of all NCAA member institutions that have drug education or drug testing programs in place.

Drug Education Programs

The NCAA sponsors programs in drug use prevention, intervention, and education that reach out to college student athletes, coaches, and athletic administrators, as well as grade school, junior high, and high school students. A speaker's grant program provides funding for speakers for athletic department drug education or wellness programs at member schools, and each year a major portion of the money ($3.5 million in 1990–91) from the NCAA basketball championship television contract is distributed to conferences that sponsor Division I men's and women's basketball, with the requirement that a portion of the money be used to establish drug education programs and services for athletes and staff. Each year, the NCAA also produces several 15- to 30-second public service videotapes about drug and alcohol abuse that are televised during NCAA championships as well as at other times on request. Full or partial funding also is provided by the NCAA for innovative research, development, and implementation of model drug education programs with special emphasis on the unique needs of college athletes.

Two major youth-oriented programs are sponsored by the NCAA: Youth Education through Sports (YES) and the National Youth Sports Program (NYSP). The YES program is directed at students aged 10–18 years, and is offered at selected NCAA championship sites throughout the year. In addition to sports skill instruction, sessions about drug abuse prevention are led by student athletes and local drug education experts. The NYSP is directed at 10- to 16-year-old economically disadvantaged youth. It is conducted at 139 institutions of higher education each summer and 45 institutions from October through April. In addition to drug abuse prevention techniques, presentation topics include nutrition, personal health, career opportunities and job responsibilities, and opportunities in higher education.

Drug Testing Program

A major component of the NCAA drug program is the drug testing program. It is far beyond the scope of this chapter to discuss this intricate program in detail. However, the preamble to the program underscores its intent.

> With their approval of Proposal No. 30 at the January 1986 Convention and Proposal Nos. 52–54 at the January 1990 Convention, NCAA member institutions reaffirmed their dedication to the ideal of fair and equitable competition at their championships and postseason certified events. At the same time, they took another step in the protection of the health and safety of the student athletes competing therein. So that no one participant might have an artificially induced advantage, so that no one participant might be pressured to use chemical substances in order to remain competitive, and to safeguard the health and safety of participants, this NCAA drug-testing program has been created.

In recognition of the pharmacodynamics of anabolic–androgenic steroids, and of the fact that the ergogenicity of these drugs may persist long after use of the drug is discontinued, the NCAA modified its drug testing program beginning in August 1990. The new program included not only testing at NCAA championship events but also random testing for anabolic–androgenic steroids in Division I football players throughout the year. More recently, this program was expanded to include Division I track and field athletes, and the intent is to gradually expand to other divisions and sports in the future. Also included in the year-round testing program are diuretics (used in an attempt to mask the presence of steroids in the urine) and other urine manipulators. The NCAA drug testing program, with its loss of championships and loss of eligibility sanctions for athletes testing positive, is designed to be a primary prevention tool. Any secondary or tertiary prevention activities (such as rehabilitation) are left to the individual member schools to develop and implement.

In addition to the national program, the NCAA has developed guidelines for NCAA member institutions wishing to implement their own drug testing programs. Within the framework of these institutional programs, the individual institutions are advised to develop, distribute, and publicize the specific policy of their institution. The policy should include such information as: "(a) a clear explanation of the purposes of the drug-testing program; (b) who will be tested and by what methods; (c) the drugs to be tested for, how often, and under what conditions (i.e., announced, unannounced or both), and (d) the actions, if any, to be taken against those who test positive." (National Collegiate Athletic Association, 1990, p. 16).

SUMMARY

This chapter has underscored the complexity of issues to be addressed when considering prevention and early intervention strategies of drug abuse within the context of organized sports. These strategies must be an integral part of sport at all levels of participation. They must commence as soon as a child begins to participate in organized sports, when the primary motivations for participation are fun, fitness, and an opportunity to relate to one's peers. Subsequently, these strategies must be integrated into every level of organized sports, including the professional level, where the motivation is primarily career-oriented.

The facts and studies cited in this chapter provide an important data base on which to build both general and sport-specific drug prevention and early intervention strategies that can be applied at all levels of organized sports. Furthermore, while society has focused on the complex issues and consequences of recreational drug abuse, sports organizations must also cope with the complexities of ergogenic drug abuse.

The development of a program of drug abuse prevention and early intervention in sports requires leadership and governance in each sport, whether at the community level or the professional level, to articulate its philosophic goals and objectives relative to drug use and abuse. Predicated on these goals and objectives, specific programs can be developed and implemented. Too often, provoked by a crisis, sports organizations and other societal institutions have responded with quick fixes and poorly conceived programs.

The information presented in this chapter provides a strong indication that a major portion of drug abuse prevention in sports must take place from the beginning of a child's participation in organized sports. Primary prevention generally is less expensive than secondary or tertiary prevention, and is the most reasonable approach for youth sports organizations and school sports programs. One focus should be training the coach in the importance and the techniques of primary drug abuse prevention, because at these levels (aside from parents) the coach is the only member of the sports organization with regular contact and with any real influence on the athletes. Effort also must be made to involve the parents of athletes. One successful approach to implementing prevention programs is through the use of preseason meetings, as described in the section on the TARGET program. This approach directly involves all members of the sports organization: athletes, parents, coaches, and administrators. The TARGET program provides complete information on organizing pre-season meetings and makes available low-cost and free educational materials to be used in these meetings, including materials produced by the NCAA. At the college level and beyond, where members of the sports medicine community become more prominent members of the sports organization, the athletic trainer and the team physician should begin to shoulder much of the responsibility for drug abuse prevention.

To be effective, the sports medicine community, as well as sports organizations, must be credible. That credibility must rest on state-of-the-art knowledge about drug use in sports, not on hearsay and anecdotes. Although sports management, coaches, athletic trainers, and sports medicine physicians may understandably feel uncomfortable with this very complex subject, they cannot escape their very real responsibilities as agents of drug abuse prevention and early intervention in sports.

REFERENCES

American Institutes for Research (1988). Studies of intercollegiate athletes—Report no. 1. Summary results from the 1987–88 national study of intercollegiate athletes. Palo Alto, CA: AIR.

Anderson, W. A., Albrecht, R. R., & McKeag, D. B. (1993). *Second replication of a national study of the substance use and abuse habits of college student-athletes.* East Lansing: College of Human Medicine, Michigan State University.

Anderson, W. A., & McKeag, D. B. (1985). *The substance use and abuse habits of college-student athletes.* East Lansing: College of Human Medicine, Michigan State University.

Anderson, W. A., & McKeag, D. B. (1989). *Replication of the national study of the substance abuse habits of college student-athletes.* East Lansing: College of Human Medicine, Michigan State University.

Benowitz, N. L., Jacob, J., III, & Yu, L. (1989). Daily use of smokeless tobacco: Systemic effects. *Annals of Internal Medicine, 111,* 112–116.

Buckley, W. E., Yesalis, C. E., Friedl, K. E., Anderson, A. L., Streit, J. E., & Wright, J. E. (1988). Estimated prevalence of anabolic steroid use among high school seniors. *JAMA, 260,* 3441–3445.

Clark, N., Nelson, M., & Evans, W. (1988). Nutrition education for elite female runners. *Phys Sportsmed, 16,* 124–136.

Connolly, G. N., Orleans, T. C., & Kogan, M. (1988). Use of smokeless tobacco in major league baseball. *New England Journal of Medicine, 318,* 1281–1285.

Cowart, V. S. (1989). Erythropoietin: A dangerous new form of blood doping? *Physician and Sports Medicine, 17* (8), 115–117.

Cowart, V. S. (1990). Blunting 'steroid epidemic' requires alternatives, innovative education. *JAMA, 264,* 1641.

Edwards, S. W., Glover, E. D., & Schroeder, K. L. (1987). The effects of smokeless tobacco on heart rate and neuromuscular reactivity in athletes and nonathletes. *Physician and Sports Medicine, 15* (7), 141.

Elite Women Athletes Survey (1987). Minneapolis, MN: Hazelden Health Promotion Services.

Ernster, V. L., Grady, D. G., Greene, J. C., Walsh, M., Robertson, P., Daniels, T. E., Benowitz, N., Siegel, D., Gerbert, B., & Hauck, W. W. (1990). Smokeless tobacco use and health effects among baseball players. *JAMA, 264,* 218–224.

Goldstein, A., & Kalant, H. (1990). Drug policy: Striking the right balance. *Science, 249,* 1513–1521.

Kashkin, K. D., & Kleber, H. D. (1989). Hooked on hormones? *JAMA, 262,* 22.

Kelly, D. (1990). Students say sports is key to college aid. *USA Today,* Nov. 26, 1A.

Kirshenbaum, D. S. (1984). Self-regulation and sport psychology: Nurturing an emerging symbiosis. *Journal of Sports Psychology, 6,* 159.

National Collegiate Athletic Association (1989). *1988 Division I academic reporting compilation.* Overland Park, KS: NCAA.

National Collegiate Athletic Association (1990). *NCAA drug testing/education programs, 1990/91.* Overland Park, KS: NCAA.

National Federation of State High School Associations (1990). *Annual report of participation in high school sports.* Kansas City, MO: NFSHSA.

Nicholl, Jr., A. M. (1987). Psychiatric consultation in professional football. *New England Journal of Medicine, 16,* 1095.

Pope, H., & Katz, D. (1988). Affective and psychotic symptoms associated with anabolic steroid use. *JAMA, 145,* 487–489.

Rosecan, J. S., Spitz, H. I., & Gross, B. (1987). In H. I. Spitz & J. S. Rosecan (Eds.), *Cocaine abuse—New directions in treatment and research.* New York: Brunner/Mazel.

Sklarek, H. M., Montavani, R. P., Erens, E., Niederman, M. S., Fein, A. M., & Heisler, D. (1984). AIDS in a bodybuilder using anabolic steroids. *New England Journal of Medicine, 31,* 1701.

Spillich, G. J. (Aug. 1987). Cigarette smoking and memory: Good news and bad news, presented at the 95th Annual Meeting of the American Psychological Association.

USA Today/NBC News Poll (1990). *USA Today,* Sept. 10–14.

U.S. General Accounting Office (Aug. 1989). Drug misuse—Anabolic steroids and human growth hormone. Report to the Chairman, Committee on the Judiciary, U.S. Senate, GAO/HRD-89-109.

Vallerand, R. J., Deci, E. L., & Ryan, R. M. (1987). Intrinsic motivation in sports. *Exercise and Sports Science Review, 15,* 389.

Wadler, G. I. (1994). Drug abuse update. *Medical Clinics of North America, 78,* 439.

Wadler, G. I., & Hainline, B. (1989). *Drugs and the athlete.* Philadelphia: F.A. Davis.

Warren, B. J., Stanton, A. L., & Blessing, D. L. (1990). Disordered eating patterns in competitive female athletes. *International Journal of Eating Disorders, 9,* 565–569.

Winn, D. M., Blot, W. J., Shy, C. M., Pickle, L. W., Toledo, A., & Fraumeni, Jr., J. F. (1981). Snuff dipping and oral cancer among women in the southern United States. *New England Journal of Medicine, 304,* 745–749.

Wright, J. E., & Cowart, V. S. (1990). *Anabolic steroids: Altered states.* Carmel IN: Benchmark Press.

Zemper, E. D. (1991). Drug testing in athletics. In R. H. Coombs & L. West (Eds.), *Drug testing: Issues and options.* New York: Oxford University Press.

CHAPTER 11

ADVERTISING INDUSTRY

ROGER G. PISANI

ADVERTISING SELLS, BUT CAN IT "UNSELL"?

The classic role of advertising is to sell a product or service by attracting new users or motivating users of another brand to switch. It is accepted in the business world that advertising sells products. Though criticized in some circles, it is instructive to see how other community segments employ this tactic—universities advertise for students, religious organizations advertise for donations, and politicians advertise for votes. We know advertising can sell, but can it also "unsell"? Can well-targeted, compelling advertisements develop and reinforce antidrug attitudes? Can they reduce demand by deglamorizing illegal drugs and those who use them?

It is important to recognize that media advertising does not exist in a precisely measurable, controlled environment. In the commercial world, sales are also affected by pricing, distribution, level of trade and consumer promotions, and competitive activity. Public service announcements have been created to affect attitudes about substance abuse, and exist in an environment of school and workplace education programs, public and private sector community programs, and major news events such as the cocaine-induced death of basketball player Len Bias.

It is difficult to measure how media advertising affects attitudes and drug use. Therefore, the intent of this chapter is not to provide solutions, but to examine and illustrate the role of advertising in substance abuse prevention.

The focus will be on the classic public service announcement (PSA) used to deliver a message (television, radio, print), as opposed to editorial or programming messages. Although reference will be made to advertising of age-legal products (tobacco and alcohol), emphasis will be placed on drugs that are illegal to all age groups. There have been a number of small-scale studies of advertising's effect on drug attitudes and usage, particularly on the public service campaigns of the late '70s and early '80s. Although lessons learned from these latter studies will be examined, focus will be on the latest, and by far most extensive antidrug advertising effort, conducted by the Partnership for a Drug-Free America. We will examine elements that appear critical to the intelligent development and placement of antidrug messages.

A BRIEF HISTORY OF PUBLIC SERVICE ADVERTISING

The power of modern media has long been recognized, from presidential fireside chats to Jimmy Conners' "Nupe It" commercials. The average American child will spend more time watching television than any other activity and research indicates that learning takes place during viewing (Pearl et al., 1982; Roberts, 1983). Studies also indicate that the media are a prime source of substance abuse information (Sheppard, 1980; Mayton et al., 1990; Mirzale et al., 1991).

It is obvious, then, that any organization seeking to influence substance abusing behavior must consider media-delivered messages that build antidrug attitudes.

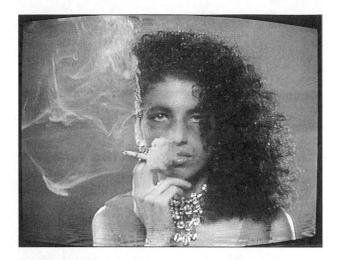

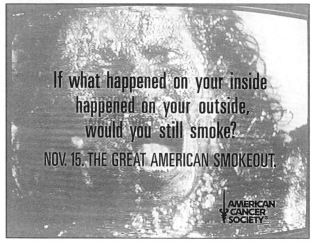

FIGURE 11.1.   These two frames from an American Cancer Society TV message clearly show its targeting of young women. Reprinted with permission of the American Cancer Society.

Cigarettes

The first broad use of modern advertising techniques to reduce substance abuse was the antismoking campaigns of the late 1960s. The social and political environment for this effort was set by media coverage of the Surgeon General's Report, constant advocacy by such groups as the American Cancer Society and the American Heart Association and, perhaps in small part, by a convert, Emerson Foote. A famous advertising executive, Foote supervised the Lucky Strike account for many years. He resigned as chair of the McCann–Erickson agency in 1964 and immediately took up the chair of the National Agency Council on Smoking and Health. Representing this antismoking organization at a November 1965 White House conference on health protection, Foote chided the American Medical Association for failing to endorse the Surgeon General's Report while accepting a $10,000 research grant from the tobacco industry.

In a public notice dated June 6, 1967, the Federal Communications Commission (FCC) stated that its Fairness Doctrine applies to cigarette advertising and ordered that stations carrying cigarette commercials provide "a significant amount of time for the other viewpoint." Encouraged by this ruling, antismoking activists mounted substantial antismoking media campaigns.

A study called *Mass Media and Smoking Cessation* (Flay, 1987) analyzed forty mass media campaigns and concluded that "the counter advertising campaign of 1967–70 under the Fairness Doctrine . . . demonstrates convincingly that mass media played an important role in changes in smoking prevalence. Our confidence in these findings is enhanced because cigarette consumption started to increase again upon the removal of counter ads after cigarette advertising was banned from radio and television" (p. 77). Several conditions contributed to this effectiveness: a number of novel spots rather than just one or two, widespread dissemination, high saturation (estimated value of the campaign in 1970 was $75,000,000), and continuity over time (almost three years).

More recent antismoking advertising includes TV messages by the American Cancer Society and a major 1990 multimedia effort in the State of California funded by a 25-cent excise tax on the sale of cigarettes. The campaign, with an estimated 1990 value of $29,000,000, addresses various age groups as well as African-Americans, Hispanics, and Asian-Americans.

Pre- and postadvertising research shows a significant increase in the percentage of smokers thinking about quitting (Popham et al., 1991). The number of California students who considered quitting went from 43.1% precampaign to 48.1% postcampaign. Adult smokers contemplating quitting went from 38.6% to 42%. There was a reduction in percentage of students smoking, from 12.8% pre- to 10.9% postcampaign.

A concurrent usage study (Burns et al., 1992), conducted during the anticigarette campaign and compared with 1987 estimates of California smoking prevalence from national studies, indicated a 17% decline in smoking prevalence.

It is unlikely that this decline can be attributed to the recent media campaign. Many people involved with the California anticigarette campaign believe that media did have a positive effect, but that the significant price increase was a greater factor in smoking cessation. Tobacco tax funds paid for this media effort. Unfortunately, the 1991–92 state budget crisis resulted in cancellation of the planned $32 million budget for 1991–92 media; excise tax, going instead, into the state's general budget.

Alcohol

The country may not have legalized alcohol for drinkers under 21, but it certainly seems to be "normalized," as Table 11.1 illustrates.

Television, the major medium affecting young people, permits wine and beer advertising. A number of studies show that young people who are aware of beer advertising generally have a more favorable attitude toward drinking (Strickland, 1982; Grube et al., 1991). These same studies state that no effect of advertising exposure on total consumption has been demonstrated (see Table 11.2).

In Canada, some provinces permit alcohol broadcast advertising, whereas others do not. Although studies show no significant difference in adult consumption of alcohol in these provinces (Horgan, 1986), fatal alcohol-related motor vehicle accidents per 100,000 population were actually lower in broadcast markets (Simpson et al., 1985).

There appears to be limited research on the effectiveness of national antialcohol campaigns. In 1982, NIAAA mounted an antialcohol campaign, but only 12 messages were produced and subsequent evaluations indicated that limited air time was given to these PSAs (Field et al., 1983). An examination of the University of Michigan High School Senior Survey for this period shows no significant increases or decreases in overall consumption or in students' perceptions of risk from trying one or two alcoholic beverages (Johnson, 1981, 1982, 1983).

Alcoholic beverages can be legally sold to, and therefore consumed by, the majority of the

TABLE 11.1   Alcohol Use (1992)

	EVER	PAST 30 DAYS
NIDA Household Survey (12–17 yr)	46.4%	24.5%
Gordon Black Survey (13–17 yr)	71.6	36.9
University of Michigan Survey (High School Seniors)	87.5	51.3

American public. When abused, alcohol physically harms the user and negatively affects the nonuser through alcohol-related accidents, higher insurance rates, lost productivity, and birth defects. Largely activated by these secondary effects, advocacy groups have formed to ban alcoholic beverages and make marketing more difficult through advertising restrictions, increased taxes, and restricted distribution.

Aware that restrictive legislation would hurt sales, the liquor industry undertook an alcohol abuse awareness and education program using the same marketing techniques they employ to sell their products. Anheuser-Busch developed the first major program in late 1982. The objective was to build responsible personal attitudes regarding underage drinking and drunk driving.

Underage Drinking

Almost uniformly, the legal drinking age in the United States is 21 years. Because manufacturers of alcoholic products want people 21 and over to be responsible consumers, it is inconceivable that the manufacturers would direct their messages to the under-21 group. Their strategy directs messages to parents of young people to remind them that parents must take personal responsibility in setting examples to be observed by the family, and to people who sell alcoholic products, the gatekeepers who are expected to deny service to underage drinkers.

Drunk Driving

"Know when to say when," the creative theme for all Anheuser-Busch educational programs, has specific relevance for potential drinking and driving situations. Five of the company's TV messages and two radio messages were specifically designed to encourage the designated driver program. National alcohol producers have joined local independent beer wholesalers to promote "don't drink and drive" messages:

TABLE 11.2   Effect of "Know When to Say When" Message

	TOTAL ADULT POPULATION	BEER DRINKERS	COLLEGE STUDENTS
Aware of "know when to say when" message	64%	76%	80%
"Know when to say when" means:			
• don't drink and drive	68	72	85
• stop drinking before you get intoxicated	68	70	74
Message is effective in encouraging responsible consumption of alcoholic beverages	68	72	81

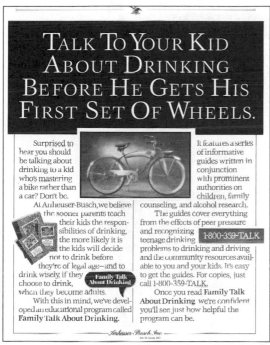

TALK TO YOUR KID ABOUT DRINKING BEFORE HE GETS HIS FIRST SET OF WHEELS.

Surprised to hear you should be talking about drinking to a kid who's mastering a bike rather than a car? Don't be.

At Anheuser-Busch, we believe the sooner parents teach their kids the responsibilities of drinking, the more likely it is the kids will decide not to drink before they're of legal age—and to drink wisely, if they choose to drink, when they become adults.

With this in mind, we've developed an educational program called Family Talk About Drinking.

It features a series of informative guides written in conjunction with prominent authorities on children, family counseling, and alcohol research.

The guides cover everything from the effects of peer pressure and recognizing teenage drinking problems to drinking and driving and the community resources available to you and your kids. It's easy to get the guides. For copies, just call 1-800-359-TALK.

Once you read Family Talk About Drinking we're confident you'll see just how helpful the program can be.

1-800-359-TALK

Anheuser-Busch, Inc.
Inc. St. Louis, MO

FIGURE 11.2. Alcohol producers and marketers are attempting to educate parents about underage drinking.
Reprinted with permission of Anheuser-Busch, Inc.

- "Alert Cab" and "I'm Driving" are two promotions that encourage responsible behavior by offering reduced price cab rides and promoting the designated-driver concept.

- Students Against Drunk Driving (SADD) undertakes educational and self-help programs for teenage students with financial help from Anheuser-Busch.

- The T.I.P.S. program has been established to train bar and liquor store sales personnel to detect and intervene in underage and alcohol abuse situations in public establishments.

The paid media value of the "Know when to say when" campaign from its inception through 1990 is approximately $75,000,000. Research undertaken in 1990 by the Roper Organization shows the enormous awareness generated by this program; 76% of beer drinkers and 80% of college students were aware of it.

Figures published in June 1990 by the U.S. Department of Transportation show that the proportion of all traffic deaths involving a drunk driver is down 16% (from 46.3% in 1982 to 41.1% in 1986 and 39.0% in 1989); the number of teenage (ages 15–19) drunk drivers in fatal crashes is down 40% (from 2,187 in 1982 to 1,711 in 1986 and 1,311 in 1989); the proportion of teenage drivers in fatal crashes who were drunk is down 39% (from 28.4% in 1982 to 21.0% in 1986 to 17.0% in 1989). These favorable trends have carried over into the '90s. Although a direct causal relationship between moderation-promoting advertising and improvements noted in DWI data is impossible to establish, logic suggests, as it does for antismoking campaigns, that sustained, frequent, and powerful advertising can affect attitude and behavior in a positive way.

HISTORICAL ANTIDRUG ADVERTISING

In 1978, the National Institute on Drug Abuse (NIDA) initiated a nationwide media campaign as part of its efforts to prevent drug abuse. The goals of the campaign were to increase public awareness that drug abuse can be prevented, to motivate segments of the population in direct contact with young people aged 8 to 20 to improve their prevention knowledge and skills, and to inform or remind organizations and individuals working with youth of their role in drug abuse prevention. The campaign used PSA announcements for radio and TV, and posters and pamphlets distributed to federal and local agencies. Campaign material was disseminated to stations through Single State Authorities (coordinated government departments) and local drug prevention organizations, with a kick-off coinciding with Drug Abuse Prevention Week (January 17, 1978). The approximate duration of the campaign was 18 weeks. The estimated media value of PSA TV time received was $2,600,000; use of other media could not be determined.

A summary evaluation of this effort (Teh-wei Hu et al., 1982) was based on research conducted via phone interviews with 5,455 respondents in

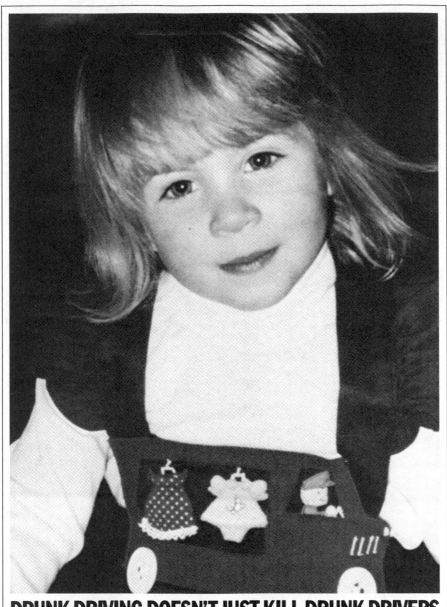

DRUNK DRIVING DOESN'T JUST KILL DRUNK DRIVERS.

Andrea Harris, killed August 26, 1991 at 6:00pm on El Camino Real, Atascadero, California.

FIGURE 11.3. Private and public sector campaigns have contributed to the declining drinking and driving accident figures. "Friends Don't Let Friends Drive Drunk" is a long-maintained effort of The Department of Transportation and the Ad Council.

10 selected cities. It concluded that an estimated 10% of the target audience (age 12–65) remembered seeing the TV messages and that 71% of respondents were extremely concerned about drug abuse; 24% expressed involvement or planned involvement. This was 6 to 10 points higher than in the control city, Seattle. It also concluded that "there is no empirical evidence and direct quantitative measurement on the effects of these indicators on the reduction in drug abuse."

An overview of this media-based antidrug effort provided useful cautions for organizations considering similar PSA campaigns:

— It can be difficult to get media to run PSA material.
— It can be difficult to know precisely when it was run.
— Media messages must have sufficient weight and duration to have any measurable effect.
— Ongoing tracking research is needed.
— The ability of broad-scale, affordable research to identify causal relationships is limited.

Furthermore, even the best PSA campaigns can make an impact only when the target public (and the media) have already been sensitized to the issue through "external" events, such as the Surgeon General's Report on smoking or the growing awareness of the illegal drug problem that occurred in the 1980s when a major antidrug effort was undertaken.

"Just Say No," a phrase summarizing Nancy Reagan's commitment to substance abuse prevention, became a rallying cry in the early '80s and formed the creative basis for a multimedia campaign launched by NIDA in October 1983. In conjunction with the Ad Council, the campaign had as its main objectives to motivate young people to resist peer pressure to try drugs, and to motivate parents to learn about drugs, to talk to their children about the drug problem, and to join with other parents in a stand against drugs in their community. The campaign consisted of two PSAs targeted to youth and one targeted to parents in TV and radio, plus magazine, newspaper, and transit ads, brochures, bumper stickers, posters, and buttons. Broadcast messages were distributed to the major networks, 800 local TV stations, and 6,000 radio stations.

Two types of research were conducted to evaluate the campaign in the phase researched (October 1983 to April 1984). The first was pre- and postcampaign attitudinal surveys among the target groups in two media and two nonmedia control markets. It was concluded that the PSAs had not been run with a sufficient weight to provide any meaningful evaluation. The second was postcampaign interviews with the public affairs directors of radio and TV stations in the surveyed markets. Again, useful conclusions can be drawn. Stations can receive more than 150 PSA spots per month; ideally, spots should be hand-delivered with an accompanying "sales pitch" or they get lost. The broadcast tape format must be known for each TV station (2-inch, 1-inch, or 3/4-inch). The campaign must be timed to accommodate broadcasters' schedules because there is less space available for PSAs in seasons of high commercial demand, such as Christmas. Furthermore, spot length is important: 10-, 15-and 30-second spots are best, and longer spots are less likely to be aired. Locally produced spots or those that can be adapted for a local reference normally get more air time than "national" messages. Finally it is important to match station format and message format. It is unproductive to send a rap spot to a country/western radio station.

There appears to be no clear statistical proof that the "Just Say No" campaign had a major impact in building widespread antidrug attitudes. However, it should be noted that during the years this phrase was widely quoted in the media, the American public became increasingly concerned about the consequences of illegal drug use. It was during this period of public concern that the first major private sector attack on illegal drugs began.

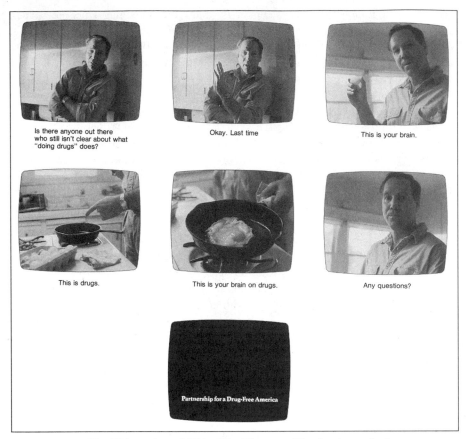

Is there anyone out there who still isn't clear about what "doing drugs" does?

Okay. Last time

This is your brain.

This is drugs.

This is your brain on drugs.

Any questions?

Partnership for a Drug-Free America

FIGURE 11.4. The TV version of "Fried Egg" is one of the best-recalled messages in the history of the medium.
Reprinted with permission of the Partnership for a Drug-Free America.

CURRENT ANTIDRUG ADVERTISING: THE PARTNERSHIP FOR A DRUG-FREE AMERICA

The most recent, and by far the largest, ongoing public service advertising effort against illegal drugs has been mounted by the Partnership for a Drug-Free America.

The Partnership for a Drug-Free America is a nonprofit private sector coalition of volunteers from advertising, public relations, production, talent guilds, research, and media companies. It was conceived in 1986 by Phil Joanou, chairman of the Dailey Advertising Agency, who believed that the disciplines used by the communications industry to sell billions of dollars worth of goods could be used to "unsell" illegal drugs. The advertising industry, through the Ad Council, has long been involved in creating public service messages, from "Loose Talk Costs Lives" during World War II to "Smokey the Bear." Because it was felt that the problem of illegal drugs was severe enough to warrant a separate industry effort, in the fall of 1986, the American Association of Advertising Agencies (AAAA) agreed to fund the startup of the partnership. Today, the Partnership is sponsored by corporations and foundations. The Partnership differs from most advocacy groups in that it is made up of communication experts rather than health, academic, government, or community experts (although these experts are called on for counsel). Under the leadership of Dick O'Reilly, a small paid staff and a large group of volunteers studied the issue of substance abuse prevention in the same way they would approach a product marketing problem. Beginning with research, they developed basic, creative, constituent, and community strategy. Salient features are an estimated $1 billion in donated media and an excellent PSA placement.

For example, in 1991 the American Broadcasting Corporation (ABC) television network ran 663 Partnership messages, 55% in prime time. A close relationship with the advertising and production community has resulted in approximately 100 advertising agencies donating creative, production, and media talent to develop more than 400 different antidrug messages that receive high recall. Of surveyed children ages 9–11, 93% recalled seeing or hearing a specific antidrug ad, as did 95% of teenagers (ages 13–17) and 97% of adults (Gordon Black Corporation National Survey, 1992).

Research

Research was undertaken with the Gordon S. Black Corporation in three broad areas: a literature review undertaken in the fall of 1986 to ascertain what can be learned from history; a qualitative research with preteens, teens, adults, and parents in the fall/winter of 1986; and quantitative research conducted in 1987 among 6,000 preteens, teens, adults, and parents. This survey provided the base by which attitude and usage changes have been subsequently tracked. Results from this survey, in addition to input from academic, government, and health care experts, formed the body of knowledge from which basic strategy was developed.

Basic Strategy to Define the Product

Based on research findings and the advertising experience of staff and volunteers, several broad strategies were agreed on, with the single overall objective of reducing demand for illegal drugs by deglamorizing drugs and those who use them. The product strategy concentrated on illegal drugs for all age groups. There were two major reasons for this decision. At the time the Partnership was founded, there were several public and private sector organizations using the media to speak out against tobacco and alcohol, but no major mass media effort against illegal drugs had been implemented. Strategically, it was felt that the credibility and hence the effectiveness of the illegal drug message could be diminished when linked to substances that are or soon will be legal for the target audience to consume. "Hell, they say marijuana is bad and beer is bad, but Dad drinks beer and he's fine, so how bad can marijuana be?"

As a second consideration, it was decided that although the Partnership should create general antidrug messages, where possible these messages would be drug-specific to marijuana, cocaine, and crack. Although the great majority of the American public considers all illegal drugs to be bad, there are degrees of perceived risk. One cannot credibly talk about marijuana in the same way as crack; therefore, drug-specific messages would enhance the credibility needed for an effective antidrug message.

Creative Strategies for the Target Audience

Target Nonusers

Research showed that the majority of young people (ages 9–12) were nonusers but that 1 in 6 had been approached to try illegal drugs. The first effort, therefore, would be to provide preteens and teens with reasons not to initiate substance use. These same messages might help the occasional user, but it was widely recognized they would have little or no impact on substance abusers. This segment of the population needs professional treatment, not media messages.

Target marketing is essential in selling products and services and is no less critical in developing effective antidrug messages. One cannot talk to an 11-year-old in the same way as a 19-year-old; to be effective, messages must recognize the problems and responses of the various age groups targeted. In addition to a 9–12 age target, research

TOP TEN MOST BOGUS THINGS ON EARTH

10. The Donut Diet.
9. Cars that can talk.
8. "Do Not Remove Under Penalty Of Law" tags on mattresses.
7. Pop quiz on Monday following major weekend.
6. 1-900-DEBBY.
5. Lawn flamingos.
4. Imitation cheese.
3. Referee in Professional wrestling.
2. Did we mention the pop quiz?
1. Drugs.

PARTNERSHIP FOR A DRUG-FREE AMERICA

FIGURE 11.5. Print is not a key medium for reaching teens, but there are some appropriate vehicles for appropriate copy.
Reprinted with permission of the Partnership for a Drug-Free America.

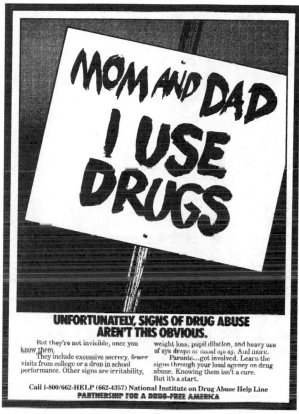

FIGURE 11.6. Many Partnership ads target influencers. Reprinted with permission of the Partnership for a Drug-Free America.

was conducted and advertising agencies briefed to create messages for teenagers 13–15, 16–18, college students, and young adults. Subsequently, 6- to 8-year-olds were added as a specific target.

A need was also recognized to target "influencers," people who, because of their position, have a significant role to play in discouraging experimentation and reducing demand. The most important influencers are parents, managers in the workplace, and healthcare professionals. Each of these groups was targeted in the media with messages appropriate to them.

Although there have been many successful advertising campaigns using famous spokespeople, the Partnership decided not to follow this route. Discussions with teenagers showed a fair

degree of cynicism; "they get paid for saying that," teenagers often respond. Spokespeople messages tend to be "talking head" messages—that is, executed in a simple, talking-to-the-camera style—not the most compelling executional format. Also, today's star spokesperson could be tomorrow's busted-in-a-raid headline. Similar conclusions regarding celebrity spokespersons have been reached by subsequent researchers (Mayton et al., 1990).

Constituent Strategies: Volunteers

The Partnership for a Drug-Free America was established as a volunteer coalition of professionals and companies in the communications industry.

"MY COMPANY'S TOO SMALL TO HAVE A DRUG PROBLEM."

No company's too small. Nearly three-fourths of all illegal drug users are employed. They could be working for you. And they'll cost you: in absenteeism, on-site accidents, higher insurance rates and lower productivity.

So call **1-800-843-4971** for a free guide on how to implement a drug-free workplace. Because unless you act, your small business could get swallowed up by something a lot bigger.

PARTNERSHIP FOR A DRUG-FREE AMERICA

FIGURE 11.7. With the majority of large corporations now having antidrug policies in place, Partnership workplace messages focus on small businesses. Reprinted with permission of the Partnership for a Drug-Free America.

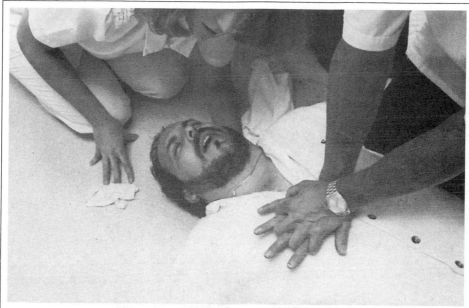

**BEFORE GIVING LIDOCAINE,
ASK ABOUT COCAINE, OR YOU MAY BE
PRESSING MORE THAN YOUR LUCK.**

We all know that cocaine kills. But who would suspect it could kill right in your office?

The effects of cocaine—increased heart rate and blood pressure due to small vessel vasoconstriction—can alone be fatal. But the potential for tragedy in your practice increases if you give a cocaine-intoxicated patient a local anesthetic. The epinephrine in local anesthetics can produce serious cardiovascular effects if inadvertently injected into the vascular system of a patient on cocaine.

So if you suspect cocaine abuse in a patient, take the first step and educate him or her on the medical risks. Or you could have more on your hands than you bargained for.

For a copy of the American Dental Association Policy Statement on Dental Care and Recovery from Chemical Dependency, write:

Drug Free America Campaign/91
c/o Council on Dental Practice
American Dental Association
211 East Chicago Avenue
Chicago, Illinois 60611

This public service message is approved by the Advisory Committee on Chemical Dependency Issues, Council on Dental Practice, American Dental Association.

Reference: 1. Gobetti JP. The chemically dependent patient: A new challenge for dentistry. *The Detroit Dental Bulletin* 1989;58(Dec):16-19.

DRUG ABUSE...
Get the truth or face the consequences.
Partnership for a Drug-Free America

MT-275

FIGURE 11.8. Workplace-oriented messages often focus on providing information rather than appealing to emotions.
Reprinted with permission of the Partnership for a Drug-Free America.

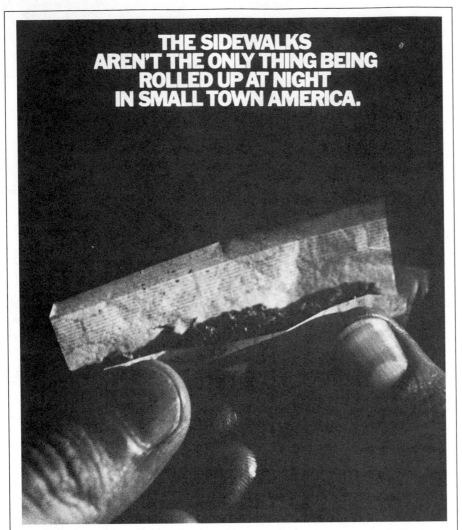

FIGURE 11.9. Awareness is the first step in prevention.
Reprinted with permission of the Partnership for a Drug-Free America.

Five principles were developed to encourage on-going participation from volunteers. First, from the beginning of the Partnership, it was agreed that if any one group or company got a commercial advantage from participation, the effort would collapse. Therefore, messages are not signed by the creating agency and no public acknowledgment is given to the participating production or talent unions. Second, initial research in the African-American and Hispanic-American communities showed that although many of the pressures for initial experimentation and occasional use of illegal drugs are similar to those faced by all Americans, there are some differences. The Partnership recognized that the sensitivity to create compelling messages for these communities lay with African-American and Hispanic advertising agencies.

Task forces were formed, but these agencies were typically small and could not readily afford to pay for the production of the messages. The Partnership raised production funds through donations from philanthropic foundations and companies.

Third, advertising agencies can be expected to volunteer their time, talent, and production dollars only if they have the freedom to exercise their creativity. This suited the Partnership objectives because it is unlikely that any one visual or phrase would serve for all targets. Therefore, the agencies were given the freedom to create rather than work around an assigned slogan. The large volume of donated media time and space also meant that there was no need to repetitively drive home a single message, as might be the case with a small-budget campaign.

Also, volunteers will contribute only if they believe that their work will be judged fairly and professionally when being considered for production. To this end, a Creative Review Committee was formed. This committee consists of leading creative directors from some of America's best-known advertising agencies. Their charge was to judge each message by the following criteria: Will it cut through the clutter of advertising in the media? Will it be compelling to the target audience? Is it credible? For this latter judgment, the committee is joined by drug experts who check the factual accuracy of the work.

Fourth, the most frequent reasons given for the failure of previous substance abuse PSA campaigns was that the media didn't run the messages. This problem is minimized by the fact that the media are actively involved in the Partnership. Nevertheless, a media strategy was essential. It embraced shared responsibility, and all media are actively encouraged to participate. The Partnership recognized the fact that we face an American crisis, not simply a crisis among television viewers. Constant personal communication is maintained between the management of national media and Partnership staff. Volunteer coordinators, working in local agencies in the largest 30 markets, regularly contacted media in those markets, and the Partnership maintained contact with all other markets through visits and regular mailing of new messages and information. The Partnership also recognized that, in addition to personal contact, outstanding creative work was the key to motivating the media to run a PSA. The quality and variety in creative work must be high. The media will not run boring messages, no matter how well-intentioned!

Fifth, accountability is crucial for continued volunteer support; volunteers need to know that their efforts are helping to make a difference. In recognition of this need, the Partnership commissioned an annual attitude and usage survey similar to the product attitude surveys familiar to all Partnership constituents. The survey, conducted each spring by the Gordon S. Black Corporation of Rochester, New York, is one of the largest attitude surveys conducted in the United States and by far the largest on drug attitudes.

The research experts advising the Partnership acknowledge that there are shortcomings in all broad-scale measures of advertising's influence on attitudes; myriad events and activities, totally separate from the Partnership messages, can have an effect on any attitude shift noted. Waiting the several years necessary to "test" and perfect research instruments would, however, let

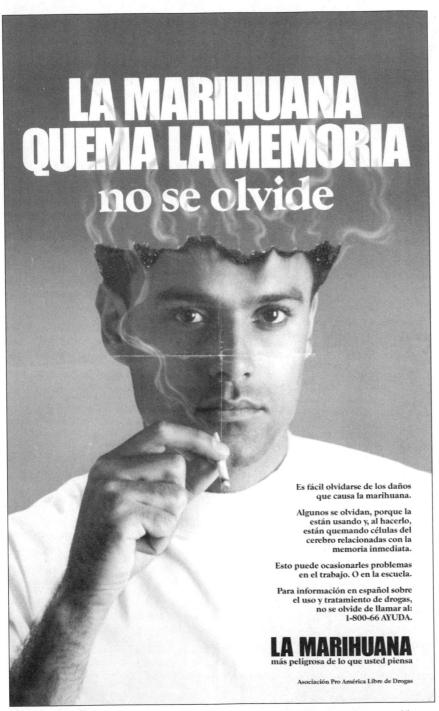

FIGURE 11.10. Spanish-language ads target Hispanic-American communities. Reprinted with permission of the Partnership for a Drug-Free America.

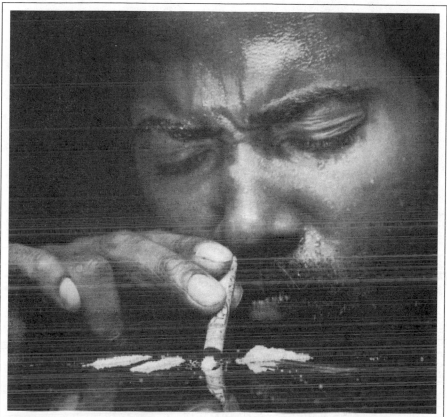

FIGURE 11.11. Controversial but consistently effective messages have been developed by African-American advertising agencies.
Reprinted with permission of the Partnership for a Drug-Free America.

Audience Profile: Preteens Ages 9–12 (Grades 4–7)

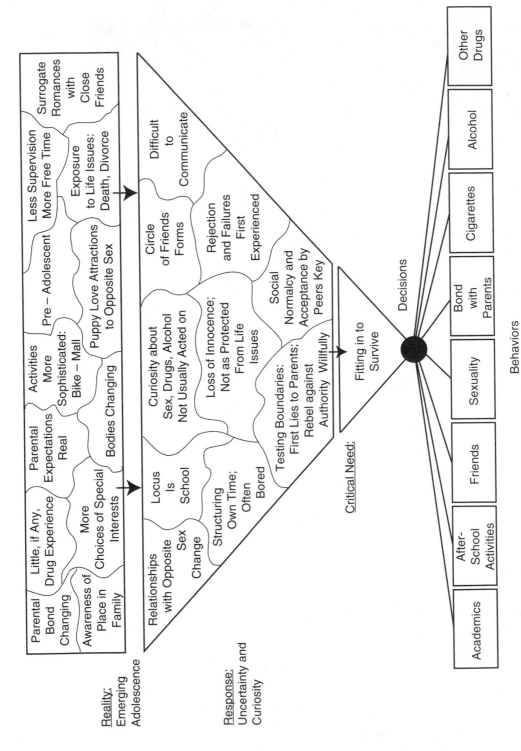

FIGURE 11.12. Audience Profile of 9- to 12-Year-Olds.

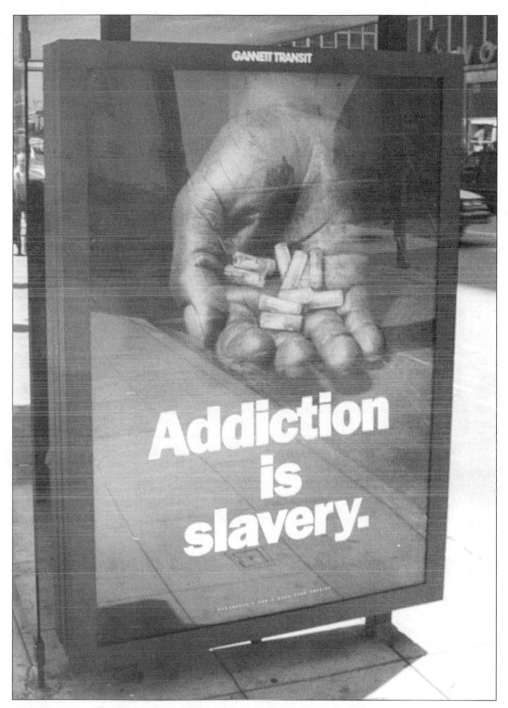

FIGURE 11.13. Public displays are used to reach a wider audience.
Reprinted with permission of the Partnership for a Drug-Free America.

the problem fester that much longer. Central location research was selected and this methodology has been successfully used since 1987 (Black et al., 1992). In 1989, the study was accepted for funding by NIDA.

Community Strategy: Local Efforts

It is believed that media-delivered messages over time can help build antidrug attitudes that will in turn affect behavior. In addition, these messages help set a national agenda, encouraging volunteers to attack the problem on a community basis. Specific local activities can be most effective in reducing demand for illegal drugs. The Partnership therefore makes its material available free of charge to state and community action groups. Ten states are adapting Partnership messages to carry information specific to their antidrug programs.

IMPLEMENTING THE PARTNERSHIP STRATEGY

In the same way that Partnership strategy development parallels commercial product promotion development, execution of the strategy is quite similar to the way a company and advertising agency would work together to execute a commercial advertising program.

Briefing the Volunteer Agency

The Partnership staff summarizes the results of qualitative and quantitative research and input from drug abuse and child development experts. The volunteer agency is then briefed on a specific age, target, and medium. Compelling messages come from the creative team "getting inside the head" of the target audience; to facilitate this creativity, focus group meetings are videotaped and tapes made available to the creative team.

A briefing scheme is developed for each age group; the purpose is simply to start the creative team thinking about what is going on in the life of the target audience, the reality of their world, how they react to that reality, the critical need in their lives, and decisions they face.

Obviously this is not an all-inclusive analysis of the target group. It is an effective idea generator for the creative teams. Together with Partnership focus groups and groups convened by the agency as they develop ideas, it has led to compelling, credible messages.

Reviewing the Agency Creative Work

Every eight weeks, the Creative Review Committee (CRC) meets to review agency creative work. Agencies come to these meetings and present their work in layout or storyboard form. Roughly half of the work presented is rejected for strategic or executional reasons, one-third is thought to be interesting but the agency is asked to make executional modifications, and the remainder is approved for immediate production. When work is approved, drug experts are consulted to resolve questions of fact. If the work is for TV, it is submitted like any commercial message to the three networks for their commercial clearance process.

Producing the Message

The agency contracts with production and acting talent to shoot the messages. The production community is supportive of the Partnership's efforts. The Screen Actors Guild (SAG) and the American Federation of TV and Radio Artists (AFTRA) have waived rights for Partnership TV messages. Performers often work without charge. Studios, directors, editors, platemakers, and photographers also work without charge or for minimal fees. It is truly an industrywide effort.

The finished ad is presented to the CRC for final approval. The Partnership stresses that the message is the product—it must break through and be compelling and credible. In the few cases where the potential impact or appropriateness of the ad is still in question, the agency or Partnership staff does post-production testing.

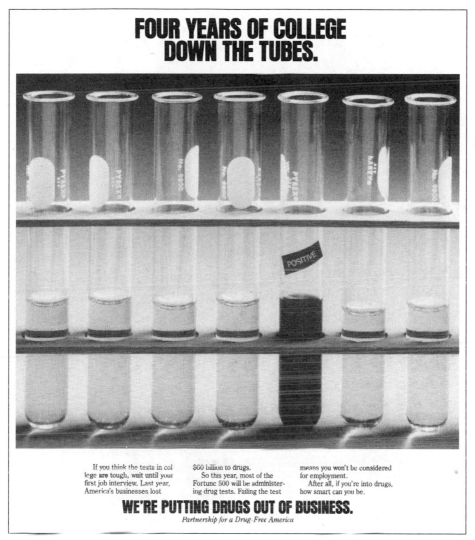

FIGURE 11.14. The increasing use of pre-employment drug testing prompted this message to high school and college students.
Reprinted with permission of the Partnership for a Drug-Free America.

Distributing the Final Product

The most compelling creative work is useless unless it is seen by the target group. Distribution of material appears to have been a weak point in previous substance abuse prevention programs. To strengthen its distribution efforts, the Partnership follows these procedures: The staff contacts national media (TV networks, national magazine and newspaper corporations, and radio networks) directly on a regular basis. Messages are delivered in person with suggested insertion schedules for broadcast and print media to reach the target audience. The Partnership's local coordinator regularly calls on local media in the top 30 markets, and headquarters-based personnel make

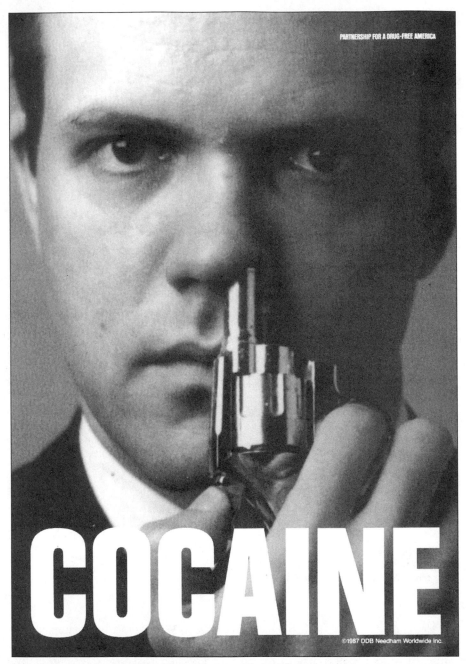

FIGURE 11.15. There is no single "Partnership style"; long copy may be appropriate in some instances, strong graphics in others.
Reprinted with permission of the Partnership for a Drug-Free America.

visits twice a year. In smaller markets, material is disseminated by American's Special Anti-Drug Priority (ASAP), a direct mail operation set up in conjunction with the Ad Council. Community Partnership task forces solicit minority-specific media such as the two Spanish TV networks and independent Spanish and African-American radio and print media. Partnership staff hold quarterly meetings with network representatives to keep them informed of Partnership activities, learn of their programming plans for drug-related stories, and solicit network input to Partnership media strategies. The Partnership makes presentations to national media associations such as Outdoor Advertising Association of America (OAAA), National Association of Black Broadcasters (NABOB), and Radio Advertising Bureau (RAB) to solicit support and input from members, to present accountability reports, and to express appreciation for their support.

RESEARCH: HOW IS THE AD AFFECTING ATTITUDES AND BEHAVIOR?

Isolating and measuring the effects of advertising on substance abuse prevention is difficult. The problems are well-known; some can be minimized, few can be totally eliminated. For example, nonadvertising programs and events affect public attitudes. Len Bias's death in 1986 was a watershed event in the declining use of cocaine, at least as important as ongoing advertising messages. Furthermore, it is difficult to obtain samples that replicate the nation as a whole, and it is impossible to precisely measure weight of advertising run by the media. Finally, it is difficult to accurately measure illegal drug use through surveys because respondents are, naturally, reluctant to admit committing a crime. Theoretically, the "lying" factor should wash out in trend information over large samples, but it is possible that the more unacceptable drug use is perceived to be, the more users will deny use.

Nevertheless, research is essential for learning and for accountability. In the spring of 1987, before the launch of the Partnership effort, the Gordon S. Black Corporation conducted some 6,000 interviews across the United States. This study has been repeated each spring through 1992. Two objectives of the study are to detect changes in attitudes about illegal drugs and to obtain some idea of drug use patterns. Use is measured with larger samples in studies conducted by NIDA among the most potentially vulnerable group, high school students. Lloyd Johnston of the University of Michigan conducted a NIDA-funded survey. The Gordon Black research has samples including subgroups of 9- to 12-year-olds, 13- to 17-year-olds, adults, and parents. African- and Hispanic-Americans were included but to date these subsamples have been too small for precise trending. Data are collected by the Central Location Sampling method in some 75 locations across the country. The primary advantage of this methodology is that it provides the respondent with complete anonymity; the identity of the respondent remains unknown to the recruiting interviewer. The respondents are asked to fill out a written questionnaire and are given a private place to do it. When finished, the respondent seals the questionnaire in an unidentified envelope and places it in a collection box. The usual demographic data are obtained for appropriate cross-tabulations.

Results from the 1992 survey indicate that street drugs such as marijuana, cocaine, and crack are readily obtainable. More than half (55%) of the adults surveyed said it is easy to obtain marijuana, 42% found it easy to get cocaine, and 37% crack. Few teenagers have difficulty obtaining these drugs (See Table 11.3).

Not only are illegal drugs easily obtainable, they are often free. Sixty-two percent of the teenagers (13–17 years old) and 38% of the adults said that these drugs were offered to them on the first approach, without charge (1990 survey). About one in seven children ages 9–12 (16% in 1992) were approached by others offering these drugs.

Fortunately, antidrug attitudes are at high levels among children. Most children ages 9–12 readily perceive the danger of illegal drugs. The

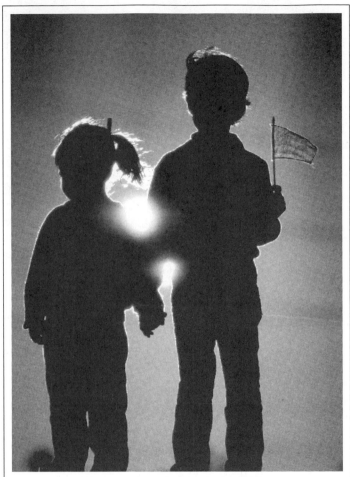

There's another tiny nation
that's worth fighting for.

Partnership for a Drug-Free America

FIGURE 11.16. Many Partnership messages appeal to
positive emotions.
Reprinted with permission of the Partnership for a Drug-Free America.

TABLE 11.3   Ease in Obtaining Illegal Drugs (Gordon S. Black 1992 Survey)

I AGREE, IT IS EASY/FAIRLY EASY TO OBTAIN:	AGES 9–12	AGES 13–17	ADULTS
Marijuana	13%	46%	55%
Cocaine	9	32	42
Crack	9	29	37

1992 survey found that 87% were "scared of taking drugs," 89% thought "crack or cocaine can kill you," 80% thought it "easy to get hooked on drugs," and 94% reported their parents "would feel really bad if they found I was using drugs." Some children feel that commercials sometimes exaggerate the danger and risk of drug use: Almost half agree that the dangers of marijuana (43%) and cocaine (42%) are overstated.

Children ages 9–12 report growing dialogue about drug use. Three-fourths (74%) have talked with their parents about this subject, and 63% with their school teachers. More than half (55%) have had these discussions with friends and 40% with their siblings (1992 data).

The majority of teenagers ages 13–17 recall antidrug commercials that made them feel less likely to use drugs. More than two thirds (67%) agreed that "an increasingly negative attitude toward illegal drugs appears to affect drug usage."

A comparison of the 1987 and 1992 survey results shows that teenagers (13–17) increasingly see great risk in using illicit drugs (Table 11.4). Between 1987 and 1992, their attitude toward drug users has become increasingly negative (Table 11.5).

These results suggest that antidrug messages shape drug attitudes and that advertising can have a beneficial impact. However, it is clear that further opportunities exist to increase antidrug attitudes among teens.

As encouraging as these historical results have been, it must be noted that the most recent research (the 1993 University of Michigan survey published February 1994) shows an increase in drug use among high school seniors but at levels still well below their peaks. For example, past-year marijuana use peaked in 1979 at 50.8%, fell steadily to 21.9% in 1992, but increased to 26% in 1993. Past-year cocaine use peaked in 1985 at 13.1%, fell to 3.1% in 1992,

TABLE 11.4   Perceived Personal Risk in Using Drugs (Gordon S. Black 1992 Survey)

I AGREE, PEOPLE RISK HARMING THEMSELVES (THEY TAKE GREAT RISK) IF THEY DO THE FOLLOWING:	1987	1992
Try marijuana once or twice	18%	21%
Smoke marijuana occasionally	31	37
Smoke marijuana regularly	65	70
Try cocaine once or twice	36	44
Do cocaine occasionally	55	66
Do cocaine regularly	81	86
Try crack once or twice	52	54
Do crack occasionally	67	71
Do crack regularly	81	87

TABLE 11.5   Image of Drug Users by 13–17 Year-Olds (Gordon S. Black Surveys)

	1987	1992
A marijuana user:		
is a loser	53%	60%
is boring	22	28
has no future	57	65
A cocaine user:		
is a loser	56	66
is boring	25	33
has no future	63	72

and increased to 3.3% in 1993. Lloyd Johnston notes, "at the same time some important attitudes and beliefs about drugs began to soften." The attitudes referred to are "perceived risk" and "disapproval of use." In 1979, only 9.4% of high school seniors felt there was a risk in using marijuana once or twice. This grew to 24.5% in 1992 but fell to 21.9% in 1993. Similarly, 34% perceived a risk for using cocaine in 1985; this grew to a high of 59.4% in 1991 and fell to 57.6% in 1993.

The attitude of "disapproval of use" is now considerably higher than in earlier years but also shows some fall-off in the last two years.

Although there is no empirical evidence to explain this increase in use and softening of attitudes, it has been noted that this has occurred in a period when the drug issue has fallen off the national political agenda. Illegal drugs were not a major issue in the 1992 elections and have been little mentioned subsequently. One result of this has been significantly less media space devoted to the subject and devoted to Partnership PSA messages.

LESSONS LEARNED

A review of substance abuse prevention campaigns suggests that they reinforce and change attitudes and behavior when two conditions are met. First, is there existing public concern? Is the issue visible and important to the public and

politicians? The best illustration is the enormous media coverage given to the Surgeon General's report sparking the anticigarette efforts of the '60s and by daily media coverage of drug-related crime that energized the public in the 1980s. Existing concern is particularly important if the advertising campaign depends on donated PSA time and space; the media will not provide such time and space for issues that are not of growing public and political interest. This, in large part, can explain the recent fall-off in media time devoted to Partnership messages. The very strength of advocacy is the passion with which the cause is embraced. However, this passion can mislead the advocate into thinking that the entire population shares the concern. A cool assessment of popular concern would probably steer many advocates away from broad PSA campaigns toward more specifically targeted actions.

Second, is the campaign mounted following commercial marketing disciplines? It seems logical to think that one would consider advertising for substance abuse prevention only if one believes that advertising for commercial products and services is effective. It seems equally logical, therefore, to follow effective commercial marketing disciplines for substance abuse prevention advertising campaigns.

Substance abuse campaigns that appear to have had the greatest success have the following features in common.

Phase I: The Basic Strategy

These questions are asked. What is our issue? Is it sufficiently important to the public to warrant PSA time and space? What public? Is any other group doing it? Are we prepared to stick to it for years? Where will the funding come from? Do we have access to the raw materials (creative talent) necessary to develop our product (the message)? Can we get and keep distribution (media time and space)? In other words, the strategy phase embraces nothing more than the basic questions any manufacturer would ask before launching and advertising a product. In the case of anticigarette advertising, the issue was important, the creative talent was available, and the Fairness Doctrine made distribution easy. With drinking responsibly, the issue was important to the sponsor and that is all that mattered because the sponsor had the funds to put the program in place. With Partnership for a Drug-Free America, the issue was important and the coalition had access to creative talent and media. In all three cases, these groups chose to work with other groups interested in the issue to extend reach. Substance abuse issues, like consumer product markets, are not static; there is constant change, so the strategy needs constant review.

Phase II: Creative Development

This phase takes a number of factors into account. It is curious that not one of the dozens of papers on advertising and substance abuse prevention reviewed for this chapter showed the creative work. The product is the message; get it wrong and at best you don't attract the attention of your intended audience; at worst, you turn them off to your issue. It is important to listen to the target audience—qualitative research is essential for developing messages that reinforce or change existing beliefs. Share your learning with creative experts and listen to them. Issue advocates such as academic and government experts and advertising agency clients usually have all the information they need. They don't know how to pre-

sent it compellingly, however, and certainly not in 30 seconds. Work with creative professionals.

Insist on high-quality products. Your message must first appeal to the media gatekeeper; who wants to give valuable time and space to amateur messages?

Your message must compel attention and action from an individual in your target audience who probably sees hundreds of advertising messages per day. The product is the message; a poor-quality message equals a poor-quality product.

Judge the creative work critically but fairly. Ask these questions: Will the message attract the attention of the intended audience? Is it credible and applicable to them? Is there new information or is the information presented in a new way that will help change attitudes?

The Partnership for a Drug-Free America, with some 400 messages directed to a variety of audiences, has learned a number of creative lessons: Don't preach; simple graphics can often be more compelling than a well-reasoned verbal message. Don't try to fit one phrase or visual to all targets. "Just Say No" may be a strong statement to the adolescent for whom it was first created. It becomes less meaningful when used with an older target where rebellion and the need for argumentation become factors.

Opinion is divided on the most effective content for substance abuse media messages. Should one depict the positive side of being drug-free or the negative effects of substance use? Focus groups conducted by the Partnership for a Drug-Free America indicate that teenagers clearly respond to the negative approach. Recent studies (Mayton et al., 1990) reach the same conclusion. In reality, the issue is one of credibility. Fear of adverse consequences can be a powerful motivator. The successful antismoking campaign of the late 1960s was almost totally negative. Perceived risk correlates closely with a drop in use of cocaine and marijuana by high school seniors (Bachman et al., 1990). It is essential, however, that the risk or consequences are credible; a bold statement such as "try pot once and you will

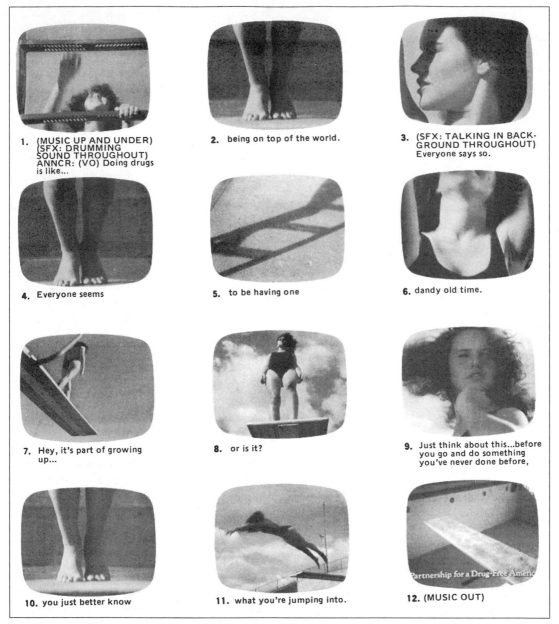

1. (MUSIC UP AND UNDER) (SFX: DRUMMING SOUND THROUGHOUT) ANNCR: (VO) Doing drugs is like...

2. being on top of the world.

3. (SFX: TALKING IN BACK-GROUND THROUGHOUT) Everyone says so.

4. Everyone seems

5. to be having one

6. dandy old time.

7. Hey, it's part of growing up...

8. or is it?

9. Just think about this...before you go and do something you've never done before,

10. you just better know

11. what you're jumping into.

12. (MUSIC OUT)

FIGURE 11.17. Partnership for a Drug-Free America "Pool Party."
Reprinted with permission of the Partnership for a Drug-Free America.

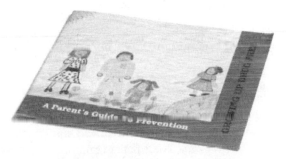

Parental guidance suggested.

Growing Up Drug Free is a parent's guide to prevention.
Call 1-800-624-0100 for your free copy. It's for parents of all ages.

Partnership For A Drug-Free America

FIGURE 11.18. Partnership messages offering a free Parents' Guide developed by the Department of Education have resulted in some 27,000,000 requests
Reprinted with permission of the Partnership for a Drug-Free America.

become a homeless addict" is incredible and thus counterproductive.

Variety is important. A well-developed substance abuse campaign should contain positive messages as well as physical and social risk messages. A word of caution: Many attempts to depict the positive side of being drug-free look like soft drink commercials. Will the message stand out? If so, is there enough money in the budget to produce it? Soft drink messages are expensive to produce.

Influencers such as parents can be asked to talk to their children about illegal drugs. Early Partnership messages did so. Newer messages have an 800 number for a free parents' guide on when, where, and how to talk to kids about drugs. Influencers are more prepared to influence if they feel they know what they are talking about. These latter messages offer help and are stronger because of it. Listen to the target audience again. They are the reason you are in business.

Phase III: The Media Strategy

This phase addresses the question of how to get the ad on the air. The majority of public health and substance abuse prevention campaigns have relied on PSA time and space. The difficulties inherent in getting any PSA time and space are well-documented. To obtain highly rated PSA time and space, well-considered media strategy and execution are imperative.

First, and often overlooked, is the necessity for creative quality and message variety. Great work has a greater chance of being used. Personal contact with the media is critical to obtaining PSA time and space. A station may receive more than one hundred PSA messages per month. Personal contact with the general manager and community affairs director permits the "selling" of the issue and provides useful guidance on technical matters. For example, PSA media is usually "remnant" time and space; what variety of message lengths and print formats stand the greatest chance of use?

Think local. Messages with a local content have a greater chance of frequent use. Initial messages created for the Partnership for a Drug-Free America were standard in format (30-second television or radio spots). More recent messages are also made available in 22-second lengths so that local, nonprofit substance abuse organizations can add information about local programs.

Plan to break through the clutter. The American public is deluged by commercial advertising messages. Creative content and excellent production help a PSA message stand out, but it also needs frequent exposure over time. A number of substance abuse prevention campaigns have not produced the desired results, in part, because their distribution has been too widespread. It may be a better tactic to concentrate effort and resources on fewer markets where constant follow-up with the media could result in more and better message placement over a longer period of time. An additional benefit of this approach is that research is easier and more affordable. Indications of positive effect can then be used with the media in "expansion" markets.

Phase IV: Community and Editorial Relations

It seems clear that frequent exposure to well-targeted, compelling advertising messages can, over time, contribute to reinforcing and changing attitudes, but it cannot accomplish this goal in a vacuum. The advocacy group, whether depending on PSA media or paid media, should enlist the support of others who can help reach the target audience or help keep the issue in front of the public. The Partnership for a Drug-Free America works with a number of private sector coalitions, as well as state and local governments, to further the national objective of reducing demand for illegal drugs; Rochester Fights Back, the Substance Abuse Initiative of Greater Cleveland and the Robert Wood Johnson Foundation-sponsored "Fighting Back" are all examples of local programs that have used Partnership material. Substance abuse prevention advertising can help set a local and national agenda and in turn become more effective as other members of the community become advocates of the issue.

WHAT TO DO IF YOU THINK YOUR CHILD IS ON DRUGS.

Take a deep breath.

You're not a failure as a parent. You're not helpless. And you're not alone.

If you think you're a failure, consider this: There are many kids with neglectful parents who never use drugs. There are also children with seemingly model parents who do use drugs.

So the first thing to accept is that drugs, while indeed dangerous, are one more problem for youngsters to handle. And they'll do it better and faster if you're aware, involved, and don't stick your head in the sand.

THE AWARE PARENT IS THE GOOD PARENT.

Part of awareness and a major deterrent to experimentation is to talk to your kids about drugs.

But even with a lot of parental involvement, there are no guarantees. So it's important to know the symptoms of drug use and to take action if you see your youngster displaying them.

THE WARNING SIGNALS.

There are no symptoms that are absolutely reliable. But there are clues (see box).

Most of these symptoms tend to be gradual which is why parental awareness is so important.

But don't jump to conclusions.

Many of the warning signs for drug use are the same as those for depression or for the ups and downs of being a teenager. There's also the possibility it's a physical or emotional problem.

But whatever the problem, we're talking about a child who needs help. Right now.

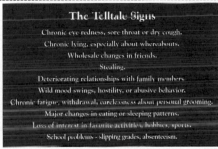

The Telltale Signs

Chronic eye redness, sore throat or dry cough.

Chronic lying, especially about whereabouts.

Wholesale changes in friends.

Stealing.

Deteriorating relationships with family members.

Wild mood swings, hostility, or abusive behavior.

Chronic fatigue, withdrawal, carelessness about personal grooming.

Major changes in eating or sleeping patterns.

Loss of interest in favorite activities, hobbies, sports.

School problems - slipping grades, absenteeism.

START WITHIN THE FAMILY.

Nothing beats the power of love and family support. That has to start with a frank discussion.

Don't make it an attack. And don't try to talk with your child if he or she seems under the influence.

Wait for a calm moment and then explain that you're worried about certain behavior (be specific) and give your child every opportunity to explain. That means really listening, not doing all the talking.

At the same time, it's important to speak frankly about the possibility of drugs. And it's particularly important to talk about your values and why you're dead set against drugs.

If your youngster seems evasive or if his or her explanations are not convincing, you may want to consult your doctor to rule out illness and to ask for advice.

You may also want to have your child visit a mental health professional to see if there are emotional problems.

FURTHER ACTION MAY BE NECESSARY

If your child seems non-responsive or belligerent, and you suspect drugs are involved, immediate action is vital.

First, you'll need an evaluation from a health professional skilled in diagnosing adolescents with alcohol or drug problems.

You may want to get involved with an intervention program to learn techniques that will help convince a drug user to accept help.

For the user, there are self-help, outpatient, day care, residency, and 24-hour hospitalization programs.

The right program depends entirely on the circumstances and the degree of drug involvement. Here, you'll need professional help to make an informed choice.

Another point: If a program is to succeed, the family needs to be part of it. This can mean personal or family counseling. It may also involve participating in a support group where you learn about co-dependency and how not to play into the problems that might prompt further drug use.

If you don't know about drug programs in your area, call your family doctor, local hospital or county mental health society or school counselor for a referral. You can also call the national helpline – 800-662-HELP – for advice and a referral.

WHATEVER YOU DO, DON'T GIVE UP.

That child who upsets you so much is the same little boy or girl who, only yesterday, gave you such joy. They're in way over their heads, and they never needed you quite as much as they need you now.

No matter what they say.

For more information on how to talk with your kids about drugs, ask for a free copy of "A Parent's Guide to Prevention." Call 1-800-624-0100.

PARTNERSHIP FOR A DRUG-FREE AMERICA

FIGURE 11.19. Parent education plays a key role in prevention.
Reprinted with permission of the Partnership for a Drug-Free America.

Phase V: Evaluation

As we have seen, isolating and evaluating advertising's contribution to substance abuse prevention is difficult. It is, however, necessary for refining the messages and building volunteer and media cooperation. Again, commercial marketing disciplines can provide guidance in developing an evaluation program. Establish before the campaign what you want to measure. In any case, pre- and postcampaign research is useful. If the objective is to affect attitudes in specific target groups in specific markets, it may be possible to compare campaign markets with other markets. If it is a national effort, tracking studies can be useful. If a key objective is to generate public or media attention, measures of the number of articles written or broadcast references to the issue can provide some evaluation. Recognize that advertising research will give only directional results. It can be argued that resources devoted to obtaining a perfectly controlled testing environment might better be invested in up-front qualitative research for the creative process, effective distribution of the messages, and constant follow-up to ensure that the messages are heavily exposed.

Phase VI: Patience and Concern

It has been said that America does not have a substance abuse problem; it has a patience problem. Once we have identified a problem, we want it solved tomorrow. There is no overnight solution to the problem of substance abuse. Just as school programs and treatment must be made widely and constantly available, so too must PSA campaigns be heavy and continuous; this can only happen in an atmosphere of public and political concern.

REFERENCES

Bachman, J. G., et al. (1990). Explaining the recent decline in cocaine use among young adults. *Journal of Health & Social Behavior, 31.*

Black, G. S., et al. (1992). *PATS: Consistency of estimates obtained through central location sampling.* Unpublished manuscript.

Burns, D., et al. (1992). *Tobacco use in California.* Sacramento: California Department of Health Services.

Field, T., et al. (1983). *Implementing public education campaigns: Lessons from alcohol abuse prevention.* Summary Report to NIAAA.

Flay, B. R. (1987). Mass media and smoking cessation: A critical review. *American Journal of Public Health, 77* (2).

Grube, J. W., et al. (1991). *The effects of television beer advertising on children.* Unpublished manuscript.

Horgan, M. M. (1986). *Does broadcast advertising of alcoholic beverages increase self-improved risk?* Unpublished manuscript.

Johnson, L. (1981, 1982, 1983). *Annual Monitoring the Future survey.* Lansing: University of Michigan.

Mayton II, D. M., et al. (1990). The perceived effects of drug messages on use patterns in adolescents. *Journal of Drug Education, 10* (4).

Mirzale, E. (1991). Sources of drug information among adolescent students. *Journal of Drug Education, 21* (2).

Pearl, D., et al. (1982). *Television and behavior—Ten years of scientific progress and implications for the eighties.* ADAMHA DHHS pub. no. (ADM) 82-1196.

Popham, W. G., et al. (1991). *Evaluating the California 1990–91 tobacco education media campaign,* Executive Reports.

Roberts, D. F. (1983). *Children and Commercials; issues, evidence interventions.* In *Rx television: Enhancing the prevention impact of TV.* Haworth Press.

Sheppard, M. A. (1980). Sources of information about drugs. *Journal of Drug Education 10* (3).

Simpson, H. M., et al. (1985). *Alcohol-specific controls: Implications for road safety.* Traffic Injury Research Foundation of Canada.

Strickland, D. E. (1982). Alcohol advertising: Orientations and influence. *Journal of Advertising, 1.*

Teh-wei-Hu et al. (1982). *Cost effectiveness evaluation; the 1978 NIDA drug abuse prevention television campaign.* University Park: Institute for Policy Research and Evaluation, Pennsylvania State University.

CHAPTER 12

MASS MEDIA

THOMAS E. BACKER

The power of the mass media to convey information, stimulate awareness, provoke debate, change attitudes, and sometimes to change important behaviors, has been confirmed time and time again. By the time they reach adulthood, American children have spent more time watching television than any other single activity except sleeping (Backer, Rogers, & Sopory, 1992). Rightly or wrongly, the media, especially television, are assumed to have an important impact on violent behavior, as reflected in highly emotional congressional hearings and a public policy "Summit Conference" on this topic in Hollywood during the summer of 1993. Many other attitudes and behaviors, from gender-based discrimination to loss of motivation and judgment, are claimed to be related to mass media exposure.

Television, radio, newspapers, magazines, and other media thus play an ongoing role of great importance for public health education on topics such as drug abuse prevention. For instance, research beginning with the work of George Gerbner and his associates at the Annenberg School for Communication at the University of Pennsylvania has demonstrated that most Americans get most of their knowledge about health issues from television (Backer, 1990; DeFleur & Dennis, 1981). In some cases, campaigns using mass media are conducted to provide information and pave the way for behavior change. Thus, mass media can have a potentially positive or negative impact on health behavior.

The bulk of mass media attention to health issues comes because they are considered newsworthy or because certain aspects of them are

seen as entertaining or as part of everyday life as seen in entertainment programs. But beyond this more passive role, played by the mass media simply "because they are there," there also have been an increasing number of media-based health communication campaigns to transmit health information and change the risk behaviors of Americans in a number of health-related areas. Empirical research shows that such campaigns, which involve use of mechanisms such as public service announcements (PSAs), can have a significant impact. This is especially true when such campaigns are part of larger social systems interventions (Backer, 1990; Backer, Rogers, & Sopory, 1992).

Few health issues have received more attention in recent years than drug abuse and its prevention, especially among America's youth. Mass media campaigns on this topic have proliferated, and some of these have been quite successful. Others have generated controversy about both their methods and their actual impact.

The Human Interaction Research Institute conducted a four-year research program supported by the Center for Substance Abuse Prevention, which examined health communication campaigns emphasizing mass media health behavior messages, with a main emphasis on substance abuse prevention for high-risk youth. The social systems in which these campaigns exist have received special attention.

Phase I of this research involved a comprehensive literature analysis and in-depth interviews with campaign designers and researchers. Study findings included a number of principles for effective campaigns that appear to have some generality across topical areas (Backer, 1990; Backer, Rogers, & Sopory, 1992). Phase II examined further the critical role of media, government, and community organizations and their collaboration in the success of health communication campaigns (Backer & Rogers, 1993).

In this chapter, the dimensions for success of mass media drug abuse prevention campaigns are explored, drawing principally on findings from this research program. The ways in which media, government, and community organizations have worked together in a sample of recent campaigns are also analyzed, and the critical role of organizations in health communication campaigns is examined. Finally, some recommendations for how campaigns using mass media can best be integrated with other systemic interventions for drug abuse prevention are presented.

OVERVIEW OF MASS MEDIA CAMPAIGNS

Television, radio, film, and the print media are increasingly being used in creative ways to present health information and to stimulate awareness, attitude change, and both individual and group behavior change. Campaigns have been undertaken in a variety of subject areas; substance abuse, AIDS, traffic safety, heart disease prevention, smoking cessation, and nutrition are just a few examples. Most large-scale mass media campaigns today depend on network television as their most important delivery system, although newspapers, magazines, radio, cable television, videotapes, and other media are also used. Health communication campaigns typically have a major mass media component, but also have community involvement, advocacy, and legislature action components as well.

Some campaigns, such as Nancy Reagan's "Just Say No" efforts to prevent drug abuse by children, have reached very high levels of public visibility, whereas others, such as the Stanford Heart Disease Prevention Project, have been much lower in public profile (though not necessarily less effective). A few have been systemati-

cally evaluated, but most campaigns have not been, so extracting what works and what does not from these various campaigns is a challenge.

Often, media campaigns involve communicating findings from medical research almost as soon as they are generated. Today, many of these research findings are about risk behaviors. In areas ranging from AIDS to smoking to weight control, Americans are bombarded with information through the mass media about what behaviors are risky. To a lesser extent, they are also bombarded by information regarding what behavioral scientists are learning about ways in which behaviors can be changed—what strategies for individual behavior change work the best and how groups (ranging from families to whole communities) can help support the change process.

Because of the mass media's endless appetite for new subjects to present, and because of the increasing public interest in health and fitness topics, the media are not a passive vehicle for such efforts. Health reporters in newspapers, radio and television are commonplace, as are "disease of the week" television movies or documentaries that concentrate on a character with a severe or life-threatening illness such as cancer or AIDS.

Portrayals of various health issues in entertainment television programming are numerous, although research indicates that these images often are in serious conflict with what health professionals agree are appropriate guidelines (Signorielli, 1988). Health matters are discussed and presented today in news, information, and entertainment programming because of their commercial viability. The mass media increasingly are taking an active role in disseminating information about risk behaviors in various areas of health and illness. There is even some perception among media professionals and institutions that they have a social responsibility to do so.

Involvements of this sort are not new. The mass media always have been concerned with social issues, so the specific involvement with health matters is not surprising. Effects of mass media campaigns have been the focus of evaluative research since the 1930s (DeFleur & Dennis, 1981).

In early research on the mass media's impact in changing attitudes or behavior, it was assumed that a message could be directly implanted in people's minds, with direct, immediate, and powerful effects. This came to be called the hypodermic needle model for mass media effects. Research during the 1940s and 1950s challenged this assumption. In particular, some critical studies by Paul Lazarsfeld and his colleagues at Columbia University showed that the model did not accurately describe the outcomes of many media campaigns. During this time, many social scientists came to believe that mass media could not be deployed effectively to change human behavior in significant ways (DeFleur & Dennis, 1981). To this day, social scientists are often skeptical about the direct impact of such campaigns because of the "complex causal chain that is presumed to mediate exposure to a message and ultimate behavioral change" (Flay, 1986, p. 1).

Then, in the 1960s and 1970s, further research studies began to show that mass media campaigns could succeed if they incorporated certain key strategies such as formative evaluation to help design a campaign; segmentation of the target audience into key groups, with differing strategies for communicating with each group; and an interpersonal network to supplement the mass media channels for more powerful effects on behavior (Rogers & Storey, 1988). Moreover, campaigns during this time started with more modest goals.

A few evaluations of mass media campaigns have been conducted with a high degree of rigor. Examples include smoking cessation programs (Flay, 1986) or heart disease prevention (Maccoby & Solomon, 1981). From these studies have emerged certain principles for success, and some strategies that clearly do not work. In other areas, even without rigorous evaluation, guidelines and examples of success or failure are available that may have potential for wider use at least on a conceptual level. An initial set of generalizations that have emerged from the present study is presented later in this chapter.

As DeJong and Winsten (1989) observe in their analytic review of mass media campaigns, current research and professional attitudes about the role mass media campaigns play in changing health behavior fall between the excessive expectations of impact of past years and more recent pessimism after evaluations of campaigns that failed to take account of some important contextual factors. They assert that the slow changes in American society—including real behavioral changes—concerning smoking are an example of how mass media campaigns can play a role in changing health behavior, but the changes are evolutionary and affected by many nonmedia factors. The Stanford Heart Disease Prevention Project and a smoking cessation campaign in Australia are cited by DeJong and Winsten (1989) as examples of long-term programs with mass media components that seem to have had powerful effects.

DEFINITION OF CAMPAIGNS

Rogers and Storey (1988) reviewed a number of definitions of health communication campaigns with mass media components, yielding the following four essential ingredients:

- A campaign is purposive and seeks to influence individuals.
- A campaign is aimed at a large audience.
- A campaign has a specifically defined time limit.
- A campaign involves an organized set of communication activities.

The analysis of definitions of mass media campaigns begun in Rogers and Storey (1988) has been extended in the research reported here by creating an analytic framework (see Table 12.1) in which mass media campaigns on any topic can be interpreted. *Mass media campaign* is used here to mean a health communication campaign with a major mass media component. The framework includes types of media components (the delivery systems for the campaign content), types of collaboration (both individuals and organizations), the context or environment in which the campaign is intended to have impact, the structure or procedural steps into which campaigns are organized, the principles for what works in a campaign (derived from the analysis in Backer, 1988a, and extended in the more comprehensive list of generalizations presented later in this chapter), and the desired levels of effects on its target audience from a campaign (derived from the analysis of Rogers & Storey, 1988).

Finally, there are some historical realities about the current emphasis on substance abuse itself, related to media coverage, that must be taken into account. Accounts such as Kerr (1986) make it clear that the "drug abuse crisis" of 1986 in fact was not due to any sudden rise in drug use or the severity of its consequences. The causes include the dramatic effect on urban neighborhoods of crack, the new and potent form of cocaine.

The death of Len Bias, a young basketball star at the University of Maryland, and the approaching November 1986 elections helped to focus attention in the U.S. Congress. There were also deeper trends having to do with an antidrug and antialcohol sentiment building among the public in the United States since the early 1980s, reflecting the end of the tolerant era of the late 1960s and 1970s.

Appearance of drug issues in the mass media also had an effect, as did the number of celebrities disclosing their problems with alcohol or drug addiction, beginning with Betty Ford in the early 1980s. The appearance of *Time* cover stories and *The New York Times* articles on substance abuse provided a focus of attention that helped to create public urgency for action, as well as providing motivation among lawmakers to legislate solutions.

These factors are important here because they provide a context for the discussion of actual and planned campaigns. Perhaps most importantly, if fighting substance abuse in America is in part a matter of resetting values and refocusing attention, then mass media health behavior

campaigns must be designed in ways that take advantage of that reality. Certainly the specific role that the mass media have played in elevating public attention to alcohol and drug abuse is important, including the extent to which media professionals and organizations may feel that this is an old issue or that message clutter has begun to occur in entertainment, news, and public service programming. Such statements have appeared in the pages of *Daily Variety* and other media trade publications beginning in 1988. Campaign designers must therefore be very careful, when approaching media organizations or celebrities, to state why a particular campaign has elements not already overdone or overexposed in the media and why it can contribute something unique.

EXAMPLES OF SUCCESSFUL DRUG ABUSE PREVENTION CAMPAIGNS

The five examples that follow are reflective of mass media campaigns concerning drug abuse prevention (in the final case, drug abuse and AIDS) launched during the 1980s. All of the campaigns involve significant partnerships between media, community, and government organizations. Their origins and funding mechanisms differ greatly, and so do their strategies, beyond certain common features such as the use of PSAs.

Just Say No

Just Say No is both the program title and the catch-phrase for one of the most widely visible prevention and education programs in history, and certainly the most visible drug abuse prevention campaign of the 1980s. Starting in 1984 with activities of the National Institute on Drug Abuse and then first lady Nancy Reagan, this effort to teach coping skills to children regarding drug abuse (in particular, how to effectively resist peer pressure) grew to significant national proportions. More than 10,000 local Just Say No clubs were started, and many celebrities and organizations lent their support to the movement.

TABLE 12.1   Mass Media Campaigns on Health Behavior: Analytic Framework

Media Components

1. PSAs—radio and TV.
2. News programs—radio and TV.
3. Information programs—radio and TV (talk shows, interview shows, documentaries).
4. Entertainment TV programs— episodic, soaps, TV movies.
5. Celebrity personal appearances.
6. Fundraising events.
7. Print media—newspapers, magazines, booklets.
8. Posters.
9. Feature films.
10. Radio—DJ discussion/interviews.
11. Educational films/video.
12. Special events—contests, awards.

Structure of Campaigns

1. Setting objectives.
2. Research.
3. Collaborating individuals/groups.
4. Design.
5. Production.
6. Ongoing operation.
7. Formative evaluation.
8. Redevelopment.
9. Outcome evaluation.

Effects

1. Awareness.
2. Factual information.
3. Attitude.
4. Intention.
5. Behavior.
6. Continued use.
7. Maintenance.

Collaborators

1. Mass media product developers.
2. Government.
3. Health care prevention.
4. Community/advocacy.
5. Media experts and expert organizations.
6. Media trade/professional organizations.

Context

1. Health care system.
2. Schools.
3. Family.
4. Workplace.
5. Government.
6. Community.

Principles for What Works

1. Use multiple media.
2. Combine media and interpersonal/community strategies.
3. Segment audience.
4. Use celebrities to get attention; entertainment programs to sustain attention.
5. Provide simple, clear message.
6. Emphasize positive behavior more than negative consequences.
7. Emphasize current rewards, not distant negative consequences.
8. Involve key power figures and organizations.
9. Take advantage of timing.
10. Use formative evaluation.

The mass media components of this multifaceted campaign were significant. Local and national television and radio PSAs, rap music videos by professional athletic teams, media appearances by Nancy Reagan and others identified with the program (including her appearances on several entertainment television programs), and extensive news coverage were among the strategies used.

Cocaine: The Big Lie

This behavioral-science-based program was initiated by the National Institute on Drug Abuse. The campaign featured print and television PSAs, with a toll-free telephone number for counseling and follow-up information, targeted to older teenagers and young adults who are currently nonusers or non-hardcore users of cocaine; a second phase was directed to high school and college students. The principal message of the campaign is that widely held views that cocaine won't hurt you and isn't addictive are simply not true.

Behavioral science consultation was used in the selection of content for the PSAs—messages oriented to debunking myths about cocaine in nonjudgmental terms, delivered by athletes, celebrities, and ex-users. The campaign was developed by Needham Harper Worldwide in conjunction with the Ad Council, a nonprofit group dedicated to public service uses of advertising.

Stop the Madness

An international campaign on drug abuse prevention, Stop the Madness, featured a music video and record with the same title. The music video followed the model established by "We Are the World" and featured music, television, sports, and political celebrities. The campaign also included a series of youth-oriented programs ("Rap for Life"), coordination with local drug abuse prevention efforts in 15 states, and international campaigns in Germany, Austria, Italy, and England. Developed by the Entertainment Industries Council (EIC) and funded in part by the National Institute on Drug Abuse (NIDA), this campaign was featured on the CBS Television Network, which donated millions of dollars worth of airtime for the PSAs the campaign generated.

The campaign was designed to hit hard on negative aspects of drug abuse, but was presented with high-concept entertainment values to hold the attention of its target audience of young teenagers. Health care professionals were involved in the selection of message content and in the development of community follow-through activities.

Facts for Life

According to the Centers for Disease Control, more than 25% of all people with AIDS in the United States are IV drug abusers; the incidence of AIDS among IV drug abusers is especially high in the black and Hispanic populations. These are difficult populations to reach; social isolation and the lifestyle and psychological characteristics of IV drug abusers and their sexual partners tend to make campaigns designed for other populations relatively ineffective. Although HIV infection rates appear to be decreasing dramatically among gay men, HIV infection is on the rise among IV drug abusers. A study by AIDS Project Los Angeles (Davis, 1988) suggest that the true rates of seropositivity amongst IV drug abusers may be much higher than previously thought and a comprehensive study by Stoneburner et al. (1988) among New York IV drug abusers confirms this finding. There have also been disturbing reports of increased incidence of HIV infection among cocaine abusers.

The nonprofit Entertainment Industries Council received a contract from the National Institute on Drug Abuse to develop a campaign directed at AIDS and IV drug abuse within the entertainment industry. The purpose of this project was to mobilize the resources of the film, television, and radio industries on behalf of AIDS education and prevention.

The project included major conferences for media professionals in New York and Los Angeles. Other activities involved EIC's collaboration on several industry-sponsored media projects in both the television and radio media. For instance, the project has worked with Spanish-language radio stations on a media campaign aimed at Hispanic men and women at risk for AIDS through IV drug abuse.

In a related effort (based on a successful previous NIDA project concerned with drug abuse), EIC and the Human Interaction Research Institute developed a multipart program that provided information and technical assistance to entertainment organizations whose own employees needed AIDS-related education or services. This included establishment of a 25-member labor–management voluntary group, the Entertainment Industry Workplace AIDS Task Force, which sponsored a conference for entertainment employers, published an information kit in notebook form, and offered a technical assistance service. This four-year effort to stimulate an industrywide AIDS policy and program development activity is documented in Backer (1992). These efforts were all ultimately intended to increase awareness and receptiveness of decision makers in the industry to public education efforts through the mass media.

The specific mass media campaign discussed here, called Facts for Life, is an offshoot of this above-described activity, and was conducted collaboratively by NIDA, EIC, and CBS Television. The result was production of 102 10-second public service announcements on AIDS and drug abuse that now air on prime time television, with an audience of many millions of people. Participating celebrities included Burt Lancaster, Whoopi Goldberg, Betty White, Melody Thomas, Theresa Ganzell, Smokey Robinson, Susan Flannery, and Marcia Wallace. Topics covered in the spots ranged from general service announcements on AIDS Awareness Month (in collaboration with the CDC national campaign) to more specific content regarding AIDS and IV drug abuse:

— The epidemiology of AIDS: It is not possible to contract AIDS through casual contact.
— The risk of contracting AIDS through needle-sharing in IV drug use.
— The risk of contracting AIDS through sexual contact with infected IV drug users.
— Women's risk of infecting their unborn babies through their IV drug use or sexual contact with infected drug users.

Forty of the 64 approved scripts were generic AIDS prevention scripts, including several that were time-limited because they were tied to October 1987 (AIDS Awareness Month). The remainder were specific to drug abuse, and mostly concentrated on IV drug abuse in particular. The latter included spots that touched on the epidemiology of AIDS among IV drug abusers, pointing out that one-quarter of all AIDS patients are IV drug abusers.

It has been estimated that CBS Television donated $10 million of air time for these PSAs, with a potential audience also in the tens of millions. Therefore, Facts for Life is one of the few mass media campaigns to have wide exposure on prime-time network television. Some critical ingredients related to the success of this campaign include the following:

— *Top Management Involvement.* From the beginning, B. Donald Grant, then president of CBS Entertainment, supported this project, as did Dr. Charles R. Schuster, Director of the National Institute on Drug Abuse. Approaching the CEOs of both organizations as a precondition of launching the campaign helped to get the go-ahead on a number of delicate issues (such as financial support from NIDA and use of the top CBS celebrities in the PSAs).
— *Financial Support.* The National Institute on Drug Abuse provided more than $50,000 in direct financial support for this project, to pay out-of-pocket production and creative expenses that could not be easily absorbed by CBS. This meant that the project did not have to be done cheaply, as so many PSA campaigns are, with resulting compromises in the content and appearance of the produced spots, and with a disproportionate amount of the campaign designers' energies going to hustling money rather than to making a good campaign.
— *Careful Attention to Scientific Content.* One of the three writers engaged to write the PSA scripts was a healthcare professional and support was provided for a thorough review of the latest scientific and medical data on AIDS and IV drug abuse in order to generate PSA content. For instance, the simple negative warning, "get AIDS and you'll die" is simply not effective with drug abusers, who already are at risk for death from overdose and who often have self-destructive personalities. Research by Dr. James Sorenson and his colleagues at the University of California–San Francisco Medical Center shows that other types of messages, such as "AIDS is very painful," are much more likely to have an impact on drug abuser's behavior. Such research was fed directly into the script development process, and scripts also were reviewed by technical experts at NIDA as a further check.

— *Focus on Direct Payoff to CBS.* The majority of mass media campaigns have concentrated on the community service and social responsibility rewards to the media for their involvement. Although such motivations clearly were relevant to the decision makers at CBS, this campaign was both easier to sell to CBS top management and easier to conduct (in terms of access to CBS production facilities and stars) because EIC designed it from the beginning to serve other, more commercial purposes as well. For instance, the spots began airing at the beginning of a new television season and CBS stars were featured. CBS was not asked to invest any money up-front, and current and former CBS personnel were directly involved in the production of the PSAs.

— *Attention to Commercial Requirements.* Even today, many mass media campaign designers do not acknowledge that PSAs longer than 10 seconds do not air in national prime time because of the high costs of commercial time at those hours. If only 30-second or 60-second PSAs are produced, they will not be seen except at off-hours or on local stations. Thus, although the 10-second format placed some strong limitations on the content of the Facts for Life spots, the result was a tremendous increase in the overall audience for the campaign.

Ironically, despite the significant success of Facts for Life, this campaign did not take advantage of all the principles for success mentioned later in this chapter. For instance, there was no coordinated community follow-through and only the 10-second PSA medium was used. Censorship also limited the success of the spots—when they were commissioned (this situation has since changed somewhat), CBS would not allow the word *condom* to be used, and NIDA did not permit mention of needle exchange programs.

Partnership for a Drug-Free America

Founded in 1986, the Partnership for a Drug-Free America is a coalition of advertising agencies, media buyers, television networks, publishers, trade associations, cable television companies, and many other organizations. The Partnership's mission is to use the power of the mass media to prevent drug abuse. In its first four years of operation, the Partnership was able to place approximately $150 million per year of pro bono public service advertising in print, radio, and television media.

The Partnership is a nonprofit corporation with a staff of more than 25 full-time employees based in New York City. Its key executives include a number of current and retired senior persons from the advertising and media industries.

The Partnership began its activities in 1986 with a careful needs assessment and review of public service advertising techniques, including dialogues with media campaign scholars and consultants in academic settings. From this review came the conviction that the most successful campaign (contrary to some of the expert opinion the Partnership's founders had received) would be one that emphasized a fear appeal in its early stages, in order to capture attention and impress the national audience about the seriousness of the problem. Out of this conviction came the famed "Fried Egg" public service announcement ("this is your brain on drugs"), which generated great acclaim and considerable controversy.

Now the Partnership has moved on to a number of follow-up campaigns, including several targeted to minority communities. A national evaluation has been conducted by the Charles Black Corporation, showing evidence of considerable awareness and attitude change among key target audiences such as teenagers. Some projections about actual impact on drug use in the United States also have been made from the evaluation results, and the Partnership's work has been commended by presidents Reagan and Bush, the U.S. Congress, and the National Institute on Drug Abuse.

The Partnership's initial campaigns were intended primarily to prevent experimentation with drugs. They were targeted to preteens, teenagers, adults, and their influencers—peers, parents, healthcare professionals, and business leaders. Special task forces have developed campaigns targeted specifically to African-American and Hispanic audiences. The first Spanish-language advertising was launched in March 1989, and the African-American campaign was released in October 1989.

Some Partnership efforts also have been directed at employers and labor unions, as part of a response to the problem of drug abuse in the workplace. For instance, the National Institute on Drug Abuse's toll-free Employer Helpline was marketed through the partnership's print ads, which resulted in a large number of telephone calls to the Helpline. The Partnership has participated in Hoffman LaRoche's efforts to organize employer responses to drug abuse in the workplace through a series of conferences and print publications.

A public relations campaign spearheaded by Fred Berger, former vice chair of PR firm Hill & Knowlton, has used public relations approaches to convey new messages about the effects of drugs on nonusers and about the progress in reducing drug abuse that has actually been made in the last several years. Another campaign element has involved tying in the Partnership's activities with those of local, city, state, and grass-roots and consumer organizations. Yet another campaign element involves working with Hollywood to help place messages on entertainment programs and to use the enormous power of the entertainment media.

The media objective for the Partnership has been reached: $365 million a year in donated media, or $1 million a day. Already, the Partnership has achieved a penetration of American media unparalleled in the history of public service campaigns:

- The three television networks broadcast more than 4,000 Partnership messages.
- Eleven cable networks ran more than 6,000 Partnership spots.
- Eleven radio networks aired more than 9,500 Partnership commercials.
- More than 1,000 newspapers have run Partnership ads.
- More than 100 magazines are supporting the Partnership with hundreds of national and regional pages.

- Medical journals ran 1,310 full-page ads created separately by 10 healthcare agencies.
- Hundreds of radio and television stations have broadcast thousands of Partnership messages to millions of Americans every day since March 1987.

There has also been a great deal of nontraditional media use of the advertising. For example, corporations use Partnership messages for employee education programs. Many schools and community prevention and treatment organizations across the country have incorporated Partnership ads into their programs, and the messages have been added to in-home video rentals and used as posters.

Some of the critical factors that account for the extraordinary success of the Partnership include the following:

- A top-level leadership coalition was developed early, consisting of some of the most influential individuals and organizations in the advertising, marketing, and media industries.
- A bandwagon effect developed early on, with organizations feeling compelled to get on board because so many of the leaders in their industry already were.
- The campaign flowered at just the time that America's national consciousness about drug abuse was at its peak.
- An early effort was made to get the CEO or other top executives of major organizations (such as Dan Burke at ABC Television) involved in the campaign to make a personal commitment, which in turn helped to overcome both organizational and individual resistance.
- Participating advertising agencies and others were eager to have their work seen by their professional peers and by potential clients, which had both an indirect professional prestige aspect and a practical business development aspect.
- The campaign was deliberately styled as an elite effort, with screening committees that actually rejected ads that were not up to very high creative standards, in striking contrast to most public service campaigns, where any donation is gratefully accepted, even if of inferior quality.
- Organizations in the participating industries are concentrated in New York City, which made communication and collaboration easier.

- Early, comprehensive attitudinal research and input from drug abuse and media campaign experts were solicited, which helped to provide a solid empirical base for the campaign's messages.
- Empirical evidence of what messages got on the air or in print, and especially empirical evidence of impact from the Gordon S. Black evaluation, were of great value both in convincing potential sponsors and collaborators to come on board, and in boosting credibility of the program with the public and with government agencies whose efforts could be coordinated with those of the Partnership.
- A deliberately low-key approach was taken, with only limited visibility for the Partnership and its members, so that the messages about drug use stand on their own.

The Partnership campaign is documented in Backer & Rogers (1993).

GENERALIZATIONS: WHAT WORKS AND WHAT DOESN'T

In Phase I of the research study for the Center for Substance Abuse Prevention, a comprehensive literature review was conducted to determine what strategies and principles had been found successful in past media campaigns. Literature reviews, analytic articles, case studies of media campaigns, and empirical research reports were analyzed for this purpose.

Next, the researchers interviewed 29 experts in mass media campaigns, ranging from campaign designers to senior media professionals to scholars conducting research on campaigns. These narrative interviews were content analyzed for principles related to what had been learned from the literature.

Following are generalizations about mass media campaigns extracted from the comprehensive literature review and 29 interviews with world experts on mass media campaigns conducted by Backer, Rogers, & Sopory (1992):

- More effective mass media campaigns use multiple media.
- More effective mass media campaigns combine mass media with community, small group, and individual action options, supported by an existing community structure (using a systems approach).
- More effective campaigns carefully target or segment the audience that the campaign is intended to affect.
- Celebrities can help to attract public attention to a campaign issue. Embedding a campaign's behavior change message in an entertainment program helps to sustain public attention.
- Repetition of a simple, clear message makes for a more effective campaign.
- Preventive mass media campaigns are more effective if they emphasize positive behavior change rather than the negative consequences of current behavior; arousing fear is rarely successful.
- Mass media campaigns are more effective if they emphasize current rewards rather than avoidance of distant negative consequences.
- More effective mass media campaigns involve in their design and operation key power figures and groups in mass communication organizations and in government bodies.
- Timing of a media campaign (when it is introduced, what else is happening during its operation, etc.) is important in determining campaign effectiveness.
- More effective communication campaigns use formative evaluation techniques to appraise the campaign and improve it as it operates.
- More effective mass media campaigns set fairly modest, attainable goals in terms of behavior change.
- Commercial marketing and social marketing techniques have potential for increasing the effectiveness of mass media campaigns.
- More effective campaigns use both entertainment and education strategies.
- More effective mass media campaigns make deliberate efforts to resolve potential conflicts between evaluation researchers and message creators.
- More effective mass media campaigns address the larger social-structural and environmental factors impinging on a health problem (such as poverty and lack of economic opportunity).
- More effective mass media campaigns are connected to a direct service delivery component so that there can be immediate follow-through if behavior change begins to occur.
- Segmentation of campaign audiences by demographics is not very effective; segmentation by psychographic variables may be more successful.

- More effective mass media campaigns direct messages to those around the targeted individual for behavior change, especially individuals in positions of interpersonal influence (peers and parents in particular).
- More effective mass media campaigns choose their role models carefully, as they can easily become tainted (such as celebrities who later are discovered to have a substance abuse problem themselves)
- If fear appeals are used, they should be coupled with mechanisms for reducing the anxiety that is created.
- Public Service Announcements (PSAs) alone generally are not effective in bringing about behavior change; they must be combined with other approaches.
- More effective mass media campaigns interact with the news media as a means of increasing the visibility of a campaign.
- The role of government in media campaigns is mainly to provide funding for campaigns and appropriate leadership on controversial issues.
- More effective mass media campaigns address existing knowledge and beliefs of the target audience that are impeding adoption of the desired behavior.
- More effective mass media campaigns communicate incentives or benefits for adopting desired behaviors that build on the existing motives, needs, and values of the target group.
- More effective mass media campaigns focus the target audience's attention on immediate, high-probability consequences of behavior.
- More effective mass media campaigns use extensive pretesting to ensure that the campaign materials are appropriate for and appeal to the target audiences.

Some additional generalizations emerged from this study that are more specific to designing mass media campaigns specifically targeted to substance abuse prevention activities with high-risk youth:

- Mass media campaigns may start as early as grades 5 and 6. "Reminder campaigns" then can be phased in as these youngsters grow into adolescence. Because research shows that substantial numbers of youth begin substance abuse in junior high or earlier, campaigns that are truly prevention-oriented must start even earlier. Campaigns that focus on gateway drugs—alcohol, tobacco, and marijuana—are especially likely to have long-term impact.
- Mass media campaigns also may include efforts to increase public awareness of broader social contexts in which substance abuse occurs. They can promote discussion of public policy options and enhance the climate for actual changes in policy. This in turn can promote individual behavior change. Debate about tobacco and alcohol advertising and use of promotions targeted to minority adolescents are among the policy issues that can be addressed in this way
- More effective mass media campaigns for high-risk youth may include components with specific educational messages to parents. Parents exert much influence over their children, so strategies such as encouraging parents to talk with children about drugs and working with parent groups that sponsor drug-free parties can have a real impact.
- More effective mass media campaigns must include campaign messages that highlight important themes in the development of adolescent identity, including freedom, autonomy, and peer group acceptance. Substance use often occurs in response to these powerful themes. Prevention campaigns that work are often those that highlight coping skills for avoiding drugs or that emphasize assertively making choices in response to pressures from advertisers or substance-using peers. Sometimes presenting older peers who display such skills can be of particularly critical importance.
- Effective mass media campaigns may be more effective if they use peer models rather than celebrity adults as campaign spokespersons. Youth who are rebellious against authority are likely to view any adult spokesperson with suspicion.
- More effective mass media campaigns may include the use of image or lifestyle advertising to promote an active, healthy lifestyle that is by its nature intolerant of substance use. Such strategies have worked well for many commercial products.
- More effective mass media campaigns for high-risk youth may include radio as a critical delivery system. Radio is much less costly as a message delivery service and plays an important role in the everyday lives of many young people.

THE IMPACT OF ORGANIZATIONS AND INTERORGANIZATIONAL NETWORKS ON MASS MEDIA CAMPAIGNS

Both the case examples and the research-based generalizations cited above make it abundantly clear that mass media campaigns are more likely to be successful if they bring to bear the combined resources of a number of organizations through strategic alliances. A critical but little-studied aspect of mass media campaigns is the impact of organizations.

Organizations get involved in media campaigns, with productive or nonproductive results, for reasons related to internal championship, organizational climate, interorganizational linkages, resistance to change, and other factors well-known to organizational theorists and management consultants. Organizational factors have been touched on in recent works such as Kathryn Montgomery's *Target Prime Time* (1989), but the critical role of organizations in mass media campaigns has been little explored to date. More importantly, organizational theory and practice have not been applied to enhancing understanding of this role and how campaign designers can learn to better inspire, design, implement, and evaluate campaigns in drug abuse and related health areas.

In Phase II of the research program for the Center for Substance Abuse Prevention, these variables were examined using a case study model in which campaign designers wrote about their work; each case study then was analyzed by a senior management scientist with expertise in organization development and change. Six mass media campaigns were selected for examination in this study, four of which focus on substance abuse prevention: the Partnership for a Drug-Free America, which has been analyzed above; the Drug Abuse Resistance Education (DARE) Program, which brings police officers into schools for prevention education in more than 600 American communities; the Harvard Alcohol Project, a foundation-funded campaign for public education that centers on depiction of alcohol use in entertainment television programs; and Project

STAR, the Kansas City–based drug abuse prevention campaign including both media and community involvement components (Backer & Rogers, 1993).

The following generalizations emerged from the case studies and organizational analyses:

— *Prestige.* The prestige of organizations involved in a health communication campaign is a factor in the campaign's success.
— *Insider–outsider relationships.* Effective relationships between outsider and insider organizations contribute to the success of health communication campaigns.
— *Reinvention.* Campaign elements are often reinvented and modified as organizations contribute experiences from other campaigns in which they have participated, and as general campaign approach is fitted to local community conditions.
— *Long-term institutional change.* Strategies for long-term institutional change in organizational culture, and for creating permanent organizations to replace temporary systems, are used by organizations involved in a campaign to facilitate long-term behavior change in their target audiences.
— *Consensus vision.* A campaign is more likely to be successful if it has an overall vision statement that represents a consensus among the organizations that collaborate in the campaign.
— *Charismatic organizational leaders.* Charismatic leaders of organizations involved in health communication campaigns help organizations collaborate in successful ways.
— *Interorganizational diffusion.* Interorganizational collaboration can speed the diffusion of a health communication campaign approach.
— *Organizational career path.* Participation in a health communication campaign can affect the career path of individuals in the collaborating organizations.
— *Organizational culture conflict.* Differences in organizational culture, such as those between government and private organizations, can limit the success of health communication campaigns unless these differences are overcome.
— *Timing.* The timing of a health communication campaign is a crucial factor in its success, and timing often rests on the activities or decisions of organizations involved in the campaign.

- *Reframing.* Reframing health communication campaign behavior in terms of organizational theory can facilitate understanding of the key factors in a campaign's success.
- *Transorganizational issues.* Transorganizational issues of collaboration, control, and resistance among groups of organizations affect the chances for success of health communication campaigns.

SUGGESTIONS FOR FUTURE CAMPAIGNS

The above two sets of generalizations may be applied to campaign design and execution in a number of ways. For instance, it may be helpful to create a checklist of desirable campaign features based on the generalizations. Any campaign design can be compared against this checklist while it is still in its earliest stages.

Reference could also be made in planning sessions to the text of these generalizations. They are meant to provoke questions as much as answer them, so not a lot of clarifying discussion has been added. However, campaign designers might want to review selected interview transcripts or literature citations listed in this report for more background.

Such a checklist might be especially useful as a strategic planning device for a campaign developer or advisory committee. Economics, special campaign circumstances, or the philosophies and values of those conducting or sponsoring a campaign might preclude addressing certain generalizations, but the evidence suggests that there is a critical mass for campaign effectiveness that can be moved forward by such a strategic planning process.

The above generalizations are by no means presented as unchanging realities about what works and what doesn't in mass media health behavior change campaigns. Though cross-validated in a number of campaigns, these principles and strategies are still only incompletely understood. They have not been analyzed in terms of their relative importance across different topical areas, although some effort was made here to

look at the mass of evidence with special attention to high-risk youth.

Other topics of considerable importance have not been addressed by researchers or campaign designers in any systematic way, yet seem highly relevant to the development of future mass media campaigns:

- Word-of-mouth and promotional messages that are pro-use, including advertising of legal (for adults) drugs such as alcohol and tobacco, are also part of the environment in which media campaigns operate. How might campaigns be designed in a way that would intercept such messages (for example, addressing street myths about drug effects or exploring the potential of counteradvertising or media advocacy opportunities)? How can the array of pro-use messages for a particular topic and target audience be taken into account in planning a mass media campaign?
- How can strategies used in advertising, public relations, and corporate public affairs campaigns be added to the array of intervention already used in campaigns? Press conferences, product placements in films and television shows, and public relations strategies such as mentions of campaigns on television and radio news shows or in print media are among the possibilities. Some fairly specific options for intervention already are available, such as getting set designers and production designers in films or TV shows to use prevention-oriented posters on their sets so that they'll appear on the screen. Such an effort could be facilitated by a union or other media-based organization.
- How do community involvement and interpersonal strategies interweave with all of the desirable campaign features included in this analysis? How does the mix of campaign strategies need to vary depending on the other components of the overall message system?
- How can strategic planning among a wide range of organizations contribute to large-scale systems change in various health behavior areas—including as components mass media campaigns, community involvement, interpersonal strategies, policy and legislative changes, and other factors that all interweave to change structures, values, and behaviors?

— How can mechanisms be developed for the pretesting and evaluation of mass media campaigns, including those that take advantage of the comparative synthesis approach used here? The federal government at one time sponsored a Health Messages Testing Service. Could such a program be productively restarted?

— What other mechanisms for evaluation of the long-term impacts of mass media health behavior campaigns should be created?

— In fast-evolving areas such as AIDS, how do mass media health behavior campaigns remain responsive to changing science and medical practice?

MEDIA CAMPAIGNS RELATED TO OTHER SYSTEMS INTERVENTIONS

Mass media campaigns to change health behavior are *systems* interventions, complex and requiring exquisite attention to detail in order to be successful. Media campaigns often pay careful attention to the principles of individual behavior change (which are, of course, quite complex, especially where matters such as drug abuse or sexual behavior are concerned). Sometimes campaigns also pay attention to the related principles for small group or community involvement. However, campaign design in organizational change terms is uncommon—often resulting in unnecessary setbacks or shortcomings in campaign effectiveness.

Backer (1988b) examined America's response to the AIDS health crisis in terms of planned organizational change, and mass media campaigns on this and other health-related topics are best seen through that framework. Organizational change principles abound in the generalizations about what works and what doesn't that were presented earlier in this chapter, and in the discussion of the five mass media drug abuse prevention campaigns given as examples. At a more general level, understanding the nature and tradition of media organizations is needed because that enables effective organizational or systemwide interventions.

With such a perspective, no mass media campaign exists in isolation. The Facts for Life campaign is an ideal example: It began with EIC's success in another, related campaign with CBS (the Stop the Madness drug abuse PSA campaign), and continued in the context of many other efforts EIC was developing under its contractual relationship with NIDA, including efforts to provide information and service directly to entertainment employers and unions dealing with AIDS in their own ranks.

The campaign was carefully orchestrated with other ongoing efforts, such as the CDC-sponsored America Responds to AIDS campaigns. Some of the principles that have already been identified as common to success in mass media campaigns are almost universally embraced, such as the need for community involvement. Yet even otherwise well-designed campaigns such as Facts for Life don't always use these strategies. Other principles, such as involving media professional societies in program design and execution, are not as well-recognized and accepted. Still others may have some real generality, but have not yet been identified at all outside the health behavior area, where they were first invented and applied. As more knowledge is accumulated about what works and what doesn't, new options will arise for the design of effective mass media campaigns to change health behavior.

REFERENCES

Backer, T. E. (1988a). Health professionals and mass media campaigns to prevent AIDS and drug abuse. *Counseling and Human Development, 20* (7), 1–10.

Backer, T. E. (1988b). Utilization, planned change and the AIDS health crisis. *The Disseminator, 2* (1), 3–4.

Backer, T. E. (1990). Comparative synthesis of mass media health behavior campaigns. *Knowledge: Creation, Diffusion, Utilization, 11* (3), 315–329.

Backer, T. E. (1992). An industry-wide OD intervention: The entertainment industry responds to AIDS. In A. M. Glassman & T. G. Cummings (Eds.), *Cases in organization development.* New York: Business Publications, Inc.

Backer, T. E., & Rogers, E. M. (Eds.). (1993). *Organizational aspects of health communication campaigns: What works?* Newbury Park, CA: Sage.

Backer, T. E., Rogers, E. M., & Sopory, P. (1992). *Designing health communication campaigns: What works?* Newbury Park, CA: Sage.

Davis, R. J. (1988). *Survey of substance abuse or misuse among clients of AIDS Project Los Angeles.* Los Angeles: AIDS Project Los Angeles.

DeFleur, M. L., & Dennis, E. E. (1981). *Understanding mass communication.* Boston: Houghton Mifflin.

DeJong, W., & Winsten, J. A. (1989). *Recommendations for future mass media campaigns to prevent preteen and adolescent substance abuse.* Unpublished paper, Center for Health Communication, Harvard School of Public Health.

Flay, B. R. (1986). *Mass media and smoking cessation.* Paper presented at the Annual Conference of the International Communication Association, Chicago.

Kerr, P. (1986). Anatomy of the drug issue: How, after years, it erupted. *New York Times,* November 17, A1.

Maccoby, N., & Solomon, D. S. (1981). Heart disease prevention: Community studies. In R. E. Rice & W. J. Paisley (Eds.), *Public Communication Campaigns.* Newbury Park, CA: Sage.

Montgomery, K. (1989). *Target prime time.* New York: Oxford University Press.

Rogers, E. M., & Storey, J. D. (1988). Communication campaigns. In S. Chafee & C. Berger (Eds.), *Handbook of communication science.* Newbury Park, CA: Sage.

Signorielli, N. (Sept. 1988). *Health and the media: Images and impact.* Paper presented at Mass Communications and Health: Complexities and Conflicts Conference, Annenberg Center, Rancho Mirage, CA.

Stoneburner, R. L., et al. (1988). A larger spectrum of severe HIV-related disease in intravenous drug users in New York City. *Science, 242,* 916–919.

PART THREE

CLIENT-ORIENTED PREVENTION STRATEGIES AND PROGRAMS

CHAPTER 13

COLLEGE STUDENTS

LEWIS D. EIGEN

Surprising as it may seem, colleges and universities are particularly risky environments for problems of alcohol and other drugs. When we compare drug use by college students with that of their noncollege counterparts, we find that college students are generally heavier drinkers of alcohol, and are more likely to use marijuana, MDMA ("ecstasy"), and inhalants. However, for other drugs such as heroin, stimulants, cigarettes, cocaine (including crack) and all other drugs, use among college students is less than among their noncollege peers[1] (Johnston et al., 1991). Colleges and universities are communities with their own cultural traditions, physical environments, and well-defined populations that are often quite different and somewhat removed from their immediate surroundings. Their alcohol and other drug problems are distinct, and approaches to prevention must be focused and often quite different from preventive approaches in the outside community.

PREVALENCE

Table 13.1 presents the 1990 full-time, undergraduate college student monthly, annual, and lifetime prevalence figures for various different drugs (Johnston et al., 1991).

If we were to apply these prevalence rates to Prototypical University, with a student body of 10,000 undergraduates, we could assume that last month 1,400 students smoked marijuana and 7,450 students drank alcohol. These two drugs accounted for the overwhelming majority of all drug use on the campus. True, 140 Prototypical U

students used stimulants, 120 ingested cocaine (including crack), 140 students tried hallucinogens (mostly LSD), and a few used many of the other drugs, but with the exception of alcohol and marijuana, campus use of drugs is limited to only about 4.4% of the student body in any given month. Although this use is serious and must be prevented, it can reasonably be defined as unusual or nonnormative on the typical campus. At the other extreme is alcohol, which is commonly used by the overwhelming majority of students. This drug use is the norm; it is expected. In-between is marijuana. It is currently used by a minority of students, but a sufficiently large minority in that marijuana is not perceived as being as aberrant as other illicit drugs. To the degree that prevention efforts are a process of denormalization of drug use, it is much more difficult to denormalize student alcohol use than to denormalize the other drugs.

Males drink more often and in heavier amounts (even corrected for body weight) than females, in college as well as elsewhere in society (Eigen, 1991). For other drugs, the lesser prevalence of female college student use is also well-established (Johnston et al., 1991). However, college women are by no means risk-free, and long-term trends indicate that the gender difference may be disappearing. There is increasing evidence that as women's gender-role orientations more closely approach those of men, their alcohol and other drug risk and behavior also move in that direction. For example, employment in a male-dominated occupation and the possession of an advanced educational degree

267

TABLE 13.1   Prevalence of College Undergraduate Drug Use

DRUG	MONTHLY	ANNUAL	LIFETIME
Marijuana	14.0%	29.4%	49.1%
Inhalants	1.0	3.9	13.9
Hallucinogens	1.4	5.4	11.1
LSD	1.1	4.3	9.1
Cocaine	1.2	5.6	11.4
Crack	.1	0.6	1.4
MDMA	0.6	2.3	3.9
Heroin	0.0	0.1	0.3
Other opiates	0.5	2.9	6.8
Stimulants	1.4	4.5	13.2
Crystal methamphetamine	0.0	0.1	1.0
Barbiturates	0.2	1.4	3.8
Tranquilizers	0.5	3.0	7.1
Alcohol	74.5	89.0	93.3

are both additional alcohol risk factors for females (S. C. Wilsnack et al., 1985). Other research has shown that women of lower educational status were much more likely to be alcohol abstainers (R. W. Wilsnack et al., 1984).

RACIAL AND ETHNIC GROUPS

The drinking patterns and associated problems of nonwhites are generally different from those of whites. Black college students are more likely to be abstainers than their white counterparts, and when they do drink it is generally not as frequently or heavily (Johnston et al., 1991). There are not a great deal of college-specific data on the drinking patterns of Hispanics, Asian Americans and Native Americans. However, drinking patterns vary by Hispanic subgroup and Native-American tribe. In all American ethnic subgroups, males are heavier and more frequent drinkers than females (Johnston et al., 1991). This is also true for illicit drugs.

THE MAJOR CAMPUS DRUG
PROBLEM: ALCOHOL

In her 1990 interview with *Time Magazine,* University of Wisconsin chancellor Donna Shalala,

later to become Secretary of Health and Human Services, was asked what the biggest problem was on her campus. The answer was alcohol. Her opinion is not atypical. In a recent Carnegie Foundation survey, college presidents classified alcohol abuse as the campus life issue of their greatest concern (Carnegie Foundation, 1990). The data support their view. Alcohol is, by far, the drug used most frequently and most heavily on most college campuses, accounts for the majority of adverse health consequences, produces the greatest risk of addiction on campus, is associated with the most property damage and the most crime, and diverts the largest amount of student funds away from more constructive purposes. Of a typical student body, 74.5% will drink some alcohol next month, whereas only 71% of their noncollege counterparts will. Forty-one percent of U.S. college students engaged in a bout of heavy drinking (five or more drinks in a row) in the last two weeks, whereas only 34% of their noncollege counterparts did so (Johnston et al., 1991). The same survey tells us that next year, only 11% of U.S. students will refrain from drinking. Perhaps most serious, almost 4% of all college students will drink every single day next month. That's 400 students every day on the Prototypical U campus. Not just a few beers at the fraternity party Saturday night, or some wine at the campus dance, but daily drinking. The college versus noncollege pattern is even stronger with women. In a recent study of New York State College women age 23 and younger (Harris, 1986), it was found that their rate of heavy drinking (17%) was more than twice the heavy drinking rate of their noncollege counterparts (8%).

DRINKING PATTERNS

The national drinking average per college student is more than 34 gallons per year. This is a very conservative estimate for college students in that it is based on averages for the general population age group, and college students are known to drink more alcohol than their noncollege counterparts. For the more than 12 million college students in the United States, the annual consumption of alcoholic beverages totals well over 430 million gallons (Johnston et al., 1991). By volume, beer represents the vast majority of campus alcoholic beverage consumption. Although beer generally has a lower ethanol content than wine or spirits, most of the college students' ethanol intake comes from beer. The annual beer consumption of American college students is just short of four billion cans. If these cans were stacked end-to-end, the stack would reach the moon and then go 70,000 miles beyond (Eigen, 1991). Compared with other drinks, the national consumption of alcoholic beverages exceeds that of soft drinks, tea, milk, juice, and even coffee (U.S. Department of Commerce, 1989).

When they do drink, college-age people tend to be more reckless and determined to get a "kick" than others. As mentioned above, more than 40% of U.S. college students will toss down 5 or more drinks in a row in the next two weeks. At a "drinking campus," the majority of students will do so. At a recent conference, many college administrators reported a growing trend in student drinking with the clear intent of intoxication (Missouri Governors' Conference, 1990). Drinking to the point of regurgitation is not uncommon in college. A 1987 survey of 56 colleges found

that 37% of the students had vomited as a result of drinking in the last year (Engs & Hanson, 1988). If one ignores the abstainers, roughly half of the drinking college students drank to the point of vomiting at least once during the year. This binge drinking represents the greatest immediate health threat to the drinker and others around the drinker.

ECONOMIC CONSEQUENCES

Former Surgeon General Antonio Novella has observed that college students spend more money on alcohol than on textbooks. Alcohol consumption, abuse, and its consequences have an economic cost to the college and the campus community. This estimate is generally conceded to be much greater than the cost estimate of non-alcoholic illicit drug use. It is not that alcohol per se is a much more deleterious drug than cocaine or heroin. The problem is that so many more college students use and abuse alcohol than use and abuse illicit drugs. Therefore, the effects and costs of alcohol use and abuse are much greater and more widespread. On a representative campus, the student body expenditure for alcohol—about $446 per student—will far exceed the operating costs for running the library. The total annual cost of the scholarships and fellowships that all the colleges and universities of America provide to students is but a fraction of the $5.5 billion college students spend yearly on alcohol (U.S. Department of Commerce, 1989).

There is simply no measure of exactly what proportion of campus vandalism and theft is alcohol- and drug-related. One estimate given in *The Chronicle of Higher Education* was that 80% of all campus vandalism was alcohol-related. A recent national study estimated that more than two-thirds were alcohol-related (Anderson & Gadaleto, 1991).

HEALTH CONSEQUENCES

The most serious health consequence of alcohol and other drug abuse is death. It occurs all too often. The most immediate death threat to the college student is an alcohol-related automobile crash. Of the 20,000 deaths that will occur in America this next year as a result of alcohol-related automobile crashes, college students will be overrepresented. For every fatality, there will be many more maimings and serious injuries. How many college students drive drunk? A poll reported in *The Wall Street Journal* (1983) disclosed that two out of every three undergraduates admitted to driving while intoxicated. A more recent study at the University of Iowa indicates that this proportion may have decreased somewhat. The Iowa study indicated a 40% annual prevalence rate of driving after drinking and the same rate of knowingly driving with a driver who had had too much to drink (Petroff & Broek, 1990).

Another cause of immediate death is the popular practice of "chug-a-lug"—the rapid ingestion of alcohol (usually beer). Students often die as a result of engaging in this traditional activity that goes back hundreds of years to the European universities. Overdoses of illicit drugs such as cocaine and heroin, though not common in colleges, also produce tragedies.

Alcohol-related suicides, drownings, and fatal falls account for many college student deaths each year (Eigen, 1991). Homicide is also a risk, as in the case of an intoxicated student who shot and killed one of his fellow students in a residence hall of Concordia College of Nebraska. Many college students also die as a result of fraternity or sorority hazing. Nine out of every 10 of these deaths are related to alcohol use (*Chronicle of Higher Education, 1982*). The president of California State University at Chico anguished, "I write a couple of letters a semester to parents of kids who have died because of something related to the use of booze" (Wilson, 1990).

Immediate alcohol- and drug-related death is actually a much lower risk than eventual alcohol-related death. If past trends continue, between 240,000 and 360,000 of the 12 million U.S. college students will eventually die of alcohol-related causes. This figure is equivalent to the entire undergraduate student body of all the schools of the Big Ten (Eigen, 1991).

Alcohol and other drugs affect memory, perception, judgment, and behavior. Young drinkers are more susceptible to drinking to the point of memory lapse than older drinkers. Among 18- to 25-year-old drinkers, 26% reported that they were unable to remember what happened at least once in the last year (National Institute on Drug Abuse, 1988). Human memory is particularly susceptible to disruption by acute doses of alcohol. The blood alcohol concentration (BAC) correlates with the extent of the amnesia. A BAC as low as .04 grams per milliliter alters memory functions, and memory impairment gets worse as the BAC increases (Parker, 1984). A BAC of .04 is far less than that of many students on a typical American campus each Saturday night, and less than the .10 level that defines legal intoxication in most states. The impaired judgment and coordination of drinking college students produces hundreds of thousands of injuries each year. Most of us are familiar with the danger of alcohol-related car crashes, but alcohol-related injuries take myriad forms. These range from the University of Idaho sorority pledge who fell from the sorority house balcony and was paralyzed (*Lewiston Tribune,* 1993) to the students who fell down the elevator shaft in Oneonta, New York.

In 1987, 91,000 18- to 25-year-olds were admitted to American hospitals with alcohol-related diagnoses (Stinson, 1987). These hospital admissions do not include any alcohol-related injuries or the results of alcohol-related accidents. They reflect only the alcohol-related diseases that are usually brought about by prolonged or heavy drinking.

How many of the students who need assistance from the student health center require it for alcohol-related conditions? It is difficult to verify. Although health center records indicate alcohol-related diseases, like hospital discharge records they tend to underestimate alcohol-related health incidents. The main reason is injuries. Is the broken finger or nose just an accident or the result of an alcohol-related incident? Is the young woman who seeks a pregnancy test simply trying to assess the damage of an alcohol-related sexual encounter she may not fully remember? The University of Iowa has estimated that 15% of its undergraduates had suffered from alcohol-related injuries in the past year (Petroff & Broek, 1990). The same study found that more than 29% of its undergraduates had engaged in unplanned sexual activity, during or after drinking, at least once in the last year.

SOCIAL CONSEQUENCES

There are a number of social consequences of drinking alcohol on campus. Some consequences are positive. There is little doubt that alcohol is a part of most college culture and tradition. In a sense, alcohol is a social lubricant that gives students, faculty, and alumni an easy, traditional way of initiating conversations, bonding, and socializing. We have our college drinking songs, our alcohol-related (sometimes dominated) events, and the alcohol-related stories. Those stories typically form the backbone of alumni reunions and other events. In one recent study of college student drinking, it was found that for males, almost all their bonding with their fellows took place with alcoholic beverages, and this was the main purpose of their drinking (Burda & Vaux, 1988). Even among campus athletes, who seem to have great social status, 87% stated that their main reason for drinking was recreational or social. The next most frequent reason, "makes me feel good," was given by only 10%, and dealing with the stress of college life and athletics was given by fewer than 3% (Anderson, 1989).

The process of forming social relationships with members of the opposite sex is also facilitated by drinking and the events that accompany it. Many students drink only in social situations. There are many female students who will never have a drink unless they are on a date or in the company of men. Many college men drink in co-ed social situations because they perceive a correlation between drinking and their prospects for social success. The relationship between drinking and social interactions is by no means limited to co-ed situations, but is a factor in the shaping of interpersonal relationship development. In a certain sense, many view this as the distinction between healthy and unhealthy drinking. The person who drinks alone is perhaps in trouble, or seems to be. In a perverse contrast with reality, those who drink in social situations are often erroneously believed to not be in trouble. Most college drinking is done in couples or in small or large groups.

This socialization function of alcoholic beverages is a fundamental benefit for which many pay the negative health and economic consequences. Imagine the findings that sociologists from Mars would report if they came to Earth and studied our college campuses. They would undoubtedly write about the primitive belief and custom that this strange liquid was needed to "bless" almost all events, social unions, and discussions. They would point to our superstition that alcohol was a necessary ingredient for much campus activity.

According to a 1987 study, there were 285,000 serious crimes committed on America's university campuses, including 31 murders, 600 reported rapes, 13,000 assaults, and more than 23,000 robberies and burglaries (*New York Times,* 1990). In addition, there were tens of thousands of incidents of brawling, fighting, rape, vandalism, and other acts of violence that were never reported or treated as crimes. A recent Carnegie Foundation study (1990) observed, "We also found a close connection between alcohol abuse and campus crime." In a recent report to Congress by the Secretary of Health and Human Services, the issue was summarized: "In both animal and human studies, alcohol, more than any other drug, has been linked with a high incidence of violence and aggression" (NIAAA, 1989).

Under the influence of alcohol and many other drugs, perception is weakened, judgment is impaired, inhibitions are reduced, and all too often, aggressiveness and hostility are increased. That was what the University of Wisconsin Chancellor was referring to when she, like so many others, linked alcohol to the problem of campus rape (*Time,* 1990). For young adults, expressing themselves clearly regarding areas of sexual desire and consent is even more troublesome than it is for their more mature elders, for whom this has always been difficult, even when sober. An intoxicated young man's perception of what he may be hearing or seeing is less reliable than normal. His judgment is flawed, compounding the problem of his misperception. If the woman has also been drinking, her judgment and ability to say "No" are also imperfect. The more drinking or other drug-taking involved, the greater the likelihood that, at best, a disagreeable misunderstanding will occur and, at worst, a violent crime. Drinking is also a factor in many gang rapes that occur on college campuses ("Gang Rape," *New York Times,* 1986). Typical is the recent rape of a Florida State student who had attended a huge fraternity party where everyone brought their own booze (*St. Petersburg Times,* 1993).

One school study indicated that 7% of its undergraduates had stolen something in the last year after drinking, almost 10% had committed acts of vandalism, and 7% had been in fights after drinking (Petroff & Broek, 1990). Theft in order to obtain alcohol or other drug money is all too common on college campuses. However, there is little specific, quantitative research to support the overwhelming anecdotal evidence on the connection of drinking with crime on campus. However, there are very good data on this relationship in society in general. More than half of the perpetrators of crimes of violence are impaired by alcohol.

Drinking alcohol also potentially increases one's chances of being a crime victim. The impairment of judgment diminishes the ability to take prudent protective actions. While "under the influence," people often place themselves in potentially dangerous situations. Also, many with criminal intent look for alcoholically impaired victims, who are easy targets and whose testimony, in case of a criminal trial, can be easily impeached. This is especially true of rape, other assaults, and robbery (NIAAA, 1987).

Only a small fraction of the socially undesirable consequences of drinking and other drug use are ever reported as crimes. There are arguments and fights; emotional relationships are destroyed; exams and courses are failed; part-time jobs are lost; and students drop out of college. Almost 30% of the 18- to 25-year-old drinkers reported that they had gotten aggressive while drinking in the last year, and 19% had been in "heated arguments." Eleven percent had been absent from school or work as a result of drinking (National Institute on Drug Abuse, 1988). More specifically, in a recent study of British college students, almost 5% admitted to having committed an assault while under the influence of alcohol. Nineteen percent of the male students and 10% of the females had been assaulted when drinking (West et al., 1990).

Some institutions are more aggressive than others in trying to solve alcohol-related problems. Often it takes courage, because acknowledging student alcohol problems exposes problems that might be suspected to exist on other campuses, but are not "officially" known. The University of Iowa Health Center has a program that assesses the alcohol problems of students who have been caught committing alcohol-related crimes and have been ordered into treatment by the courts. In 1989, more than 240 Hawkeyes were convicted for alcohol-related crimes (*Iowa City Press Citizen,* 1990), more students than play on the Iowa varsity football, baseball, and basketball teams put together. The difference between Iowa and most other universities is that Iowa knows something about the magnitude of its alcohol crime problem and is doing something about it.

An environment of drunkenness and the consequent rowdiness and violence on college campuses is not a new phenomenon. Hundreds of years ago, the provost of the University of Paris rode around with a mounted squad of archers to discipline unruly students. In 1858, the president of the University of Alabama appealed to the state legislature to obtain authority to deal with the "dissipation and rowdyism."[2] The history of academic institutions here and in Europe is replete with attempts to deal with the campus alcohol problem. In a sense, these early attempts saw the problem as a discipline or moral problem, as opposed to a health, educational, informational, and cultural problem.

EDUCATIONAL CONSEQUENCES

There are a host of studies that demonstrate the relationship between drinking and academics, painting a bleak picture. The studies take different approaches. Two separate studies found that college students of high academic standing drink less in almost all contexts than do their peers of low academic standing (Hughes & Dodder, 1983). First-year students on probation at Kansas State University drank much more than those of good academic standing (Brown, 1989). Several studies have shown the negative relationship between college grades and the amount of alcohol consumed (Hill & Bugen, 1979). However, recent results of the U.S. Department of Education–FIPSE-funded CORE national survey of more than 50,000 college students demonstrate not only that there is such a negative relationship, but that it is a very strong one (Presley &

Meilman, 1992). This is dramatically illustrated by Figure 13.1.

The same study shows that more than 30% of college students have missed one or more classes in the past year as a consequence of drinking or ingesting illicit drugs; 23% admit having performed poorly on a test as a consequence of drinking or drug use. In a recent series of longitudinal surveys, college administrators indicated that alcohol is a factor in 40.8% of all academic problems and 28.3% of the dropouts (Anderson & Gadaleto, 1991). These 1991 percentages represent statistically significant increases over the estimates of 1985 and 1988. Examine the latest incoming class. It has been estimated that more than 7% of these young men and women will become dropouts for alcohol-related reasons. That's more than 120,000 students of this year's first-year students, more than there are in Montana, Idaho, Wyoming, New Mexico, Colorado, Utah, and Nevada colleges combined, and three times as many as in Tennessee colleges (U.S. Department of Commerce, 1989).[3] Those alcohol-related dropouts will not earn what their graduating counterparts will, and their loss in lifetime earnings will be about $33 billion.[4] There will be defaulted student loans

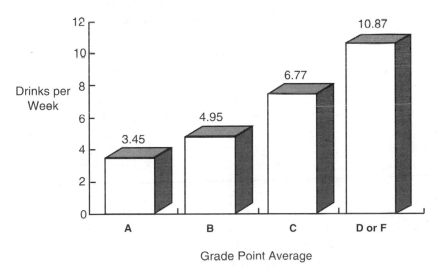

FIGURE 13.1.   Academic Achievement and Alcohol Use

and unreached potentials and aspirations. This year's freshman class will pay $3.1 billion less over their lifetime in taxes alone[5] than they would if there were no alcohol-related dropouts. That $3.1 billion in annual lost tax revenue is more than the federal outlay for all the guaranteed student loans in the nation.[6] The same will happen next year, and the year after that, until there is a profound change in the environment on our campuses.

Although the relationship between alcohol consumption and academic performance is clear, the causal dynamics are not. The time spent drinking or taking other drugs and its occasional aftermath may well subtract from potential studying time. At one large Midwestern university, more than 25% of the undergraduates had cut class after drinking during the year, and 14% of the student body does so in any given month (Petroff & Broek, 1990). The drinking—especially heavy drinking—may impair a student's intellectual functions sufficiently to hurt academic performance. It is also true that the stress of poor academic performance might cause students with such troubles to have more anxiety and drink more than other students. There may well be other personality or previous environmental factors that cause both increased drinking and poor academic performance. The bottom line is that a college is primarily an academic institution, and the relationship between drinking or use of other drugs and academics is clearly a negative one.

There is almost no facet of college life that is not negatively affected by alcohol problems. Student athletes are generally considered to be highly motivated to succeed, especially in their chosen sports. Studies sponsored by the National Collegiate Athletic Association revealed that there was a decrease between 1985 and 1989 of the use of illicit, nonalcoholic drugs on the part of American student athletes. The combination of all the substance abuse prevention efforts of our society appears to be turning the tide for other drugs, but not for alcohol. It is the one drug whose use by student athletes appears to have gone up slightly (Anderson, 1989). What is most surprising is that almost half of the student athletes who drink admit that their use of alcohol has had a harmful or slightly harmful effect on their athletic performance, yet most continue to drink.

INSTITUTIONAL VARIABLES

As a direct result of the CORE study (Presley et al., 1993) we now understand some of the institutional variables associated with alcohol and other drug use. For example, students drink more at small schools than at large institutions, although the drinking is substantial throughout academia. Drinking is heaviest in Northeastern schools and lightest in West Coast institutions; the same is true for illicit drugs in general, but cocaine use is highest in East Coast schools. Students in upper-Midwestern schools reported the highest rate of drinking and driving, however.

THE REASONS FOR ALCOHOL AND OTHER DRUG USE

The college alcohol environment is particularly risky, but it is unclear why. Perhaps the risky environment is caused by the high concentration of young men and women at a point in their lives when risk taking is common and peer acceptance is particularly important. Perhaps it is the cultural traditions of the institutions. Perhaps it is the fact that the various forces of society target colleges for particularly heavy marketing of alcoholic beverages (Ryan & Mosher, 1991). Perhaps it is because there are few alternatives to drinking on campus. It is likely that all these are factors, as well as many other influences.

Most college drinkers started drinking in high school, and for them the college alcohol problem is just a continuation of a previously existing problem. But some drinkers do not start until they reach college, and many students increase the amount they drink in their first year over their high school pattern (Moos, 1977); very few reduce it. Research shows that the proportion of heavy-drinking students jumps sharply from the senior year in high school to the first year of college (Bachman & O'Malley, 1980).

The culture of the campus, the opportunity to be independent of daily parental control, the need to conform, and the insecurity of a new and intimidating setting all make new students particularly vulnerable. Another indicator of the greater risk on the college campus is the difference that was found in New York State in the rates of heavy drinking between college students who lived at home with their families and those who lived on campus or in off-campus apartments. The latter had a heavy drinking rate (23%) that was more than twice the rate of the former (11%) (Harris, 1986).[7]

Normative Environment

In most inquiries regarding high-risk behavior, the question is usually asked, "Why do they do it?" The prevention assumption is that an understanding of the reasons for high-risk behavior is a necessary precursor to designing prevention programs. It also frequently presupposes that the high-risk behavior is not typical and is aberrant in some sense. However, in the college environment, we have found it more constructive to ask the question, "Why don't college students use drugs?" For it is the unusual student who has passed through college without using alcohol or illicit drugs. It is the atypical student who has not violated the law in the process, either by participating in underage drinking or the use of illegal drugs or both. Furthermore, even those few students who avoid this behavior have observed it in their fellow students and in effect have condoned the behavior by their presence.

The key is that the college environment is, on most college campuses, a drug-supportive environment. This is not to say that it is intended to be by the administrators, trustees, faculty, alumni, or the students themselves. But they do not have total control over their environment any more than a particular town or community has total control over its environment. They do, however, have influence over the college environment. In the case of many colleges, that influence is not being brought to bear as effectively as it might. It is these environmental factors that form

and sustain the campus norms and traditions, and these norms and traditions support alcohol and other drug-using behavior.

In the extensive literature on the subject, college students assert a host of reasons for drinking and taking illicit drugs. These include wanting to fit in, be popular, and reduce tension, and having nothing else to do. Almost all of these reasons are consequences of the school environment. If there are few recreational alternatives in the school environment or they are promoted badly or they are not what students prefer, then there is "nothing else to do." If it appears that most of the popular and successful people on campus drink or smoke marijuana, then it is not irrational to believe that abstinence might not lead to popularity. Otis Singletary, former chancellor of the University of Kentucky, has observed that "whatever people think, is." The college environment produces these images, and although those images are not necessarily reality, they might as well be, for the same influences result.

Sensation Seeking and Performance Enhancement

Generally, young people are more likely to be thrill- or sensation-seekers. Many drive too fast even when unimpaired by alcohol or other drugs, and engage in other high-risk behavior. There is a correlation of students' sensation-seeking intensity with use of alcohol and other drugs. Typically, measures of sensation seeking correlate more highly with alcohol and other drug use than do other instruments. Some research shows that female college students who drink heavily have a greater fear of failure and possess greater desire for sensation seeking than their lighter-drinking female counterparts (Jason, 1989).

Some Purposive Athletic Drug Use

There is one dramatic exception to the points made above. College athletes, in addition to their exposure to the "normal" college environment, have additional pressures and norms within their campus subculture. There, anabolic steroids are not taken recreationally or for social reasons, but for the purpose of improving athletic performance, usually effectively, albeit at great and often tragic health cost. Likewise, unauthorized use of pain medicines is purposive; they are used to enable athletes to practice, make the team, or play in a big game. A recent study of NCAA college athletes shows that generally college athletes, like their nonathletic peers, have reduced their illicit drug use over the last several years, but their use of steroids and alcohol has remained constant and their use of drugs to relieve pain has increased (W. A. Anderson, 1991).

CURRENT AND PAST PREVENTION STRATEGIES

There are a wide variety of prevention programs in place on campuses throughout the country. The Center for Substance Abuse Prevention of the United States Public Health Service "Put on the Brakes" college initiative has identified 30 different current operational strategies (Eigen et al., 1993).

Here we describe a few of the recent prevention strategies that have been attempted in recent years. We examine these in light of their effect on the college environment.

Campus Regulation

Although any use of illicit drugs is illegal on a college campus, alcohol presents a more ambiguous situation. The most common prevention strategy American colleges have used over the last decade is regulation of drinking activities, often brought about by U.S. Department of Education Regulations or the legal liability associated with dram shop laws and other legislation. This places disciplinary sanctions on certain impermissible activities, requires other activities, and makes symbolic statements that presumably affect the college environment. Campus regulation is often an area of philosophical, if not political, controversy.

The most traditional form of regulation on a college campus is the regulation of times and places of drinking. Some institutions have banned entirely the use of alcohol on campus, both for campus events and for students personally. Others have banned alcohol at campus-sponsored events. There is virtually no college campus in America on which drinking is not, to one degree or another, regulated. Twenty-five percent of the campuses ban beer and 32% do not allow hard liquor on campus (Anderson & Gadaleto, 1991).

Almost all campuses specifically prohibit drunken and disorderly behavior on the part of students and other members of the university community. However, the efficacy of the rules lies more in the school's enforcement practices and policies than in their existence. Many campuses that have rules against drunken and disorderly behavior often do not enforce them or enforce them extremely selectively.

Some schools have formalized the time differentials allowed for drinking. At the College Park Campus of the University of Maryland, the serving of alcoholic beverages at parties was restricted to weekends only (*Washington Post,* 1990). A special provision allows Thursday night beer parties for campus organization whose student grade point average is higher than the previous year. This policy, incidentally, was first suggested and initiated by students.

One of the most creative methods of influencing student drinking times was implemented at California State University at Chico. Thursday nights were the traditional party nights at Chico, until the president suggested that faculty schedule quizzes, examinations, and critical classes on Friday mornings. Friday attendance improved dramatically and there are now far fewer parties on Thursday evenings at Chico State (Wilson, 1990).

Whenever the serving of alcoholic beverages is allowed on the campuses, two types of regulations have been very helpful in ameliorating alcohol-related problems. First is the requirement that nonalcoholic beverages be readily available at all functions where alcohol is served. Fully

95% of American institutions of higher education now have this requirement (Anderson & Gadeleto, 1991). Another more recent innovation is the requirement of server training whenever alcohol is served. With this form of regulation, the institution sets up training programs for individuals who will serve alcohol on the campus to ensure the health and safety of the patrons.

Another condition of use that has recently been regulated on college campuses is the method of beer service. Specifically, some campuses have prohibited dispensing beer from kegs. This policy was instituted by Colorado State University in the early 1980s, and many others have followed suit. The logic of the keg ban was outlined by William Thomas, vice president of Student Affairs of the University of Maryland, when he announced his campus policy in 1990. "The availability of a non-incremental source of alcohol contributes to the abuse of alcohol. If alcohol is dispensed differently, it has a better chance of not being abused" (*Washington Post*, Oct. 8, 1990). In a study at Virginia Polytechnic Institute and State University, it was shown that when bartenders serve alcohol to college students, both males and females actually drink less than in a self-service drinking environment (Kalisher, 1989).

In reaction to a rise in alcohol-related violence and vandalism on campus, Northwestern University adopted a policy of controlling the amount of alcohol that may be served at any campus party. Specifically, they allow the party sponsors to have available a maximum of six beers for every legal-aged drinker. Other schools have similar rules.

Many campuses are dry. In 1985, slightly more than 20% claimed to be (Anderson & Gadaleto, 1991). Even beer was not allowed on campus. However, when one looks carefully at many of these dry campuses, there is often a little "moisture." For example, on many of these dry campuses, drinking in fraternity houses is as rampant as drinking on many "wet" campuses. The fraternity houses are often owned by the fraternities and are not, strictly speaking, on the

campus grounds. In some institutions, the school regulates all activities of any organizations that are in any way affiliated with the school. At other institutions, the campus is more narrowly defined. At the University of Missouri at Rolla, a dry campus, many students form informal groups and rent nearby off-campus apartments just for the purpose of having parties at which alcohol may be served. The campus policy didn't help the young UM student who died of acute alcohol poisoning in late 1991. At one large urban university where the president boasted that he had a dry campus, the prohibition rules were so flagrantly violated that students had installed winches to hoist beer through back windows and avoid the package checking and inspections that took place at the entrances to the residence halls.

Because fraternities are the locus of so much alcohol and other drug activity, the attention of the campus regulators is frequently focused on the Greek system. Requiring dry rush periods and prohibiting drinking at initiations are the most common measures taken. Some schools, such as Colgate, eliminate rushing entirely. The fraternity role in campus alcohol and other drug use is perhaps the most contentious issue on most campuses. Many "Greeks" resent the fact that they are singled out for more criticism, regulation, oversight, and sometimes blame. The data are very clear however that, in general, living in a fraternity house is a huge risk factor. Until recently, these data were gathered on a campus-by-campus basis, showing heavier and more frequent drinking in fraternities. But these studies were not conducted at all campuses, or even most campuses. The typical reaction was that "it may be true on some other campus, but not here." However, as a result of the U.S. Department of Education–funded CORE survey conducted by Cheryl Presley and her colleagues at Southern Illinois University, we now have national data. Essentially, students who live in fraternity houses consume more alcohol than other students do—a lot more. Findings from a national sample of the CORE study for a 1989–1991 cohort of students (Core Institute) show that the Greek residents of both sexes averaged almost 15 drinks a week compared to students not living in Greek residences, who only averaged 5 drinks a week. For men, it was more than 20 drinks per week, compared to 7.5. The same study also found that Greek residents binged more than twice as often, missed class more than twice as often, and had a host of other more negative health consequences. Fraternity enthusiasts are in institutional denial, as many educators put it. One hypothesized that although the fraternities are a disproportionate part of the problem, they come in for even more than their disproportionate share of criticism and control attempts. Therefore, they become more defensive (David Anderson, personal interview, June 1991). However, there is little doubt that a very large part of the college drinking problem could be solved if a prevention program were initiated that would reduce the fraternity drinking to the same level as the remainder of the student body.

In all forms of campus regulation, two key factors are the definition of the extent of the campus and the degree of enforcement. Clearly, the most troublesome regulation issue for most college campuses is the enforcement of the minimum-drinking-age requirements. The now-universal age limit of 21 splits the student body. The decision, however, is no longer the school's to make. This issue has been decided by law. It is illegal to serve beer to people under the age of 21. However, the degree of enforcement on the campus is the crucial issue for most institutions. Will a 19-year-old who is caught drinking at a campus function be disciplined, and if so, to what degree? Is he or she to be treated as a criminal? In most jurisdictions, the student would be. Littering is a criminal offense in many communities and the student who litters is generally not considered to have committed a serious infraction, even though it be criminal. Speeding is a crime committed by many of us, though few regard speeders as criminals. The fundamental issue is, How serious an infraction is underage drinking on a particular campus? Many schools have rules on the subject of underage drinking

and some require elaborate means of implementing them. Identification requirements and hand stamping at campus functions surely help, but most students report that these controls are easy to evade. Underage drinking is, unfortunately, quite common on almost any college campus today. Professor Earl Rubington of Northeastern University conducted a study of residence hall advisors (RAs) at an anonymous university. He concluded, "In effect, RAs teach residents how to break drinking rules" (Rubington, 1990).

The drinking laws prohibiting alcohol use by anyone under age 21 have had some very positive effects. The most dramatic is the significant reduction of alcohol-related automobile crashes among the 18- to 20-year-old age group (U.S. General Accounting Office, 1987). However, there is little evidence that underage drinking in college has substantially changed. For example, no reduction of underage drinking occurred at The State University of New York at Buffalo (George et al., 1989). The drinking law did, however, alter the locations of underage drinking, with more students reporting drinking in cars as opposed to bars or taverns. The flouting of the underage drinking laws has also been observed at Hobart College (Perkins & Berkowitz, 1989). The University of Iowa Student Health Service surveyed the 30-day drinking prevalence of its undergraduates. There was no apparent significant difference between students over and under 21 (Petroff & Broek, 1990).

One of the biggest changes brought about by the new drinking age limits is the student use of false IDs. In a 1991 national survey (Anderson & Gadaleto, 1991), more than twice as many college administrators believed that this practice had increased than believed that it had decreased over the last few years.

One of the biggest evasions of underage drinking rules occurs when older students obtain alcohol for younger ones. This may be at a party, in the fraternity house, the residence hall, or at a football game. Any 21-year-old can go to a nearby convenience store or other legal outlet, buy a six-pack or two, and return to the campus to share it with friends under age 21. In many communities, legal alcohol outlets in the vicinity of a campus are often the worst offenders. Underage students can often easily obtain drinks in bars and restaurants, buy beer in supermarkets or convenience stores, and even obtain alcoholic beverages in liquor stores. The Chief of Police of Iowa City, Iowa, has observed that bars and taverns around the university not only regularly serve minors, but when the police arrive to check for underage drinking, the bartenders turn the music way up or down and the underage students refrain from drinking until the coast is clear (*Iowa City Press Citizen*, 1990). At the University of Maryland, the local off-campus stores used to make beer, liquor, and wine deliveries to the campus. The age of the recipient was rarely checked. Even when the deliverer was concerned about age, the alcohol would be turned over to anyone at the delivery site who was over age 21 and had the money to pay. The situation got so bad that the local county, with support from the university administration, banned all deliveries of alcoholic beverages to the campus (*Washington Post*, Sept. 20, 1990).

This raises the question of how serious an offense the institution considers a student under age 21 obtaining alcohol for his or her younger classmates. What signal does the answer send to the student body? The Alpha Epsilon Pi fraternity at Cornell had a party at which a group of underage students was served alcohol. There were some arguments and then a fight. When it was over, a student was dead. Alpha Epsilon Pi was placed on probation for two years (*New York Times*, 1989).

What should the school's response be to a student who is caught using a false ID to purchase alcohol? In a 1991 study, it was found that 58% of the schools impose a fine or probation, 9% suspend the student, and 22% report the offense to law enforcement authorities or the motor vehicles bureau (Anderson & Gadaleto, 1991). In early 1990, four Texas Tech students were arrested and charged with felonies for counterfeiting driver licenses and providing them to other students for evasion of the drinking laws (*New York Times*, 1990).

Often, the school is hampered in its efforts by existing state or local laws. Consider the plight of the University of Iowa when it issued its policy on a drug-free environment. The section on "Applicable Criminal Sanctions" includes the following: "A person found guilty of giving or selling an alcoholic beverage to a 19- or 20 year-old may be fined up to $50." The school is not responsible for the fact that the penalty for selling or giving alcohol to students aged 19 or 20 is only $50. The State of Iowa complied with the federal law mandating a minimum drinking age of 21, but was not too serious about the sanction for violation. The typical faculty member or student (or anyone else) will reasonably get the following message: "The university is telling us that we don't have to worry too much about providing alcoholic beverages to underage students. If you get caught, the fine is very small, and the school hasn't added any administrative or disciplinary sanctions. So the institution doesn't really take this seriously either. Everyone is going through the motions, but no one is serious" (University of Iowa, 1990).

The university could have added administrative sanctions to their policy, could have made a moral statement, or they could have simply stated that the provision of alcohol to underage students was against state law. By quoting the specific penalties of a state law that trivializes the activity, the school gave a message—not necessarily intended—that the offense is in a class with spitting on the sidewalk or not cutting the grass often enough.

Consider the difficulty if the university attempts to place serious academic and administrative sanctions on the provision of alcohol to underage students. Would the average faculty member or administrative employee, such as a residence hall staff member, be willing to jeopardize the entire academic career of an older student whose infraction was only worth a $50 fine to the Iowa State legislature? Should the school attempt to enforce the society's criminal law in a more zealous manner than the state itself? Should it have stiffer sanctions?

Conversely, some schools use state criminal sanctions to apply social pressure to alter student behavior. Chico State scans the local newspapers for any alcohol-related criminal arrests of students. When they find one, they send a letter to the address of record (usually the home of the student's parents) stating that the local police had performed the arrest, and if further information was desired, to please contact the dean of students (Wilson, 1990).

College Newspaper Advertising

Approximately 35% of all the college newspaper advertising revenue comes from alcohol advertisements (Breed, in press). A study conducted during 1984–1985 found that the average college newspaper had more than 40 column inches of alcohol advertising per issue. This average, incidentally, includes the roughly 20% of the college newspapers that do not accept alcohol advertising at all (CASS Student Advertising 1981-1992), and many that, because of the small size of the campus, get no advertising from the national alcohol companies. There is 20 times more alcohol advertising in college newspapers than book advertising, and more than 40 times more alcoholic beverage advertising than soft drink advertising. What is perhaps even more astounding is the fact that these incredible ratios hold despite the fact that alcoholic beverage advertising is decreasing in college newspapers. College students are major targets of breweries, alcohol distilleries, and wineries. College students are heavy consumers of the products and, much more importantly, they are at the age when brand name identification can really have a payoff for the manufacturer. The Miller Brewing Company lectures its marketers, "25% of all beer drinkers stay with their first regular brand choice for life" (Miller Brewing Company, 1989). The brewers do have a problem. Theirs is a legal product, and their marketers function in a very competitive environment. Because so many young people

under the age of 21 are drinking beer illegally, many brand selections will be made for life before the youngster even reaches the age where he or she may drink legally. The responsible brewer who eschews any marketing to the under-21 age group cedes the field to his less principled competitor. The result for a large proportion of underage drinkers is permanent brand loyalty.

Students appear to be primary targets of a huge, skilled, and wealthy alcoholic beverage industry and its advertising industry. It is not a large, disaggregated industry made up of many small companies. In 1987, there were only 120 breweries and 102 distilleries operating a multibillion-dollar industry in the United States. Students are the targets of extremely large, well-financed corporations that make the athletic shoe companies appear small by comparison. The primary vehicle that the alcoholic beverage companies use is not an industry secret. "The college newspaper is the key," is the way Bill Schmidt of the Pabst Brewing Company put it several years ago (Jacobson, 1983).

In recent years, there has been extensive public pressure on the marketing of alcohol to students under 21 in general and at colleges in particular. Many campuses now severely restrict various alcohol marketing methodologies. Also, the industry has taken a much lower profile, maintaining that they no longer target the college market to the same degree, and has in many cases actively opposed underage drinking. A 1991 Center for Substance Abuse Prevention financed study by the Marin Institute found that "[t]he alcohol industry has moderated its aggressive marketing efforts on college campuses in the last two years" (Ryan & Mosher, 1991), although not as much as Marin would like. A good example of this was the decision by beer brewers not to sponsor activities at the Fort Lauderdale 1991 Spring Break. However, table placards and other beer advertising directed at young people were in evidence throughout Fort Lauderdale stores and restaurants, including many that served no alcoholic beverages. Perhaps the originators of these placards and posters intended them only for young adults over 21, but the display was prominent in locations known to be heavily frequented by under-21 students and other young people. A more successful moderating approach taken by the alcohol industry has been the decision of the liquor distillers to voluntarily refrain from television and radio advertising because there was no practical way to ensure that advertisements would not be viewed by youth under 21.

Men are by no means the only target. As a matter of fact, the evidence indicates that a large proportion of alcohol advertising is now being targeted to female students. In the 1991–1992 football TV season, there was a heavy emphasis on young women, not merely as the "bimbos" of previous years, serving beer to the boys and ogling the drinkers. The females are "fellow mountain men" and drinking participants in the alcohol lifestyle portrayed by the ads. In addition to the factors that cause companies to target male students, there is much more payoff to the advertiser if females can be induced to drink with the same frequency and in the same amounts because females start with a lower drinking base. If this and other perversions of equal opportunity were to be successful, American females would soon have the opportunity to lose as many years of productive life due to alcohol problems as their average male counterpart.

A fundamental issue for every college is whether it should regulate the advertising of alcoholic beverages in the college newspapers. Also at issue is the extent of the regulation, which could range from outright prohibition, a practice on many campuses, to a *laissez faire* position that allows any advertising whatsoever. Assuming the institution wishes to take a position somewhere in between the two extremes, there are a wide variety of considerations. Consider the following three categories of advertising slogans that have appeared in college newspapers.

1. "Dining, drinking, and dancing."
   "Hoist a brew and celebrate after the game."
   "More than thirty brands of beer."
2. "Monday nights are pre-week party nights."

"Tuesday 25-cent draft, 75-cent kamikazes."
"Ladies night—ladies drink free."
3. "Every Thursday ladies night. $1.00 cover, first six drinks free."
   "Friday 4–6:30 P.M. $4.00 all you can drink."
   "Fraternity chugging contest. We furnish the beer, you furnish the team. $24.00 to winning frat."

The first category of advertisements represents the least potentially harmful one. These advertisements, in effect, inform students where they may drink and describe something of the context of the drinking setting. In effect, they say, "If you want to drink, drink in our place." Arguments for restricting the type of advertisement in the first category generally hang on the implicit message of endorsement or approval of a lifestyle that includes drinking. Counterarguments would say that the advertisements in category one simply recognize that drinking is part of our culture, and a legal part at that. They are not encouraging drinking except by implication. They are certainly not encouraging more drinking or more time devoted to drinking. The second category of advertisements is potentially more dangerous. These advertisements, in effect, seek to persuade students to drink more or drink earlier than they otherwise would. In contrast to the advertisements in the first category, they are advocating more drinking in the lifestyle of the student. They say, "Start your partying Monday instead of Friday." If this type of ad is successful, there will be more drinking on the campus, at times that are not conducive to the academic objectives of the institution and fundamentally do not support the social objectives. They differ profoundly from the advertisements in the first category.

The third category of advertisements is the most harmful and potentially devastating of all. In this category, students are not only being asked to increase the amount they drink or their time devoted to drinking, but they are specifically being asked to engage in behavior that creates a danger to their health and the health of others around them. This is totally independent of the deleterious effect that it might have on their academic performance. For a college newspaper to advertise a chug-a-lug contest is the moral equivalent of advertising a contest for Russian roulette. The only difference is that the odds aren't quite as bad. Alcohol is virtually the only drug that a small part of our culture actually practices imbibing as much as possible in as short a period of time as possible. Even the worst crack addicts do not try to ingest as much cocaine as they possibly can within a fixed period of time. No cigarette smoker would ever try to see how many cigarettes he or she could smoke in a fixed period of time, much less call this "fun and recreation."

Advertising a fixed price for "all you can drink" is almost as reprehensible as the chug-a-lug contest. The ad that encourages women to come in and offers them the first six drinks free is clearly not just offering a place for someone to have a drink, but specifically encourages and provides financial incentives for them to have a number of drinks, which immediately puts them into the heavy-drinking class with much greater risk. This particular ad generally is characteristic of a type of alcohol advertising in which women are solicited at greatly reduced prices under the well-known marketing technique for young men—namely that if you convince them that "that's where the women hang out," they will come also. Tragically, the sexual exploitation of this type of ad is compounded by potentially endangering female students' lives and subjecting them to moral degradation. Holding college women out as bait for getting drinking men into a bar is ethically offensive and may lead to them being victims of alcohol-related violence or rape.

The third category of advertisements represent clear and present dangers to health and safety. The ads in the second category advocate unhealthy behavior, but the danger is neither as clear nor as immediate. The first category of ads does not advocate any increased drinking or any specific unhealthy or dangerous drinking practices. Are the more dangerous ads in categories two and three rare? Unfortunately not. One study found that 37% of college newspaper ads encouraged excessive drinking (Walfish et al., 1981), as opposed to simply extolling the virtues of a brand.

Sponsorship of Events and Other Campus Marketing

— A tennis tournament at the University of Oregon is sponsored by Budweiser.
— A rock concert on the University of Colorado campus is sponsored by Miller.
— Free Anheuser-Busch beer is provided in front of the University of California Student Union before big football games.
— The Budweiser Sorority Volleyball Tournament is held at the University of Tennessee.
— The Charlie Daniels Band in concert at Southern Illinois University was sponsored by Busch beer. (Jacobson, 1983)

Although the University of Michigan at Ann Arbor and some other schools ban campus representatives of alcohol firms (Roth, 1989), their presence and sponsorship is pervasive at hundreds of campuses and the students are generally very appreciative.

Beer companies sponsor senior class picnics, postgame dances, pep rallies, and tailgate parties that precede the games. The beer companies promote their brands, promote drinking, and all too often promote dangerous activities. Budweiser, for example, sponsored a beer drinking contest at the Chi Psi fraternity at Berkeley. The following is part of an eyewitness account: "[T]eam members gulped and choked, red-faced, trying to get the beer down. Three or four guys vomited in the bushes after chugging the beer" (Roth, 1989).

What should be the policy of schools toward sponsorship by alcoholic beverage companies? What is the implication of a private organization's sponsorship of a campus event? Does the allowance of the sponsorship imply anything to the student body and the community, such as concurrence of the university with the purposes, goals, and methods of the sponsoring organization? These are not simple questions, but ones that must be addressed. Clearly, most academic institutions would give much more latitude to sponsorship of campus speakers than to sponsorship of campus events. Speakers are an integral part of the free exchange of ideas. But are dances? Football parties? Volleyball tournaments? Chugging contests? Surely, the school has some responsibility to see to it that the activity to be sponsored is not dangerous. A wide range of sponsorship regulations is possible. Each institution must create its own policies and make its own decisions. One of the major promotional methodologies of the alcoholic beverage companies on college campuses is the sponsorship of events. Events sponsored include athletic tournaments, concerts, parties, contests, almost anything. Although the practice is discouraged by many schools, many beer companies actually have an official campus representative assigned to most major and many smaller campuses. When representatives hear that an organization is going to have a party, they make contact and offer free publicity, free trophies, free prizes, and financial assistance. The following ad (not atypical) appeared in the campus newspaper of the University of Hawaii:

> *Having a Party? See Chuck Parker, Your Budweiser Campus Representative. Call Chuck at 123-4567 for your beer needs right on campus.* (Jacobson et al., 1983)

The economics of sponsorship cannot be ignored. There is no accurate estimate of the total economic value of all the sponsorship of college campus activities. Many of the activities are worthwhile and not dangerous or unhealthy. Where would the funds for signs for a student dance come from if not for the beer companies? Who would provide the trophies for intramural athletic events? But what is the alcohol-related cost of the status quo and who is paying it?

Sponsorship is not the only campus marketing technique used by the alcoholic beverage manufacturers. There are a wide variety of others. Posters for student residence halls, fraternities, and sororities are extremely popular. These posters, like alcohol-related advertising in campus newspapers, range from brand recognition material to the encouragement of unhealthy, dangerous behavior. Many perpetuate myths and falsehoods regarding alcohol and drinking. Others make fun of or degrade education. Many

show scantily clad young women and handsome young men. Typically they show one of the latter holding a beer can, surrounded by a dozen or so of the former. The few that treat anything academic are noteworthy. Here are contents of three of these posters:

> *Studyin' with the Real Taste of Beer.*
> *Great Writing Starts with a Little Listening,*
>   *a Little Beer, and a Lot of Legwork.*
> *No College Education Is Complete without*
>   *Triple Sec.*

The first was used by Pabst. The second, by Miller, quotes author Mickey Spillane. Unfortunately, the "legwork" referred to is not of the library or research variety, but a shapely female leg in a net stocking, which is the largest visual object in the poster. The third, used by Hiram Walker, goes on to say, "Secs won't lead to better grades. Just better times." One of the themes of a Michelob ad campaign was "Put a Little Weekend in Your Week," encouraging students not to limit their beer drinking to weekends.

Then there are T-shirts, caps, boxer shorts, and other articles of clothing. One leading alcohol marketer observes that alcohol companies like to use the students as walking billboards. The campus provides the concentration of potential customers and, inadvertently, is the vehicle by which the alcohol companies use the students to sell to each other.

It is not only the alcohol companies that market the culture of drinking on the campus. The university itself often does also! The university insignia, logos, and mascots are elements that are inextricably connected with the campus alcohol issue. Examine any campus bookstore. Typically you will find the college logo on all kinds of drinking paraphernalia—most typically beer mugs, steins, and drinking and shot glasses. But the computers sold in the bookstore do not have the school logo, nor do the books, pads, pens and other tools of academia. For what purposes should the symbols of the institution be used? What symbolic messages are sent by the use of the school's symbols? Recently, a counteradvertising campus health poster showed a beer stein with the caption on the stein, "Most campus rapes start here!!!" How many schools would want their logo to appear on the beer stein if it also had that caption? Many schools, such as California State University at Chico, have eliminated the sale of drinking paraphernalia at their bookstores.

A recent dramatic situation occurred at the University of Nebraska. At the same time that one part of the university was wrestling with the campus alcohol problem, the athletic department sold the rights to the Nebraska Cornhusker mascot image to the Coors brewing company. Coors plans to put it on the six-packs and beer cans they will sell in Nebraska, both on campus and off, where following Cornhusker football is almost a religion (Malcolm Heard, personal communication, October 17, 1990).

Attitudes toward Regulation

There is a core of libertarian values in almost every academic institution. Therefore, any form of regulation on campus—on virtually any subject—is rarely welcomed without opposition. Students come to the university with a strong opposition to serious alcohol regulation. In 1986, less than 20% of high school seniors thought that getting drunk in private should be prohibited by law. Only about half felt that public drunkenness should be prohibited by law (National Institute on Drug Abuse, 1987). These attitudes are reinforced in college.

Campus attitudes toward regulation of drinking are very much related to the drinking behavior. At the University of California at Berkeley, it was found that the heavier drinkers in fraternities and sororities tended to express more opposition to campus alcohol regulation than their lighter-drinking fraternity and sorority counterparts. Leonard Goodwin of the Prevention Research Center on that campus observes that "women are significantly more in favor of external [campus] control over drinking than men," and that "nonwhite individuals are significantly

more in favor than are whites" (Goodwin, 1984). There is, on almost any campus, a solid, core group of students who resent the drinking culture. They are among the most proactive forces for aggressive campus regulation. In the middle are the bulk of the students and faculty, and it is this group that will influence any proposed regulatory activity and will be instrumental in the enforcement of and compliance with any regulations that are instituted.

Reasonable regulation, if deemed appropriate on a particular campus, would be facilitated considerably if faculty would get involved in policy making and enforcement instead of leaving the administration to fight it out with the students. Indeed, on many campuses, it is the faculty senate that has taken leadership on campus. Chico State experienced drunken riots. The faculty senate passed a resolution requesting that the president withdraw campus recognition from any student organization that is involved in alcohol-related violence (Wilson, 1990).

Regulation and the Campus Culture

A simple illustration of how far our campus cultural norms have moved in undesirable directions is the Stanford University band. Most of us have done some improper or even illegal things in our lifetimes, and many when we were young. Generally, these are things that we were not proud of and did not manifest in the spotlight of public scrutiny. Yet The Incomparable Leland Stanford Jr. University Marching Band had to be reprimanded for arriving at football games drunk and urinating on the field. This behavior was exhibited in front of tens of thousands of people—students, parents, and alumni—with the activities also being observed by the press and TV cameras. These were not a few troublemakers or campus iconoclasts representing counterculture behavior in obscure corners of the campus. This was a typical subset of the student body of one of our finest institutions of higher education exhibiting what has become normal behavior in front of the world. This collegiate norm that makes such gross and absurd behavior acceptable, if not worthy of emulation, is not a problem we will solve only by ferreting out the troublemakers and making examples of them, or by making rules and regulations, although regulation and disciplinary enforcement are typical elements of most overall normative change processes.

Rules and regulations may be effective control mechanisms when those strictures reflect cultural norms and societal and community values, but a change in norms will require more.

Campus Regulation Enforcement Dilemmas

Campus regulation of alcohol use involves certain inherent dilemmas that face the campus community beyond the libertarian and free speech issues already discussed. Foremost among those is a point of view that appears to be commonly held but rarely surfaced for attribution. Specifically, the more effectively the university regulates alcohol use, the more the students' drinking will be driven off-campus, but the campus is, in almost all cases, a safer and more benign atmosphere. Friends, other students, and staff are almost always in the immediate vicinity. An intoxicated student is less likely to be assaulted or robbed on campus, among other students, than off campus. Impaired students who are on the campus are much less likely to drive. This latter point is of particular concern to rural or isolated schools, where there are few establishments within walking distance and going off-campus to drink involves driving some distance to roadhouses and taverns.

Another major dilemma is the reality that alcohol abuse is so culturally ingrained on the typical American campus that it is unlikely that the problem can be substantially improved in a short time frame. If this is true, the campus leader who takes on this issue as a major element of his or her agenda risks the classic political hazard of calling attention to a problem that he or she will not likely be able to solve within his or her tenure. When University of Wisconsin chancellor Shalala took her stand, she risked being asked at every faculty meeting, every press conference, and every state appropriations hearing whether she had solved the problem yet. There is no panacea and few policy and programmatic solutions that will change campus norms instantly.

Programs and Policies

Many campuses have instituted comprehensive alcohol and other drug prevention programs with some success (NIAAA, 1987). They're no panacea, and they don't work for everyone, but most college alcohol prevention programs show positive changes in student knowledge and attitudes about alcohol use and its potential problems. Several evaluations demonstrate fewer alcohol problems at post-test follow-up. Successful college programs tend to be longer (20 to 36 hours) than the unsuccessful shorter ones (2 to 20 hours). Also, field experiences (in addition to classroom work) tend to improve the effectiveness. Field experiences that appear to be helpful are police ride-alongs, visits to treatment centers, planning and implementing campus alcohol awareness programs, advocating campus alcohol regulation changes, and acting as peer counselors.

Sometimes there are very creative campus policies regarding alcohol education. For example, in order to have a party and serve alcohol at Willamette College of Salem, Oregon, a fraternity or other campus organization must obtain a qualified speaker and require its students to attend an educational seminar on the problems related to the use of alcohol and other drugs. Although fraternities are, in general, disproportionate contributors to the campus alcohol problem, some fraternities have taken a major leadership role in implementing preventive education programs (Cruz & Bubl, 1990).

The process of making the various decisions as to whether there will be alcohol education programs, and which combination of variables would be used, can be a part of the campus debate and dialogue. At Luther College in Iowa, student athletes and coaches were exposed to a formal educational program and then allowed to set their own rules, regulations, and standards for alcohol and other drug use (Johnson, 1989).

Educational efforts do not guarantee success with all subgroups of the campus population. A study by the Fordham University Counseling Center observed that there was a stable core of heavy-drinking students who were not influenced into moderation by their education efforts (Tryon, 1989).

Designated Driver Programs

One of the most popular and successful programs on college campuses (as well as elsewhere) over the last few years has been designated driver programs. The consciousness-raising potential and the behavioral change involved in selecting drivers who will not drink are obviously extremely helpful, basic steps to be taken to reduce the carnage on the nation's roads caused by some alcohol-impaired drivers. But there is a subtle caution that must be observed by the many institutions that have or are considering designated driver programs. Specifically, the designated driver program may, if care is not taken, overshadow all other efforts and actually give students the wrong impression of the balanced dangers. It is critical that we examine not the intention of the program designers and implementers, but the results in terms of student perception. From the designated driver program and the publicity that surrounds it, students may receive the message that it's okay to get drunk as long as you don't drive.

There are also many other alcohol-related health risks. We would not, for instance, consider such a program related to alcohol-related suicide, assaults, date rape, and vandalism. A fraternity or other organization would not have a designated nonvandalizer or a designated nonrapist. To the degree that a designated driver program singles out one danger of drinking to the exclusion of others, it may be of limited value, especially on a college campus. To the degree that the designated driver program is part of a larger, more comprehensive program that makes students aware of all the risks of drinking and takes care not to promote intoxication, it may be helpful.

Responsible Drinking

The conceptual linchpin of many formal educational efforts is the notion of responsible drinking. At first inspection, it is hard to fault a program with a responsible drinking theme. However, the concept of responsible drinking turns out to be much more complicated than it appears. There is considerably more consensus as to its desirability than its definition. Many of us would see responsible drinking as imbibing in moderation, so as not to produce any negative health, social, economic, or educational consequences, as was articulated thousands of years ago by Aristotle. Most AA advocates would say that for a recovering alcoholic, a single drink is irresponsible. They and others might argue that responsible drinking in many cases is an oxymoron. A Native American alcohol educator recently put it this way: "Responsible drinking might be a nice concept, but I've never seen it for my people" (Cruz & Bubl, 1990). Also, a part of the population has chosen to define responsible drinking by being nondrinkers.

It is hard for most of us to tell exactly how much alcohol is a responsible amount on any given occasion or for any particular person. There are so many factors involved, including what and how fast we've drunk, the social setting, what we've eaten recently, heredity disposition, environmental and psychological factors, and the like. The additional complication is that, as we drink and reach points of critical decision making, our ability to make an unimpaired judgment is decreased by the alcohol we have already consumed. Most undergraduates are at the "immortal" stage of life. Intellectually, most know about many risks, but they take them anyway. They drive too fast, drink too much, and engage in other risk-taking behavior that older people might not, certainly not with such frequency. That was the thinking of many advocates of increasing the minimum drinking age to 21.

The concept of responsible drinking places virtually the entire public health burden on the individual student as opposed to the environment and the community. Someone who drinks too much is somehow stigmatized as irresponsible. Is anyone else responsible, such as the host of the party, the sellers and distributors of the alcohol, the advertisers and promoters, and the university that creates the climate? Under the concept of responsible drinking, only the drinker seems to bear the responsibility. As the "responsible" student drinks, his or her ability to make responsible decisions and judgment is constantly eroded. Thus, in the responsible drinking model, society generally blames only the drinker, and the drinker often blames the booze. It is not surprising that so many elements of our society are enthusiastic about the responsible drinking model—it takes us all off the hook. Many hosts and manufacturers may not feel any sense of responsibility for irresponsible drinking, but consider the parallel when someone is harmed by other legal drugs. If a college student had a medical emergency as a result of taking a prescription medicine, most of us would first look to the health center or physician to determine whether it were properly prescribed; to the pharmacist to see whether proper instructions had been provided with the sale; and to the pharmaceutical company to determine whether the drug had been properly manufactured, labeled, and packaged. We would rarely look first to the consumer. Under the responsible drinking concept, however, all the negative consequence to society associated with alcohol can be attributed to a minority of "irresponsible" individuals.

Responsible drinking program models have been operational for a while, and may be helpful, but are not at all sufficient. As has been observed by one college president, "there is just too much booze" (Wilson, 1990). There must also be initiatives on-campus to alter significantly the alcohol culture and environment and to reduce the amount of alcohol that is consumed. This does not necessarily mean requiring on-campus abstinence by all students. It does mean making sure that there are a culture and atmosphere that realistically support and allow abstinence on the part of those students who prefer it or for those who should be abstinent as a result of past personal history or current circumstances, such as pregnancy. It does mean leveling the alcohol infor-

mation playing field. It does mean countering the incessant drum of prodrinking messages. It does mean regulating the conditions of use. At the bottom line, it does mean reducing the total amount of booze.

The U.S. Department of Health and Human Services convened a consortium of 300 national health organizations and all state health agencies to identify national health opportunities and objectives to be achieved by the year 2000. One major goal is to reduce by 20% the total intake of alcohol by Americans (U.S. Department of Health and Human Services, 1990). Another is to reduce and restrict the promotion of alcoholic beverages that is focused principally on young audiences. These national goals transcend responsible drinking. To the degree that designated driver programs function in place of responsible drinking programs or divert efforts away from reducing campus alcohol consumption, they do a partial disservice. If responsible drinking programs function in lieu of, or crowd out, environmental and cultural normative efforts, they will be counterproductive. It is politically very easy to institute a designated driver program. It's slightly more complicated to operate responsible drinking programs. It takes much more community and institutional courage and wit to alter the college drinking environment. But that is exactly what it's going to take.

Counteradvertising

Advertising and promotion are extremely powerful, dynamic forces in our society in terms of altering the behavior of our citizens. America is the most advanced nation with regard to advertising and promotion. Its combination of art and skill has helped to develop its rising economy and the high standard of living. However, there is a potential shortcoming. Specifically, most advertising and promotion is organized, developed, and placed by private organizations that have specific economic benefits to gain from the desired changes in the consumers' behavior. In general, if there is no entity with a potential financial benefit from the advertising and promotion of an area, there is no advertising and promotion in that particular area. One idea is that the same communication techniques can be applied to producing healthy behavior and avoiding dangerous practices and products. The theory is certainly sound. In practice, the problem is knowing who has the vested interest to pay for the use of the techniques.

Humor is a very powerful force in alcohol counteradvertising. One leading proponent at the University of Houston has a presentation titled "Laughing the Drug Dealers out of Town" (Blum, 1990). The "drug dealers" are the alcohol and tobacco companies, and humorous and sarcastic parodies of successful alcoholic beverage ads are prominently presented to show how absurd are the claims and associations of the ads. In Canada, the Ontario universities have a Campus Alcohol Education Initiative. A main focus of this program is the production and printing of advertising parodies of beer ads in the campus newspapers and on posters. "The satirical strategy allows us to build on typical visuals and themes popularized by beverage producers," observes one of the designers of that program (Robert Simpson, letter to Robert Denniston, September 21, 1990).

Sometimes, counteradvertising involves more than just using the same techniques as the advertisers, often more than showing irony and contrast. In 1990, in Harlem, New York, the Reverend Calvin Butts led a group of protesters with cans of paint; they painted over a number of billboards that targeted the black community with regard to alcohol products. Similar tactics have been used successfully in other communities.

THE FUTURE

Alternative Activities and Use of Campus Facilities

The majority of student drinking is done in the evenings and on weekends. Because the majority of the drinking is for social and recreational purposes, ary strategy directed at reducing the amount of campus drinking must realistically consider social and recreational alternatives. This consideration often starts with the use of campus facilities. There are numerous campuses where many, if not the majority, of the recreational and social facilities on campus close at the very hours when students are most apt to want to socialize and recreate. As David Burns, vice president of the American College Health Association, puts it, "we sleep when the students are awake" (personal communication, Jan. 28, 1991). The bars and off-campus taverns become the de facto inheritors and are often the only social game in town. How many campus swimming pools, basketball courts, or movie theaters are open after midnight? How many off-campus taverns and bars are? What time does the library close? On one campus, the library was a major locus of social activity until 10:00 P.M., when it closed. Then the students went to the bars, not necessarily because they wanted to drink, but because they had nowhere else to go (Eigen, 1991).

Every campus will soon, if it has not already done so, examine its own facilities to ask the question, "What is available to groups of students who spontaneously would like someplace to go?" The groups may be as small as a couple or up to 8 or 10 people. Surrounding most campuses are bars, taverns, and bistros. These entities solicit patronage and advertise their late-night availability. Except on extreme occasions of overcrowding, students need not plan in advance. Each academic institution must ask, "Are there spontaneously available, attractive alternatives? Where on the campus can students get a hamburger and argue politics or philosophy at 2:00 A.M.?" On some campuses, it has been said that there is not a single campus facility where young couples can have any sense of real intimacy. It does not take much: low lighting, a little background music, and booths or corners where couples can have the sense that they are alone. Almost every college community has many such places off-campus, and they almost inevitably serve and promote alcoholic beverages. Many of these establishments have two- or three-drink minimums.

It is not necessarily the case that every campus should maintain an all-night, comprehensive, parallel recreational facility, completely ignoring the resources of the community surrounding the campus. It is important, however, that each institution conduct a realistic assessment of the social and recreational alternatives available to students at various times of the night and day, on weekends and weekdays. If at all possible, activities should be regular, frequent, planned by the students, varied, and should involve as many student groups as possible. Indeed, the college or university can help support activities on or surrounding the campus that do not serve alcoholic beverages by offering them free listings in the campus newspaper; free poster space in the student union, residence halls, and fraternity and sorority houses; or advertisements and announcements on the campus radio. This information is just as important and useful, perhaps, as the listings of places of worship, which most colleges actively promulgate.

There are many campuses that have virtually no off-campus community resources of any kind. The campus is the community. These remote schools, such as Dartmouth and Bucknell, have often had the reputation of being heavy-drinking schools. These institutions have a particularly difficult recreational burden and realistically must do more to produce the same level of recreational opportunity as campuses in more densely populated and developed communities.

There is also the relationship between recreational economics and drinking. As a practical matter, sitting around and drinking beer is a relatively inexpensive recreational activity, typically costing about a dollar an hour. Movies at a commercial theater might cost two or three times that amount. Eating out is still more expensive. What about typical campus activities? Some, with fees, may well be more expensive than drinking. Check a varsity basketball game. You'll often find that it's much more expensive per hour to attend a game than it is to drink.

Though certainly a complex issue, the recreational facilities, activities, policies, and practices of any college and its surrounding community are inextricably tied to the drinking problem, and it is unlikely that any comprehensive school program will be successful if it does not address such recreational opportunities.

Leveling the Intellectual and Informational Playing Field

Virtually every college student has to make a personal decision as to whether to drink alcohol, and this decision is faced continuously. If this decision is affirmative, the student will have to make another set of decisions as to how frequently, how much, what kind, and under what circumstances to drink. Even students who are too young to legally drink must decide whether to obey the law, and in any event, the decision whether to do so legally will face them in a year or so, usually while they are still students. Where do college and university students get the information to make such decisions? Is it accurate, complete, and unbiased?

Consider the information and impressions college students obtain on campus. There are references to alcohol throughout the curriculum. There are the great creators, such as the artist Jackson Pollack and the writer Dylan Thomas, who were alcoholics. In a philosophy class, students may encounter Bertrand Russell's famous humorous quote, "I am as drunk as a lord, but then, I am one, so what does it matter." "What's drinking? A mere pause from thinking!" and "Man, being reasonable, must get drunk" are two well-known lines of Lord Byron from *The Deformed Transformed* and *Don Juan*. Fielding's "Today it is our pleasure to be drunk," from *Tom Thumb* is another example. They are typical of the thousands of lines from our greatest literature that place drinking and drunkenness in a positive light. In American history, we learn that George Washington in his first campaign supplied each voter in his Virginia district with over a quart of alcoholic beverage. It should not be surprising that alcohol, drinking, and even drunkenness are referenced positively, if not romantically, throughout our historical, philosophical, or literary tradition. Drinking has been an integral part of Western culture and history. However, just as the full negative health consequences of smoking were not understood until relatively recently, the totality of the problems associated with alcohol and drinking are still emerging from current science.

Certainly, we don't want to make any literary, artistic, or historical decisions about the propriety of including material in courses on the basis of how the alcohol issue is treated, but it is important to appreciate that what might be classified as prodrinking messages are frequently conveyed throughout the typical college curriculum. There are also literary selections that might be classified as antidrinking, but these are naturally less common because the literature reflects a historically prodrinking society.

Next, consider the noncurricular campus information sources. The college newspaper contains a large amount of advertising for alcoholic beverages. Occasionally, there is a news item about alcohol-related problems on campus, but most of the copy related to drinking in a typical college newspaper is unabashedly prodrinking.

What of the other messages on campus? Consider the signs and announcements of the beer bashes, the posters in the student residence hall rooms, the sponsorship of campus events, the fraternity parties, and other social functions at which alcohol is an attraction, if not the prime draw.

One of the biggest and most influential sources of information on a college campus is word of mouth. The views and opinions of other students rebound between classes, in residence halls, and at meals. On a typical campus, most of this information not only encourages drinking, but almost glorifies and romanticizes it. The alcohol marketers, particularly, take advantage of this situation. In the words of one marketing executive, "The campus lifestyle is one that encourages camaraderie and interaction, and is a fertile area for word-of-mouth to get going. It's a great place for promotion" (Rose, 1982). The word-of-mouth information is generally biased toward promoting alcohol; it is often inaccurate, and it is sometimes dangerous. Our culture drives much of it, but the marketers steer the rest.

The campus is not an island isolated from the rest of society. Students watch television like most other Americans. There is not only the sampling of positive (and some negative) images of alcohol and drinking embedded in the story lines of the programs, but the heavy, explicit advertising of the alcoholic beverage industry. A study by the National Institute of Mental Health has estimated that there are approximately 10 episodes per hour of typical television that involve drinking. Some are advertisements, some are major components of the story line, and most are incidental. Most show drinking in a positive light and associated with desirable activities.

Pro-alcohol messages are everywhere: newspapers, radio, magazines, billboards, and television. Research has demonstrated that exposure to beer advertising is second only to peer influence in predicting adolescent beer drinking (Atkin et al., 1984).

Where is the information that modern medicine and the physical and social sciences have brought us? On most campuses, much of it is in the library, in pamphlets, in the heads of professionals at the health or counseling centers, and in the knowledge base of a few of the faculty, who may well have been the major contributors to this rapidly increasing scientific body of knowledge. It is not in most of the classes, not usually in the campus newspaper, and not in the signs advertising campus social events. More than half of our schools have an undergraduate course on alcohol and alcoholism (Anderson & Gadaleto, 1991), but only a small fraction of the students attend these courses. How are students to make mature, informed decisions with this incredible imbalance of information? What intellectual, if not moral, obligation does the university have to try to level the playing field? Jean Mayer, the president of Tufts University, articulated the difficulty: "You have to go across-current of an entire civilization" (Jacobson et al., 1983). To do so, he has recently spoken at new-student orientation himself, observing that each year he must write letters to parents of dead students explaining the circumstances of their alcohol-related deaths.

Consider the following dramatic example. The typical student has seen literally tens of thousands of images associating alcohol with attractive members of the opposite sex and their social and sexual interactions. Couple this with the romantic poetry in the curriculum, the almost endless discussions about socializing and sex in which students are expected to engage, and the observation of other students in social and sexual situations involving alcohol.

> *Drinking will make you attractive to the opposite sex.*
> *Drinking will facilitate and enhance sexual activity.*
> *People who have successful careers drink.*
> *Drinking will promote and enhance your friendships.*
> *Drinking will relax you and make you better able to cope.*
> *Drinking will enhance your creativity.*
> *Everybody else is drinking.*

Every student gets these messages virtually every day on a typical college campus. They help to create and enhance the normative drinking culture found on most campuses—a culture in which most social, and indeed much intellectual, activity revolves around alcohol. How do the members of the college community receive any anti-alcohol messages?

In the United States, the image held of people is influenced by whether they use alcohol and other drugs. This, together with the societal images of alcohol and alcohol users, is a potent combination. Therefore, it should be no surprise that, although 66% of adult Americans describe a person who does not use any drugs as "intelligent," only 40% describe that person as "having many friends," and a bare 18% associate the term *sexy* with that person (Black et al., 1989). That is the image that alcoholic beverage advertisers and promoters have helped to create: Abstainers may be

smart but they have few friends and are not very sexy. It is the one that we must all work to erase.

> *There are lots of successful nondrinkers.*
> *Creativity and productivity are reduced by alcohol.*
> *The alcoholic beverage industry targets college students.*
> *Sexual function and sensation are impaired and reduced by drinking.*
> *Many drinking practices are dangerous.*
> *Drinking is associated with lower grades and dropouts.*
> *Alcohol problems run in the family.*
> *Alcohol interferes with personal relationships and harms many.*
> *Large numbers of Americans die or are injured every day from alcohol-related causes.*

Sex and sexuality are of great interest and concern to most college students. One of the major implications and messages of these massive advertising campaigns is that alcohol facilitates and enhances sex. Thousands of variants of this message reach college students each year. In contrast, how can they find out that "although alcohol has been regarded as an aphrodisiac, it actually induces sexual dysfunction" (Shuster, 1988) or that short-term alcohol effects include both erection dysfunction and ejaculation incompetence in males and reduced sensation and stimulus in both sexes (Mandell & Miller, 1983; Fahrner, 1987; Blum, 1984)?

In 1987, an Illinois appellate judge wrote a legal opinion in a case involving a Beta Theta Pi initiate who was required to go through a ceremony involving dangerous drinking practices. The judge opined that a fraternity had a legal duty to refrain from requiring participation in continuous drinking after intoxication (*William Quinn v. Sigma Rho Chapter of Beta Theta Pi Fraternity,* 1987). In retrospect, the amazing thing about this opinion is the other duties it implicitly calls into question:

— The intellectual duty of the university to teach those Beta Theta Pi members, and presumably others on the campus, that drinking after the point of intoxication is dangerous and potentially deadly.

- The ethical duty of the school community not to allow such activity.
- The social duty of the fraternity and the university to provide healthy social settings.

Class Scheduling

It is not openly discussed very often, but in most gatherings of college faculty and staff discussing the campus alcohol problem, the subject of class schedules soon comes up. In most schools, Friday and Saturday classes are fewer and farther between than in the past. If most students have no Saturday classes, there is less reason for drinking moderation on Friday night. If a student's last class is on Thursday at 2 P.M., why not start the weekend Thursday at 4 P.M.? It is ironic, but it may well be that one of the best campus prevention strategies is classes and other academic activities such as colloquia, labs, conferences, and the like on Thursdays, Fridays, and even Saturday mornings.

Extracurricular Activities

Surprising to many in our society who see the campus as a vibrant, dynamic place with a universe of activity choices, one of the most common reasons college students give for drinking and drugging is "there's not much else to do." Although it can be demonstrated to the satisfaction of most college administrators that the complaint is objectively unfounded, there is a harsh reality that what these students are saying is, "The choices I am offered here are not very attractive to me. They're no better, and usually a lot worse than swilling beer."

Go to Pasadena in the weeks before the Rose Parade and watch the students work on their float designs and construction. You won't see a lot of drinking or drugging. Watch the Young Democrats and Young Republicans in an election year. Their energy and passion find interesting, creative, and constructive outlets. One of the most fascinating observations of all the students, black and white, who were so involved in the Civil Rights marches of the 1960s is the fact that there was so little drinking and illicit drug use (at a time when both were generally heavy in the age group). There was little time for such things when there were worlds to be changed and societies to be reformed. There are common elements: a goal or cause, relatively loose structure, creative outlet, passion, a real need for the student efforts, and contact with the opposite sex. During the 1991 spring break, so infamous for excessive drinking, one group of students in the Midwest involved a substantial number of students in spending their time and money helping the homeless instead.

Local Research and Dissemination Efforts

Manhattan College of New York, the University of Indiana, University of Iowa, Penn State, Central Missouri State, and many other schools use the intellectual resources on their campus to learn more about their own student body and its relationships to alcohol. Consider the prevention possibilities of the following:

- Mobilizing the intellectual capabilities of students and faculty to direct term papers and masters and doctoral dissertations toward this problem.
- Organizing the art students to design posters and the business and economics majors to analyze the local economics of alcohol use.
- Using social scientists to survey the real attitudes of the students and faculty and the philosophers and ethicists to structure the ethical debate.
- Using management and law students to propose appropriate campus rules and regulations.
- Encouraging literature students to find the many literary references to the problems of drinking.
- Encouraging biologists and physiologists to explain the truth about alcohol and sexual function in language the rest of the campus will understand.
- Encouraging the journalists, poets, and communications students to use the campus newspapers, radio stations, and closed circuit and cable TV to broadcast appropriate information about alcohol.
- Having cheerleaders and student athletes include messages about alcohol at pep rallies.

— Having marketing majors analyze and keep track of the number and kind of messages related to alcohol use that reach the student body.

There is virtually no department of the modern college or university that could not make a major contribution to a campus prevention effort. The opportunity is there to use and practice the skills the students are being taught every day and improve the quality of campus life in the most profound way—by preserving it. The college and the student body can take back control from the various economic, legal, and social forces in society, and the students can shape their own destinies and control their own behavior rather than simply being the target and market of special interests who have no interest in the students other than as current and potential customers.

Change in Campus Community Norms

Norms change all the time in America. Historically, it is probably one of the things that is most unique about our country when compared with the rest of the world: the rapid rate of change within our society. The most rapid and visible normative changes are fashion and entertainment. The white buck shoes and "rep" ties of the college male of yesteryear have been replaced by Nikes and no ties at all on the modern college campus. Popular music and music groups of today were, for the most part, unheard of three or four years ago. Even curricular preferences of college students radically change over relatively short periods of time, as witnessed by the inability of many schools to keep up with the number of students that wanted to major in business and computer science in the late '80s.

These normative changes didn't just happen: they are the result of forces that were put into play on the campus community by advertisers, health officials, campus representatives, students, administrators, faculty, promoters, and others. Although these forces that produce the normative changes don't always coordinate with each other, change represents the cumulative effect of a host

of environmental forces working on society in general and the campus in particular.

Alcohol and other drug abuse prevention lies in harnessing these forces to produce a critical mass of social dynamics to bring about change in the desired direction.

In the health arena there has probably been no more dramatic, normative change in our society in general, and on the campuses in particular, than behavior and attitudes toward smoking. Although too many college students still smoke cigarettes, the prevalence is now far less than in former years, and the norm is not to smoke at all. If anything, there is a hostility to smoking as being somewhat antisocial. This did not occur by accident. A massive number of forces acted over a period of years to alter the campus environment.

The same fraternity social dynamics that can take a pledge who never before drank alcohol and persuade him to chug to the point of passing out or death can certainly produce other behavior that is more healthy, safe, and constructive. It is a matter of will. Fraternities and sororities on many campuses are the social trendsetters. They have been a disproportionate part of the problem; they have the capacity to contribute disproportionately to solutions involving normative change. All the other elements of the campus can be similarly directed to the problem of altering the environment.

Program Size and Scale

For campus programs that have as their objective a change of environment, the culture and the norms of the campus community make individual, isolated, programmatic forays—regardless of how creative, clever, and effective—unlikely to produce a discernible change. Normative behavior change does not take place with a sudden gestalt of collective insight leading to group consensus about behavior change. Politicians recognize that, advertisers recognize that, fashion designers recognize that, and we in public health and education must also appreciate that reality.

Recently, some advertising experts were reviewing a government-sponsored public service antidrug campaign, and it was observed that if the ads are not run repeatedly and communicated in a variety of forms, they are not likely to have a significant effect on behavior. This principle is what advertising personnel refer to as the scale of the campaign or a critical mass. There is a rough rule in the advertising world that unless you can get three to five impressions of your message, you can't even begin to get the attention of the target, much less alter behavior. In this light, orientation of incoming students is unlikely to have any significant effect. However, that same orientation, as the first impression of an orchestrated set that will prevail and be repeated for the first semester of school, will probably have much more success.

The designer with a new fashion trend he or she wants the world to adopt does not announce it at an intellectual convention of fashion designers or even display it at a fashion show and leave it at that. It is but one impression of a series of orchestrated efforts that will include advertising, public relations, intellectual persuasion, training, and emotional appeals. The designer will find high-visibility stars to wear the new design in public, give interviews, write articles, and appear in public. Often, a promoter will not only welcome controversy but will seek to produce it under the theory that the criticism that will probably take place will be more than offset by the additional number of impressions.

In college communities, we will probably see parallel efforts on a large enough scale to produce change—massively parallel communications. The central issues of our prevention programming must not only be what message, but how often, how frequent, and from how many different sources. The college campus is ideal for these parallel efforts in that it is a community that encompasses a wide variety of customs, moralities, ideas, politics, religions, and philosophies that can approach a problem from a variety of different perspectives. They can form a coalition, like the community partnerships, around the shared desire to eliminate the adverse consequences of alcohol and other drug use. At the same time, there can be wide diversity with regard to abstention versus moderate drinking, campus regulation, legalization issues, science, and the like. Each individual or organization can, if galvanized, contribute its unique perspective and contribute to the massively parallel communications to the campus community as a whole. The interfraternity competition might be to see which Greek society produces the most positive campus impressions. At the central leadership level of the campus, coordination of the message is not nearly so important as empowering and stimulating campus activity, recognizing that it will probably take many forms and faces.

THE PRESENT TO THE FUTURE

The government has provided much help and stimulation. The Center for Substance Abuse Prevention of the U.S. Public Health Service has for several years maintained a *Put On The Brakes* campaign that provides materials, research, and other assistance to campuses throughout the country. It sponsors a national contest for development of campus prevention materials. Through its National Clearinghouse for Alcohol and Drug Information and its RADAR Network, it provides an information resource available to college students, teachers, and administrators throughout the country. The U.S. Department of Education provides grants through its FIPSE program, research, a network of campus mutual assistance, and policy guidelines. Many states have their own initiatives, such as the Missouri governor's convocation of all the colleges in the state to address the campus alcohol and other drug problems. In the final analysis, the college, like any other community, must galvanize itself, mobilize its resources, and take control of its own community norms. That is what campuses throughout the country have been starting in the last few years. With continued public and community support, these efforts will increase in the coming years. The campus and the nation will be healthier, safer, and more productive as a result.

NOTES

1. College students' daily drinking prevalence is not higher than that of their noncollege counterparts, as are monthly, weekly, and other prevalence figures. Most important, however, is that their heavier drinking and more dangerous drinking prevalence is higher.

2. Landon C. Garland was the president. The Alabama legislature responded by converting the university to a military school to restore discipline (*The New York Times,* Oct 28, 1990).

3. Based on 1986 data, there were 2,642,000 high school graduates in America and 54.8% (1,447,816) then enrolled in college. Seven percent of this number is more than 101,000.

4. The annual earnings differential between a college graduate and a nongraduate is approximately $7,200. Over a typical 40-year work life, that amounts to $288,000 for each alcohol-related dropout.

5. Based on a 9% average personal tax payment.

6. The 1988 federal outlay for student loans was $2.6 billion (U.S. Department of Commerce, 1989).

7. The implication of causality should be made cautiously in this case. The students living at home with family are often not as affluent as those living on or near campus; with less disposable income, they cannot afford to drink as much. Furthermore, heavier drinkers may well want to be more independent of family influences so that they may continue or increase their heavy drinking without interference.

REFERENCES

Anderson, W. A., et al. (Oct. 1989). *Replication of the national study of the substance use and abuse habits of college student athletes.* East Lansing: Michigan State University College of Human Medicine.

Anderson, W. A., et al. (1991). National survey of alcohol and drug use by college athletes. *Physician and Sportsmedicine, 19* (2), 104.

Anderson, D. S., & Gadaleto, A. F. (1991). *The college alcohol survey.* Fairfax, VA: George Mason University.

Atkin, C., et al. (1984). Teenage drinking: Does advertising make a difference. *Journal of Communication, 34,* 157–167.

Bachman, J. G., & O'Malley, P. M. (1980). *When four months equal a year.* Ann Arbor: University of Michigan Institute for Social Research.

Black, G. S., et al. (1989). *The attitudinal basis of drug abuse: The third year.* Rochester, NY: Gordon S. Black Corporation, Table 41.

Blum, K. (1984). Influence of psychopharmacological agents on sexual function. *Handbook of Abusable Drugs.* Gardner Press, pp. 645–661.

Blum, A. (1990). *Laughing the drug dealers out of town.* Presentation at the Oregon Seventh Annual Prevention Conference, Sunriver, October 21.

Breed, W., et al. (in press). *Alcohol advertising in college newspapers: A seven-year follow-up.*

Brown, J. L. (1989). Alcohol consumption among Kansas State University freshmen by probation and non-probation status. *Journal of Alcohol and Drug Education, 34* (3), 14–21.

Burda, P. C., & Vaux, A. C. (1988). Social drinking in supportive contexts among college males. *Journal of Youth and Adolescence, 17* (2), 165–171.

The Carnegie Foundation for the Advancement of Teaching (1990). *Campus life: In search of community.* Princeton, NJ: Princeton University Press.

CASS Student Advertising, Inc. (1992). *1981-92 national rate book and college newspaper directory.* Evanston, IL.

Chronicle of Higher Education, July 21, 1982.

Cruz, C., & Bubl, J. (1990). Promotion and price: How the alcohol industry targets youth. Paper presented at the Oregon Seventh Annual Prevention Conference, Sunriver, October 21.

Eigen, L. D. (1991). *Alcohol practices, policies, and potentials of American Colleges and Universities Center.* Washington, DC: Office for Substance Abuse Prevention (OSAP), National Clearinghouse for Drug and Alcohol Information.

Eigen, L. D., et al. (1993). *College alcohol and other drug prevention strategies.* Rockville, MD: National Clearinghouse for Alcohol and Drug Information.

Engs, R. C., & Hanson, D. J. (1988). University students' drinking patterns and problems: Examining the effects of raising the purchase age. *Public Health Reports, 103* (6), 667–673.

Fahrner, E. M. (1987). Sexual dysfunction in male alcohol addicts: Prevalence and treatment. *Archives of Sexual Behavior, 16* (3), 247–257.

Gang Rape: A Rising Campus Concern. *The New York Times,* February 17, 1986.

George, W. H., et al. (1989). Effects of raising the drinking age to 21 years in New York State on self-reported college students. *Journal of Applied Social Psychology, 19* (8), 623–635.

Goodwin, L. (1984). Explaining alcohol consumption and related experiences among fraternity and sorority members. *Journal of College Student Development, 30* (5), 448–458.

Harris, L. (1986). Telephone survey. New York State Research Institute on Alcoholism.

Hill, F. E., & Bugen, L. A. (1979). A survey of drinking patterns among college students. *Journal of College Student Personnel, 20,* 236–243.

Hughes, S., & Dodder, R. (1983). Alcohol consumption patterns among college students. *Journal of College Student Personnel, 20,* 257–264.

Iowa City Press Citizen, October 3, 1990.

Jacobson, M., et al. (1983). *The booze merchants: The inebriating of America.* Center for Science in the Public Interest, pp. 57–58.

Jason, P. B. (1989). Personality correlates of heavy and light drinking female college students. *Journal of Alcohol Education, 34* (2), 33–37.

Johnson, J. (Aug. 1989). Comparison of alcohol use by college students, 1983 and 1988. Conference paper presented in New Orleans.

Johnston, L. D., et al. (1991). *Drug use among American high school seniors, college students and young adults, 1975–1990.* Washington, DC: National Institute on Drug Abuse.

Kalisher, M. J. (1989). *Behavior analysis of alcohol consumption and impairment at university parties.* Doctoral dissertation, Virginia Polytechnic Institute and State University.

Lewiston Tribune, August 27, 1993.

Mandell, W., & Miller, C. M. (1983). Male sexual dysfunction as related to alcohol consumption. *Alcoholism, 7* (1), 65–69.

Miller Brewing Company (1989). *Miller notes on contemporary marketing.*

Missouri Governor's Conference on Issues of Substance Abuse and Higher Education, December 4–5, 1990, Lake Ozark, Missouri.

Moos, R. H. (1977). *Evaluating educational environments.* San Francisco: Jossey-Bass.

The New York Times, Oct. 28, 1990.

The New York Times, Dec. 17, 1989.

The New York Times, Jan. 7, 1990.

The New York Times, Nov. 11, 1990.

The New York Times, Sept. 23, 1990.

NIAAA (1987). *Alcohol and health: Sixth special report to Congress on alcohol and health from the Secretary of Health and Human Services.* Washington, DC: U.S. Department of Health and Human Services.

NIAAA (1989). *Seventh special report to the U.S. Congress on alcohol and health from the Secre-tary of Health and Human Services.* U.S. Department of Health and Human Services, p. 144.

National Institute on Drug Abuse (1987). *National trends in drug use and related factors among American high school students and young adults, 1975–1986.* DHHS pub. no. (ADM)87-1535.

National Institute on Drug Abuse (1988). *National household survey on drug abuse: Main findings 1985.* DHHS pub. no. (ADM)88-1586.

Parker, E. S. (1984). Alcohol and cognition. *Psychopharmacology Bulletin, 20,* 494–496.

Perkins, H. W., & Berkowitz, A. D. (1989). Stability and contradiction in college students' drinking following a drinking-age law change. *Journal of Alcohol and Drug Education, 35* (1), 60–77.

Petroff, B., & Broek, L. (1990). *The University of Iowa alcohol and other drug use assessment: Spring semester, 1990.* Iowa City: University of Iowa Student Health Service.

Presley, C. A., & Meilman, P. (1992). *Alcohol and drugs on American college campuses: A report to college presidents.* Carbondale: Southern Illinois University.

Presley, C. A., et al. (1993). *Alcohol and drugs on American college campuses.* Carbondale: The Core Institute, Student Health Program, Southern Illinois University.

Rose, M., (1982). Quoted in *Advertising Age,* August 2, 1982.

Roth, R. (1989). The impact of liquor liability on colleges and universities. *Journal of College and University Law, 13* (1), 45–64.

Rubington, E. (1990). Drinking in the dorms: A study of the etiquette of RA–resident relations. *The Journal of Drug Issues, 20,* (3), 451–461.

Ryan, B. E., & Mosher, J. F. (1991). *Progress report: Alcohol promotion on campus.* The Marin Institute.

St. Petersburg Times, Sept. 2, 1993.

Shuster, C. (1988). *Alcohol and sexuality.* New York: Praeger.

Stinson, F., CSR Inc. (1990). Alcohol epidemiological data system. Special computer analysis of 1987 unpublished hospital discharge data from the National Center for Health Statistics.

Time, April 23, 1990.

Tryon, G. S. (Aug. 1989). Comparison of alcohol use by college students, 1983 and 1988. Conference Paper, 97th Annual Convention of the American Psychological Association, New Orleans.

U.S. Department of Commerce (1989). *Statistical abstracts of the United States.* Washington, DC: U.S. Government Printing Office.

U.S. General Accounting Office (1987). *Drinking-age laws: An evaluation synthesis of their impact on highway safety.* Washington, DC: General Accounting Office.

University of Iowa (1990). *The University of Iowa faculty and staff policy on a drug-free environment.* September 10, 3.

Walfish, S., et al. (1981). *International Journal of Addictions, 16,* 941–945.

The Wall Street Journal, Feb. 8, 1983.

The Washington Post, Oct. 8, 1990.

The Washington Post, Sept. 20, 1990.

West, R., et al. (1990). Alcohol consumption, problem drinking and anti-social behavior in a sample of college students. *British Journal of Addiction, 85,* 479–486.

William Quinn v. Sigma Rho Chapter of Beta Theta Pi Fraternity, no. 4-86-0538, Appellate Court of Illinois, April 8, 1987.

Wilsnack, R. W., et al. (1984). Women's drinking and drinking problems: Patterns from a 1981 national survey. *American Journal of Public Health, 74,* 1231–1238.

Wilsnack, S. C., et al. (1985). Gender-role orientations and drinking among women in a U.S. national survey. *Alcohol, Drugs and Tobacco: An International Perspective. Past Present and Future: Proceedings of the 34th International Congress on Alcoholism and Drug Dependence,* Calgary, Alberta, Canada, International Council on Alcohol and Addictions, 242–255.

Wilson, R. (1990). Better times at Chico State. *Prevention File.* San Diego: University of California at San Diego, Fall.

CHAPTER 14

HELPING PROFESSIONALS

ROBERT H. COOMBS
BERNARD B. VIRSHUP

Helping professionals, especially health professionals, are the last people most of us would suspect of being drug abusers. But training in the health sciences and helping professions does not immunize a person against substance abuse or other debilitating problems. On the contrary, addiction, an equal-opportunity destroyer, may be an occupational hazard for those in the professions (Vaillant, Brighton, & McArthur 1970; Talbott, 1986).

The impact of substance abuse on professionals and those they serve can be devastating. Compulsive drug use undermines the user's health, well-being, and job performance. It also adversely affects family health and places patients or clients at great risk. Colleagues who rely on their professional competence also suffer.

PREVALENCE OF CHEMICALLY IMPAIRED PROFESSIONALS

About 13.5% of the U.S. population are alcoholic and another 6.1% abuse other drugs (Regier et al., 1990). Chemical dependency may be even higher among helping professionals. The National Council on Alcoholism estimates that the percentage of alcoholic professionals is 1.5 times greater than among nonprofessionals (Busch, 1982; Normark, et al., 1985). Talbott (1986), who runs a treatment program for addicted professionals, suggests that "the rate of alcoholism is thirty-five times higher among medical people than among laymen." These high estimates were challenged by Brewster (1986), who noted that when alcohol and other drugs are considered together, the prevalence of such problems among physicians is not unusually high. Reality probably lies somewhere between these widely varying estimates.

Statistics about chemically impaired professionals generally come from three sources, disciplinary actions, treatment populations, and research surveys. With regard to the former, the president of the California State Bar notes that at least one in seven California lawyers has a serious substance abuse problem. Half of the 5,000 legal misconduct cases investigated each year by the California Bar were linked to substance abuse (Haldane, 1990). Forty percent is the lowest figure reported in other states for all disciplinary cases that involve drug abuse, but the New York Bar Association indicates that as many as 75% of those coming before their grievance committee are substance abusers (Dowell, 1988).

Other professions report similar statistics. During the past decade, for example, about 1% of the licensed physicians in California (695 of about 76,000 doctors) participated in a state-sponsored monitoring program for the treatment and aftercare of chemically impaired physicians

Much of this chapter is condensed from *Drug Impaired Professionals* by R. H. Coombs, Harvard University Press, 1995. We acknowledge with appreciation the contributions of Wendy Kohatsu, Carla Vera, and Carol Jean Coombs.

(Ikeda & Pelton, 1990; Joan Gladden, personal communication, Dec. 1994). The program director estimates that a nearly equal number received help for chemical addiction in other treatment programs (Chet Pelton, personal communication, Feb. 1992). Still others, no doubt, have avoided identification and treatment altogether. California doctors represent about 10% of the nation's physicians.

With regard to treatment populations, Alcoholics Anonymous' 1980 survey of 24,950 members found that 17% of the men and 18% of the women identified themselves as professionals (Bissell & Haberman, 1984). Hazelden, an inpatient addiction treatment program, reports that in any year, admissions statistics show a relatively stable pattern: About 15% of all admissions are professionals; physicians are the only profession showing an increased incidence over time (Spicer, Barnett, & Kliner, 1978).

Research studies also indicate widespread abuse. A 20-year longitudinal study of 45 physicians compared with 90 nonphysicians found that the former took significantly more tranquilizers, sedatives, and stimulants than the latter (Vaillant, Brighton, & McArthur, 1970). Thirty-six percent of the physicians, compared to 22% of the nonphysicians, were in a high drug-use group that included heavy drinking or trouble with control of alcohol.

A national survey of 9,600 randomly selected physicians (Hughes et al., 1992), compared their drug and alcohol use with results from the National Household Survey of Drug Abuse. Physicians were significantly more likely to use alcohol and prescription medications—especially minor opiates (such as codeine and Darvon), and benzodiazepine tranquilizers—and less likely to use cigarettes and illicit substances such as heroin, cocaine, and marijuana. Ten percent reported daily use of alcohol, with 9.3% consuming five or more drinks per day at least once in the past month. One in nine (11%) had treated themselves in the past year with benzodiazepines and one in six with minor opiates. Younger physicians showed significantly higher rates of illicit drug use in the past year than older physi-

cians and were also more likely to have used alcohol. Few gender differences were found except that young male doctors compared to female physicians of the same age had significantly higher rates of tobacco and marijuana use.

About 1.6% of physicians responding to this survey defined themselves as having abused or been dependent on alcohol in the past year. As Hughes and colleagues (1992) report, the lifetime rate of self-defined alcohol abuse revealed by these respondents, 6.0%, is higher than that found by McAuliffe (1984) for New England physicians (4.1%) and much lower than those reported for Johns Hopkins Medical graduates age 52–68 (12.9%) and for 100 physicians in a New York county (14%). These latter studies, suggesting rates of alcohol abuse for physicians ranging between 13% and 14%, are consistent with the 13.5% rate of alcohol disorders in the adult population recently reported by the National Institute of Mental Health. These studies used different survey methods and criteria for defining alcohol abuse (Hughes et al., 1992).

A national survey of resident physicians in training (Hughes et al., 1991) reported that, when compared with young adults of similar age, residents had higher rates of past-month use of alcohol (5% drank alcoholic beverages daily) and benzodiazepines but lower rates of other drugs such as marijuana, cigarettes, cocaine, barbiturates, and heroin.

A longitudinal study of an entire class of medical students (Clark & Daugherty, 1990) disclosed that, during the four years of medical school, 11% of the students had been involved in excessive drinking for at least one six-month period and 18% were identified as alcohol abusers during medical school. Interestingly, alcohol abusers had better first-year grades and overall scores on the National Board of Medical Examiners test, Part I, than their classmates (Clark, 1988).

Similar statistics can be cited for other professionals. A 1984 survey mailed to all licensed pharmacists in North Carolina, for example, revealed that nearly half (43%) of the 1,370 respondents knew at least one pharmacist who had personal problems severe enough to interfere with everyday activities (Normark et al., 1985). More than 28% had worked with someone addicted to alcohol or other drugs.

In a national survey of pharmacy faculty, alcohol use was reported by 89% of respondents (Baldwin, 1990). A 1987 survey of pharmacy students at two midwestern schools found that 89% of the students used alcohol. This number is significantly more than the 68% of young adults in the general population who drink (Tucker et al., 1988).

A survey of randomly selected attorneys in Washington State revealed that 18% were problem drinkers and one in four attorneys had tried cocaine (Benjamin, Darling, & Sales, 1990). An Oregon Bar study disclosed that 15% of attorneys were addicted to alcohol (Hickey, 1990). These statistics suggest that between 72,000 and 130,000 attorneys drink beyond their control (Hickey, 1990).

EXPLAINING SUBSTANCE ABUSE AMONG PROFESSIONALS

A number of interrelated factors account for chemical abuse among professionals: easy access to drugs, pharmacological optimism, an environment that encourages recreational drug use, stressful working conditions, dysfunctional family origins, feelings of immunity, and a training system that rewards self-sacrifice and discourages self-care and the affective aspects of personal growth.

Easy Access to Drugs

Alcoholic beverages and other drugs are readily accessible to most people, but professionals have much easier access to controlled substances. Pharmacists, nurses, dentists, anesthesiologists, and emergency room physicians have particularly easy access to workplace drugs: the drugs prescribed for patients, the free samples provided to physicians, and the stocked supplies kept on

some patient units. "It's like working in a candy store," a physician remarked (AAAS Conference, 1992).

Street drugs, particularly cocaine, are readily available to criminal trial lawyers, who may barter their services for drugs (Silas, 1987). "Everywhere I went, it [cocaine] was there," a lawyer explained.

Pharmacological Optimism

The emphasis on drug therapy in the training of health professionals reinforces the belief that there is a chemical remedy for every physical and emotional problem. Medicating oneself is a small step from medicating others. Nitrous oxide, for example, used by dentists to calm an anxious patient, can also relax and uplift an overworked professional.

Accustomed to "miracle drugs," health professionals and the patients they serve often develop an uncritical acceptance of drug therapy. "Much of our population is conditioned to think that the first moment of mental, physical, or emotional discomfort is a signal for instant pharmaceutical treatment," a pharmacist remarked (Spierer, 1986).

Recognizing that physicians are the difference between their drug product line profiting or perishing, pharmaceutical companies woo physicians, gatekeepers of the legal drug industry, with several mailings a day and frequent visits by pharmaceutical representatives bearing free samples. Each year, the pharmaceutical industry spends more than $5 billion marketing drugs to physicians—about $8,000 for every doctor in the United States (Whitaker, 1991).

Informal Encouragement to Use Recreational Drugs

A survey of senior dental students in a midwestern dental school found that all of the students used alcoholic beverages and 45% used marijuana occasionally (Bowermaster, 1988). Coming from the ranks of college students, professional trainees have developed permissive attitudes about the recreational use of alcohol and other substances such as marijuana and cocaine. Social events featuring alcoholic beverages and other addictive drugs are common in professional training and incoming students are often welcomed by the preceding class with an alcohol party. After exams, they gather to unwind with alcoholic drinks and other drugs, just as they did in college.

A typology of addictive origins (McAuliffe, Rohman, Feldman, & Launer, 1985) includes recreational addicts who begin at parties and other socials to go along with friends and to satisfy their curiosity about drug effects; therapeutic addicts who begin drug use as treatment, usually for physical pain, most often at the direction of a physician or dentist, but in some cases as self-treatment, especially to deal with emotional pain; and instrumental addicts who begin using stimulants to relieve fatigue and to enhance performance. Helping professionals may use drugs for all three purposes, but recreational use of drugs other than alcohol has recently become pronounced. In the past, addicted health professionals began opiate use as self-treatment for physical pain, fatigue, emotional disorders, insomnia, and other problems. "Today, for the first time," McAuliffe (1984) notes, "Young health professionals have grown up during an era marked by tolerance of drug abuse" (p. 2). Consequently, a new type of professional addict has emerged, one addicted to so-called recreational drugs such as marijuana and cocaine.

Dysfunctional Family Origins

There are at least 10.5 million alcoholics in the United States and 76 million Americans have an alcoholic family member. Nearly one in five (18%) spent their childhood with an alcoholic (Schoenborn, 1991). An inordinately high percentage of health professionals come from such families (Peters, 1990). A South Carolina study of nurses, social workers, and medical students found that 22–30% were raised in families dominated by alcohol abuse (Peter Johnson, personal communication, June 13, 1990). A New England survey of about 500 physicians and nearly equal numbers of medical students, pharmacists, and pharmacy students revealed that 22% of the physicians and 27% of the medical students had family histories of substance abuse, as did a similar number (22% and 25% respectively) of pharmacists and pharmacy students (McAuliffe et al., 1987). Surveys at various dental schools have found that more than 35% of the dental students come from families with a history of chemical dependency (Bowermaster, 1988).

Vaillant, Brighton, and McArthur (1970) postulate that a lack of parental support and concern during childhood leads professionals to dedicate themselves to the care of others. They seek emotional gratification from their clients and patients to compensate for the dismal lack of parental care during their formative years. "Individuals with low self-esteem tend to be attracted to professions that make them feel powerful and make their egos feel big," an impaired attorney observed. "[The legal profession] puts you in a situation where you can financially afford to do crazy things and the stress gives you an excuse for doing them" (Haldane, 1990, p. E2).

Stammer's (1988) study found that many nurses (59%) develop an exaggerated idea of their role as caretaker; most (85%) feel a strong need to care for others and measure their self-worth by how much they meet others' needs. Characteristic of those who grow up in the families of alcoholics, they are eager to gain the approval and acceptance they did not receive at home. The caretaker role offers a continuation of familiar patterns, and because they are often perfectionists, many compete successfully for places in professional schools (Smith, Mangelsdorf, Louderbough, & Piland, 1989; Smith, 1989).

Impaired professionals are often high academic achievers. Bissell and Jones (1981) and Cross (1985) note that addicted nurses in recovery are often in the top third of their graduating classes, earn degrees beyond their basic training, and are viewed as very able by their colleagues.

Anxiety about self-worth propels the impaired professional into an unbalanced lifestyle of overwork and superhuman achievement. Anderson (1990) notes that the most emotionally abused medical students tend to favor the most demanding programs. "It is the only reward system they know. They develop work addiction, the subtle yet definitely numbing anesthetic for the pain of loss of control" (p. 6).

The school environment is skewed in favor of those most verbal and willing to work the hardest for grades. Students from chemically dependent homes often do well here, despite or perhaps because of the psychological difficulties of their home life. They see school and professional training as their ticket out of these difficulties.

Emotional Neglect During Training

Professional training programs that neglect the affective development of trainees heighten vulnerability to substance abuse. Professional school curricula skillfully teach the basic sciences and technical skills, but give woefully little emphasis to emotional development. Not surprisingly, anxious and depressed trainees sometimes turn to chemical solutions for relief. Some drugs enable them to work longer and more intensively; others help them unwind and relax.

Wolf and Kissling (1984) describe lifestyle changes that occur during the first seven months of medical school: Students become less physically active, sleep fewer hours, and report increased stress. Students describe their training environments as rigid, dehumanizing, depressing, and even abusive (Wolf, Randall, & Faucett, 1988). Small wonder that their physical health and emotional well-being decrease.

Sleep deprivation is common among professional trainees expected to work excessively long hours. In law school, for example, first-year students are generally overwhelmed with a workload that leaves them with little time to sleep, relax, and enjoy friends and relatives (Benjamin, Kaszniak, Sales, & Shanfield, 1986). First-year grades determine the distribution of honors, law

review, job placement, and consequently the students' sense of personal self-worth. Third-year students, many of whom work part-time while trying to keep up with demanding course work, feel continually pressed for time; they often complain about insufficient rest and sleep. When graduation and the bar exam are behind them, the neophyte professional's lifestyle remains imbalanced due to work demands and the need to impress critical colleagues.

A resident physician's training, with work weeks of 90–140 hours, requires great physical and emotional stamina at a time of profound change in role, responsibilities, and self-image. All too often, they use substances to cope.

Stressful Career Circumstances

The professional environment encourages professionals to be workaholics, a situation complicated by a poor support network and few recreational outlets. Professionals in such stressful circumstances often use alcoholic drinks and other drugs for a pick-up. Others help them relax and sleep or offer short-term relief from the stress caused by their demanding work. A conspiracy of silence in the workplace and the enabling behavior of colleagues and family members exacerbate the situation.

Many physicians find their work stressful and emotionally unrewarding. Burnout, cynicism, disillusionment, and financial problems are rife. Their days are often time-pressured with excessive and unmanageable caseloads (Hilfiker, 1985). They must stay current with exploding technical knowledge and worry about malpractice suits. Many carry large debts from their medical education.

Increased governmental control and the emergence of health maintenance organizations (HMOs) have eroded traditional medical ideals, undercut independence, and diminished the physician's sense of being special. HMO physicians feel pressured to see more and more patients. When overworked, they tend to drift unconsciously into personal syndromes characterized by ritualized behavior, irritability, and neglect of self and family. They experience frustration over endless paperwork and worry about the possibilities of making mistakes that could seriously harm a patient (Coombs, May, & Small, 1986).

Job satisfaction in dentistry also leaves something to be desired. According to a dental management survey (Pfifferling & Corbin, 1988), 42% of dentists would switch to another career if an opportunity arose. Dentists complain of tight scheduling, physical confinement, patient anxiety, lack of regular interaction with peers, office management problems, boredom, and panic in emergency situations. Some dentists feel tension from causing patients pain. Because dental education is one of the most expensive of all professional training programs, many dentists are under heavy financial pressures.

A survey of North Carolina pharmacists found that 6-16% of the respondents lacked such important health ingredients as time alone, an exercise program, good time-management practices, and someone with whom they could share their problems, needs, and accomplishments. Ciaccio, Jang, and Caiola (1982) report that 8–25% of pharmacists are at high risk for burnout. Pharmacists in chain and hospital pharmacies, found to be twice as likely to experience burnout, have lower well-being scores than pharmacists who are managers or work in independent pharmacies.

Nurses often suffer from emotional exhaustion caused by the psychologically demanding nature of their work and the technical tasks they must perform. Nearly a third quit within the first two years after nursing school (Haack, 1988). Because nursing achievement usually lacks institutional recognition, nurses often believe that the public neither understands nor appreciates their contribution (Clark, 1988). The resulting self-pity and a sense of powerlessness underpins depression (Green, 1989).

The North Carolina Quality of Life Study of 2,570 attorneys reported that 43% feel that work demands deny them sufficient time for a satisfying life outside of work. Although 81% say that they are "mostly satisfied," only 53.9% would encourage their children to become attorneys and more than 24% reported depression symptoms at least three times a month during the past year (North Carolina Bar Association, 1991).

Feelings of Immunity

Elitist attitudes, common among professionals, also contribute to substance abuse. Feeling too smart and too well-educated to become addicted, professionals sometimes develop a false sense of security. Vaillant, Brighton, and McArthur (1970) observe that they tend to disassociate themselves from the dangers of drugs and adopt the attitude, "It can't happen to me."

The addicted health practitioners studied by McAuliffe (1984) were knowledgeable about the possible adverse effects of drugs and some had treated patients for addiction. Unfortunately, this knowledge did not deter their own harmful use. Being in a controlling position of power facilitates denial and rationalization. Professional pride hampers a recognition of warning signs and willingness to seek help. Even if a professional admits to herself that she has lost control of her life, she would "rather die" than admit to colleagues she is floundering.

The attorney's well-developed ability to argue helps him rationalize or deny drug-related problems. Paid large fees to be defensive, they become skillful in minimizing problems, finding loopholes, blaming others, and thinking up excuses. This helps them cover up their own problems.

TERTIARY PREVENTION

Typically slow to seek help for their addictions (Bissell & Haberman, 1984), professionals may go undetected longer than other groups. Their relative affluence and prestigious status cushions them from the consequences of their dependence. Those closest to them—family members, office staff, and professional colleagues—typically protect them from the consequences of their addiction because they too are vulnerable to loss and embarrassment.

Usually, their abuse is exposed when an outside agency forces the issue. In Bissell and Haberman's (1984) study of alcoholic professionals, more than three-fourths of the nurses, two-fifths of the physicians, and two-thirds of the other professionals could not remember a superior or colleague who ever said anything to them about their drinking. Yet 62% reported drinking during working hours (ranging from 37% of the nurses to 80% of the attorneys), 60% reported regular morning drinking, and 76% acknowledged drinking to relieve withdrawal symptoms.

Identification and Intervention

Because professionals and trainees with drug problems rarely seek help on their own, someone else must identify the problem and encourage them to get help. Colleagues are reluctant to reach out to impaired associates; professional training has taught them to wait for the patient or client to come to them. Moreover, with a growing increase in lawsuits, professionals are reluctant to take additional risks by intervening in the personal lives of their colleagues.

An effective intervention can greatly improve the chances that a chemically dependent peer will accept treatment. This approach consists of a compassionate group of concerned family members, friends, and associates confronting the addict. Acting in concert, the team carefully documents the impairment, participates in group confrontation, and assists in monitoring and follow-up. This is particularly effective when backed by licensing board sanctions.

Interventions Sponsored by Training Institutions

A consortium of more than 20 medical schools, begun at the Memphis branch of the University of Tennessee, organized a system to identify and intervene with substance abusers in their ranks. Called Aid to Impaired Medical Students (AIMS), the program seeks to reduce the number of impaired medical trainees and physicians by identifying, treating, and preventing emotional impair-

ments that lead to substance abuse (Edelman, 1990). The program rationale is that young professionals and future physicians have a moral, albeit painful, responsibility to report a classmate's impairment. "Once colleagues become impaired," their guidelines state, "they may literally be unable to help themselves" (AIMS brochure, University of Tennessee).

Interventions Sponsored by Hospitals

Hospitals have recently recognized that it is in their best interest to identify and confront health-care professionals whose impairment may adversely affect patient care (Fisher & Weisman, 1988). Landmark legal decisions have made hospitals responsible for impaired practitioners' mistakes. As a result, physicians' aid committees have been widely implemented to provide practical information about how to monitor chemically dependent clinicians and help implement strategies for treatment and recovery. These committees monitor the release of information, testing of body fluids, and evaluation.

Interventions Sponsored by Professional Societies

Professional organizations have traditionally taken a lax approach to peer review. Clinging to a code of silent loyalty, they unwittingly enable addicted colleagues. To avoid erosion of public confidence, however, professional associations have recently been forced to address the problem. State and county organizations now seek to identify and provide effective treatment and aftercare to impaired colleagues, diverting them from the criminal justice system.

These diversion programs, typically supervised by state regulatory boards, are clearly coercive. The impaired professional is allowed to practice with a restricted license and all record of action against his or her license is removed as long as he or she abides by the provisions of the treatment program. If relapse occurs, the license is suspended or revoked (Green, 1989; Ackerman & Wall, in press).

In 1970, only seven state medical societies had active programs for impaired physicians (Carmichael & Herlihy, 1981). However, an explosive response occurred when a 1972 conference sponsored by the American Medical Association called on physicians to report debilitated colleagues and urged states to oversee treatment. Twelve years later (1984), all 50 state medical societies reportedly had impaired-physician committees. However, as Bissell (1989) notes, some programs exist only on paper; some are little more than cosmetic, and others have fallen into disrepair or inactivity.

Other professional organizations followed the AMA lead. In 1985, the American Dental Association and its Council on Dental Practice formed the Advisory Committee on Chemical Dependency Issues (ACCDI) and sponsored the first national conference on chemical dependency in the dental profession. Additional conferences were held in 1987, 1988, and 1990 (Bowermaster, 1988).

The American Nursing Association (ANA) sponsored its first Conference on Impaired Nurses in 1985, more than a decade after the first AMA conference (Sullivan, Bissell, & Williams, 1988). A resolution addressing the impaired nurses issue was defeated at a 1980 Houston ANA meeting. "Evidently," Bissell and Jones (1981) lament, "organized nursing is not yet sure how to address this problem and some nurses continue to be needlessly lost to the profession and to treatment and care" (p. 101) However, since the 1979 initiation of the Maryland State Nurse's Association Peer Assistance Program, other states have instituted similar programs, and recently more than half of the country's state nurse's associations have passed resolutions to address the problem.

In 1988, the American Bar Association created the Commission on Impaired Attorneys and charged it with the development and implementation of a program to address lawyer addiction problems. The commission provides a directory and survey of state and local lawyers' assistance programs as well as videotapes on addiction, substance abuse, and intervention techniques. It annually sponsors a national workshop for lawyers' assistance programs (Spilis, 1992).

In 1982, the American Pharmaceutical Association's (APhA) House of Delegates adopted a resolution to establish counseling, treatment, prevention, and rehabilitation programs for impaired pharmacists and pharmacy students. They resolved to plan educational sessions for the American Pharmaceutical Association's annual meeting, develop guidelines to help state boards of pharmacy deal with impaired pharmacists, published a handbook and established an informal Impaired Pharmacist Program Network (Nickel & Briske, 1985).

In 1983, the APhA assumed sponsorship of the pharmacists' section of the annual University of Utah School of Alcoholism and Other Drug Dependencies. Growing from one of the smallest of the school's 21 sections, it has become the largest. This forum, involving pharmacy students, faculty, and state board members, has led to the development of peer assistance programs for pharmacists and students whose competence has become compromised by chemical dependence. Scholarships and other encouragement provided by the American Association of Colleges of Pharmacies, the National Association of Boards of Pharmacy, the National Association of Chain Drug Stores, and the APhA Academy of Students of Pharmacy have swelled participation (American Pharmaceutical Association, 1993).

Treatment and Aftercare

The oldest residential treatment program for chemically impaired professionals is the Georgia Medical Society's Impaired Physician Program (IPP). This residential treatment stresses the disease concept of chemical dependence, emphasizes family therapy, Alcoholics Anonymous (AA), Narcotics Anonymous (NA), spiritual development, group therapy, coping skills training, and detailed education on the psychosocial and biogenetic characteristics of alcoholism and drug addiction. Group therapy sessions involve participants from the same profession. After completing the inpatient phase, professionals move to a halfway home. The final phase is an aftercare contract that includes a clear plan of action in case of relapse (Talbott, 1984).

Only a few methodologically rigorous evaluations have been made about treatment outcomes of drug-impaired professionals. California treatment facilities report recovery rates that are impressively high. More than half of relapsed professionals return to treatment. Three-fourths (74%) of the physicians who participate in the California Diversion Program successfully complete the program (California Physician's Diversion Program, 1992). The Michigan State director of the Physician Recovery Network (Skutar, 1990) reports that treatment centers that track patients two years after treatment find that 95% remain clean and sober. Of the 140 professionals treated at the Parkside Recovery Center, an intervention program modeled after the Georgia Recovery Program, 90% maintained continuous sobriety for one year and 80% for two years (Angres, 1990).

Eugene Willis states, "I have been involved with the treatment of 230 dentists from 29 states and three Canadians. To the best of our knowledge, the recovery rate is about 90%" (personal correspondence, June 20, 1990). Similarly, Spicer, Barnett, and Kliner (1978) report that the year after discharge from treatment at Hazelden, 91% of the professionals remained free of mood-altering drugs and 74% were attending AA meetings at least once a month. Professionals as a group showed more improvement than nonprofessionals.

These outcome statistics, profoundly higher than for nonprofessional addicts (Hubbard et al., 1989), indicate that professionals are highly advantaged in the recovery process. This advantage is their motivation to keep their licenses. Intervention efforts and follow-up monitoring get professionals into treatment (rather than jail) and ensure that they remain abstinent. In California, for example, addicted physicians in the substance abuse diversion program are followed for five years. To continue practicing and retain their licensure during this time, they must submit to random drug testing and consistently participate

in other aftercare activities such as weekly group therapy sessions and numerous 12-step meetings. This rigorous and long-term monitoring enhances compliance and greatly improves the chances for a long-term recovery.

Helping professionals are no more immune to addiction than the clients they serve, but they clearly have greater access to treatment and preventive resources. Growing awareness of the legal liability and detrimental image of chemically impaired colleagues is forcing training and practice centers to implement preventive and remedial interventions. These centers are usually endowed with ample treatment, evaluation, and follow-up resources.

SECONDARY PREVENTION

Secondary prevention programs, aimed at early recognition and treatment, are intended to keep budding problems from escalating and becoming chronic. They include effective identification, confrontation, and, when necessary, treatment.

Professional Counseling Services

Individual counseling has been the customary way to deal with emerging drug problems. A survey of 114 medical schools discovered that all of the 85 responding schools provided counseling services, but one-third were perceived by students as inadequate; counseling services are underused due to poor advertising and student concern about confidentiality (Seigle, Schuckit, & Plumb, 1983).

A model program, the UCLA Mental Health Program for Physicians-in-Training, addresses trainees' reluctance by providing well-advertised counseling at an off-campus location where confidential, high-quality evaluation and treatment are provided at a nominal cost (Borenstein & Cook, 1982).

Snow (1969) points out that counseling services are cost-effective. Even if the training institution absorbs the total therapy expense at private rates, the cost per trainee represents less than 10% of the investment made by the school for each incoming student. If treatment is successful in only half of the cases, the institution will still reduce its economic losses from dropouts by 80%. More important, as Borenstein and Cook (1982) note, human costs far outweigh financial losses. Besides the losses that result from suicide, substance abuse, and mental disorders is the subtler but equally disturbing "hardening of the spirit." The latter is manifest with increasing frequency in a litany of complaints about helping professionals.

Peer Counseling and Advocacy

A peer advocacy committee at the University of South Carolina teaches interested students how to reach out to fellow students before severe problems develop (Johnson, personal communication, June 13, 1990). Although the effectiveness of this program waxes and wanes as students come and go, the concept of collegial assistance is of constant importance to students during their training. A similar peer-counseling program at the Bowman Gray School of Medicine offers formal certification (McGann, 1990). The curriculum includes substance abuse education and counseling intervention skills.

The Medical College of Wisconsin offers peer-counseling training to second-, third- and fourth-year medical students. It consists of a 12-hour Saturday session followed by four two-hour sessions during succeeding weeks, with additional supervision provided on request (Spiro, Roenneburg, & Maly, 1978). During the first 18 months of the program, peer counselors spent 1,185 hours assisting their peers. More than half (56%) of these sessions were formal appointments, 29% were casual (meeting with peer counselors in hallways between classes or at lunch), and 13% were conducted over the telephone (1% were anonymous telephone calls).

Employee Assistance Programs

Employee assistance programs (EAPs), employer-sponsored programs (called lawyer assistance programs among attorneys), are designed to help employees with problems that interfere with their job performance. EAPs train work supervisors how to use constructive confrontation with an employee, cite evidence of impaired performance (such as absenteeism or behavior problems), and offer assistance to resolve the problem. EAP referrals may also be made by co-workers, trade unions, or employees themselves. EAP staff evaluate the problem and either provide the appropriate treatment or refer the employee to another service provider (McCrady, 1989).

Services are typically offered to employees free or at minimal charge. The company recovers their costs in savings from reduced absenteeism and personnel turnover, decreased use of health benefits, and improved job performance.

Currently, more than 60% of Fortune 500 companies and a growing number of smaller companies provide counseling services to employees. Recently, large law firms in Georgia have implemented EAPs (Elzea, 1989).

Hospitals, clinics and other health-service settings represent the last frontier for the EAP movement (Solursh, 1989). "If workers in centers of commerce, transportation and education can benefit from the services provided by an EAP," Solursh asks, "why cannot professional health-care providers similarly benefit?" (p. 105).

Resistance to EAPs by physicians and other healthcare professionals presumably stems from professional pride; although their wages are paid by a healthcare institution, they do not consider themselves employees (Solursh, 1989). Physicians may feel superior to EAP personnel—usually social workers, addiction counselors, or psychometricians—because the latter usually have less professional training and stature. They also worry about the paper trail created by application forms, medical records, and insurance claims and the humiliation of being a patient. Solursh (1989) notes that even the most desperate health professional is not likely to risk being seen in a busy waiting room full of support staff and patients.

Orioli (1986) points out that "EAPs are uniquely suited to the hospitals as centers of healing and health care." A successful program at the Medical College of Georgia in Augusta serves more than 6,000 employees—faculty and administrative personnel, support staff, interns, residents, fellows, and postdoctoral and graduate students (Solursh, 1989). Evaluative records based on the first nine months found that 92% of client contacts were self-referrals; 108 consultation phone calls were received. Alcohol was the most frequently cited drug of abuse by physicians and other healthcare professionals (about 20% of participants). Consequently, this EAP sponsors a drug abuse awareness program for all health profession trainees. According to Solursh (1989), this demonstrates that the EAP approach is a workable and viable model for medical colleges, hospitals, and other healthcare facilities.

Other EAP evaluations support this conclusion. EAPs have a positive impact on work performance and reduce absenteeism, disciplinary actions, accidental injuries, and turnover rates. However, poor recordkeeping and possible biases in perceptions and recollections have hindered research.

PRIMARY PREVENTION

Rehabilitation rather than prevention is the usual approach of health professionals to drug problems. Very few training institutions and professional societies have programs to benefit personal development and well-being; even fewer have systematically evaluated these programs. Action is rarely taken until after problems become embarrassingly obvious.

The rationale for primary prevention is that people use drugs to feel good and to deal with painful feelings of inadequacy and fear. The goal of primary prevention is to help potential drug abusers meet these needs in healthy ways.

A survey of 143 accredited medical schools in the United States, Canada, and Puerto Rico found that of 120 responding schools, only 29 offer health promotion programs and 19 others plan to begin soon; 48% had a budget to support organized health promotion and wellness activities for medical students. About half of these programs (52%) had a systematic evaluation component that included feedback, mostly from first-year student participants (Wolf, Randall, & Faucett, 1988).

The first health promotion program in medical school was introduced in 1975. Physical well-being (including exercise and nutrition) have been most frequently emphasized, and spiritual well-being the least. The well-being components most frequently offered are study skills (offered by 62% of reporting medical schools), support groups (62%), time-management training (59%), aerobics (55%), intramural sports (55%), and financial planning (52%) (Wolf, Randall, & Faucett, 1988).

Substance Abuse Education

Although alcohol and other drugs are involved in the illnesses of 20–50% of hospitalized patients, curriculum time devoted to substance abuse in the health professions has been minimal or nil. "Contrary to what may be expected," Miller and Gold (n.d.) note, "education and curricula in medical schools are gravely and dangerously inadequate regarding alcohol and drug problems" (p. 46). Similar neglect has been documented in the training of other professionals. Undergraduate nursing programs, for example, usually offer only two to four clock hours on addictions, and some offer no information at all (Haack & Harford, 1984).

Fewer than two thirds (63%) of 61 surveyed dental schools offer instruction about alcoholism and addiction, and those that do usually offer only an occasional lecture (Sandoval, 1988). About half of those providing instruction offer a maximum of three lecture hours. "It is imperative that dental schools establish an adequate, uniform chemical dependency curriculum to address the needs of students, both while in school and after graduation" (Bowermaster, 1988, p. 18).

The negative stereotypes about addicted patients held by many health practitioners is reinforced by unpleasant emergency-room experiences with chronic, late-stage "skid-row" alcoholics. Derogatory slang terms for these patients include "dirt ball," "scumbag," "slime dog," and "alky-bum" (Coombs, Chopra, Schenk, & Yutan, 1993). Moreover, an addicted physician is not likely to challenge a patient with the same (untreated) problem.

Most embarrassing of all, Miller and Gold (n.d.) note, health professionals have not taken a leadership role in dealing with substance abuse problems. Although the American Medical Association and the American Psychiatric Association regard alcoholism as a disease, attention and concern about chemical dependency have originated mostly from newspaper and magazine reports. The health professions have looked to journalistic sources for the most current and complete information on this subject.

In the 1970s, a movement began to rectify this educational deficiency from, as Lewis (1986) notes, "almost total neglect to general inadequacy" (p. 827). An AMA position paper emphasized that the neglect of alcoholism education in medical training had reached "a point of urgency" (Galanter, 1987, p. v). Federally initiated career teaching grants in 61 professional schools (59 medical, one dental, and one public health) resulted in a tripling of elective courses on drug and alcohol abuse in 10 years and the formation of a new national organization, The Association for Medical Education and Research in Substance Abuse (AMERSA; Lewis, 1989). More recently (1988), the Pharmacology and Therapeutics Section of the American Association of Dental Schools appointed a committee to develop curricular guidelines for alcoholism and other chemical dependencies (American Association of Dental Schools, 1989).

DuPont (1991) suggests that guidelines to prevent self-medication should be included in the curricula of those who handle prescription medications. A national survey of 9,600 randomly selected physicians (Hughes et al., 1992) found that in the past year, 11% had treated themselves with benzodiazepines and 18% with minor opiates. The investigators warn, "Self-treatment with controlled substances poses a risk not present when prescribing for a patient, where the prescriber can be objective in determining drug, dose and duration" (p. 2339).

Exemplary substance abuse education programs have recently been developed at a number of medical schools. Model small-group experiential seminars are offered at the UCLA School of Medicine. In small self-teaching groups of 12–14, medical students meet two hours weekly for eight weeks to explore substance abuse issues. Each student visits a 12-step program (such as Alcoholics Anonymous) and other sites such as the police department's drug education program, a walk-along with an outreach team to the homeless, an inpatient detoxification center, an adolescent residential facility, an outpatient treatment facility, or a methadone maintenance center. Students recount their experiences in class and debate topics such as the disease concept of alcoholism, the pros and cons of random urine testing, the policy implications of drug legalization versus zero tolerance, and the merits of incarceration versus treatment for mothers of "crack babies." Students also report on selected reading and personal interviews with resource professionals. Course-end evaluations are consistently enthusiastic.

Medical students at the University of New Mexico School of Medicine learn about chemical dependence by serving as mentors to high school students. They coordinate visits by high-risk teenagers to teaching hospitals and jails to interview chemically dependent patients, inmates, and their families. Medical students also conduct four 4-hour sessions imparting information to teenagers about alcohol and other drugs. During a four-year period, 39 medical students contributed more than 7,500 hours of time as peer educators. An evaluation found that participating students experienced great satisfaction and reported that their knowledge about substance abuse had become extensive and well-integrated (Wallerstein & Bernstein, 1988).

First-year medical students at the University of South Carolina are required to anonymously complete two short paper-and-pencil tests. The first test, the Michigan Alcohol Screening Test, provides a convenient, reliable way to detect alcohol abuse. The second, the Children of Alcoholics Screening Test, measures a wide array of behavioral, emotional, and psychosomatic dysfunctions. These tests enable students to assess their drinking status and background. Personal information about one's risk for chemical dependency has led more than half of those students seriously at risk to seek therapy (Johnson, Michaels, & Thomas, 1990).

Students at the Emory University School of Medicine (Talbott, 1982) learn about drug abuse by interacting with impaired physicians during weekly clinical rounds at a drug treatment center. Seminars are also held in the medical school, where impaired physicians relate their personal addiction stories. Each physician addresses the topic "It Couldn't Have Happened to Me as a Medical Student." Groups of medical students and their spouses also meet with recent graduates from the drug treatment center and their spouses. Recovering addicts address the topic "Things I Wish They Had Taught Me in Medical School." Talbott (1982) reports "tremendous bilateral gains and reward to both the student and the impaired physician" (p. 275).

Policy to Protect Trainee Well-Being

Policies to encourage healthy lifestyles and discourage drug abuse, defining a standard of professional knowledge and acceptable behavior, can have a preventive impact. Unfortunately, however, few professional organizations and training establishments have developed policies about alcohol and other substances except as pertaining to the most extreme behaviors. An AMA-sponsored study of fourth-year medical students at 23 regionally distributed schools found that only one-fourth (25.7%) were aware of any substance abuse policy at their own schools (Baldwin et al., 1991).

The need for policy has become increasingly clear. The American Association for Colleges of Pharmacy Special Interest Group on Student and Faculty Impairment developed 10 policy guidelines that were later adopted by the Association of American Medical Colleges and its group on student affairs. In 1986, the American Dental Association House of Delegates adopted a five-part policy statement on chemical dependency (Peters, 1990).

Most policies arise in response to crisis, as illustrated by the debate about the work hours of resident physicians in training. Legislation in some states to limit the length of shifts hospital officials may require trainees to work was precipitated by the death of Libby Zion, a young New York woman admitted to the hospital with a high fever. She was treated by exhausted and sleep-deprived house staff. Her father, influential with New York politicians, brought her death to the attention of the Manhattan U.S. District Attorney, where charges of criminal neglect–homicide were filed and a grand jury convened in December 1986. The grand jury concluded that although there was insufficient evidence for a criminal indictment because the conditions implicated in Zion's death were not confined to the hospital to which she was admitted, contributing factors in her death were the prescribed drugs, failure to alleviate her fever, and a resident's refusal to see her. The New York State Department of Health reacted by drafting legislation to limit working days to 12-hour shifts in emergency rooms and 24-hour limits elsewhere in the hospital, with at least one 24-hour shift off each week.

A continuing nationwide debate on the nature of graduate medical education ensued and several more states are now contemplating significant changes. Major national medical organizations have been forced to review their policies on house staff hours and supervision.

Well-Being Committees

Well-being committees provide a proactive rather than reactive approach to personal well-being. Emphasizing self-care, balanced lifestyles, and emotional expressiveness, they initiate activities to reduce the emotional isolation many professional trainees experience that, all too often, is relieved with drugs.

Well-being committees help professional trainees get support from one another and develop such skills as listening, reflecting, affirming, emphasizing, and summarizing, not only with their clients and patients, but with each other. They learn to recognize and share their feelings and build self-esteem on factors other than school grades and performance. Committees sponsor activities that maximize stress-management skills, address ways to deal with painful feelings, use criticism constructively, accept failure and less-than-perfect results. They also help trainees develop intimate relationships.

Stanford University School of Medicine was one of the first to form a well-being committee in 1980, in response to the disturbing finding that almost a third of the graduating class had sought counseling at the Student Health Services during their training. This number did not include those who sought counseling elsewhere (Weinstein, 1983). Consisting of faculty, administrators, and students, the committee first surveyed students to ascertain needs and concerns about emotional issues. Among the programs instituted were appointment of an ombudsman, establishment of a resource center for exchange of information, a support group for partners of house officers, a course on the psychosocial issues in medical training, and arrangements to provide better access to counseling for residents.

A well-being committee at the UCLA School of Medicine offers more than 20 activities to enhance emotional well-being (Coombs & Virshup, 1994). On the first day of school, each entering medical student receives a printed menu of well-being activities to choose from and, if willing, to help plan specific functions. Standing members of this committee include the class president, vice-president, and an elected representative from each class, but the committee is open to all students who wish to play a leadership role on one of the well-being activities. Faculty and staff members act only as advisors to ensure continuity from year to year and to provide encouragement and logistic support. Most of the energy comes from the students. Their enthusiasm creates a generalized climate of emotional support and an awareness of the importance of self-care. Committee-sponsored activities include well-being seminars regularly held in faculty homes; lunchtime discussions about coping skills, substance abuse, and cultural diversity; support groups for those with special needs such as couples, parents, city newcomers, older students, ethnic groups, and gays and lesbians; service opportunities that help students experience "helper's high"; and student publications such as student newsletters, a well-being resource handbook, and survivors' manuals.

Programs to Provide Realistic Expectations

Prospective professionals often have unrealistic expectations about the profession and its training. Not surprisingly, many are quickly disillusioned and sometimes depressed when confronted by harsh realities. A study of first-year medical students found that 40% considered withdrawing (Coombs, 1978). This is remarkable considering how hard they worked to gain admission.

Advance exposure to the socioemotional realities of training and practice that await them may prevent debilitating adjustment problems. Ideally this is done early before trainees are so caught up in the fast-paced track that they have little time to reflect or reconsider. The University of Maryland School of Medicine holds a four-day orientation retreat for incoming medical students. Upperclassmen and faculty members plan and organize the retreat using a small-group format to encourage discussion about the human dimension in medical education. A program evaluation found that participants valued the experience and derived an enhanced sense of self-awareness. They gained a more personal relationship with faculty advisors and, compared to nonparticipants, were more at ease in approaching them with personal problems (Plaut et al., 1982).

Some training institutions foster realistic expectations by assigning students to preceptors, clinicians in their chosen career. Students develop clearer views of their futures by accompanying their preceptors as they go about their work.

In 1983, a preceptorship program for women in premed programs was initiated in Philadelphia by the American Medical Women's Association. In addition, some of these students were given summer jobs in physicians' offices. Understandably, students were very enthusiastic (Koprowska & Wheeler, 1986).

At the UCLA School of Medicine, interested students are matched with a physician preceptor; women and ethnic minorities are paired with preceptors of the same sex and ethnicity. Personalized interaction with a caring professional provides an advisor, role model, and friend.

Premedical students at UCLA are offered an 11-week seminar to prepare them with realistic expectations about a physician's career (Coombs, Perell, & Ruckh, 1990). Titled "Professional Socialization of the Physician," the course meets weekly for three hours to explore the socioemotional challenges that occur at various stages in the physician's development. Invited discussants (two or three representatives each session representing a different career stage) respond to student questions. Students are also assigned to preceptors recruited from the clinical faculty, who meet weekly with them in clinical situations.

Course-end evaluations revealed great enthusiasm: "It taught me more than I could ever begin to express and profoundly influenced my expectations of medical school and the profession," one said. Those who changed their medical career plans (one in five participants) were also grateful: "It saved time and the trauma of planning for a career that would have been a mistake" (Coombs, Perell, & Ruckh, 1990, p. 578).

This format is also used in an elective course for first-year UCLA medical students informally called "Well-Being Dinner Seminars" (Coombs & Virshup, 1994). Groups of six or seven first-year students (the same group each session) and two or three invited discussants (different people each session) meet in the homes of faculty hosts five times during the year. The host provides dinner and orchestrates the proceedings so that stu-

dents do most of the talking. Two or three expert discussants, physicians at various stages of their careers, answer student questions about stress and coping. Student evaluations have been extraordinarily enthusiastic. Said one: "This program is the one that has kept me in medical school. I had a difficult time adjusting to medical school life. The reassurance I received from all participants was *invaluable!* I learned that I wasn't the only one with these anxieties."

Similar elective courses for first-year students are offered at Stanford, Albert Einstein, New Jersey Medical School, and Wright State University. The Stanford course, called "Approaching Medicine: What Is Happening To Me And Why?," is a one-quarter course of 90-minute lecture and demonstration sessions followed by one-hour small group meetings. Feedback from students has been extremely positive (Weinstein, 1983).

First-year students at the Albert Einstein College of Medicine are offered an elective seminar about physician socialization (Goetzel et al., 1984). The course compares sociological literature with the personal experiences of the students. Originally scheduled as a six-week experience, the course has been extended to the full academic year due to student enthusiasm.

First-year medical students at the University of Medicine and Dentistry of New Jersey are offered an elective course called "Parenting and Professionalism." This nine-session course, designed to raise student's consciousness concerning the challenges that lie ahead, devotes considerable time to child rearing in two-career families. An evaluation found that participants felt greater satisfaction and less loneliness than their nonparticipating classmates (Brodkin et al., 1983).

A two-week elective is offered to first-year medical students at the Wright State University School of Medicine on physician lifestyle management. To enhance the quality of life planning and to prevent emotional impairment, each participating student spends afternoon office sessions with a physician. Students familiarize themselves with the workings of an office practice, see a physician interact with patients, staff, and community, and participate in the clinical practice as time permits. This course received high ratings from the participants and helped medical students develop concepts about satisfying life roles (Rudisill & Painter, 1982).

Similar opportunities have been offered to medical school graduates. Residents at the Letterman Army Medical Center in San Francisco can participate in a course titled "Transition to Residency Seminar." Four or five evening meetings each year are held in participant homes using a question and discussion format. Participants describe the seminars as a nonthreatening forum where they can discuss their feelings and experiences and learn what lies ahead. After one year, the participants reported that the seminar had provided anticipatory guidance, eased their transition, and helped them develop closer relationships with colleagues and faculty (Jensen, 1983).

Health Enhancement and Stress Management Workshops and Classes

A health awareness workshop at the University of Louisville School of Medicine for incoming medical students and their significant others is part of an orientation program offered in four half-day workshops. The goal is to teach students ways to promote their own health (Dickstein & Elkes, 1983).

More extensive health promotion courses, each lasting 12 weeks, are offered at Stanford and Louisiana State University Schools of Medicine. Offered since 1983, the Stanford course (John Farquhar, personal communication, 1990) meets weekly at noon plus two longer evening sessions. An evaluation found that compared with nonparticipating classmates, participants experienced significant, positive, immediate improvement in health-promoting behaviors, attitudes, and knowledge; gains were also better after three years.

Farquhar (personal communication, 1990) notes that a physician's personal health is a prerequisite for optimal patient care and that, ironically, health-enhancing behaviors tend to deteriorate appreciably during medical training; the rigorous academic demands teach students to care for other people at the expense of their own health. Can physicians who are unable to manage their own well-being perform at their best and make optimal decisions in patient management?

The LSU course teaches medical students to attend to their personal health habits while learning preventive medicine skills to help patients (Wolf, Randall, & Faucett, 1990). At the course conclusion, participants demonstrated significantly improved preventive health behaviors, attitudes, and knowledge as compared with a control group.

Similar to health enhancement courses, stress management courses focus primarily on coping skills. Kelly et al. (1986) note that stress-management education is an effective way to provide these skills. A behavior modification program at the University of Washington School of Medicine (Holtzworth-Munroe, Munroe, & Smith, 1985) consists of six weekly one-hour meetings. The objective is to help students identify stress responses during the initial stages and to apply appropriate coping skills. Compared with a control group, participants reported greater tension awareness, experienced less test anxiety and other stressors, and coped better with school-related stress.

At the University of Mississippi Medical Center, a similar stress-management training seminar is offered to all medical school classes (Kelly, Bradlyn, Dubbert, & St. Lawrence, 1982). A clinical psychologist conducts 60- to 90-minute sessions over a three-week period. A comparison of participants and nonparticipants on a battery of stress indices, including a self-monitoring log, found that this training was effective in bringing about significant personal improvements.

Support Groups

Many training institutions organize support groups to facilitate student adjustment. Voluntary participants who share common interests and life situations benefit greatly from meeting together at a scheduled time, with or without a leader, to discuss common problems, share feelings, and give mutual support. Unlike therapy groups, whose participants are identified as patients in need of therapy, support groups consist of ordinary people in similar life situations.

The need for social support is felt by all professional students, but is most acute for those from emotionally deprived homes. Noting the emotional support given to patients on an alcoholic rehabilitation unit, one such student remarked, "It's too bad that you have to be an alcoholic to get this kind of support!" (Coombs, 1995).

Support groups have been described for medical students (Goetzel et al., 1984; Ficklin, Hazelwood, Carter, & Shellhamer, 1983; Plaut, Hunt, Johnson et al., 1982), house staff (Blackwell, 1986; Martin, 1986; Brashear, 1987; Siegel & Donnelly, 1978; Ziegler, Kanas, Strull, & Bennet, 1984), women (Calkins et al., 1987; Hilberman et al., 1975), and spouses of medical trainees (Bergman, 1980). At some institutions, these groups are extracurricular; participants meet in members' homes or other locations on their own time. Other institutions use social support in their curricula. At the University of Southern California School of Medicine, first-year students participate in a course called "Introduction to Clinical Medicine." Groups of six students meet with a physician leader four hours every Tuesday morning and every other Thursday afternoon to interview patients, and then discuss the experience. The approach is less structured at the UCLA School of Medicine. Students are invited to form groups and offered membership in a variety of groups to ensure that every student has an opportunity to be involved.

Evaluations of support group effectiveness have been unanimously positive. Ficklin, Hazelwood, Carter, and Shellhamer (1983) report high ratings from first-year medical students who participated in a support group. Participants strongly encouraged program continuation because it helped them become acquainted with classmates and develop close friendships. Participation decreased their sense of personal anonymity and lessened their anxieties.

Three-fourths of the medical student participants at the Albert Einstein College of Medicine benefitted by "getting together with people I like and feel close to" (75%) and "receiving support and help from fellow students and faculty; not feeling alone and unique with my problems" (74%) (Goetzel et al., 1984).

Support groups for women at the University of Missouri–Kansas City School of Medicine were effective in reducing attrition. During the five years preceding implementation, more than half of the medical school dropouts were women. Afterwards, the attrition rate for women dropped to 29% (Calkins et al., 1987).

An evaluation of a support group for house officers (Strahilevitz et al., 1982) noted diminished feelings of isolation. Similarly, a support group for medical interns found that the most helpful benefits were getting to know and understand one another, having the opportunity to talk and listen, discovering that many anxieties and fearful fantasies were shared by others, and laughing and yelling together. One said, "The group allowed us to share those feelings of fear, excitement, fatigue, despair, loneliness, burden of responsibility, and anger not usually discussed because of the need to maintain a professional attitude" (Siegel & Donnelly, 1978).

Couples-Strengthening Programs

Contrary to the view that marriage and professional training do not mix, studies show that married trainees, compared with their single classmates, cope better with the stresses of professional training. In a longitudinal study of an entire class of medical students, Coombs and Fawzy (1982) found statistically significant evidence that medical school is a more stressful experience for unmarried medical students than for married ones. Another study, a five-year retrospective study of medical students seen for psychiatric evaluation or treatment, found that emotionally impaired students were likely to be unmarried (Niccolini & Thomas, 1985). A survey of 281 house staff at a university medical center found that, compared with their unmarried associates, married house staff had stronger support systems and less substance abuse, anxiety, and depression. Twice as many unmarried as married residents felt isolated (Koran & Litt, 1988).

The University of Maryland School of Medicine offers a support group for medical students and their partners. Called "The Other Half," it provides social activities and supportive networks to enhance couple relationships (Plaut et al., 1982).

At the UCLA School of Medicine, medical students in couple relationships are offered an opportunity to participate in a couples strengthening group called PAIR (Practice at Improving Relationships). Held during dinner hours, each session begins with food provided by the dean's office, followed by an interactive exercise and group discussion designed to enhance couple relationships.

Bergman (1980) conducted a support group for the spouses of medical house staff that met for one year at two-week intervals. The objectives were to ventilate feelings, provide emotional support, and exchange information. Although these meetings had no particular agenda, themes of depression, anger, frustration, and powerlessness in the training experience emerged. An evaluative questionnaire several months after the group ended found that the support group had been a positive experience for all participants. The group gave them a forum, a safe environment to express their frustrations, thereby deflecting anger from their marital partner.

SUMMARY

Helping professionals are at high risk for substance abuse. Coming from the ranks of college students where recreational drug use is the norm, many fail to recognize their vulnerability. They are surrounded by drugs designed to alleviate physical and emotional problems and encouraged to prescribe them for others. Professional training

and status encourage a feeling of immunity to chemical dependence and give a ready rationale for denial.

Many helping professionals come from family backgrounds where they have played a caretaking role with alcoholic parents. Moreover, professional training sometimes mimics these parental homes by emotional abuse and neglects the development of healthy affect. Drugs provide an easy escape from the resulting fatigue and depression.

Compleat professionals develop three interdependent areas of disciplined competence symbolized by three overlapping circles: the intellect (head), professionals skills (hands), and affect (heart). Chemically impaired professionals typically develop only the first two: the head and the hands. The emotional aspects of their development are retarded by neglect. When painful experiences create uncomfortable feelings, these professionals often turn to drugs for temporary relief.

The challenge of professional schools is to help trainees develop into compleat professionals who get their highs from healthy, balanced lifestyles rather than chemicals. Training institutions and professional organizations that encourage self-care help not only their professional colleagues but also the patients and clients they serve. It is critical that well-being policies and committees be established to promote healthy emotional development. Substance abuse education must also be an integral part of the ongoing training program at every institution.

Professional training will come of age when there is a recognition that emotionally malnourished professionals are at risk for addiction. The emphasis on rehabilitating chemically dependent professionals must be expanded to provide effective programs of secondary and primary prevention.

REFERENCES

Ackerman, T. F., & Wall, H. P. (in press). A program for treating chemically impaired medical students. *Medical Education.*

AIMS brochure. Memphis: The University of Tennessee College of Medicine, the Health Science Center.

American Association for the Advancement of Science, personal communication, Feb. 1992.

American Association of Dental Schools (1989). *Curriculum guidelines for education in alcoholism and other chemical dependencies.* Chicago: American Dental Association, American Student Dental Association.

American Pharmaceutical Association, Pharmacist Recovery Network (1993). *PRN Memo, 36.* Washington, DC.

Anderson, C. T. (1990). The doctor, naked. *Bulletin of the Society for Professional Well-Being, 2* (June), 1–6.

Angres, D. H. (1990). *Regionalization of chemical dependency treatment for health care professionals.* Maywood, IL: Loyola University Medical Center.

Baldwin, D. C., Hughes, P. H., Conard, S. E., Storr, C. L., & Sheehan, D. V. (1991). Substance use among senior medical students. *Journal of the American Medical Association, 265* (April), 2074–2078.

Baldwin, J. N. (1990). *Student impairment—The college perspective.* Salt Lake City: University of Utah School on Alcoholism and Other Drug Dependencies, Pharmacist Section, College Programs.

Benjamin, A., Darling, E. J., & Sales, B. (1990). The prevalence of depression, alcohol abuse, and cocaine abuse among United States lawyers. *International Journal of Law and Psychiatry, 13,* 233–246.

Benjamin, A., Kaszniak, A., Sales, B., & Shanfield, S. B. (1986). The role of legal education in producing psychological distress among law students and lawyers. *American Bar Foundation Research Journal* (Spring), 225–252.

Bergman, A. S. (1980). Marital stress and medical training: An experience with a support group for medical housestaff wives. *Pediatrics, 65* (May), 944–946.

Bissell, L. (1989). An historical review: Alcohol and drugs in the professions. In T. W. Nester (Ed.), *Professionals and their addictions.* Macon, GA: Charter Medical Corp., 3–23.

Bissell, L., & Haberman, P. W. (1984). *Alcoholism in the professions.* New York: Oxford University Press.

Bissell, L., Haberman, P. W., & Williams, R. L. (1989). Pharmacists recovering from alcohol and other drug addictions: An interview study. *American Pharmacy, NS29* (June), 391–402.

Bissell, L., & Jones, R. W. (1981). The alcoholic nurse. *Nursing Outlook* (Feb.), 96–101.

Blackwell, B. (1986). Prevention of impairment among residents in training. *Journal of the American Medical Association, 155* (March), 1177–1178.

Borenstein, D. B., & Cook, C. (1982). Impairment prevention in the training years, A new mental health program at UCLA. *Journal of the American Medical Association, 247* (May 21), 2700–2703.

Bowermaster, D. P. (1988). Chemical dependency and the dental student, *Dentistry, 88* (Dec.), 16–19.

Brashear, D. (1987). Support groups and other supportive efforts in residency programs. *Journal of Medical Education, 62,* 418–207.

Brewster, J. M. (1986). Prevalence of alcohol and other drug problems among physicians. *Journal of the American Medical Association, 255* (April), 1913–1919.

Brodkin, A. M., Shrier, D., Alger, E., Layman, W., & Buxton, M. (1983). Allaying loneliness in freshman medical students: An outcome of an elective course. *Journal of Medical Education, 58* (Sept.), 722–727.

Busch, L. (1982). Rehabilitating the impaired dentist: A look at what the profession is doing to help. *Journal of the American Dental Association, 105* (Nov.), 781–787.

California Physician's Diversion Program (1992). Sacramento, CA: Board of Medical Quality Assurance (brochure).

Calkins, E. V., Arnold, L. M., Margolin, R. L., Siridge, M. S., & Reaner, R. G. (1987). Functions of a women's support group in a school of medicine. *Journal of the American Medical Women's Association, 42* (March/April), 51–53.

Carmichael, S. M., & Herlihy, C.E. (1981). The impaired physician: Medical school and physician approaches. *Alabama Journal of Medical Science, 18* (1981), 192–195.

Ciaccio, E. A., Jang, R., & Caiola, S. (1982). Well-being: A North Carolina study. *American Pharmacy, NS22* (May), 20–22.

Clark, D. C., & Daugherty, S. R. (1990). A norm-referenced longitudinal study of medical student drinking patterns. *Journal of Substance Abuse, 2,* 15–27.

Clark, M. D. (1988). Preventing drug dependency: Part I, recognizing risk factors. *Journal of Nursing Administration, 18* (Dec.), 12–15.

Coombs, R. H. (1978). *Mastering medicine.* New York: The Free Press.

Coombs, R. H. (1995). *Drug-impaired professionals.* Cambridge, MA: Harvard University Press.

Coombs, R. H., Chopra, S., Schenk, D., & Yutan, E. (1993). Medical slang and its functions. *Social Science and Medicine: An International Journal, 36,* 987–998.

Coombs, R. H., & Fawzy, F. I. (1982). Medical marriage as preventive for physician impairment. *California Family Practice, 33* (July/Aug.), 14–18.

Coombs, R. H., May, S., & Small, G. (1986). *Inside doctoring: Stages and outcomes in the professional development of physicians.* New York: Praeger.

Coombs, R. H., Perell, K., & Ruckh, J. (1990). Primary prevention of emotional impairment among medical trainees. *Academic Medicine: Journal of the Association of American Medical Colleges, 65,* 567–581.

Coombs, R. H., & Virshup, B. (1994). Enhancing the psychological health of medical students: The student well-being committee, special issue on medical student well-being. *Medical Education* (United Kingdom), *28,* 47–54.

Cross, L. (1985). Chemical dependency in our ranks: Managing a nurse in crisis. *Nursing Management, 16* (Nov.), 15–16.

Dickstein, L. J. & Elkes, J. (1983). Health awareness workshops for freshmen medical students. *Canadian Journal of Psychiatry, 28* (April), 236.

Dowell, L. B. (1988). Attorneys and alcoholism: An alternative approach to a serious problem. *North Kentucky Law Review, 16,* 169–189.

DuPont, R. L. (1991). *Preventing chemical abuse among physicians.* Speech given at the Annual Meetings of the American Psychiatric Association.

Edelman, H. (1990). Shot full of pain. *The New Physician* (Sept.), 14–20.

Elzea, D. (1989). Employee assistance programs. *Georgia State Bar Journal, 25,* 118.

Ficklin, F. L., Hazelwood, J. D., Carter, J. E., & Shellhamer, R. H. (1983). Evaluation of a small-group support program for first-year medical students. *Journal of Medical Education, 58* (Oct.), 817–819.

Fisher, K., & Weisman, E. (1988). Special issue on impaired health care professionals. *Quarterly Review Bulletin, 14,* 98–99.

Galanter, M. (1987). In D. M. Gallant, *Alcoholism, A guide to diagnosis, intervention and treatment.* New York: W.W. Norton and Company.

Goetzel, R. Z., Croen, L. G., Shelov, S., Boufford, J. I., & Levin, G. (1984). Evaluating self-help support groups for medical students. *Journal of Medical Education, 59* (April), 331–340.

Green, P. (1989). The chemically dependent nurse. *Nursing Clinics of North America, 24* (March), 81–94.

Haack, M. R. (1988). Stress and impairment among nursing students. *Research in Nursing & Health, 11,* 125–143.

Haack, M. R., & Harford, T. C. (1984). Drinking patterns among student nurses. *International Journal of the Addictions, 19,* 577–583.

Haldane, D. (1990). Legal remedies. *Los Angeles Times,* Section E (June 7), 1–2.

Hickey, M. C. (1990). Attorney alcoholism. *The Washington Lawyer,* (March/April), 32–42.

Hilberman, E., Konanc, J., Perez-Reyes, M., Hunter, R., Scagnelli, J., & Sanders, S. (1975). Support groups for women in medical school: A first-year program. *Journal of Medical Education, 50* (Sept.), 867–875.

Hilfiker, D. (1985). *Healing the wounds: A physician looks at his work.* New York: Pantheon.

Holtzworth-Munroe, A., Munroe, M. S., & Smith, R. (1985). Effects of a stress-management training program on first- and second-year medical students. *Journal of Medical Education, 60* (May), 417–419.

Hubbard, R. L., Marsden, M. E., Rachal, J. V., et al. (1989). *Drug abuse treatment: A national study of effectiveness.* Chapel Hill: University of North Carolina Press.

Hughes, P. H., Brandenberg, N., Baldwin, D., Storr, C. L., Williams, K. M., Anthony, J. C., & Sheehan, D. V. (1992). Prevalence of substance abuse among U.S. physicians. *Journal of the American Medical Association, 267* (May 6), 2333–2339.

Hughes, P. H., Conard, S. E., Baldwin, D. C., Storr, C. L., & Sheehan, D. (1991). Resident physician substance use in the U.S. *Journal of the American Medical Association, 265* (April 24), 2069–2073.

Ikeda, R., & Pelton, C. (1990). Diversion programs for impaired physicians. *Western Journal of Medicine, 152,* 617–621.

Jensen, P. S. (1983). The transition to residency seminar. *Journal of Psychiatric Education, 7,* 261–263.

Johnson, N. P., Michaels, P. J., & Thomas, J. C. (1990). Screening tests identify the prevalence of alcohol use among freshman medical students and among students' family of origin. *The Journal of the South Carolina Medical Association* (Jan.), 13–14.

Kelly, J. A., Bradlyn, A. S., Dubbert, P. M., & St. Lawrence, J. S. (1982). Stress management training in medical school. *Journal of Medical Education, 57* (Feb.), 91–98.

Kelly, J. A., Hansen, D. J., Plienis, A., Stark, L. J., Smith, S., Ford, F. D., & Draper, E. (1986). *Stress management training for medical students, A training procedures manual.* Jackson: University of Mississippi Medical Center.

Koprowska, I., & Wheeler, J. (1986). Preceptorships for premedical students with women physicians. *Journal of the American Women's Association, 41* (5), 160–161.

Koran, L. M., & Litt, I. F. (1988). House staff well-being. *The Western Journal of Medicine, 148* (Jan.), 97–101.

Lewis, D. C. (1986). Doctors and drugs. *New England Journal of Medicine, 315,* 826–828.

Lewis, D. C. (1989). Putting training about alcohol and other drugs into the mainstream of medical education. *Alcohol Health and Research World, 13* (1), 8–13.

Martin, A. R. (1986). Stress in residency: A challenge to personal growth. *Journal of General Internal Medicine, 1* (July/Aug.), 252–257.

McAuliffe, W. E. (1984). Non-therapeutic opiate addiction in health professionals: A new form of impairment. *American Journal of Drug and Alcohol Abuse, 10,* 1–22.

McAuliffe, W. E., Rohman, M., Feldman, B., & Launer, E. K. (1985). The role of euphoric effects in the opiate addictions of heroin addicts, medical patients and impaired health professionals. *Journal of Drug Issues* (Spring), 203–224.

McAuliffe, W. E., Santangelo, S. L., Gingras, J., Rohman, M., Sobol, A., & Magnuson, E. (1987). Use and abuse of controlled substances by pharmacists and pharmacy students. *American Journal of Hospital Pharmacy, 44* (Feb.), 311–317.

McCrady, B. S. (1989). The distressed or impaired professional: From retribution to rehabilitation. *The Journal of Drug Issues, 19,* 337–349.

McGann, K. P. (1990). *AIMS Council report for 1989–90.* Winston-Salem, NC: Wake Forest University, The Bowman Gray School of Medicine.

Miller, N. S., & Gold, M. S. (n.d.). Alcoholism and drug addiction among physicians: Humanitarian approach. *Psychiatry Letter,* 43–46.

Niccolini, R., & Thomas, J. (1985). The extent of impairment at one Michigan medical school. *Michigan Medicine* (Aug.), 433–434.

Nickel, R. O., & Briske, K. (1985). Aiding impaired pharmacists: What's being done today? *American Pharmacy* (June), 40–43.

Normark, J. W., Eckel, F. M., Pfifferling, J.-H., et al. (1985). Impairment risk in North Carolina pharmacists. *American Pharmacy, 25* (June), 373–376.

North Carolina Bar Association (1991). Report of the Quality of Life Task Force and recommendations, June 20.

Orioli, E. M. (1986). Caring for the health and wellness of the healer within the healthcare institution. In C. D. Scott & J. Hawks (Eds.), *Heal thyself: The health of health care professionals.* New York: Brunner/Mazel Publishers.

Peters, A. C. (1990). ADA policy statement on chemical dependency. *CDA Journal, 18* (Feb.).

Pfifferling, J.-H., & Corbin, R. W. (1988). The stress of dental life. *The Bulletin of the Society for Professional Well-Being, 1* (Dec.), 6.

Plaut, M. S., Hunt, G. J., Johnson, F. P., Brown, R. M., & Hobbins, T. E. (1982). Intensive medical student support groups: Format, outcome, and leadership guidelines. *Journal of Medical Education, 57* (Oct.), 778–786.

Regier, D. A., Farmer, M. E., Rae, D. S., Locke, B. Z., Keith, S. J., Judd, L. L., & Goodwin, F. K. (1990). Co-morbidity of mental disorders with alcohol and other drug abuse: Results from the epidemiologic catchment area (ECA) study. *Journal of the American Medical Association, 264* (Nov. 21), 2511–2518.

Rudisill, J. R. & Painter, A. F. (1982). Physician lifestyle management: A selective for first-year medical students. *Journal of Medical Education, 57* (May), 367–371.

Sandoval, V. A. (1988). A survey of substance abuse in North American dental schools. *Journal of Dental Education, 52* (3), 167–169.

Schoenborn, C. (1991). Exposure to alcoholism in the family: United States, 1988. In *Advance Data.* Hyattsville, MD: U.S. Department of Health and Human Services, 205 (Sept. 30), 1–7.

Seigle, R., Schuckit, M., & Plumb, D. (1983). Availability of personal counseling in medical schools. *Journal of Medical Education, 58* (July), 542–546.

Siegel, B. & Donnelly, J. C. (1978). Enriching personal and professional development: The experience of a support group for interns. *Journal of Medical Education, 53* (Nov.), 908–914.

Silas, F. A. (1987). A profession's scourge: Lawyers on drugs, bar programs offer help to those in despair. *Bar Leader, 13* (Nov./Dec.), 12–15.

Skutar, C. (1990). Physician recovery network. *Michigan Medicine* (Dec.), 30–32.

Smith, D. (1989). Current issues: Physicians. In T. W. Hester (Ed.), *Professionals and their addictions.* Macon, GA: Charter Medical Corporation, 159–166.

Smith, H. L., Mangelsdorf, K. L., Louderbough, A. W., & Piland, N. F. (1989). Substance abuse among nurses: Types of drugs. *Dimensions of Critical Care Nursing, 8* (May/June), 159–168.

Snow, L. H. (1969). Preliminary observations of the psychotherapy of medical students. *American Journal of Psychotherapy, 23,* 293–302.

Solursh, D. S. (1989). An EAP program for the health profession. In T. W. Hester (Ed.), *Professionals and their addictions.* Macon, GA: Charter Medical Corporation, 105–114.

Spicer, J., Barnett, P., & Kliner, D. (1978). *Characteristics and outcomes of professionals admitted to the Hazelden Rehabilitation Center, 1973–1976.* Center City, MN: Hazelden Educational Services.

Spierer, D. (1986). Testimony to San Diego hearing, Attorney General's Commission on the Prevention of Drug and Alcohol Abuse, January 9, 72.

Spilis, D. (1992). *Informational report to the House of Delegates.* San Diego, CA: American Bar Association, Commission on Impaired Attorneys, June 9.

Spiro, J. H., Roenneburg M., & Maly, B. (1978). Teaching doctors to treat doctors: Medical student peer counseling. *Journal of Medical Education, 53* (Dec.), 997.

Stammer, M. E. (1988). Understanding alcoholism and drug dependency in nurses. *QPB* (March), 75–80.

Strahilevitz, A., Yunker, R., Pichanick, A. M., Smith, L., & Richardson, J. (1982). Initiating support groups for pediatric house officers. *Clinical Pediatrics, 21* (Sept.), 529–531.

Sullivan, E., Bissell, L., & Williams, E. (1988). *Chemical dependency in nursing.* Menlo Park, CA: Addison-Wesley.

Talbott, G. D. (1982). The impaired physician and intervention: A key to recovery. *The Journal of the Florida Medical Association* (Sept.), 793–797.

Talbott, G. D. (1984). Elements of the Impaired Physicians Program. *Journal of the Medical Association of Georgia* (Nov.), 749–751.

Talbott, G. D. (1986). In D. Wholey, *The Courage to Change.* New York: Warner Books.

Tucker, D. R., Gurnee, M. C., Sylvestri, M. F., Baldwin, J. N., & Roche, E. B. (1988). Psychoactive drug use and impairment markers in pharmacy students. *American Journal of Pharmaceutical Education, 52,* 42–47.

Vaillant, G. E. (1982). Adaptation of a lecture: When doctors fail to care for themselves. *Harvard Medical Alumni Bulletin, 56* (Winter), 18–21.

Vaillant, G. E., Brighton, J. R., & McArthur, C. (1970). Physicians' use of mood-altering drugs: A twenty-year follow-up report. *The New England Journal of Medicine, 282,* 365–370.

Vaillant, G. E., Sobowale, N. C., & McArthur, C. (1972). Some psychologic vulnerabilities of physicians. *New England Journal of Medicine, 287,* 372–375.

Wallerstein, N., & Bernstein, E. (1988). Empowerment education: Freire's ideas adapted to health education. *Health Education Quarterly, 15* (Winter), 379–394.

Weinstein, H. M. (1983). A committee on well-being of medical students and house staff. *Journal of Medical Education, 58* (May), 373–381.

Whitaker, E. (1991). Ethics of a donut. *The New Physician* (Sept.), p. 48.

Wolf, T. M., & Kissling, G. E. (1984). Changes in life-style characteristics, health, and mood of freshman medical students. *Journal of Medical Education, 59,* 806–814.

Wolf, T. M., Randall, H. M., & Faucett, J. M. (1988). A survey of health promotion programs in U.S. and Canadian medical schools. *American Journal of Health Promotion, 3,* 33–36.

Wolf, T. M., Randall, H. M., & Faucett, J. M. (1990). A health promotion program for medical students. *American Journal of Health Promotion, 4* (Jan./Feb.), 193–201.

Ziegler, J. L., Kanas, N., Strull, W., & Bennet, N. E. (1984). A stress discussion group for medical interns. *Journal of Medical Education, 59* (March), 205–207.

CHAPTER 15

CHILDREN AND ADOLESCENTS

CHRISTOPH M. HEINICKE
SHIRAH VOLLMER

It has repeatedly been concluded that to be effective and sustained, preventive intervention must be focused not only on the child but on the family system with which he or she interacts. Thus, interventions directed at infant development (Heinicke, Beckwith, & Thompson, 1988) or preschool development (Bronfenbrenner, 1974) have been shown to be effective and sustained if the family functioning is also the explicit target of change and if the family improves its impact on the child.

In this chapter, we argue similarly that child and adolescent drug abuse must be seen in the context of the development of other socially deviant behaviors and that this deviant behavior is in turn in part a product of the child's inadequate caretaking environment. It follows that both the early onset and the excessive use of drugs (not experimentation) are not likely to change unless the associated care environment is also changed. Once the substance abuse disorder is firmly established, interventions must be intense, are costly, and may not be effective. We argue that intervention designed to promote the type of family functioning that nurtures and guides the child is cost-effective and may be one of the few ways of preventing the development of socially deviant behavior and drug abuse.

To illustrate, we present the following case: Celia is an 11-year-old half-caucasian and half-black female who was brought to the clinic because her mother was concerned that "she never listened." After psychological testing, it was discovered that Celia had an IQ of 70. In addition, her mother reported that she often left Celia home alone. When the therapist explained to the mother that her daughter was functioning as a six-year-old and should not be left home alone, the mother resisted the idea. After frequent episodes of Celia again being home alone, she began to steal from her mother's purse. Celia also started to play with children down the street who were involved with drugs. The mother found out about the drugs and felt that Celia was a "bad kid."

During the meetings with the mother, the therapist tried to reframe her concept of Celia as "bad" to the idea that her daughter could not be expected to exhibit good judgment when left unmonitored. Eventually, the mother arranged for a babysitter for her daughter and Celia's behavior was no longer a problem. This example illustrates how teaching parents the value of monitoring their children can prevent drug-seeking behaviors.

To elaborate and provide support for these primary prevention assumptions, we first summarize four different models of how family functioning influences antisocial behavior and drug abuse. These models are designed to guide intervention with school-aged children. Accordingly

This research was supported by the Ahmanson Foundation of Los Angeles; the Lita Annenberg Hazen Charitable Trust, New York; the National Institute of Child Health and Human Development, Grant #HD13186; and the National Institute of Mental Health, Grant #MH45722.

we also describe the family-oriented interventions that have been used to reduce the incidence of school-age drug abuse. From these studies, socially deviant behavior in early and late adolescence, including drug abuse, emerges as a central outcome linked to specific family and school conditions.

We examine whether these socially deviant late childhood trends can be linked to earlier family and child developments. For example, does the nonresponsiveness of the mother to her five-year-old increase the child's difficulty in forming relationships and propel the child to social deviance?

Further setting the stage for primary prevention, we summarize what is known about the aspects of the earliest family and parent–infant development that are likely to affect preschool and kindergarten status. Is the mother's nonresponsiveness to her five-year-old anticipated by family developments in the first five years of the child's life? If so, what early family-oriented interventions can be used to alter the developmental sequence to prevent socially deviant behavior and drug abuse?

SECONDARY PREVENTION IN THE SCHOOL YEARS

In the following sections, we summarize the etiological models for adolescent drug abuse and the results of family-oriented treatment programs of four research teams led by the following investigators: Gerald Patterson, David Hawkins, Karol Kumpfer, and Peter Bentler. Our purpose is not to provide an exhaustive review but to focus on family determinants of the emergence of socially deviant behavior and the associated drug abuse.

Patterson et al.: The Family Management Model of Adolescent Substance Abuse

Throughout their published research, Patterson and his colleagues have stressed the influence of family management skills such as discipline and monitoring on the child's membership in deviant peer groups and the development of antisocial behavior, drug abuse, and ultimately delinquency. Where a breakdown in family discipline and monitoring occurs in the early school grades and there is already evidence of the child's negative peer relations and antisocial behavior, this "early start" is likely to lead to delinquency, including drug abuse.

The model is first expanded to show that both paternal and maternal antisocial personality traits are affected by stress, which in turn increases the frequency of irritable discipline.

Another expansion of the model cites the possible influence of parental rejection on the further development of child's antisocial behavior. That is, the rejection of the child as well as the breakdown of discipline and monitoring may enhance the development of antisocial behavior.

In the further search for the determinants of antisocial behavior, the authors examine the evidence for nonmediational and mediational mechanisms. In regard to the first, they indicate that there is little evidence for the direct inherited contribution of parental antisocial traits to adolescent delinquency, but suggest that adult crime may be so influenced. By contrast, the authors again emphasize the strong influence of the mediational mechanism of irritable family interaction styles in enhancing the development of delinquency (Patterson & Dishion, 1988).

This presentation of the Patterson et al. findings has emphasized the general determinants of antisocial behavior and delinquency. Like many other investigators, this research group makes the assumption that early drug use and delinquency are somewhat different aspects of a unified behavioral process. The interrelation has been outlined by Dishion, Reid, and Patterson (1988). They demonstrate, first of all, that parents who are highly proficient in the family management skills of discipline, monitoring, problem solving, parent involvement, and positive reinforcement tended to have children who were not antisocial, showed little drug experimentation, were less depressed, and were more adequate in their academic skills, peer relations, and self-esteem. The central assumption is that coercive family processes serve as training for youngsters to practice coercive, antisocial, and rule-breaking behaviors, including drug abuse in other settings. The primary process underlying the child's training is hypothesized to be negative reinforcement. For antisocial children, it has been found that about 70% of the time the child's counterattack on a family member was followed by the attacker withdrawing or by a positive or neutral outcome. Noting the importance of deviant peer groups in initiating drug use, the authors emphasize that membership in the group and antisocial behavior are themselves determined by inadequate parental monitoring and discipline.

In further discussing the etiology of adolescent drug abuse, Dishion, Reid, and Patterson (1988) develop separate models for preadolescent drug experimentation and later adolescent drug use. Child drug experimentation was derived from a composite of both the parents' and child's report. The child characteristics that covaried with preadolescent drug experimentation were the child's antisocial behavior, observed coercive behavior in the home, the extent to which the child's peers were characterized as antisocial, and low self-esteem. Family management, such as parental monitoring and discipline, as well as a composite index of parent drug use also correlated with the child's drug sampling. Further statistical analysis (structural equation models) allowed the authors to show that parent monitoring did not have a direct effect on drug experimentation but its absence did have an indirect effect through allowing the child increased exposure to deviant peer influences. In considering possible interventions, the authors suggest that parent monitoring may be influenced by parental stress, parent drug use, marital discord, and single-parent status.

In their analysis of adolescent drug use, both alcohol and marijuana use were correlated with measures of deviant peer membership and parent monitoring and discipline. It was hypothesized that as opposed to preadolescent drug sampling, adolescent drug use would be affected by monitoring both directly and indirectly via deviant

peer membership. This turned out to be true for self-reported marijuana use. However, for alcohol use, only the membership in deviant peer groups was associated with abuse.

These findings support the assumption that negative adolescent outcomes, such as delinquency and drug use, arise within the family and are later exacerbated by the influence of membership in deviant peer groups.

Patterson et al.: Parent-Training Treatment

The above results stress the potential impact of parent–child transactions and, in particular, inept monitoring and discipline on the antisocial behavior and drug use of the child. Several questions arise: What is the impact of parent training on child outcome variables? If changes in child outcome occur as a function of treatment, do family management skills changes also occur? Are differences in the parental reaction to the treatment program (process variable) related to child outcome?

Child and Parent Outcome

To assess the effect of intervention programs on childhood behavior, Patterson and Chamberlain (1988) developed an outcome measure of a composite of behaviors called Total Aversive Behavior (TAB). This TAB score is based on home observations of 16 behaviors selected to measure negative microsocial interactions. Included are behaviors with a negative content and those with a neutral content but a negative affect. TAB scores can be thought of as reflecting how deviant a child is on these 16 behaviors compared with a normal distribution of children.

The preliminary results are based on the first portion of the sample to complete the parent treatment. The treated sample ($n = 16$) showed significant reductions in the child TAB score from baseline to termination ($p = .03$), whereas comparison group cases ($n = 9$) showed no change ($p = .69$).

The preliminary conclusion is that parent-training treatment changes the problem behavior of antisocial children. It was also found that all three parent management scores—monitoring, discipline, and problem solving—covaried significantly with the termination TAB score.

Parent Process: The Parental Reaction to Treatment

Patterson and Chamberlain (1988) also studied the effects of parent struggle during the treatment sessions on the child's behavior. Parent struggle included challenging and confronting, hopelessness and blaming, and interfamily conflict. Daily stress, marital discord, and parental depression were found to influence struggle within a session. They conclude, based on these preliminary results, that therapy is best served if part of the focus is on reducing stressors and the accompanying depression.

Indices of conflict within the treatment session were related to changes in both the parent management skills and the child's antisocial behavior. One such index of conflict, the parental "I won't" reaction to the expectations of the parent training, was seen as an index of active involvement. The occurrence of this reaction in mothers during the closing quarter of the treatment was correlated with a positive change in monitoring practices. Similarly, there was an association between the occurrence of the mother's within-session conflict and the child's behavior. Mothers who could express their conflict within a session had children whose aversive behavior decreased. In summary, involvement or noninvolvement in the parent-training treatment influences both the parent monitoring and the child's antisocial behavior (Patterson & Chamberlain, 1988).

Hawkins et al.: Intensive Family Prevention Services

In its emphasis on the importance of family discipline and monitoring, the approach to prevention developed by Hawkins, Lishner, Catalano, and Howard (1986) and Hawkins, Catalano, Jones and Fire (1987) is very consistent with the Patterson et al. family management model. Their research has also established several family-related factors as antecedents of teenage problem behaviors. Among these are poor family management practices, as indicated by unclear or inconsistent expectations for children's behaviors, poor parental monitoring of children, and negligent or excessively severe and inconsistent discipline; high levels of conflict within the family; and extreme family disorganization as indicated by simultaneous entrapment in conditions of extreme poverty, poor housing, single parenthood, and below-average parental educational, occupational, and social skills.

This knowledge suggests that interventions that successfully strengthen high-risk families by improving parents' family management skills, reducing family conflict, and empowering multiply-entrapped parents to overcome extreme family disorganization hold promise for preventing teenage delinquency, drug abuse, and school misbehavior.

Parent-training programs have shown some effectiveness in reducing conduct problems, but they also present some serious implementation problems. There is some evidence (Hawkins & Salisbury, 1983) that parent-training programs are disproportionately available to white rather than minority families nationwide, and that white, middle-class, two-parent families participate in parent training more readily than do minority, low-income, single parents (Hawkins, Catalano, Jones, & Fire, 1987). High dropout rates for parent training are common. Families experiencing disruption and disorganization are particularly difficult to enlist and maintain in parent training.

Intense family preservation involves in-home intervention. This model is called *Homebuilders*. The Homebuilders group provides line staff with training in 21 specific training modules including defusing, engaging, and confronting clients; teaching such family skills as anger management and other problem-solving skills; and dealing with termination issues. This familiarization of the intervention, by training therapists to assess what specific intervention modules may be of most immediate use, is one of the most important achievements of the Homebuilders group.

The service is time-limited and is available for 30 days. From an implementation perspective, the Homebuilders approach shows some promise for reaching and retaining high-risk families in an intensive intervention without creating dependence. To date, the effectiveness of this model has not been subjected to experimental investigation.

Hawkins, Catalano, and Kent (1991) also designed and conducted a television-assisted parent-training campaign consisting of a one-hour TV special and nine series of four two-hour parenting workshops conducted at weekly intervals and offered simultaneously at 87 sites. The parent workshops were from the "Preparing for the Drug (Free) Years" parenting curriculum that is part of the Hawkins, Lishner, Catalano, and Howard (1986) study of the prevention of teenage drug abuse. The content and learning format of the program are designed to generate motivation and behavioral skills to implement risk-reduction strategies in the family. These changes in the family should reduce the influence of the following drug abuse risk factors: poor family management, parental acceptance of teen drug abuse, friends who use drugs, low family bonding, high family conflict, and early first use of drugs. The program seeks to increase protective factors against drug abuse by strengthening bonding to the family and by establishing clear family norms against drug use by teenagers. The results of this program support the combined use of broadcast media and parent skills training in a workshop format to reach and train relatively large numbers of parents. The data suggest that workshops led by trained volunteers were effective in generating significant knowledge, attitude, and behavior change in the majority of participants. A more rigorous evaluation of media/workshop is needed.

Kumpfer et al.: A Social Ecological Model of Adolescent Substance Abuse

The social ecology model of adolescent substance abuse hypothesizes that the family and the school climate affect a youth's self-esteem, which in turn influences whether he or she will turn to nonconventional (antisocial) peer groups and frequent drug use. The underlying associated process is hypothesized to be the balance between stressors and the young person's ability to cope with them. Youths with more environmental stressors than individual coping abilities or resources are hypothesized to be at higher risk for drug use. Restating their goal, Kumpfer and Turner (1990) set out to verify an extension of the Hawkins and Weiss (1985) social development model by adding the variables of family environment, self-esteem, and school climate. The Effective School Battery (Gottfredson, 1985) and various other self-report inventories were filled out by approximately 1,600 high school students. The data were reduced to 22 variables to measure family climate, school climate, self-esteem, school bonding, peer influence, and substance abuse.

A structural equations approach was used to examine the hypothesized causal relations among these variables. These hypotheses were stated as follows: A favorable *school* and *family* climate improves a student's *self-esteem*, and this facilitates the establishment of *positive bonds to the school*. A positive connection to the school facilitates *positive peer relations* and these associations reduce the likelihood of the student becoming involved in delinquent and *drug-using behavior*. Data analysis revealed that the above six latent variables (italicized) were intercorrelated rather than orthogonal; in particular, the self-esteem and school bonding latent variables were highly associated. Accordingly, in subsequent analyses these two variables were collapsed.

Results of the analyses of the cluster variables within the models indicates that the primary direct predictor of illegal alcohol and drug use in male and female high school students is association with antisocial peers and involvement in their antisocial acts. Whether students choose positive or negative peers is influenced directly by their self-esteem and school bonding for both males and females. The school bonding–self-esteem variable is in turn predicted by both the family and school climate variables. Although the research is designed as a prospective two-year study, the data analyses are based on the student's view of all of the domains as assessed at one time.

The Kumpfer and De Marsh Strengthening Families Program

Based on the above results, Kumpfer and Turner (1990) conclude that family and school environments must be improved to enhance the student's self-esteem, which in turn enhances school bonding and decreases the choice of negative peers and drug use. The authors have developed three different types of family-oriented prevention programs: a parent training program, a family skills training program, and a children's social skills training program. Preliminary analyses of the pretest and posttest data suggest that each of the three programs was successful in reducing children's risk factors as well as their alcohol and tobacco use, but only when the three approaches were combined (i.e., a comprehensive approach) did drug use decrease in the older children (De Marsh & Kumpfer, 1986).

The results of two of the programs are as follows: Parent training improved parent discipline effectiveness, which had a direct impact on the children. The children screamed less, had fewer temper tantrums, got angry less, improved their home behaviors, and displayed fewer problems. Parents reported that their children were happier, liked school better, and increased their outside activities (De Marsh & Kumpfer, 1986).

A second component, the Kumpfer Family Skills Training Program, affected family functioning, children's behavior problems, and children's expressiveness. For example, family communication increased and relations improved. Moreover, parents reported that their children were less impulsive, better behaved at home, and showed fewer problem behaviors in general. Finally, the family skills training improved the children's ability to express themselves (asking for help with homework, talking to people when they were sad, seeking more attention from their parents, and crying more). As the author notes, these results are promising but they must be tested on other high-risk populations and the outcome results reported above must be assessed in a follow-up study (De Marsh & Kumpfer, 1986).

Bentler et al.: The Interactive Developmental Domain Model of Adolescent Substance Abuse

Peter Bentler and Michael Newcomb have developed and tested statistical (structural) models depicting constructs that anticipate child drug use at two time points: early adolescence (seventh, eighth, and ninth grade) and late adolescence (four years later). Measures were in the form of scales derived from inventories filled out by the adolescents and their mothers (Newcomb & Bentler, 1988). Three latent child constructs derived from several measures were available for both time points as follows: child emotional distress, child socially deviant attitudes, and child drug use. There were four family context variables: one measured variable (family disruption) and three derived constructs (mothers' drug use, mothers' somatic complaints, and mothers' emotional distress). Data analysis was carried out on a sample of 557 subjects.

A statistical (structural) model is presented to show the interrelation of these variables in a comprehensive and economical manner. Highlights of the findings are that family disruption and all of the mother constructs were significantly correlated in a positive direction. Mothers' somatic complaints and emotional distress did not influence childrens' behavior directly but their impact was mediated via family disruption and mothers' drug use.

Mothers' drug use was significantly associated with their children's drug use, socially deviant attitudes, and emotional distress during early adolescence. Mothers' drug use did not directly influence the child's qualities or behavior in late adolescence; these effects were mediated through the early adolescent constructs of child drug use and socially deviant attitudes.

Family disruption was significantly related to the child's drug use and socially deviant attitudes during early adolescence and had a significant impact on emotional distress in late adolescence.

When all effects were considered simultaneously in a theoretically driven model, socially deviant attitudes (as opposed to conformity) had the largest impact on early drug use, whereas the impact of family context and the other child constructs on drug use was mediated through these deviant attitudes. An alternate, competing hypothesis that child drug use generates child deviant attitudes was rejected empirically (Newcomb & Bentler, 1988).

Other publications have traced the impact of the child's social conformity, perceived adult drug use, and the child's drug use in late adolescence on the drug use, disruptive drug use, and problems with drug use four years later in early adulthood (Stein, Newcomb, & Bentler, 1987). In the final statistical (structural) model, social conformity strongly influenced other latent variables across time. As assessed in late adolescence, the absence of social conformity (i.e., social deviance) anticipated problems with drug use in early adulthood. For the same time interval (late adolescence to early adulthood), early drug use and perceived adult drug use predicted young adult drug use, whereas prior drug use anticipated disruptive drug use. The implication of these findings for prevention have been outlined (Bentler, 1992) but have so far not been translated into intervention programs.

Although the findings of the above four models depicting the antecedents of drug abuse differ, certain commonalities are noteworthy. Most important, socially deviant attitudes and deviant peer group membership are the mediating conditions for drug abuse. Family variables affect these socially deviant outcomes, so it is relevant to ask what earlier family and child characteristics anticipate these adolescent outcomes. We turn next to the findings of three longitudinal studies relevant to these questions and to issues of primary prevention.

PRIMARY PREVENTION

Very few projects have studied the impact of family and child characteristics during the first five years on the emerging family and child characteristics that influence drug use in the later elementary school years. Even less has been conceptualized in terms of possible effective primary prevention efforts, partly because it is difficult to successfully target families and children who are very likely to develop antisocial and drug abusing behavior. However, those considerations must be balanced against the strong possibility that intervention directed at negative patterns of behavior established by early school age may already be very resistant to change.

In delineating a possible primary prevention approach beginning in early childhood, we summarize three studies linking child and family status at 5–6 years to adolescent drug use. We then show how this earliest school status is in turn anticipated by child and family antecedents making an impact from birth on and describe what early intervention methods have been shown to be effective in promoting positive child and family development in the first five years.

Child and Family System Characteristics that Anticipate Later Drug Abuse

There are three known longitudinal studies linking child and family development at ages 5–7 to adolescent drug abuse: the Woodlawn study (Kellam, Brown, Rubin, & Ensminger, 1983), the Berkeley longitudinal study (Shedler & Block, 1990), and studies by Brooks et al (such as Brooks, Whiteman, Cohen & Tanaka, 1991).

The Woodlawn Study

Kellam, Brown, Rubin, and Ensminger (1983) followed an entire first grade population until they were 16-17 years old. Frequency of drug use was determined from a questionnaire administered to the teenagers in a group setting; in this population, use centered heavily on alcohol, marijuana, and cigarettes. Rate of use of marijuana and alcohol was broken into three categories: never used, used 1 to 19 times, and used 20 times or more. Measures of teenage psychiatric symptoms are also reported.

Focus in this presentation is on the first grade antecedents of frequent drug use. The authors cite previous research showing that aggressive or antisocial behavior is the most frequently replicated predictor of substance use. Thus, Robins (1978) found that across all study populations, there was a reliable association of early fighting, truancy, arrests, and drinking with adult alcoholism and drug abuse.

The findings of the Woodlawn study indicate the following:

1. First grade aggressiveness without shyness increased the likelihood of males' (not females') use of all four substances (beer, hard liquor, marijuana, and cigarettes).
2. Shyness among first grade males (but not females) inhibits substance use at age 16 or 17.
3. The combination of shyness and aggressiveness in first grade males is associated with even more frequent use of substances (especially of cigarettes) than aggressiveness alone.
4. The developmental paths leading to psychiatric symptoms and substance use in adolescents are distinct.
5. First grade readiness and higher IQ lead to more teenage substance use.
6. Social maladaptation to school generally is strongly related to the characteristics of family structure and atmosphere but the specific characteristics of shyness, aggressiveness, or learning problems in the classroom were not found to be clearly associated with any specific characteristics of the current social context.

In a subsequent publication, Kellam et al. (1991) report that teenage delinquency, including physical assault, was also predicted by the pattern of antecedents listed for substance abuse under the first three conclusions of the Woodlawn Study. The link of antisocial behavior and substance abuse found by many other investigators is thus supported.

Further qualifying these findings on the current social context (see conclusion 6), Kellam et al. (1991) also report that lower-risk family structures such as mother/father, mother/grandmother, and mother/aunt lead to less aggressive first-grade children. However, among children from such families who do behave aggressively in the first grade classroom, there is an increased risk of substance abuse and delinquency later on in adolescence.

The Berkeley Longitudinal Study

Our summary of this longitudinal study (Shedler & Block, 1990) will characterize the personality profile of the frequent drug user at 18 years, show the similarity of that profile to previous independent assessments at 7 and 11 years of age, and contrast the frequent vs. experimental 18-year-old users in terms of the quality of parent–child interaction observed earlier in their life during the preschool period.

The Q-sort personality profile of the 18-year-olds was factor-analyzed to yield three factors. Their labels and highest loadings are as follows: quality of interpersonal relations (has warmth and capacity for close relationships), subjective distress (concerned with own adequacy as a person), and ego control (undercontrols needs and impulses and is unable to delay gratification). Linking to the Woodlawn assessments of aggression and shyness in the first grade children, the first factor was also loaded negatively on "has hostility toward others" whereas the second factor (subjective distress) also loads negatively on "has social poise and presence"; that is, the child is socially at ease and not shy. Further Q-sort descriptions of the users as opposed to experimenters are as follows: not responsible, not productive, deceitful, opportunistic, unpredictable, unable to delay gratification, rebellious, prone to push limits, self-indulgent, not ethically consistent, not having aspirations, critical, ungiving, not sympathetic, not liked by others, not having capacity for relationships, overreactive to minor frustrations, self-defeating, and feeling cheated and victimized by life. Using the factors and these Q-sort descriptions, the authors conclude that frequent adolescent users are interpersonally alienated, emotionally withdrawn, and manifestly unhappy, and

express their maladjustment through undercontrolled, overtly antisocial behavior.

Examination of analogous profiles at eleven and seven years of age suggest that by seven years of age, the frequent users were unable to form good relationships, were insecure, and showed various signs of emotional distress including being indecisive and unable to plan ahead. That is, the relative social and psychological maladjustment of the frequent users predates initiation of drug use. Moreover, the profile of the seven-year-old stresses the negative outcome of developments that are central to the development of the first years of life: capacity for relationships, security in autonomy, and the ability to define goals and take pride in their achievements (task orientation).

Given this relatively stable profile of the personality characteristics of the frequent users, what type of interaction with their parents did they tend to experience at the earlier age of five? Mothers of frequent users were perceived as cold, unresponsive, nonsupportive, and nonencouraging. This turned a potentially enjoyable interaction into a grim and unpleasant one.

In certain respects, the personality profile of the adolescent frequent drug user and particularly the five- to seven-year antecedents that emerge from the two prospective studies cited here are similar. Both studies describe the frequent adolescent user as expressing maladjustment through undercontrolled overtly antisocial behavior. That is, the frequent users (as opposed to experimenters) are also likely to be categorized as delinquent. Childhood antecedents of this profile stress the inability to form close relationships and, in this context, the display of interpersonal aggression. Early-school-age children who were characterized as both aggressive (hostile) and shy (socially uneasy) were most vulnerable to later frequent drug use. Unlike the Berkeley study, in the Woodlawn study these findings held only for the boys.

Both studies also isolated family conditions that are likely to anticipate frequent drug use: Mothers of frequent users were perceived as cold, unresponsive, nonsupportive, and nonencourag-

ing with their five-year-olds (Shedler & Block, 1990), and six-year-olds were more likely to be aggressive if their mothers had neither partner or family of origin support (Kellam et al. 1991).

Childhood Antecedents of Adolescent Drug Use: Brooks et al.

To study the antecedents of adolescent drug use, Brooks, Whiteman, Cohen, and Tanaka (1991), and Brooks, Whiteman, and Finch (1991) analyzed the complete interview and questionnaire data available for a sample of 420 families at three time points: T1 (ages 5 to 10), T2 (ages 13 to 18), and T3 (ages 15 to 20). Certain latent variables (underlying constructs) are best thought of as early- and late-adolescent outcome measures. Thus, for both T2 and T3, there were measures of their own drug use, perceived peer drug use, delinquency, and unconventionality. Not surprisingly, measures of these qualities at T2 (ages 13 to 18) anticipated variations of them at T3 (ages 15 to 20). Stability in these functions can therefore be inferred.

Most relevant to this review of longitudinal studies, measures of aggression at T1 (ages 5 to 10) were directly associated with drug use (for both males and females) at T2 and indirectly affected the rate of delinquency at T3 (ages 15 to 20) via this drug use at T2. That is, there was no direct association between aggression at T1 and delinquency at T3. Cross-sectional analyses, or correlations within time periods, showed that if a child was using drugs during both early and late adolescence, he or she also tended to be delinquent. Aggression at T1 also anticipated unconventionality at T2. Unconventionality at T2 in turn influenced their own drug use at T3. That is, early signs of aggression (5 to 10) affected drug use in late adolescence by way of the drug use and unconventionality seen in early adolescence.

Perceived peer drug use in late adolescence was anticipated by the perceived peer drug use in earlier adolescence and the youngster's own unconventionality. Approaching these developments from a protective or risk point of view, conventionality when combined with low peer drug use and low self-drug use in early adolescence led to the least amount of self-drug use in late adolescence.

Finally, parent sociopathy (such as illicit drug use and involvement with the police) was *negatively* associated with drug use at T2 but *positively* associated with drug use at T3. The authors suggest that in early adolescence, children listen to their parent's admonition "not to do what they do," but that in late adolescence, these admonitions are not as effective.

To summarize, self-drug use in late adolescence is directly affected by parental sociopathy and self-drug use and unconventionality in *early* adolescence. Aggression as measured at age 5 to 10 affects late adolescent drug use via early adolescent self-drug use and unconventionality. The adolescent's tendency toward delinquency as measured in late adolescence is also significantly associated with self-drug use at that time.

Findings on the parents' attitudes and quality of interaction with their children reported by Brooks, Whiteman, Nomura, and Cohen (1988) are particularly relevant to this review. Looking first at the mother–adolescent relationship variables, it was found that the mother's satisfaction and more time spent with the adolescent, a nonconflictual mother–adolescent relationship, and the adolescent's identification with the mother were negatively related to the adolescent's use of both legal and illegal drugs. Although data on the early mother–child relationship were not available, the authors assume that the quality of the mother–adolescent relationship largely reflects a continuum of interchange from infancy onward.

The Brooks, Whiteman, Nomura, and Cohen (1988) findings are similar to those reported for the Shadler & Block (1990) and Kellam, Brown, Rubin, and Ensminger (1983) studies. Frequent users are likely to be categorized as delinquent, and childhood antecedents stress the inability to form close relationships and, in this context, the display of interpersonal aggression.

Before turning to the intervention projects designed to affect the above profile of child and parent–child characteristics, and to set the stage for preventive intervention beginning as early as the postnatal period, we discuss what is known about the earliest antecedents of the preschool and parent–child transactions that have been shown to affect drug use in adolescence.

Antecedents of Preschool Parent–Child Responsiveness to Need (Parent Stimulates Cognitive and Verbal Experiences and Parent Promotes Effective Autonomy)

Various longitudinal studies of family development from birth to preschool have identified three major transactions between parent and child: parents' responsiveness to need, interacting with the child, modulates aggression (Heinicke & Lampl, 1988); parent stimulates cognitive and verbal experiences, interacting with the child's task orientation (Heinicke & Lampl, 1988); and parent promotes effective autonomy, interacting with the child's sense of separate self (Heinicke & Guthrie, 1992). The child's modulation of aggression is in turn associated with warmth and the capacity for close relationships and by ratings of a sense of positive self (security).

Given the above clusters of parent and child behaviors, which seem clearly relevant to the findings of the Woodlawn and Berkeley studies pinpointing the antecedents of later drug abuse, what in turn are the antecedents of these parent–child interactions? Moreover, what are the implications of these clusters of variables for the design of preventive interventions in the first four years of life?

We will focus on the preschool status of parent responsiveness to need interacting with the child's aggression modulation. As already suggested, the capacity for relationships, warmth, self-control, and sense of positive self-dimensions are absent in the profile that characterizes the frequent adolescent drug user (Shedler & Block, 1990). We note first of all that the transaction under discussion is significantly correlated with concurrent (four-year) measures of the mother's positive view of her marriage, her capacity for warmth, and her general adaptation-competence (Heinicke & Lampl, 1988). These three variables, as well as parent responsiveness to need and aggression modulation as measured at both 36 and 24 months, are also correlated with the 48-month transaction. The early emergence and relative stability of this profile of five correlated variables is further underlined by the finding that prebirth measures of the three maternal variables each significantly anticipate parent responsiveness to need at one month. See Heinicke (1994) for further review of the research on the prebirth determinants of parenting. These findings do not ignore the findings that variations in early stable infant characteristics such as one-month soothability and visual attention also affect parents' responsiveness to the needs of the infant. It does emphasize that early postnatal intervention directed at the crucial parent responsiveness to need must also address the associated parent and marital characteristics. What evidence exists that effective early interventions are characterized by the theoretically guided and actual changes in these parent and marital characteristics?

Postnatal Family-System-Oriented Intervention

Review of existing research shows that effective controlled interventions initiated in the first three months after birth and including a follow-up assessment are characterized by a theoretically guided intervention not just with the child but with some aspect of the parental, marital, and support system functioning (Heinicke, Beckwith, & Thompson, 1988; Heinicke, 1991). The significant impact of intervention on early family development is well-documented.

Although clearly dealing with aspects of family functioning such as parent responsiveness to need, which is relevant to later relationship capacity and sense of security and thus to the presence or absence of frequent drug abuse, there are no known longitudinal studies explicitly tracing the impact of such postnatal interventions on measured drug abuse in childhood and adolescence. However, had differential drug abuse or early onset of the use of drugs such as tobacco been assessed, in three of the existing early inter-

vention studies the beneficial impact of the comprehensive interventions might well have been established in this area of functioning. Examination of these three studies is done in detail and informs the recommendations made at the conclusion of this chapter.

The first of these intervention studies designed comprehensive family services for mostly single, inner-city poverty-level mothers with full-term infants (Seitz, Rosenbaum, & Apfel, 1985). The goal was to enhance the mother's adaptation, the quality of her relationship with her child, and the child's development. An ongoing relationship with a home visitor, pediatric care, high-quality day care, and developmental examinations were provided. A series of follow-ups attested to the efficacy of the intervention. The last follow-up, at 10 years of age, suggests that children who had not experienced the intervention were more likely to be described as disobedient, not getting along with other children, and as unhappy, sad, or depressed. More important in terms of the efficacy of the intervention affecting both the mother's functioning and the mother–child relationship, it was found that the mothers in the experimental group completed more years of education, waited longer to have a second child, were more often part of a nuclear family, were more often self-supporting, often initiated contacts with teachers, and made greater use of remedial and supportive services. Most relevant to the dimensions of affection and responsiveness, the mothers experiencing the intervention showed a better relationship with their child, who was seen as pleasing them and giving them pleasure.

Two other projects have reported findings on the impact of early family-focused intervention on the children and adolescents of multirisk families. The prevention of antisocial behavior often associated with frequent drug abuse is documented in these projects. Thus, Wieder, Poisson, Lourie, and Greenspan (1988) have reported the five-year follow-up of 32 multirisk families who received intensive, comprehensive services through the Clinical Infant Development

Program (CIDP). Three components made up this intervention:

- Organizing basic services for adequate food, housing, medical care, and educational opportunities, to deal with day-to-day survival and future family stability
- Providing a constant emotional relationship with the family through which trust could be established with the parents and the infant
- Providing specialized services to the infant and parents geared to meet the challenges at each stage of development, given each infant's and parent's individual vulnerabilities and strengths.

The follow-up assessments were relevant to these three goals. Because the first goal was to deal with basic survival and sustenance, when compared with both the beginning and the end of intervention point, both the adult and especially the adolescent mothers had made striking gains in their work status and independence from public assistance. The increased freedom to work outside the home probably resulted from the avoidance of repeat pregnancies, which in the past further drained the limited resources.

The provision of an ongoing relationship opportunity by the CIDP staff was reflected in the mother's increasing capacity to form mutually satisfying partner relationships. Five years after the intervention ended, 42% of adult mothers were married or had sustained relationships. There was a striking decline in the abusive aspects of these relationships as well as in their relationships with their children. Thus, abuse for the older mothers decreased from 60% to 5.3% and from 50% to 18% for the adolescents.

Wieder, Poisson, Lourie, and Greenspan (1988) also cite findings on the children that indicate average IQ performance (103), placement in regular as opposed to special education classes, and active involvement in team sports and local youth organizations.

Although it seems clear that the persistent, clinically skilled, comprehensive program outlined above did indeed produce sustained gains in parent and child functioning, some reservation is introduced by the fact that a comparison group was not available to highlight which positive changes were a function of the intervention and which might have occurred without intervention.

Another major project, the Syracuse University Family Development Program, has also published dramatic follow-up results (Lally, Mangione, Honig, & Wittner, 1988). The intervention was designed to influence the permanent environment of the child, the family, and the home. Poor, largely black, young, mostly single women were recruited in late pregnancy. The contact with the parent was viewed as primary and child care as supplementary.

A cadre of paraprofessional home visitors, called Child Development Trainers (CDTs), was recruited and trained intensively to encourage strong, nurturing mother–child relationships that involved giving affectionate bodily contact, respecting children's needs, and responding positively to young children's efforts to learn. CDTs offered positive support and encouragement to mothers as they interacted with their children and also responded positively and actively to the mother's need to fulfill her aspirations for herself. Many mothers came to rely on the CDT as an advisor and confidante on personal relations, finances, career changes, and education. CDTs served as liaisons between the families and community support services, including the child care component of FDRP; in addition, they helped families to learn to find and use neighborhood resources on their own (by giving families specific practice in learning how to make and maintain contact with school personnel as children reached school age, for example).

In addition, parent associations were encouraged and the Children's Center provided child and preschool education to three age groups: 6 to 15 months, 15 to 18 months, and 18 to 60 months.

The follow-up conducted ten years after the end of the program revealed that the program children showed a significantly lower rate of delinquency (6% vs. 22%) and showed that the offenses they did commit were less severe than those reported for the control group.

Girls in the program group, but not boys, were performing significantly better in school than their counterparts in the control group. Interestingly, these positive findings began to appear only during early adolescence; information on the elementary school years indicated no differences between the program and control group. Teachers rated girls from the program group as having more positive attitudes toward themselves and other people.

Compared with control group parents, parents who had been in the program reported feeling proud about the positive social attitudes and behaviors of their children and the degree of unity in their families. They were also more likely to advise young people to learn something about themselves and accomplish all they could, whereas control parents were more inclined to counsel young people to concentrate just on "getting by."

Compared with control group children, those in the program group felt more positively about themselves in early adolescence and were more likely to expect education to be a continuing part of their lives. Fifty three percent of the program group but only 28% of the controls anticipated that they would be in school at age 17 or 18.

An example of early family intervention designed to break the generational continuity of inadequate parenting, drug use, and future inadequate parenting comes from the UCLA Family Development Project (Heinicke, 1991). During the weekly home visits with Jessica, it became clear that this first-time mother had little consistent and responsive mothering from her own childlike, drug-using mother. Although Jessica renounced her heroin use when she became pregnant and participated in a methadone drug prevention as well as a weekly home visit and mother–infant program, at a certain point the current demands for mothering from her own mother and her sister as well as the lack of support from her partner led to a temporary return to drug use. She was not available to her eight-month-old son and was in danger of having to give him up to foster care. A variety of empathic and confrontive techniques were used by the home visitor to stop the continuing drug abuse and to return Jessica to her more than adequate natural ability to mother her baby boy. At 12 months, her son was secure in his relationship with her and showed good task orientation.

SUMMARY

We have shown that drug abuse, as opposed to experimentation, is mediated through socially deviant attitudes and deviant peer group membership and that these adolescent developments are influenced by, among other things, recent or concurrent family conditions and parent management practices.

We have also shown that drug abuse and the associated undercontrolled overtly antisocial behavior was anticipated by the young (five- to six-year-old) child's inability to form close relationships and a tendency to express uncontrolled aggression or be excessively shy. Early family predictors included parental unresponsiveness and the mother's lack of partner or family support.

Given the demonstration that these early (five- to six-year-old) antecedents are anticipated by earlier parent personality, marital, and parent–child relationship variables, one of the implications of the findings of this chapter is that early family primary intervention must be added to the secondary prevention approaches now being used. The efficacy of intervention with school-aged drug-abusing antisocial children, as opposed to experimental users, has been limited and certainly needs further documentation. The most recent review of existing outcome studies has found very few positive results (Bangert-Drowns, 1988). By contrast, early family intervention has been shown to make a difference, especially if also directed at parent personality and marital functioning. Although the long-term relevance of early family intervention for adolescent drug abuse and delinquency needs further demonstration, the Syracuse University Family Development Program is particularly impressive in this regard. Both the rate of delinquency and the severity of the offenses were less than those reported for the control group.

As the other chapters of this book document, socially deviant behavior, including adolescent drug abuse, is highly overdetermined. Peers clearly provide a setting and encouragement of drug use. Educational programs using group settings and peer counselors may well be effective under certain circumstances. Problem drug use must be seen as part of a developmental profile focusing on the emergence of security in relationships, preparedness and autonomy in adapting, and commitment to goals that, when achieved, lead to pride and pleasure.

This positive profile is likely to be associated with caretaking systems involving positive parent partnerships and other support systems that promote responsiveness to the needs of the infant, preparation for autonomous functioning, encouragement and guidance to tasks (Heinicke, 1994), and appropriate limit setting (Patterson & Dishion, 1988).

Although it is necessarily a long-term solution, we believe that a national family policy supporting the functioning of parenting from the child's conception on is necessary to combat drug abuse. The following questions must be addressed and resolved with new and especially integrated services: Have the expectant parents been sufficiently counseled to ensure the commitment to the infant? Are adequate prenatal medical care systems available? How can the basic problems of the housing and the financial support of the new parents be addressed? What services are available, such as home visiting, to improve the support experienced within the caretaking system and to make the best use of support available outside the family?

Although the continuing support of the caretaking system and the influence of new environments (school and peers) are significant, the need for an early nurturing and guiding environment must be addressed in any effort to affect frequent drug use. It is in this earliest period that the groundwork for the child's involvement in relationships and meaningful tasks is laid. Character

formations and family systems that foster commitments to love and work are the best antidote to the alienation, impulsiveness, and false sense of quietude and pleasure that accompany drug abuse.

REFERENCES

Bangert-Drowns, R. L. (1988). The effects of school-based substance abuse education: A meta-analysis. *Journal of Drug Education, 18,* 243–264.

Bentler, P. M. (1992). Etiologies and consequences of adolescent drug use: Implications for prevention. *Journal of Addictive Diseases, 11* (3), 47–61.

Bronfenbrenner, V. (1974). Is early intervention effective? *Columbia Teacher's College Record, 76,* 279–303.

Brooks, J. S., Whiteman, M., Cohen, P., & Tanaka, J. S. (1991). Childhood precursors of adolescent drug use: A longitudinal analysis. *Genetic, Social, and General Psychology Monographs, 118* (2), 195–213.

Brooks, J. S., Whiteman, M., & Finch, S. (1991). Childhood aggression, adolescent delinquency, and drug use: A longitudinal study. *Journal Genetic Psychology, 153* (4), 369–383.

Brooks, J. S., Whiteman, M., Nomura, C., & Cohen, P. (1988). Parental, perinatal, and early childhood risk factors and drug involvement in adolescence. *Genetic, Social, and General Psychology Monographs, 115* (2), 221–241.

De Marsh, J., & Kumpfer, K. L. (1986). Family-oriented interventions for the prevention of chemical dependency in children and adolescents. In S. Ezekoye, K. Kumpfer, and W. Bukoski (Eds.), *Childhood and chemical abuse: Prevention and intervention.* New York: Haworth Press, 117–151.

Dishion, T. J., Reid, J. B., & Patterson, G. R. (1988). Empirical guidelines for a family intervention for adolescent drug use. *Journal of Chemical Dependency Treatment, 1,* 189–224.

Gottfredson, G. D. (1985). *The effective school battery, student survey.* Odessa, FL: Psychological Assessment Resources.

Hawkins, J. D., Catalano, R. F., Jones, A., & Fire, D. N. (1987). Delinquency prevention through parent training: Results and issues from work in progress. In J. Q. Wilson & G. C. Lang (Eds.), *From children to citizens: Families, schools, and delinquency prevention,* vol.3, 186–204. New York: Springer-Leakey.

Hawkins, J. D., Catalano, R. F., & Kent, L. A. (1991). Combining broadcast media and parent education to prevent teenage drug abuse. In L. Donchow, H. E. Sypher & W. J. Nunushi (Eds.), *Persuasive communication and drug abuse prevention.* Hillsdale, NJ: Lawrence Erlbaum Associates, 283–294.

Hawkins, J. D., Lishner, D. M., Catalano, R. F., & Howard, M. O. (1986). Childhood predictors of adolescent substance abuse: Toward an empirically grounded theory. *Journal of Children in Contemporary Society, 8,* 11–48.

Hawkins, J. D., Lishner, D. M., Jenson, J. M., & Catalano, R. F. (1987). Delinquents and drugs: What the evidence suggests about prevention and treatment programming. In B. S. Brown and A. R. Mills (Eds.), *Youth at high risk for substance abuse.* Washington, DC: NIDA (ADM 87-1537).

Hawkins, J. D., & Salisbury, B. R. (1983). Delinquency prevention programs for minorities of color. *Social Work Research and Abstracts, 19,* 5–12.

Hawkins, J. D., & Weiss, J. G. (1985). The social development model: An integrated approach to delinquency prevention. *Journal of Primary Prevention, 6,* 73–97.

Heinicke, C. M. (1991). Early family intervention: Focusing on the mother's adaptation-competence and quality of partnership. In D. G. Unger and D. R. Powell (Eds.), *Families as nurturing systems: Support across the life span.* New York: The Haworth Press.

Heinicke, C. (1994). Determinants of the transition to parenting. In M. H. Bornstein (Ed.), *Handbook of parenting vol. II: Biology and ecology of parenting.* New Jersey: Lawrence Erlbaum Associates.

Heinicke, C. M., Beckwith, L., & Thompson, A. (1988). Early intervention in the family system: A framework and review. *Infant Mental Health Journal, 9* (2).

Heinicke, C. M., & Guthrie, D. (1992). Stability and change in husband–wife adaptation and the development of the positive parent–child relationship. *Infant Behavior and Development, 15,* 109–127.

Heinicke, C. M., & Lampl, E. (1988). Pre- and postbirth antecedents of three- and four-year-old attention, I.Q., verbal expressiveness, task orientation and capacity for relationships. *Infant Behavior and Development, 11* 381–410.

Kellam, S. G., Brown, C. H., Rubin, B. R., & Ensminger, M. E. (1983). Paths leading to teenage psychiatric symptoms and substance use: Developmental epidemiological studies in Woodlawn. In S. B. Guze, F. J. Earls, & J. E. Barrett (Eds.), *Childhood psychopathology and development.* New York: Raven, 17–47.

Kellam, S. G., Werthamer-Larsson, L., Dolan, L. J., Brown, C. H., Mayer, L. S., Rebok, G. W., Anthony, J. C., Laudolff, J., & Edelsohn, G. (1991). *Developmental epidemiologically-based preventive trials: Baseline modeling of early target behaviors and depressive symptoms.* Department of Mental Hygiene, the Johns Hopkins School of Hygiene & Public Health (unpublished manuscript).

Kumpfer, K. L., & Turner, C. W. (1990). The social ecology model of adolescent substance abuse: Implications for prevention. *International Journal of Addiction, 25* (4A), 435–463.

Lally, R. J., Mangione, P. L., Honig, A. S., & Wittner, D. S. (1988). More pride, less delinquency: Findings from the 10-year follow-up study of the Syracuse University Family Development Research program. *Zero to Three, 8,* 13–18.

Newcomb, M. D., & Bentler, P. M. (1988). The impact of family context, deviant attitudes, and emotional distress on adolescent drug use: Longitudinal latent-variable analyses of mothers and their children. *Journal of Research in Personality, 22,* 154–176.

Patterson, G. R., & Chamberlain, P. (1988). Treatment process: A problem at three levels. In L. C. Wynne (Ed.), *The state of the art in family therapy research: Controversies and recommendation.* New York: Family Process Press.

Patterson, G. R., & Dishion, T. J. (1986). Multilevel family process models: Traits, interactions, and relationships. In R. Hinde & J. Stevenson-Hinde (Eds.), *Relationship within families: Mutual influences.* Oxford: Clarendon Press.

Robins, L. N. (1978). Sturdy childhood predictors of adult antisocial behavior: Replications from longitudinal studies. *Psychological Medicine, 8,* 611–622.

Seitz, V., Rosenbaum, L. K. & Apfel, N. H. (1985). Effects of family support intervention: A ten-year follow-up. *Child Development, 56,* 376–191.

Shedler, J., & Block, J. (1990). Adolescent drug use and psychological health: A longitudinal inquiry. *American Psychologist, 45,* 612–630.

Stein, J. D., Newcomb, M. D., & Bentler, P. M. (1987). An 8-year study of multiple influences on drug use and drug use consequences. *Journal of Personality and Social Psychology, 53,* 1094–1105.

Wieder, S., Poisson, S., Lourie, R. S., & Greenspan, S. I. (1988). Enduring gains: A five-year follow-up report on a clinical infant development program. *Zero to Three, 8,* 6–11.

CHAPTER 16

PREGNANT WOMEN AND
THEIR NEWBORNS

JUDY HOWARD

It is estimated that in the United States, five million women of childbearing age currently use illicit drugs (General Accounting Office, 1990). Typically, drug-abusing women report polysubstance abuse, and alcohol generally is included among the substances used. The exact number of drug-affected infants born each year has been more difficult to determine. Estimates of the number of cocaine-exposed neonates range from 91,500 to 240,000 nationally (Besharov, 1989; General Accounting Office, 1990; Gomby & Shiono, 1991). However, these figures exclude information relating to the numbers of infants exposed prenatally to heroin, methamphetamine, phencyclidine (PCP), and other substances of abuse. In individual cities, estimates of the percentage of drug-involved births range from 7% in San Francisco and 7.5% in Washington, D.C., to 10–15% in Milwaukee and 16% in Philadelphia. More startling are the statistics emanating from individual hospitals, such as Hutzel Hospital in Detroit, where 43% of newborns recently tested positive for prenatal substance exposure (Feig, 1990). Furthermore, it is estimated that more than 7,000 children each year are born with fetal alcohol syndrome, a consequence of maternal alcohol use during pregnancy (Abel & Sokol, 1987).

At this time, we are unable to estimate the long-term cost to society for the health and mental health care as well as the special education services that many prenatally substance-exposed children require. A recent report examining the neonatal costs of babies whose mothers used cocaine during pregnancy illustrates only one as-

pect of this problem, the monetary expense of prenatal substance abuse. In this study, neonatal hospital costs for prenatally cocaine-exposed infants were shown to be three to four times more than for nonexposed infants. Furthermore, the costs for infants of polysubstance abusers who used cocaine in addition to other illicit substances averaged $8,450, as compared with $1,283 for non-substance-exposed infants. Extrapolating from these findings, the authors estimate that $500 million will be spent on an annual basis to cover neonatal hospital expenses alone (Phibbs, Bateman, & Schwartz, 1991).

Before the 1960s, the types of illicit drugs available in the marketplace were limited in number, and the typical abuser was male. Heroin was the most common drug of abuse after World War II, and cocaine, which had been more widely used at the turn of the century, declined in popularity during the '60s. The '60s were a time of breaking loose from the conventional postwar lifestyle and emphasizing experimentation in the areas of relationships, freedom of speech, and of "instant pleasure-seeking with sex and drugs" (Taylor & Gold, 1990, p. 573). During this decade, psychedelic and mood-altering drugs became popular as young men and women sought new experiences. By the time of the Woodstock music festival, the media had begun to regularly publish stories about large-scale use of mind-altering substances. The entertainment industry, especially in the areas of film and music, also began to highlight use of drugs in story lines and song lyrics. Thus, this decade of experimentation evolved into the 1970s, when polysubstance abuse seemed to be the trend and there were reports of an increasing incidence of addiction and use of drugs to escape from life's problems.

Due to the growing numbers of children born to substance-abusing women, recent national interest has shifted from a focus on the adult user to a focus on the children of substance abusers. As early as fifteen years ago, a small group of researchers and clinicians expressed many of the same concerns we are voicing today about the deleterious effects of drugs and alcohol on family functioning. In 1976, the National Institute on Drug Abuse published the results of a symposium on comprehensive health care for addicted parents and their children, at which some of the leading investigators working with chemically dependent families presented their research findings. Their closing remarks reflected concern about the high rate of infant mortality and parental problems in this population, the increased incidence of obstetrical and medical complications in women who abuse substances during pregnancy, and the high rate of low-birth-weight infants. Furthermore, one developmental pediatrician commented, "I have observed the growth and development of narcotic addicts' infants for the past ten years. . . . We are concerned that narcotic-affected infants, even when raised in stable environments, have behavioral, neurologic, and growth characteristics different from those of other high-risk babies" (Wilson, 1976, p. 74).

THE CHEMICALLY DEPENDENT MOTHER

This author's familiarity with chemically dependent parents is based on years of clinical experience as well as the literature regarding families of lower socioeconomic status. Very little, if anything, has been published to describe large samples of middle- or upper-middle-class substance-abusing parents and their treatment needs. It cannot be denied that the problem of alcohol and other drug abuse crosses all social and economic boundaries, and much remains to be learned about chemical dependency among families who have access to resources and social supports.

The following discussion is based on what is known about only one member of the parenting dyad: pregnant women who are chemically dependent and who come from families where there are few social and financial supports. Research results addressing the addicted father's contribution to the lifestyle of the spouse or significant other, as well as to the developing fetus and child, are not yet available.

Relationships and Parenting Skills

Given the escalating incidence of identified substance abuse among pregnant women, the issue of parenting skills within this population has become a major focus of research. Drug treatment programs originating in the 1960s, when heroin was the major substance of abuse, routinely were designed to treat the physiological symptoms of dependence. It was rare for pediatricians or other health care professionals treating family members to consider the unique needs of the parent who also happens to be an addict.

However, in 1977 Escamilla-Mondanaro graphically reported the clinical characteristics of pregnant addicts who had few social and economic resources, addressing their relationships with husbands or significant others, the guilt they experienced following their babies' delivery, the unrealistic expectations many of them had of their offspring, and the parenting relationships they developed with their growing children. In this study of 60 pregnant heroin addicts who sought prenatal care and drug treatment, a startling finding was these women's diminished capacity to experience non-drug-induced joy and playfulness, which interfered with their quality of life before the babies' birth (Escamilla-Mondanaro, 1977).

Most of these heroin-addicted women—like those we are following today who abuse cocaine, methamphetamine, heroin, and other drugs—did not plan their pregnancies. Because all of these substances of abuse can interfere with a woman's normal ovulation and menstruation, frequently resulting in missed periods, many chemically dependent women may believe they are unable to become pregnant. Of course, this is not true and, unfortunately, the late discovery of pregnancy can interfere with a woman's available options for prenatal health care and family planning.

When a chemically dependent woman suddenly discovers that she is pregnant, she may take an interest in her pending motherhood and appear to develop a bond with her unborn child. However, support from her husband or significant other, who also may be a substance abuser, commonly is lacking. Some pregnant addicts report that the fathers also respond positively to the pending birth of their babies, yet still are unable to physically, emotionally, or financially provide for their families. Other fathers initially may find the stresses related to an unplanned pregnancy more burdensome. In some instances, fathers who have been unable to cope with this responsibility have intensified their drug use and criminal activity, resulting in incarceration or hospitalization for overdose (Escamilla-Mondanaro, 1977).

When this occurs, some women may be able to tolerate the distancing behavior on the part of the child's father by harboring unrealistic expectations about the eventual relationship that will develop once the baby is born. Many chemically dependent women state their belief that, when they become pregnant, their own family members will behave more lovingly toward them and their partners will find employment in order to provide appropriate housing. Women often believe that parenthood, in and of itself, will diminish their craving for drugs (Carr, 1975).

Unfortunately, a variety of factors can mar these expectations. As her delivery date approaches, an addicted woman may experience anxiety about the delivery process and consequently increase her drug use. However, many substances of abuse can precipitate preterm delivery, exacerbating the mother's feelings of guilt. Following delivery, additional mechanisms can interfere with the new mother's relationship with her child. If the infant exhibits behavioral withdrawal symptoms, such as high-pitched cries, extreme irritability, or tremulousness, a mother may deny that these behaviors are associated with drug withdrawal and attribute them to a colic problem or her own poor caretaking abilities. In a study of 170 females in drug treatment, Colten found that chemically dependent women were more likely to feel inadequate as mothers and expressed greater concern about their children becoming addicted, dropping out, or going to jail (Colten, 1980).

Chemically dependent mothers, like many women with low self-esteem, often express the hope that their children will show them affection from very early on. Again, like other women with negative self-images, addicted women commonly want to hurry the process of infancy and toddlerhood with respect to two significant areas. First, they tend to be concerned about spoiling their children by giving them too much attention, and second, they want their children to be independent with regard to self-help skills, particularly in the areas of eating and toilet training. By making such unrealistic demands on a toddler, who is only beginning to learn about autonomy, the mother risks establishing an adversarial relationship. In such cases, a toddler's outward behavior may reflect conflict rather than the love his or her mother so desires. Finally, it is not unusual for these mothers to become authoritarian, excessively trying to control their children's developmental course as they attempt to maintain control of their own lives (Wellisch & Steinberg, 1980). These maternal behaviors— though commonly seen in women who lack support systems or who have had dysfunctional relationships with their own parents—on a clinical level are more resistent to change when the mother is addicted and unable to prioritize the child's needs over her own.

Childhood History

Professionals who serve chemically dependent clients must understand that substance-abusing individuals' behaviors and feelings about parenthood, pregnancy, and child-rearing do not exist in a vacuum. During the past decade, we have increasingly come to realize the importance of identifying the substance abuser's personal history in order to develop appropriate treatment plans (Wallace, 1991). Childhood experiences, parental use or abuse of drugs or alcohol, and educational background all are significant factors. It is not surprising to learn from the majority of parents who abuse drugs and alcohol that their own family backgrounds involved parental substance abuse (Cuskey & Wathey, 1982). As we have begun to ask questions about female addicts' childhood experiences, we have learned that many of these individuals also endured physical, sexual, or emotional abuse as children (Howard, Beckwith, Rodning, & Kropenske, 1989). Once again, the body of knowledge regarding the backgrounds of adult addicts pertains more to women's negative experiences during childhood than to men's. There is limited information about the extent to which physical and sexual abuse occur within the addict male population (Friedrich, Beilke, & Urquiza, 1988).

To understand how new this kind of information is to healthcare providers, one has to look at the history of child abuse research. In 1962, Henry Kempe and colleagues published the first major article for pediatricians describing the battered child syndrome (Kempe et al., 1962). Before this report, children who were battered often were felt to have rare bone or hematological diseases. As the types of physical abuse and severe neglect became more clearly delineated (such as fractures, burns, shaken baby syndrome, and failure to thrive), another area of abuse emerged. In 1983, we learned that 25% of young women had been sexually abused before reaching adulthood (Russell, 1983). During the 1990s, we will learn more about emotional abuse and its impact on child development and behavior.

In a current project in which researchers are making a concentrated effort to interview pregnant addicts individually before their initiation into treatment programs, my colleagues and I are learning that more than 80% of these women have histories of parental substance abuse, child physical abuse, or sexual abuse. Furthermore, the women state that very few professionals they have encountered have inquired about their childhood experiences. Once they have divulged this information about their backgrounds, we

find that it can take as long as six months in counseling before the women are able to actively grieve about the abuse they suffered during childhood.

Low Self-Esteem, Educational Deficits, and Unemployment

It is rare to find individuals with abusive backgrounds who do not have low self-esteem; this, in turn, influences their educational achievements and social support networks (Tucker, 1979). Chemically dependent women report having fewer friends and more intense feelings of loneliness than non-drug-abusing women (Tucker, 1979). The majority of adult women who are substance abusers and who grew up in homes where parents used alcohol or drugs report difficulties in attending to educational tasks as well as low motivation to seek high school diplomas or college degrees. From clinical experience, this author has found that many of these women question whether their learning difficulties in school may be related to their own parents' use of alcohol or drugs at the time of conception or during pregnancy.

Job performance parallels educational success in this population. Many chemically dependent women lack job skills and remain unemployed. Those who find work often are unable to sustain a position for more than several months, many reporting that their substance abuse activities interfere with regular employment.

Altered Mental Status

Today's addicted parents tend to be polysubstance abusers. Their pattern of drug abuse, or addiction, is compulsive, lacks internal control, and continues even in the face of adverse consequences (Smith, 1986). The primary drugs of choice are cocaine, methamphetamine, heroin, and phencyclidine (PCP), any of which may be used in combination with alcohol or marijuana to help the user sleep or relax. However, the polysubstance abusers who are being served today generally are not primarily alcoholics who have added illicit drugs to their repertoires.

The addict's abuse of stimulant compounds, such as cocaine and methamphetamine, produces a neurochemical magnification of pleasure. Users report feelings of alertness and elevated energy levels, with decreased anxiety and social inhibitions. They also experience a sense of well-being, heightened self-esteem and sexuality, and a few incidences of hallucinations. Concomitant with these subjective experiences, the user's physiological responses include tachycardia, hypertension, vasoconstriction, mydriasis, diaphoresis, and tremor (Gawin & Ellinwood, 1988).

It is currently unknown whether any predispositions to stimulant abuse exist. However, a family history of alcoholism has been noted to increase the probability of cocaine addiction when an individual is exposed to the drug (Smith, 1986). Additionally, despite professionals' general inability to identify risk factors for addiction to stimulants, once binge use occurs, dependency with increasing tolerance is an issue. Binge patterns generally are manifested when the highs become progressively briefer in duration. During a cocaine binge, a user may administer the drug as often as every ten minutes, with subsequent rapid and frequent mood fluctuations. As the binge episode proceeds, for instance, euphoria may alternate with feelings of anxiety, hyperactivity, and irritability. In some cases, a paranoid state may occur. The average length of a cocaine binge is twelve hours. In contrast, an amphetamine binge may last as long as 24 hours or more, with the user readministering the drug every one to several hours (Gawin & Ellinwood, 1988).

Eventually, when the binge episode comes to an end, a crash ensues. Users commonly become unable to experience pleasure, take limited interest in their environments, and have very low energy levels. During the crash, the user's norepinephrine and dopamine neurotransmitters are depleted, and sleep dysfunction, depression, and drug hunger can occur (Gold, Washton, & Dackis, 1985). Users who experience sleep disturbances may turn to sedatives, opiates, marijuana, or alcohol to ease agitation and induce slumber.

Over time, the memory of the more hedonistic state and the craving for drugs become so strong that another hit is virtually inevitable unless treatment is obtained. Clearly, the cost of addiction to cocaine and methamphetamine is high. Given the typical pattern of dependency, it is not difficult to understand why parents who are addicts may sell household belongings, engage in prostitution, commit other illegal acts, and even experience periods of incarceration.

Heroin, unlike cocaine and methamphetamine, is a depressant that produces a feeling of well-being in the user, along with episodes of drowsiness. Other symptoms include analgesia and respiratory depression (Ling, 1990). Heroin withdrawal symptoms are more violent physiologically than those associated with the stimulants. They may include strong muscle contractions, intense perspiration, writhing, and nausea (Finnegan & Wapner, 1987). The classic opiate withdrawal is a continuing state during which the user experiences an ongoing desire to alleviate the symptoms through repeated administration of the drug. This differs significantly from the withdrawal or crash state associated with stimulants, during which the user experiences an intense craving to sleep off the acute drug effects.

Another substance of abuse, PCP, has gained popularity in certain areas of the United States (such as parts of Los Angeles and Washington, D.C.). PCP, or angel dust, is an inexpensive synthetic drug that commonly is made in home laboratories. Smoking "Sherman" cigarettes that have been laced with PCP is the most common method of use.

Acute PCP intoxication can present in a wide spectrum of behaviors, ranging from delirium tremens and acute psychiatric illness to sedation, superhuman strength, violent acts, aggression, or a heightened state of euphoria (Fauman & Fauman, 1980; McNamara, Kimura, & Wiles, 1960; Pearlson, 1981; Pradhan, 1984; Rawson, Tennant, & McCann, 1981). In fact,

PCP was used early on in research to elicit schizophrenic behaviors in normal volunteers (Burns et al., 1975; Domino, 1980; Javitt, 1987; Lerner & Burns, 1978). Chronic PCP use seems to interfere with higher cortical function, causing problems with organizing conceptual information, auditory sequencing, and short-term memory loss (Lewis & Hordan, 1986).

Given the behavioral effects of the various substances described above, it is clear that use of any of these drugs must have a profound impact on an individual's interactions with others as well as on his or her parenting ability. The complexities of day-to-day responsive parenting are incongruent with the altered mental status seen in chronic addicts. Not only is it difficult for a chemically dependent parent to sustain a meaningful and caring relationship with a significant other, but such a person cannot meet the ongoing life-supporting and emotional needs of a newborn infant and dependent child.

In a longitudinal study examining the parenting behaviors of 47 amphetamine users, the environmental experiences of children of mothers who continued to use after pregnancy were disturbing (Billing, Eriksson, Larsson, & Zetterström, 1979). This Swedish research project showed that infants who were discharged home with mothers who had used amphetamine throughout pregnancy suffered the most adverse infancies during the 12 months of follow-up, as compared with infants whose mothers had discontinued drug use on becoming aware of pregnancy and infants who were placed in institutions or foster homes following birth. One-third had been removed from the care of their mothers because of parental neglect, approximately 40% had been hospitalized one or more times, and more than 50% had developmental or emotional problems.

The often-stated phrase "the lifestyle of the addict" evokes an image of an individual whose daily experiences revolve around the procurement and use of drugs. However, when the addict happens to be a pregnant woman or a father-to-be, that image becomes more complex. The focus shifts to the unborn child and how those parents will manage the responsibilities of caring for their offspring. A combination of circumstances that we often take for granted must be present in order to foster the growth of a baby. The mother-to-be, for instance, has a responsibility to seek prenatal care and ensure adequate nutrition. The father-to-be has a responsibility to support the mother's care of herself and the unborn child. Together, they must secure housing, dependable income, preparations for the baby's arrival, and, if the parents are addicts, drug treatment for themselves.

HEALTH PROBLEMS OF CHILDREN OF CHEMICALLY DEPENDENT PARENTS

Substance abusers commonly neglect their own healthcare needs. Compounding this problem, women who abuse drugs during pregnancy have an increased risk of medical complications including anemia, cardiac disease, hepatitis, urinary tract infections, toxemia, abruptio placenta, and postpartum hemorrhage (Finnegan, 1976, 1982; Suffet & Brotman, 1981). In addition to these medical complications, women who are addicts and who feel compelled to procure drugs to satisfy their physiological craving often resort to illegal activities, such as prostitution and theft, to sustain their habits. Increased sexual activity brings increased risk of exposure to sexually transmitted diseases such as gonorrhea, syphilis, herpes, hepatitis B virus, and acquired immune deficiency syndrome (AIDS). These diseases can be passed on to the newborn, either congenitally or during the birth process.

Gonorrhea, congenital syphilis, and hepatitis B virus are treatable when recognized in the mother and the newborn. Congenital herpes can present with a variety of symptoms ranging from blisters on the skin to full-blown central nervous system involvement by the virus. Some of the lesser problems can be treated with medication. However, when the brain is involved, the child often suffers mental retardation, seizures, or physical disability.

Pediatric AIDS is a devastating disease process, just as this virus is in the adult. Research indicates that at least two-thirds of infants exposed prenatally to the AIDS virus are asymptomatic at 18 months of age. The long-term prognosis for these children is unknown. However, children who become HIV-positive early on during infancy have a debilitating medical course ranging from early death to slow deterioration over many years (Blanche et al., 1989).

Such complications during pregnancy, combined with lack of prenatal care, poor nutrition, the toxic effects of drugs and alcohol on the placental/fetal unit, and maternal drug withdrawal, have been associated with a continuum of reproductive casualty for the fetus ranging from spontaneous abortion and stillbirth to preterm delivery, intrauterine growth retardation, or full-term delivery without complications (Finnegan, 1976; Finnegan, 1982). About one-third of drug-affected children are born preterm, which makes them biologically vulnerable on two fronts. First, they may have complications related to their prematurity, which can include intracranial bleeds, visual handicaps, cerebral palsy, and learning problems; second, they may have biological complications stemming from the effects of their mothers' prenatal drug use on the developing organ systems of the fetus. The remaining two-thirds of this group, born full-term, are also at risk for developmental problems resulting from the effects of prenatal drug exposure.

A further health risk that seems to be unique to newborns who were exposed prenatally to cocaine and methamphetamine is the occurrence of hemorrhagic infarctions in the central nervous system. Dixon and Bejar observed a group of full-term infants who had uncomplicated deliveries and who had been exposed prenatally to cocaine and methamphetamine (Dixon & Bejar, 1989). In one-third of these neonates, small central nervous system bleeds or infarctions were seen on cranial ultrasound examination. More rarely, antenatal cerebral infarction has been described in infants exposed prenatally to cocaine (Chasnoff, Bussey, Savich, & Stack, 1986). In addition to the vascular changes seen in the central nervous system, electroencephalogram abnormalities also have been noted, particularly in the temporal and frontal lobes (Dixon & Bejar,

1989; Doberczak, Shanzer, Senie, & Kandall, 1988; Hoyme et al., 1990). There have been reports of interferences in other organ systems as well, including limb development and kidney structure (Bingol et al., 1987).

Yet another health concern in infants exposed prenatally to drugs is the increased incidence of sudden infant death syndrome, or SIDS (Chavez, Ostrea, Stryker, & Smialek, 1979; Davidson Ward et al., 1990; Householder, Hatcher, Burns, & Chasnoff, 1982). The etiology of SIDS is unknown, but it is felt to have multiple causes. Exposure to toxic substances such as cocaine, methamphetamine, and heroin may interfere with an infant's normal physiological mechanisms. It is unclear at whether some early deaths from SIDS may have the same etiology as the overdose deaths of adults, who, in most cases, die from the complications of respiratory tachypnea, followed by seizures or cardiac arrhythmia (Smith, 1986).

Failure to thrive is yet another health disorder seen in infants who were prenatally exposed to drugs. It is a syndrome of disordered growth and development characterized by a marked deceleration in weight gain and a slowing in acquisition of developmental milestones (Rudolph, 1991). There are many reasons why an infant may not gain weight. Medical reasons resulting from biological causes include vomiting, excessive diarrhea, poor swallowing, cystic fibrosis, and congenital heart disease. Of course, infants also fail to gain weight if they are given insufficient protein and calories. This may occur if the caregiver mixes formula improperly, does not feed frequently enough, or fails to respond to the infant's signals when he or she is hungry.

In infants who were prenatally exposed to drugs and alcohol, failure to thrive may be due to both medical and environmental factors. A pattern of poor sucking, swallowing difficulties, and distractibility has been observed in many of these infants. In addition, children who live in dysfunctional, chemically dependent families are at increased risk for receiving inadequate nutrition on a consistent basis. Another cause of insufficient weight gain is related to emotional neglect.

Not infrequently, drug-exposed infants do not receive adequate nurturing and may actually turn away when food is offered.

Neonatal Neurobehavioral Status

Not only is the prenatally drug-exposed infant's health status of concern, pediatricians also must assess the newborn's neurological responses, which may be altered by the effects of prenatal substance abuse. We cannot address the effects of paternal substance abuse on the developing fetus at this time, as most research on this topic has been conducted with rats and mice. These animal studies, however, have shown that the offspring of males who are given morphine, methadone, or marijuana before mating are affected, even when drugs are not administered to the females (Dalterio & De Rooji, 1986; Jofee, Peterson, Smith, & Soyka, 1976; Sonderegger, O'Shea, & Zimmerman, 1979). Furthermore, researchers using human subjects have demonstrated that the children of alcoholic fathers are more likely to have lower birth weights, and their sons are more likely to perform less well in school than their sisters or children of nonalcoholics (Little & Sing, 1988; Tarter, Jacob, & Bremer, 1990).

During the past ten years, the bulk of the research has focused on maternal substance abuse and the effects of in-utero exposure to illicit drugs of abuse such as cocaine, methamphetamine, heroin, and PCP. There is extensive documentation of the early withdrawal syndrome commonly seen in infants prenatally exposed to heroin and the synthetic opiate methadone. These newborns typically are tremulous, irritable, and hypertonic, and suffer problems of vomiting and diarrhea (Finnegan, 1975; Wilson, Desmond, & Verniaud, 1973). They have poor motor control, attend less well to visual stimuli, and have increased responses to auditory sounds in the environment (Hans, Marcus, Jeremy, & Auerbach, 1984).

Cocaine and methamphetamine, once believed to be harmless recreational drugs, now have been shown to have serious and severe effects on adults as well as on infants exposed to these substances in utero. Studies have cited a higher incidence of decreased birth weight and small head circumference (Chasnoff et al., 1989; Cherukuri et al., 1988; MacGregor et al., 1987; Yonekura, Inkelis, & Smith-Wallace, 1987; Zuckerman et al., 1989). Unlike the hyperirritable infant withdrawing from prenatal exposure to heroin or methadone, the cocaine-exposed newborn tends to be lethargic and poorly responsive, has fluctuating muscle tone ranging from hypotonia to a hypertonia state with mild tremors, and has difficulty organizing a coordinated sucking mechanism and sleeping patterns (Oro & Dixon, 1987). Furthermore, these infants have rapid emotional state changes that can range from quiet sleep to irritable crying within an extremely brief span of time.

Finally, studies of infants prenatally exposed to the synthetic anesthetic and hallucinogen PCP have documented irritability, tremors, darting eye movements, and increased sensitivity to environmental stimuli (Howard, Kropenske, & Tyler, 1986; Strauss, Modanlou, & Bosu, 1981).

Developmental Patterns During the First Twelve Months

The majority of substance-affected infants have significant feeding and sleeping problems throughout their first six months of life (Deren, 1986). Protracted, high-pitched cries, frantic sucking of fists, tremors, and inability to organize normal sleep–wake cycles also continue to be observed. Infants exposed prenatally to heroin or methadone may suffer ongoing vomiting and diarrhea and exhibit excessive movements that burn up calories and contribute to poor growth and weight gain during the first half year. More recently, it has been noted that infants exposed prenatally to cocaine and methamphetamine demonstrate a different pattern of feeding and sleeping difficulties. They often have hyperphagia (excessive sucking and swallowing as if from extreme hunger), uncoordinated sucking, and poor weight gain. These prolonged withdrawal patterns can disrupt family life and exhaust care-givers. When a caregiver is thus frustrated by a demanding and irritable infant and is unfamiliar with how to provide the practical care needed, the infant may be neglected, demonstrate poor weight gain, or be physically abused.

During the second half of the first year, the majority of these infants begin to organize their sleep–wake cycles, have more success with feeding, become less irritable, attend visually to their caregivers, and, more often than not, look as if they have recovered from the developmental effects of their prenatal substance exposure. When standardized developmental evaluations are administered and the motor, cognitive, language, and personal-social areas of behavior are assessed, as a group these children score within the low normal range, as compared with non-drug-exposed groups, who score within the median normal range (Hans, Marcus, Jeremy, & Auerbach, 1984; Kaltenbach & Finnegan, 1984; Rosen & Johnson, 1982; Sowder & Burt, 1980).

The Early Childhood Years

During the second and third years of life, a child's developmental patterns become more complex and easier to assess. For instance, problem-solving, personal-social skills, and speech and receptive language evolve during this time period to the extent where the professional can determine smaller increments of progress (such as the number of words in a two-year-old child's vocabulary, as compared with cooing sounds in a six-month-old child's vocabulary).

Clinical researchers who have followed children exposed prenatally to heroin and methadone report developmental outcomes that continue within the low-to-normal range (Johnson, Diano, & Rosen, 1984; Kaltenbach & Finnegan, 1984; Wilson, Desmond, & Verniaud, 1973). However, concerns begin to emerge about the more subtle behaviors that may influence successful learning experiences and eventual productive adult life. Attention deficits, hyperactivity, impulsive behaviors, aggressiveness, poor language skills,

and difficulties in making friends and in social interactions have caught the attention of researchers in this field. In a recent longitudinal study, Griffith (1990) reported that 30–40% of preschool children exposed prenatally to cocaine demonstrated learning difficulties as assessed by standardized developmental measures. At UCLA, we have noted that preschool-aged children who were exposed prenatally to PCP, along with cocaine, marijuana, or alcohol, also present with low normal scores in the areas of language and personal-social development, as compared with a non-drug-exposed control group (Beckwith, Crawford, Moore, & Howard, in press). Thus, current studies of children who have been exposed to multiple substances show that they are similar in their developmental course to the children who were examined during the 1970s who had primary exposure to heroin or methadone. In summary, the majority of preschool-aged children demonstrate low normal to normal intelligence, do not exhibit neurological dysfunction as seen in cerebral palsy, and do not present with obvious mental retardation (IQ below 70).

Our group at UCLA has had findings similar to those described above when using structured evaluations to elicit children's developmental responses. However, as Wilson stated many years ago, the quality of these children's interactions with toys and with people in their environments is different from that of children who were not prenatally exposed to drugs (Wilson, 1976). In order to quantify these children's play behaviors in situations where there is no adult supervision, our researchers videotaped a group of toddlers who had had uncomplicated births and who had been exposed prenatally to heroin, methadone, cocaine, amphetamine, or PCP, and compared their activities with those of a group of preterm toddlers who had weighed less than 1,500 grams at birth and who had been respirator-dependent. The findings showed that the preterm toddlers played purposefully with dolls, baby bottles, beds, trucks, pots, and pans, organizing their play into meaningful patterns of interaction (for example, they pretended to cook with the pots and pans and fed themselves and the baby dolls). The toddlers who had been prenatally exposed to drugs showed practically no organized play behavior and often chewed or threw the toys in a purposeless fashion (Rodning, Beckwith, & Howard, 1989). These results add to the growing body of knowledge about these infants' high-risk status in terms of successfully functioning as independent, well-organized students in elementary school (Lodge, 1976).

The biological risk resulting from prenatal substance exposure on the developmental abilities of these children must be considered in light of the environmental factors, which also can exercise a significant effect on the development of prenatally substance-exposed children. The disorganized drug lifestyle, compounded by the multiple social and health problems associated with addiction, often hampers parents' ability to provide care and adequately supervise their children's daily activities. As noted previously, substance-abusing parents often are intermittent caregivers whose own physical need for drugs and altered mental status make them emotionally and physically inaccessible to their children.

From a research point of view, investigators are attempting to disentangle the biological effects of drugs on the developing fetus and child from the ongoing environmental impact of the chemically dependent lifestyle. For example, our team at UCLA began to examine this issue more closely in light of the possible causes of the children's poor play organization. Our goal was to clarify as much as possible whether the deviant behaviors were due to a biological cause interfering with higher cortical function, or whether they were responses to environmental conditions. It is known, for instance, that children who are raised in caring home environments and who are comfortable in their relationships with their parents or caregivers have a better social adjustment later in life (Sroufe & Fleeson, 1986). Thus, with this particular group of toddlers, we evaluated the children's attachment behaviors to their caregivers using a research paradigm that measures environmental impact.

Children who had been exposed to drugs who appeared to feel secure in the presence of their caregivers had better scores in their play attempts, but still did not score as high as the non-drug-exposed preterm group. Thus, from a clinical point of view, both biological and environmental factors affected these children's behaviors, and both must be considered if treatment programs are to be successful in alleviating some of the difficulties these children may have in their developmental outcomes.

Childhood and Adolescence

Only one reported longitudinal study has evaluated the impact of prenatal substance abuse into adolescence. This research project has followed from birth white, middle-class children who were exposed prenatally to alcohol. The majority of children whose mothers consumed alcohol throughout pregnancy have learning and behavioral difficulties in school, have difficulty making and maintaining friendships, and will need special assistance if they are to successfully enter the job market (Streissguth et al., 1991).

There have been some studies of older children and teenagers being raised by parents in drug treatment, but these children's prenatal exposure to drugs has not been ascertained. These youngsters have demonstrated behavioral and school adjustment problems (Herjanic, Barredo, Herjanic, & Tomelleri, 1979; Sowder & Burt, 1980).

In another study of older children living with addicted parents, Sowder and Burt found that 57% of the children between three and seven years of age performed poorly on tests measuring IQ and perceptual motor performance (Sowder & Burt, 1980). The children also had greater anxiety, more insecurity, and shorter attention spans. In addition, these researchers looked at the school performance of eight- to seventeen-year-old children of addicted parents. They found that teachers reported more behavior problems, repeated grades, and absences. Furthermore, the children of addicts exhibited an increased number of delinquent acts, and these acts were more serious than those of children in the control group. Finally, these children were more likely to abuse drugs and be in drug treatment programs themselves.

A few studies have examined the behaviors of children who were exposed to drugs and placed in out-of-home care (Fanshel, 1975; Nichtern, 1973; Sowder, Carnes, & Sherman, 1981). The children included in these studies have demonstrated learning difficulties in school, poor school adjustment, and problems in their relationships with adults and peers. Additionally, mental health problems were more frequent in this population.

LEGAL ISSUES

With respect to its legal implications, prenatal substance abuse presents professionals with a complex dilemma (Cole, 1990; Moore, 1990). At one end of the continuum of opinions about child abuse is the viewpoint that the unborn child may be entitled to protection under state child abuse and neglect status. During the past two decades, a number of legal conditions have been established to protect the fetus, including the fetus's right to sue for personal injury, to be protected by criminal law, and to inherit property (Johnsen, 1986). Additionally, unborn children have been granted independent legal rights ("Negligent Hiring and Retention of Babysitter," 1984, *Roussey v. Roussey,* 1985; "Suing Mom," 1985). At the other end of the continuum, some have taken the stand that the legal principles embodied in *Roe v. Wade* (1973) imply that the unborn are not persons entitled to protection under the Constitution's Fourteenth Amendment (Jessup & Roth, 1988). The answers to the question about child abuse and neglect in the prenatal situation lie beyond the scope of this chapter.

However, the postnatal status of prenatally drug-exposed infants with respect to legal implications may not be as controversial as the prenatal status. The stance proposed by Douglas J. Besharov, resident scholar at the American Enterprise Institute for Public Policy Research,

gives us a common-sense approach for addressing this issue at the time of birth. Besharov notes that unless the child is or will be seriously harmed thereby, chemically dependent parents should not be reported. However, he makes the point that chronic severe substance abuse does interfere with the adult's alert state. Thus, if a dependent child is under the care of a chronic substance abuser, imminent harm is a real consideration (Besharov, 1990).

All health care providers are required to report reasonable suspicion of child abuse and neglect according to child abuse reporting statutes in every state (English, 1990). During the newborn period, the overriding reason for suspecting child abuse and neglect traditionally has not been parental involvement in illegal activities but rather concern about the parent's ability to provide a safe environment for the baby. The terms *endangerment, safe environment,* and *safety from harm* all have been used by reporters of suspected child abuse and neglect to describe conditions under which a report should or should not be made. Is it justified for a physician to assume that parental chemical dependency is grounds for filing a child abuse report? The altered mental status associated with addiction may impair a parent's capacity to provide adequate protection for a dependent child. Thus, does chronic parental substance abuse provide the professional with reasonable cause to suspect that the child is at risk of imminent harm? If this is the case, the filing of a report initiates a process of evaluation to determine whether the child is safe from harm. Further, filing a report also provides a means for the health care provider to urge parents to seek drug rehabilitation and other necessary services to support family needs.

Under these conditions of reporting, the civil courts—not the criminal courts—become involved. During the civil court process, the child's safety is assessed, followed by a judicial ruling. The guilt or innocence of the child's parent is not at issue (Bross, 1988). This view does not support criminal sanctions, but instead advocates treatment for children and families, backed by the legal clout of the civil court. In *The Harvard Mental Health Letter*, Richard S. Schottenfeld, a physician with subspecialty training in addictionology, has stated that there is considerable evidence that some kind of leverage is almost always needed to counter the denial that is often present in drug and alcohol addiction (Schottenfeld, 1990).

During the past decade, states have begun to move away from viewing a newborn's positive toxicology screen as the single indicator that the infant is at risk of imminent harm (English, 1990). What is far more important than a positive screen is the parent's lifestyle and capacity to provide a safe environment for the child (Wilker, 1990). We know that chemically dependent families have complex problems and comprehensive service needs. A positive or negative urine toxicology screen—which tells us only what substances the mother may have ingested during the 72 hours before the screen—does not provide professionals with the kinds of information they need to develop an appropriate treatment plan that includes all family members.

Professionals must develop the skills to elicit a history from the parents that provides information about their capacity to parent a child (such as preparations for the infant's arrival, income to support the parent and child, appropriate shelter, family and community support systems, and alcohol or drug abuse). This history, corroborated by the professional's observations, is the key to establishing an individual family treatment plan.

PREVENTION AND TREATMENT STRATEGIES

The increase in the numbers of teenagers and adults, including women of childbearing age, who abuse illicit substances has resulted in a burgeoning industry of primary, secondary, and tertiary approaches to prevention and treatment. To understand the advancements that have been made in this area, one need only look at the restricted scope of treatment programs available until recent years.

Methadone maintenance was introduced as an option for long-term treatment of opioid dependency thirty years ago, when heroin was the most commonly abused drug. These programs were established by a few forward-thinking professionals who specialized in treating opioid dependency and who recognized that this was a chronic, relapsing health disorder. However, with a few exceptions, most methadone programs did not have a family emphasis and, instead, focused primarily on the adult male user (Finnegan, 1975). Furthermore, because of the relatively small number of heroin addicts, prevention efforts did not gain national attention.

Today, with polysubstance abuse becoming more and more prevalent, the issue is even more complex. Methadone, for instance, is known not to be effective in the treatment of cocaine, methamphetamine, phencyclidine (PCP), and many other addictions. Research is being done to evaluate the use of other medications to counter the addictive qualities of these substances, but to date nothing has proven successful. Besides these efforts to control addiction through medical modalities, we now recognize the importance of diverse social and cultural factors that can have a profound influence on recovery. If chemical dependency treatment is to be effective, it is critical that these issues form the underpinning of the overall treatment approach.

Concomitant with the emergence of methadone maintenance as a treatment option for heroin addicts in the '60s, the medical community had barely begun to consider the effects of parental substance abuse upon the fetus. For instance, the diagnosis of fetal alcohol syndrome had not yet been generally recognized as a consequence of maternal ethanol abuse (Clarren & Smith, 1978), despite the fact that the deleterious effects of alcohol on the fetus had been described since biblical times and more thoroughly in the mid-1800s by William Carpenter, an examiner in physiology at the University of London (Carpenter, 1851). For unknown reasons, these descriptions were largely ignored, and prevention efforts were minimal. It would be two decades before prevention activities related to the impact of illicit substances on the health of the pregnant woman and the fetus gained national attention.

Since that time, studies to formally evaluate the toxic effects of various substances of abuse have been undertaken. Researchers working in the field of addictionology have made progress in recognizing what is needed in the areas of prevention and treatment, but much still remains unknown about specific programs that will produce positive results. Through the efforts of professionals, the media, and—most importantly—members of chemically dependent families to educate the executive and legislative branches of the federal government regarding this societal problem, creation of new programs has been made possible.

The Executive Office of the President has established the Office of National Drug Control Policy, with the responsibility for setting a national agenda to combat substance abuse. In addition, Congress has established specific agencies within the Department of Health and Human Services (including the National Institute on Drug Abuse, Center for Substance Abuse Prevention, and Center for Substance Abuse Treatment) to direct national research and the development of prevention and treatment programs and has allocated large sums of money to move these programs forward. We are now entering an era of large-scale demonstration and research projects examining specific components that are critical to ensuring the success of prevention and treatment programs.

Primary Prevention

Efforts to prevent drug use on a national scale have been multifaceted. During the 1980s, "Just Say No to Drugs" became a national and international theme in substance abuse prevention. The program encompassed a variety of approaches, ranging from grass-roots campaigns using buttons and posters to organized educational programs with sessions for the children and their family members, to gala media events. Although

there were and remain many critics of this simplistic approach to addiction, it is unquestionable that large-scale efforts must be directed toward primary prevention and education.

Another program, called DARE (drug awareness, resistance, education), had its origins in Southern California during the early 1980s and has become adopted by many other states since its inception. The DARE program uses law enforcement personnel to educate elementary and junior high school-aged children about drugs and their impact on the user's functioning.

In addition to this specific program stemming from law enforcement, national sports associations, including the National Football League and the National Basketball Association, have presented a strong media message using well-known sports figures to advise children to stay off drugs.

These are examples of some of the most prominent primary prevention programs that have received national attention. However, various organizations within individual communities also have targeted prevention efforts toward specific groups—not only children. State health departments, for example, commonly distribute a variety of brochures and other educational materials discussing the risks of prenatal substance exposure.

Secondary Prevention

Substantial energy and resources have been invested in secondary prevention efforts during the past few years. The National Institute on Drug Abuse (NIDA) has funded 20 research projects, at an approximate cost of $100 million, to study the effectiveness of decreasing alcohol and drug use through sensitive and comprehensive treatment programs for pregnant women. In contrast to the narrow scope of services offered to addicts in the 1960s, these projects include many components: prenatal health care; drug treatment; pediatric care; nutritional, vocational, and educational training for mothers; parenting education; and home- and center-based services for families that include procurement of housing, financial counseling, referral to local food banks and shelters, and early intervention services for children in the household. By the mid-1990s, these projects will have collected data to help determine the specific components of treatment programs that are useful for chemically dependent families.

The effectiveness of current treatment programs directed at chemically dependent pregnant women and their offspring is unknown because this is a new area of intervention (with drugs such as cocaine, methamphetamine, and phencyclidine). In addition, we have entered a new era of understanding about the influence of genetics, cultural background, and family history (including child abuse and neglect) on the behavior of substance abusers.

In 1986, the Anti-Drug Abuse Act mandated an independent study of substance abuse treatment programs. The Institute of Medicine (IOM), along with the National Academy of Sciences, compiled a report describing state-of-the-art knowledge in this area. In this report on non-methadone treatment programs, out of 1,600 outpatient clients, 17% remained in the programs for a six-month period. Furthermore, in a residential, therapeutic setting, there was no significant improvement in substance abuse for clients who stayed less than 90 days. However, for clients who remained in treatment for longer than three months, outcome correlated significantly with total length of stay. The outcome measures for the majority of secondary prevention programs address drug use, criminal behavior, and employability. Because the majority of clients studied were males between 20 and 40 years of age, parenting behaviors were not evaluated (Kumpfer, 1991). Still, we can infer from this study that short-term treatment programs will not be as effective as longer-term programs for women as well as for men.

This author has been involved with several small, comprehensive treatment programs for pregnant addicts and their offspring. In one study involving 20 prenatally substance-exposed infants, a professional team composed of pediatricians, social workers, and public health nurses provided comprehensive services to these children and their families (Howard & Kropenske, 1990). Family composition among this group included 25 biological parents, 28 siblings, 16 extended family members, and 20 foster parents who also served as surrogate parents for some of the infants. The two primary goals of this program were to promote a stable and nurturing environment for the children and to provide consistent, ongoing health care.

In order to provide professional help based on family needs, program staff recognized the importance of learning about the parents' own backgrounds and current lifestyle. From a social perspective, 75% of the mothers had grown up in households where there was parental drug or alcohol abuse and 40% had experienced physical or sexual abuse. In addition, 100% were polydrug abusers and 55% gave a history of intravenous drug use. Eighty percent of the women had chosen a spouse or partner who also abused drugs or alcohol, and only 15% of the mothers reported a supportive relationship with the infants' fathers at the time of the babies' birth. Of the 15 mothers who had older children, 45% had a child in foster care or in the care of a relative.

The mothers' healthcare during the current pregnancy was also inadequate, with one-third of the women seeking no prenatal care. Finally, 50% of these women had obstetrical complications during delivery. In addition to these maternal issues that needed to be incorporated into the family treatment plans, project staff had to address a variety of health concerns with regard to the babies.

There were nine preterm and eleven full-term infants, all of whom demonstrated neurobehavioral symptoms such as tremors, irritability, and increased muscle tone. Significant medical complications were seen in 50% of the infants, including chronic lung disease, intraventricular hemorrhage, seizure disorders, and retinal detachment. Once the infants' medical status had stabilized and they were ready for discharge from the nursery, project staff collaborated with other agencies that are not typically involved in formulating family treatment plans.

Because all of the mothers had a history of chronic substance abuse and all infants had been exposed prenatally to drugs and were symptomatic following delivery, hospital protocol required that children's protective services (CPS) investigate the parents' ability to provide a safe home environment. In some instances, CPS determined that the parental home did not provide adequate safety. In those cases, the family court system became involved and participated in the family treatment plan. Before discharge, through the efforts of interdisciplinary personnel, 25% of the infants were discharged to their biological parents, 35% were placed with relatives, and 40% were placed in foster care. In all of these cases, project staff, working closely with community agencies, encouraged the parents to participate in drug treatment, offered support to temporary caregivers, and moved toward family reunification for children who were in out-of-home placement.

Intervention for each identified infant had three areas of emphasis. These were developmental assessment of the infant and siblings, as well as coordination of their health care and services; provision of information to the parents, foster parents, and extended family members about children's developmental, health, and immunization needs, safety, and nutrition; and assistance to all adults involved with the children regarding referrals for needed services, counseling, and help during crises.

At the completion of this two-year project funded by the U.S. Department of Education, project staff completed their work with the families, not because the families no longer required their support, but because the funding period had ended. At this time, cases were transferred to community agencies, including CPS, public health, programs for the developmentally disabled, the public schools, and substance abuse treatment programs. In reviewing the salient outcomes of this service program, we determined the following: all of the infants had received ongoing health care, timely immunizations, and adequate nutrition; at twelve months of age, 50% of the children demonstrated developmental disabilities and were referred to a federally and state-funded community agency for further assessment and early education services; all of the infants' caregivers received extensive education regarding the clinical manifestations of prenatal substance exposure and the special care needs of these infants, resulting in only two changes in placement per child during the first twelve months rather than the five that occurred without this early support; and all of the siblings received healthcare and developmental evaluations, and almost 50% required supplemental treatment from health and educational agencies. Notably, following discharge and throughout the project period, there were no reports of suspected child abuse or neglect in connection with the twenty infants.

In contrast to this hospital-based program, innovative family preservation projects targeting substance-abusing parents and their children are becoming highly visible in large urban areas. Typically, these programs are associated with public agencies such as child welfare. However, they also focus on the family as a unit, with the goal of providing short-term, highly concentrated social work intervention with the family. The unique aspects of these programs include extremely small staff caseloads, 24-hour availability, and the family home as primary site for the delivery of services.

An example of a family preservation project is "Families First," located in Detroit. Counselors work with only two families at a time, spending 20 to 30 hours each week in a family's home. They provide assistance with household tasks, child care, counseling, parent education, and assistance with obtaining health care, substance abuse treatment, and needed community services. During the first 16 months of this project, these intensive services enabled children to remain with their biologic families in 75% of cases.

Secondary prevention is critical because, unlike a primary form of prevention, it targets a specific individual or family unit. Professionals key in on strategies that are uniquely grounded both in a solid general knowledge of their discipline and in thorough and specific information about the individual who will receive the services.

Tertiary Prevention

Within the domain of perinatal substance abuse, tertiary prevention addresses the lifelong physical, healthcare, educational, social, employment, and, in some cases, total dependency needs of prenatally drug-exposed children. Because this epidemic peaked only in the mid-'80s, for the first wave of children who experienced chronic exposure to drugs and alcohol throughout their mothers' pregnancies and whose fathers' sperm may have been affected by substance abuse, the range of services these children will require is unknown. However, the reader should refer to Chapter 17 of this volume, which discusses programs that have been successfully developed and implemented for offspring of alcoholics. These models will no doubt be similar to those that will be needed to adequately serve the needs of drug-exposed children.

The educational system will play an important longitudinal role in overseeing many of the components that will be needed to serve these children. For instance, children's general healthcare is addressed by school nurses. Nutritional programs also are an integral part of the daily school routine. School counselors, psychologists, and social workers will be involved in monitoring the children's unique learning styles and in ensuring that their home environments are safe and relatively stable. Issues related to child abuse and neglect also fall under the aegis of school personnel, who are mandated reporters.

It is anticipated that 30–50% of the children who have been chronically exposed to drugs prenatally will require educational services above and beyond those provided for the general school population, based on the biological impact of their prenatal experiences on the central nervous system. For this group of children, the disabilities will range from cerebral palsy or sensory deficits, to mental retardation, to learning problems associated with normal intelligence. The time of identification of this group's disabilities will vary because certain presenting difficulties may occur during infancy (such as cerebral palsy, sensory deficits, and mental retardation) whereas others may not become diagnostically apparent until late preschool or early elementary school years (such as learning disabilities and hyperactivity).

Children who escape the biological impact of prenatal substance exposure may not escape the deleterious effects of growing up in dysfunctional and chaotic households. The environment plays a significant role in promoting a child's success or failure in life. In addition, the environment can temper some of the problems caused by biological interference, including some of the symptoms described in the preceding paragraph. Thus, schools will have a key part in addressing the social and emotional difficulties that may arise when children are living in nonnurturing, unstable environments (such as crack houses or multiple caregiving environments that lack continuity and support).

However, the schools alone cannot provide all of the services these children will require during their years of traditional education. Educational systems will need to collaborate with many agencies, including healthcare and mental health providers, community programs (including recreation and parks), after-school programs for the disabled, drug and alcohol treatment programs, and vocational training programs.

A tertiary prevention model developed by the Los Angeles Unified School District took a dynamic approach to this relatively new situation. In 1987, in response to this author's presentation to the Los Angeles School Board, a birth-to-five preschool day program was established to serve prenatally drug-exposed children and their parents. The infants and toddlers program included attendance by parents, with a focus on improving the parents' enjoyment of their children's progress and helping with general parent issues, including the importance of attending drug treatment programs. The preschool class-room the three- to five-year-olds attended was more typical of a nursery school program. It was held five days a week, and the children were bused to the school. Parents were invited to observe their children in the classroom, and school staff members made home visits. The emphasis of this program was on readying the children for entrance into elementary school. This required the children to learn school routines, pay attention to directions, demonstrate appropriate social interactions with their peers and adults, and have a chance to be creative in play and language activities in order to enhance self-esteem.

A third component of this program was the transition from preschool into elementary school. The uniqueness of this aspect of the program stemmed from teachers' observations in the preschool program that many of these children have emotional and behavioral difficulty when faced with a new situation. Thus, the teachers prepared the children for the transition from the preschool program, introduced the new teachers to the children, and accompanied the children as they moved into their new kindergarten classrooms. Besides easing the transition for the children, this program acquainted the new teachers with the children's developmental strengths and problem areas. Through teacher–teacher and teacher–student support systems, the children were set up to succeed.

A further component that was considered involved the use of more school-based social workers working collaboratively with the teachers. This team effort would have served the entire family. The specific role of the social worker was to enhance the teacher's understanding of the child's role within the family. For instance, the social worker would make home visits, provide counseling sessions, and refer family members to community agencies, with the aim of ensuring that there was a healthy, functioning family unit behind the child. This team effort, which also would have included the parents, no doubt would have led to the establishment of other not-yet-identified components to help these children become productive citizens. Unfortunately, however, this model program was discontinued.

AN OPTIMAL INTERVENTION PLAN

Substance-abusing families present unique challenges to professionals providing health, educational, social welfare, mental health, and legal services. In order for a parent to ensure that a child is in the best of health and has educational opportunities that will foster his or her individual abilities, that parent must be able to locate and secure appropriate services. Based on our knowledge of chemically dependent parents (such as their altered mental status, the nature of addiction, and the illegal activities revolving around drug use), healthcare providers, educators, and other involved professionals must be informed about the disorder of addiction and its impact on the daily life of the substance abuser. We cannot assume that chemically dependent parents will be able to advocate effectively for their children, work as team members in providing for their children's health and educational needs, and follow through with professional recommendations on a consistent basis.

If we want these "special-needs parents" to participate in community programs serving their needs, we must ensure that the parents themselves receive treatment for their addiction as well as parenting education and mental health services, if required. Furthermore, in cases where children have been temporarily removed from their biologic parents' custody because of suspected child abuse or neglect and are under the care of extended family members or foster parents, we must coordinate our efforts to ensure that information about the children is shared not only with the court-assigned caregivers, but also with the biological parents. Further, we must provide information to the temporary caregivers to help them obtain appropriate health and educational services for the children.

Providing these services will require the cooperation of professionals who traditionally have not been involved in meeting the health and educational needs of developmentally disabled children. Drug and alcohol treatment counselors, child protective services workers, law enforcement professionals, and members of the judicial system must join forces with medical and educational professionals to provide chemically dependent families with coordinated treatment services that promote a family unit that is physically and emotionally healthy. Training programs for graduate and postgraduate students from the disciplines of medicine, law, psychology, nursing, social work, education, drug treatment, special education, and other relevant areas must be developed so that these professionals will have the expertise to address these families' special needs and work collaboratively in providing coordinated and comprehensive services.

The ultimate prevention for the problems associated with chemical dependency in families is curtailment of all substance abuse. However, this appears to lie well beyond the scope of current prevention efforts. Therefore, the agencies that serve these families—whether from the healthcare, social services, or legal field—must develop formal interagency agreements if they are to provide the comprehensive and coordinated services that are so critical for this population. Only with such interdisciplinary collaboration will these children be able to grow up in safe, nurturing, and healthy environments that encourage education and productive involvement in society.

A new player in the arena of providing family services, from the healthcare perspective, is the legal system. Within our society, courts, judges, defense attorneys, prosecutors, and law enforcement officials are not usually viewed as functioning in the realm of family well-being. In fact, within the area of child abuse and neglect, the legal system may have much to offer in terms of providing incentives for maintaining safe environments for children. In order for the legal system to function effectively in this way, role definition and delineation of responsibilities among the various disciplines that serve these families are essential.

The following is an example of how physicians, nurses, social workers, and psychologists can work together with the judicial system to improve communication and understanding. An interdisciplinary team of professionals who had worked extensively with this population in conjunction with major community agencies (child welfare and public health) met with the supervising judge of the Los Angeles County family courts. From the outset, there was mutual interest and respect in each other's work with chemically dependent families.

Through this two-way communication, information was shared about the health and welfare concerns of these children within the current system. There were children, for instance, who were placed in foster homes that were miles from the residences of their biological families, thus impeding eventual family reunification. Many chemically dependent parents seeking drug treatment, whether court-ordered or not, were unable to find openings, thus making them unable to meet the conditions for regaining custody laid out by the court. Other addicted parents who had promised to enter drug rehabilitation made no efforts to pursue treatment.

Once the judge became more familiar with the multiple health and social problems of chemically dependent families, as well as the high-risk status for developmental disabilities of their children, he proceeded to learn more about the details of cases currently passing through the court system. Two major accomplishments came out of this collaboration. The first was a protocol developed to assist family court judges in making informed decisions regarding these cases. The second was the publication of an article titled "Child Abuse, Substance Abuse, and the Role of the Dependency Court" in the *Harvard BlackLetter Journal* by a law student who completed a field placement with the presiding judge (Wilker, 1990).

Community prevention efforts to improve the situation for chemically dependent families must involve not only the dependency court system, but also the health, social welfare, developmental disabilities, drug treatment, and education fields. Training programs offering specialized information about the field of substance abuse are necessary to enable various professionals to develop services for chemically dependent families, as well as to implement effective prevention programs at every level and within every related discipline.

These prevention efforts are the responsibility of professionals from many disciplines. Physicians can provide children, adolescents, pregnant women, and parents with information about the impact of substance abuse on health. Nurses in community health clinics also are responsible for educating their clients about the deleterious effects of chemical dependency on families. Social workers in hospital clinics, community programs, and child protective services agencies should incorporate information about substance abuse into counseling efforts. Teachers in both public and private school settings can address this topic with their students. Psychologists, mental health counselors, drug and alcohol treatment counselors, and developmental disabilities specialists also should inform their clients about the effects of various substances of abuse and how they interfere with mental processing and family life. Legal professionals have the responsibility of providing anticipatory guidance about the legal consequences that often are related to addiction.

REFERENCES

Abel, E. L., & Sokol, R. J. (1987). Incidence of fetal alcohol syndrome and economic impact of FAS-related anomalies. *Drug and Alcohol Dependency, 19,* 51–70.

Beckwith, L., Crawford, S., Moore, J. A., & Howard, J. (in press). Attentional and social functioning of preschool-age children exposed to PCP and cocaine in utero. In M. Lewis, M. Bendersky, & Taft (Eds.), *Cocaine Mothers and Cocaine Babies: The Role of Toxins in Development.* Hillsdale, N.J.: Erlbaum Associates.

Besharov, D. J. (1989). The children of crack: Will we protect them? *Public Welfare* (Fall), 6–11.

Besharov, D. J. (1990). *Mandatory reporting of child abuse and research on the effects of prenatal drug exposure.* Presentation given before the National Institute on Drug Abuse Technical Review Meeting on Methodological Issues in Epidemiological, Prevention, and Treatment Research on the Effects of Prenatal Drug Exposure on Women and Children, July. Currently in press as a NIDA research monograph.

Billing, L., Eriksson, M., Larsson, G., & Zetterström, R. (1979). Occurrence of abuse and neglect of children born to amphetamine addicted mothers. *Child Abuse and Neglect, 3,* 205–211.

Bingol, N., Fuchs, M., Diaz, V., Stone, R. K., & Gromisch, D. S. (1987). Teratogenicity of cocaine in humans. *Journal of Pediatrics, 110,* 93–96.

Blanche, S., Rouzioux, C., Moscato, M. L., Veber, F., Mayaux, M. J., Jacomet, C., Tricoire, J., DeVille, A., Vial, F., & Firtion, G. (1989). A prospective study of infants born to women seropositive for human immunodeficiency virus type 1. *New England Journal of Medicine, 320* (25), 1643–1648.

Bross, D. (1988). Medical diagnosis as a gateway to the child welfare system: A legal review for physicians, lawyers, and social workers. *Denver University Law Review, 65* (2–3), 213–253.

Burns, R., Lerner, S. E., Corrado, R., James, S. H., Schnoll, S. H. (1975). Phencyclidine: States of acute intoxication and fatalities. *Western Journal of Medicine, 123,* 345.

Carpenter, W. V. (1851). *Use and abuse of alcoholic liquors.* Boston: Crosby and Nichols, for the Massachusetts Temperance Society.

Carr, J. N. (1975). Drug patterns among drug-addicted mothers: Incidence, variance in use, and effects on children. *Pediatric Annals, 4* (7), 408–417.

Chasnoff, I. J., Bussey, M. E., Savich, R., & Stack, C. M. (1986). Perinatal cerebral infarction and maternal cocaine use. *Journal of Pediatrics, 108* (3), 456–459.

Chasnoff, I. J., Griffith, D. R., MacGregor, S., Dirkes, K., & Burns, K. A. (1989). Temporal patterns of cocaine use in pregnancy: Perinatal outcome. *Journal of the American Medical Association, 261* (12), 1741–1744.

Chavez, C. J., Ostrea, E. M., Jr., Stryker, J. C., & Smialek, Z. (1979). Sudden infant death syndrome among infants of drug-dependent mothers. *Journal of Pediatrics, 95* (3), 407–409.

Cherukuri, R., Minkoff, H., Feldman, J., Parekh, A., & Glass, L. (1988). A cohort study of alkaloidal cocaine ("crack") in pregnancy. *Obstetrics and Gynecology, 72* (2), 147–151.

Clarren, S. K., & Smith, D. W. (1978). The fetal alcohol syndrome. *New England Journal of Medicine, 298* (19), 1063–1067.

Cole, H. M. (1990). Legal interventions during pregnancy: Court-ordered medical treatments and legal penalties for potentially harmful behavior by pregnant women. *Journal of the American Medical Association, 264* (20), 2663–2670.

Colten, M. E. (1980). A comparison of heroin-addicted and non-addicted mothers: Their attitudes, beliefs and parenting experiences. In *NIDA, Services Research Report. Heroin-Addicted Parents and Their Children: Two Reports,* Department of Health and Human Services publication no. ADM 81-1028. Rockville, MD: National Institute on Drug Abuse.

Cuskey, W. R., & Wathey, B. (1982). *Female addiction.* Lexington, MA: Lexington Books.

Dalterio, S. L., & De Rooji, D. C. (1986). Maternal cannabinoid exposure: Effects on spermatogenesis in male offspring. *International Journal of Andrology, 9,* 250–258.

Davidson Ward, S. L., Bautista, D., Chan, L., Derry, M., Lisbin, A., Durfee, M., Mills, K., & Keens, T. (1990). Sudden infant death syndrome in infants of substance-abusing mothers. *Journal of Pediatrics, 117* (6), 876–881.

Deren, S. (1986). Children of substance abusers: A review of the literature. *Journal of Substance Abuse Treatment, 3,* 77–94.

Dixon, S. D., & Bejar, R. (1989). Echoencephalographic findings in neonates associated with maternal cocaine and methamphetamine use: Incidence and clinical correlates. *Journal of Pediatrics, 115* (5, part 1), 770–778.

Doberczak, T. M., Shanzer, S., Senie, R. T., & Kandall, S. R. (1988). Neonatal neurologic and electroencephalographic effects of intrauterine cocaine exposure. *Journal of Pediatrics, 113* (2), 354–358.

Domino, E. F. (1980). History and pharmacology of PCP and PCP-related analogs. *Journal of Psychedelic Drugs, 12* (3–4), 223–227.

English, A. (1990). Prenatal drug exposure: Grounds for mandatory child abuse reports? *Youth Law News (Journal of the National Center for Youth Law) 11* (1), 3–8.

Escamilla-Mondanaro, J. (1977). Women: Pregnancy, children and addiction. *Journal of Psychedelic Drugs, 9* (1), 59–68.

Fanshel, D. (1975). Parental failure and consequences for children: The drug-abusing mother whose children are in foster care. *American Journal of Public Health, 65* (6), 604–612.

Fauman, M. A., & Fauman, B. J. (1980). Chronic phencyclidine (PCP) abuse: A psychiatric perspective. *Journal of Psychedelic Drugs, 12* (3–4), 307–315.

Feig, L. (Jan. 1990). Drug-exposed infants and children: Service needs and policy questions. Executive summary for the U.S. Department of Health and Human Services, Office of the Assistant Secretary for Planning and Evaluation, Division of Children and Youth Policy.

Finnegan, L. P. (1975). Narcotics dependence in pregnancy. *Journal of Psychedelic Drugs, 7* (3), 299–311.

Finnegan, L. P. (1976). Clinical effects of pharmacologic agents on pregnancy, the fetus and the neonate. *Annals of the New York Academy of Sciences, 182,* 74–89.

Finnegan, L. P. (1982). Outcome of children born to women dependent on narcotics. In B. Stimmel (Ed.), *The effects of maternal alcohol and drug abuse on the newborn.* New York: Haworth Press, pp. 55–102.

Finnegan, L. P., & Wapner, R. J. (1987). Narcotic addiction in pregnancy. In J. R. Neibyl (Ed.), *Drug use in pregnancy.* Philadelphia: Lea and Febiger, pp. 203–222.

Friedrich, W. N., Beilke, R., & Urquiza, A. (1988). Behavior problems in young sexually abused boys. *Journal of Interpersonal Violence, 3,* 21–27.

Gawin, F. H., & Ellinwood, Jr., E. H. (1988). Cocaine and other stimulants: Actions, abuse, and treatment. *New England Journal of Medicine, 318* (18), 1173–1182.

General Accounting Office (June 1990). *Drug-exposed infants: A generation at risk.* Publication GAO/HRD-90-138. Washington, DC: U.S. General Accounting Office, Human Resources Division.

Gold, M. S., Washton, A. M., & Dackis, C. A. (1985). Cocaine abuse: Neurochemistry, phenomenology and treatment. In N. J. Kozel & E. H. Adams (Eds.), *Cocaine use in America: Epidemiological and clinical perspectives.* NIDA Research Monograph 61. Rockville, MD: National Institute on Drug Abuse.

Gomby, A., & Shiono, P. H. (1991). Estimating the number of substance-exposed infants. *Future Child, 1,* 17–25.

Hans, S. L., Marcus, J., Jeremy, R., & Auerbach, J. (1984). Neurobehavioral development of children exposed in utero to opioid drugs. *Neurobehavioral Teratology,* 249–273.

Herjanic, B. M., Barredo, V. H., Herjanic, M., & Tomelleri, C. J. (1979). Children of heroin addicts. *International Journal of the Addictions, 14,* 919–931.

Householder, J., Hatcher, R., Burns, W., & Chasnoff, I. (1982). Infants born to narcotic-addicted mothers. *Psychological Bulletin, 92,* 453–468.

Howard, J., Beckwith, L., Rodning, C., & Kropenske, V. (1989). The development of young children of substance-abusing parents: Insights from seven years of intervention and research. *Zero to Three, IX* (5), 8–12.

Howard, J., & Kropenske, V. (1990). A preventive intervention model for chemically dependent parents and their offspring. In S. E. Goldston, C. M. Heinicke, R. S. Pynoos, & J. Yager (Eds.), *Preventing mental health disturbances in childhood.* Washington, DC: American Psychiatric Press, 71–84

Howard, J., Kropenske, V., & Tyler, R. (1986). The long-term effects on neurodevelopment in infants exposed prenatally to PCP. In D. H. Clouet (Ed.), *Phencyclidine: An update.* National Institute on Drug Abuse Research Monograph Series 64. Rockville, MD: National Institute on Drug Abuse, pp. 237–251.

Hoyme, H. E., Jones, K. L., Dixson, S. D., Jewett, T., Hanson, J. W., Robinson, L. K., Msall, M. E., & Allanson, J. E. (1990). Prenatal cocaine exposure and fetal vascular disruption. *Pediatrics, 85* (5), 743–747.

Javitt, D. C. (1987). Negative schizophrenic symptomatology and the PCP (phencyclidine) model of schizophrenia. *Hillside Journal of Clinical Psychiatry* 9 (1), 12 35.

Jessup, M., & Roth, R. (1988). Clinical perspectives on prenatal drug and alcohol use: Guidelines for individual and community response. *Medicine and Law, 7,* 377–389.

Jofee, T. J., Peterson, J., Smith, D., & Soyka, L. (1976). Sub-lethal effects in offspring of male rats treated with methadone before mating. *Research Communications in Chemistry, Pathology and Pharmacology, 13,* 611–621.

Johnsen, D. E. (1986). The creation of fetal rights: Conflicts with women's constitutional rights to liberty, privacy and equal protection. *Yale Law Journal, 95,* 599.

Johnson, H. L., Diano, A. & Rosen, T. S. (1984). 24-month neurobehavioral follow-up of children of methadone-maintained mothers. *Infant Behavior and Development, 7,* 115–123.

Kaltenbach, K., & Finnegan, L. P. (1984). Developmental outcome of children born to methadone maintained women: A review of longitudinal studies. *Neurobehavioral Toxicology and Teratology, 6,* 271–275.

Kempe, C. H., Silverman, F., Steele, B., Droegemueller, W., & Silver, H. (1962). The battered-child syndrome. *Journal of the American Medical Association, 181,* 17–24.

Kumpfer, K. L. (1991). Treatment programs for drug-abusing women. *The Future of Children, 1* (1), 50–59.

Lerner, S. E., & Burns, R. S. (1978). Phencyclidine use among youth: History, epidemiology and acute and chronic intoxication. In R. Peterson & R. Stillman (Eds.), *Phencyclidine (PCP) abuse: An appraisal.* Washington, DC: USGPO, 66–188.

Lewis, J. E., & Hordan, R. B. (1986). Neuropsychological assessment of phencyclidine abusers. In D. H. Clouet (Ed.), *Phencyclidine: An update.* NIDA Research Monograph Series 64. Rockville, MD: National Institute on Drug Abuse, 190–208.

Ling, W. (1990). Drugs of Abuse—Opiates. *Addiction Medicine and the Primary Care Physician.* Special Issue of the *Western Journal of Medicine, 152,* 565–72.

Little, R. E., & Sing, S. F. (1988). High proof paternity: Dads who drink conceive low birth weight infants. *Health* (June), 20.

Lodge, A. (1976). Developmental findings with infants born to mothers on methadone maintenance. A preliminary report. In G. Beschner & R. Brotman (Eds.), *NIDA research report.* Symposium on Comprehensive Health Care for Addicted Families and Their Children, May 20 and 21, 1976, New York. Rockville, MD: National Institute on Drug Abuse, 79–85.

MacGregor, S. N., Keith, L. G., Chasnoff, I. J., Rosner, M. A., Chisum, G. M., Shaw, P., & Minogue, J. P. (1987). Cocaine use during pregnancy: Adverse perinatal outcome. *American Journal of Obstetric Gynecology, 157* (3), 686–690.

McNamara, B. P., Kimura, K. K., & Wiles, J. H. (Nov. 1960). Summary report on Project New Year: Section III. *U.S. Army Chemical Warfare Laboratory special publication,* 4–17.

Moore, K. G. (Ed.). (1990). Substance abuse and pregnancy: State lawmakers respond with punitive and public health measures. *The American Col-*

lege of Obstetricians and Gynecologists Legis-Letter, 9 (3), 1–7.

Negligent Hiring and Retention of Babysitter (Dec. 1984). 27 ATLA L. Rep. 438.

Nichtern, S. (1973). The children of drug users. *Journal of the American Academy of Child Psychiatry, 12* (24), 24–31.

Oro, A. S., & Dixon, S. D. (1987). Perinatal cocaine and methamphetamine exposure: Maternal and neonatal correlates. *Journal of Pediatrics, 111* (4), 571–578.

Pearlson, G. D. (1981). Psychiatric and medical syndromes associated with phencyclidine (PCP) abuse. *Johns Hopkins Medical Journal, 148,* 25–33.

Phibbs, C. S., Bateman, D. A. & Schwartz, R. M. (1991). The neonatal costs of maternal cocaine use. *Journal of the American Medical Association, 266* (11), 1521–1526.

Pradhan, S. N. (1984). Phencyclidine (PCP): Some human studies. *Neuroscience and Biobehavioral Reviews, 8,* 493–501.

Rawson, R. A., Tennant, F. & McCann, M. A. (1981). Characteristics of 68 chronic phencyclidine abusers who sought treatment. *Drug and Alcohol Dependency, 8,* 223–227.

Rodning, C., Beckwith, L. & Howard, J. (1989). Characteristics of attachment organization and play organization in prenatally drug-exposed toddlers. *Development and Psychopathology, 1,* 277–289.

Roe v. Wade, 410 U.S. 113 (1973).

Rosen, T. S., & Johnson, H. L. (1982). Children of methadone-maintained mothers: Follow-up to 18 months of age. *Journal of Pediatrics, 101* (2), 192–196.

Roussey v. Roussey, 499 A.2 d 1199 (1985).

Rudolph, A. M. (1991). Neglect: Failure to provide essentials. In *Rudolph's pediatrics, 19th edition.* San Mateo, CA: Appleton and Lange, 844–845.

Russell, D. E. (1983). The incidence and prevalence of intrafamilial and extrafamilial sexual abuse of female children. *Child Abuse and Neglect, 7,* 133–146.

Schottenfeld, R. S. (1990). How effective is coercive treatment for alcohol and drug dependence? *Harvard Mental Health Letter, 7* (1), 8.

Smith, D. E. (1986). Cocaine-alcohol abuse: Epidemiological, diagnostic and treatment considerations. *Journal of Psychoactive Drugs, 18* (2), 117–129.

Sonderegger, T. B., O'Shea, S., & Zimmerman, E. (1979). Progeny of male rats treated neonatally with morphine pellets. *Proceedings of the Western Pharmacology Society, 11,* 137–139.

Sowder, B. J., & Burt, M. R. (1980). Children of addicts and nonaddicts: A comparative investigation in five urban sites. In *Heroin-addicted parents and their children: Two reports.* DHHS publication ADM 81-1028. Rockville, MD: National Institute on Drug Abuse, pp. 19–35.

Sowder, B. J., Carnes, Y. M., & Sherman, S. N. (April 1981). *Children of addicts in surrogate care.* Unpublished manuscript prepared for Services Resource Branch, National Institute on Drug Abuse, Institute for Human Resources Research.

Sroufe, L. A., & Fleeson, J. (1986). Attachment and the construction of relationships. In W. W. Hartup & Z. Rubin (Eds.), *Relationships and development.* Hillsdale, NJ: Erlbaum and Associates, 51–72.

Strauss, A. A., Modanlou, H. D., & Bosu, S. K. (1981). Neonatal manifestations of maternal phencyclidine (PCP) abuse. *Pediatrics, 68* (4), 550–552.

Streissguth, A. P., Aase, J. M., Clarren, S. K., Randels, S. P., LaDue, R. A., & Smith, D. F. (1991). Fetal alcohol syndrome in adolescents and adults. *Journal of the American Medical Association, 265* (15), 1961–1967.

Suffet, F., & Brotman, R. (1981). Maternal addiction and child development program. In *Final Report to the National Institute on Drug Abuse,* Center for Comprehensive Health Practice, New York Medical College.

Suing Mom. (May 1985). *A.B.A. Journal, 33.*

Tarter, R. F., Jacob, T., & Bremer, D. L. (1990). Specific cognitive impairment in sons of early onset alcoholics. *Alcoholism: Clinical and Experimental Research, 13,* 786–789.

Taylor, W. A., & Gold, M. S. (1990). Pharmacologic approaches to the treatment of cocaine dependence. *Addiction Medicine and the Primary Care Physician.* Special Issue of the *Western Journal of Medicine, 152,* 573–577.

Tucker, M. B. (1979). A descriptive and comparative analysis of the social support structure of heroin addicted women. In *Addicted women: Family dynamics, self-perceptions, and support systems.* Washington, DC: National Institute on Drug Abuse, 37–76.

Wallace, B. C. (1991). Chemical dependency treatment for the pregnant crack addict: Beyond the criminal-sanctions perspective. *Psychology of Addictive Behavior, 5* (1), 23–35.

Wellisch, D. K., & Steinberg, M. R. (1980). Parenting attitudes of addict mothers. *International Journal of the Addictions, 15,* 809–819.

Wilker, S. (1990). Child abuse, substance abuse, and the role of the dependency court. *Harvard Black-Letter Journal, 7* (Spring), 1–32.

Wilson, G. (1976). Management of pediatric medical problems in the addicted household. In G. Beschner & R. Brotman (Eds.), *National Institute on Drug Abuse Symposium on Comprehensive Health Care for Addicted Families and their Children, 20–21 May 1976.* Services Research Report 017-024-00598-3. Washington, DC: USGPO, 74.

Wilson, G., Desmond, M. M., & Verniaud, W. M. (1973). Early development of infants of heroin-addicted mothers. *American Journal of Diseases in Children, 126,* 457–462.

Yonekura, M. L., Inkelis, S. H., & Smith-Wallace, T. (1987). *Cocaine intoxication during parturition: Maternal and neonatal complications.* Paper presented at the 7th Annual Meeting of the Society of Perinatal Obstetricians, Feb. 6.

Zuckerman, B., Frank, D. A., Hingson, R., Amaro, H., Levenson, S. M., Kayne, H., Parker, S., Vinci, R., Aboasye, K., Fried, L. E., and others (1989). Effects of maternal marijuana and cocaine use on fetal growth. *New England Journal of Medicine, 320* (March 23), 762–768.

CHAPTER 17

OFFSPRING OF ALCOHOLICS AND OTHER ADDICTS

TIMMEN LEE CERMAK
WALTER BECKMAN

With the advent of family systems theory and the research it has stimulated (Steinglass, Bennett, Wolin, & Reiss, 1987), our conceptualization of chemical dependence has been broadened to include not only physical, emotional, and spiritual aspects, but family aspects as well. Chemical dependence is a family disease. The family, through a combination of its gene pool and the micro- and macroculture it transmits, is the primary vector by which chemical dependence is passed from one generation to the next. This chapter explores the multiple effects of parental alcoholism and other drug addiction on offspring, with special emphasis on how this perspective should affect prevention efforts.

The sheer number of children of substance abusers (COSAs) is staggering. The latest available estimates place the number of children of alcoholics in the United States at 28 million, with nearly 7 million of these under the age of 18 (Hindman, 1975). NIAAA's estimate is 20 years old now, and therefore almost certainly low. Given the generally accepted estimate that there are twice as many alcoholics as all other drug abusers, the total number of COSAs under 18 years old has been estimated to be between 9 and 10 million (NCPCA Fact Sheet, 1989). A more accurate assessment of the number of children of alcoholics (COAs) today would clearly be useful for guiding prevention efforts.

COSAs represent an identifiable population, not a diagnostic category (Fulton & Yates, 1990). From the standpoint of public health policy, however, COSAs are a very high-risk population, in part because of their numbers, and in part because research has clearly documented their increased incidence of chemical dependence. Roughly 25% of COSAs may eventually become addicted to alcohol or other drugs (Goodwin, 1976). From a different perspective, surveys of recovering alcoholics and cocaine addicts have found that 50% were offspring of alcoholics. Prevention should clearly target the children of substance abusers as its number-one concern.

THE IMPACT OF PARENTAL SUBSTANCE ABUSE ON DEVELOPING CHILDREN

Not all children of alcoholics are affected with equal intensity or in the same manner. There is great heterogeneity within this population. In particular, it should never be assumed that the entire impact of growing up with a chronically intoxicated parent is negative. Many strengths may be developed by children who are resilient enough to develop effective intrapsychic and interpersonal coping mechanisms (Wolin, 1993). Whether the impact is positive or negative, it is valuable, both professionally and personally, to understand the details of developmental influences affecting any given individual.

The National Institute on Alcohol Abuse and Alcoholism (NIAAA) has recently summarized and validated research that documents this impact (Alcohol Alert, 1990). On a cognitive level, various measures of verbal and performance intelligence have shown either no difference between COSAs and control groups or slightly decreased capabilities among COSAs (Ervin, Little, Streissguth, and Beck, 1984; Gabrielli et al., 1982; Bennett, Wolin, & Reiss, 1988). On the other hand, both COSAs and their mothers have been found to significantly underestimate their competence at school (Johnson & Rolf, 1988). Such perceptions may have an impact on a child's motivation, self-esteem, future performance, and teacher expectations. Data support the finding that COSAs repeat grades more often, drop out of school before graduation, and are referred to school psychologists more often (Miller & Jang, 1977; Knop, Teasdale, Schulsinger, & Goodwin, 1985).

On an emotional level, research has found that COSAs exhibit more symptoms of generalized stress, including lowered self-esteem, higher levels of depression, and greater anxiety (Schuckit, 1982, 1985a; Anderson & Quast, 1983; Prewett, Spence, & Chaknis, 1981; Moos & Billings, 1982). Behaviorally, COSAs exhibit more lying, stealing, fighting, truancy, and school behavioral problems. As a result, they are more likely to receive a diagnosis of conduct disorder (West & Prinz, 1987). The fact that parental alcohol and other drug addiction is the source of these cognitive, emotional, and behavioral problems is supported by findings that such symptoms tend to lessen in recovering families (Moos & Billings, 1982); however, the question of whether these impacts are specific to alcoholism or to general parental dysfunction remains open. For example, the work of Margaret Cork (1969) shows that children of alcoholics focus their concern almost exclusively on parental fighting, arguing, and unavailability rather than on the drinking per se.

One hypothesis holds that the low levels of family cohesiveness, expressiveness, independence, and intellectual orientation, and the higher levels of conflict produced by parental chemical dependence (Moos & Billings, 1982; Clair & Genest, 1987; Steinglass, 1980; Wolin, Bennet, & Noonan, 1979) are alleviated when drinking ceases. Studies of children who have demonstrated particularly high levels of resiliency (Werner, 1986) document four central characteristics that counteract the impact of parental dysfunction: an active, evocative approach toward solving problems (including the ability to ask for help when needed), a tendency to perceive experiences constructively, the ability to gain other people's positive attention (which makes them adept at recruiting surrogate parents), and the use of faith to maintain a positive sense of meaning about life. These resiliency characteristics are fostered by a close bond with at least one caregiver during the first year, situations that require helpfulness on the COSAs part without overwhelming the child's ability to make effective contributions, and the refuge of creative hobbies.

If the last century of psychology tells us anything, it is that early childhood experiences have a critical impact on a person's lifelong personality. It is only logical, therefore, to assume that the affects on children of growing up with an alcoholic or other drug addicted parent does not disappear with the advent of adulthood. The recent grass-roots development of interest in adult children of alcoholics (ACAs) is testimony to this fact.

Our work with adults from substance abusing families has taught us that four independent factors (modified from Millon, 1981) enter into generating the final impact on any particular COSA of growing up with a substance abusing parent. Each of the following four axes must be evaluated separately:

- Biology
- The wound (stress/trauma)
- Woundcare (codependence)
- Underlearning

Biology/Genetics

The mere fact that a client has a substance abusing parent is sufficient to justify undertaking a full pharmacohistory. One of the frequent but not inevitable legacies of being a COSA is the biology that underlies much of chemical dependence.

Studies of animals successfully bred as models of human chemical dependence (Li, 1987; Li et al., 1979), of the familial incidence of alcoholism (Cotton, 1979), concordance rates among twins (Schuckit, 1981), alcoholism among adoptees who are family history positive vs. family history negative for alcoholism (Goodwin, 1976), and intriguing findings in the search for markers of alcoholism (Schuckit, 1985b; Begleiter, 1984) all point to a biological factor as one important factor in the production of alcoholism. It is the therapist's responsibility to be aware of the increased risk for chemical dependence among COSAs, to be able to recognize early and often subtle signs of incipient problems, and to have the ability to explore this issue with clients in a manner that simultaneously gathers data and educates.

The Wound

The *wound* refers to the sheer level of stress that children in substance abusing families are subjected to, and thus describes characteristics that, by definition, are exhibited by any child of trauma. Sometimes the stress is overt, such as physical abuse, and can be easily pointed to years later (although people have a remarkable capacity to minimize the intensity of the experience in their memories). At other times the stress is more covert, such as the tension of living in a family that energetically avoids acknowledging the anger and sadness that permeates everyone's experience beneath the facade each maintains. In either case, stress leaves its mark. Sometimes this mark is left by the development of defensive armor that becomes a lifelong aspect of one's character. At other times, the mark is left when the level of stress broaches one's defenses and creates the experience of overwhelming anxiety. Full blown post-traumatic stress disorder (PTSD) exists in some adult children of alcoholics, but not in the vast majority. However, some elements of PTSD can be found in enough ACAs that it becomes necessary to evaluate the degree to which each patient is suffering during adult life from stress-induced phenomena. The conclusions of such an evaluation have extremely important implications for developing effective treatment plans.

The most common stress related characteristics are psychic numbing, re-experiencing the trauma, and hypervigilance. Psychic numbing is characterized by a constriction of emotions (not knowing what one feels) and a tendency to depersonalize or dissociate during times of increased anxiety. Re-experiencing the trauma leads many COSAs to be hyperreactive to stimuli that symbolically represent earlier traumas. The result is a continuous sense of being overwhelmed emotionally. Hypervigilance is manifested by easy startle response, chronic anxiety, and an underlying distrust of the surrounding environment. A sense of impending doom suffuses one's experience.

Poor Woundcare

The term *codependence* arose in the chemical dependence field to describe the pattern of dysfunctional coping strategies typically seen in alcoholic families. Because the ineffectiveness of these defenses ultimately increases the damaging effects of stress, it constitutes very poor woundcare. Codependence refers both to the quality of interactions that govern alcoholic family systems and to the intrapsychic dynamics within each of the family members. Although the chemical dependency (CD) field does not routinely deal with characterological diagnoses, the concept of codependence clearly fits into the same arena as more traditional personality disorders. Like other character disorders, codependence is a pervasive, underlying stance toward the self and others that is expressed in an individual's every attitude and action. Although codependence is not restricted to members of chemically dependent families (it exists throughout the range of family dysfunctions), it achieves its quintessential form with great frequency in this setting. This is because the use of denial and an omnipotent, unrealistic relationship to willpower found at the core of codependence are totally consistent with, and indistinguishable from, the substance abuser's psychological makeup during active stages of addiction.

It is important to emphasize that codependence constitutes far more than dysfunctional coping strategies and problem-solving techniques. It is an entire character structure induced in many COSAs of which the characteristic coping strategies are simply overt expressions. This character structure is complementary to narcissism. Whereas narcissism arises from parents' failure to gratify, and then mature, children's normal need to be unconditionally regarded and validated, codependence arises from the failure of parents to adequately gratify, and then mature, children's normal need to see their parents as godlike figures, capable of providing infinite safety and happiness (Cermak, 1990, 1991). Cermak has recently reframed these two needs, initially called normal narcissistic needs by Heinz Kohut (1971), as normal "interpersonal needs"; the first one is the normal narcissistic need and the second is the normal echoistic need (following the myth of Narcissus and Echo).

Narcissistic parents tend to produce codependent children by rejecting their children's normal narcissistic needs and stimulating (but not maturing) their normal echoistic needs. This behavior causes children to disown their own normal narcissism and abort maturation of their echoistic impulses. When echoistic needs remain in their archaic, childhood forms during adulthood, they become pathologic echoism, or codependence.

Codependent parents tend to produce narcissistic children by stimulating (but not maturing) their children's normal narcissistic needs and rejecting their normal echoistic needs. This behavior causes children to abort maturation of their normal narcissism and disown their echoistic impulses. When narcissistic needs remain in their archaic, childhood forms during adulthood, they become pathologic narcissism.

The timing of these wounds during child development is very early, and it is prudent to assume that no age is too young to be affected.

Underlearning

The category of underlearning points to the existence of gaps in learning that result from lack of experience with mature adult role models and healthy family dynamics. It is common for COSAs to complain that they do not know what is normal. Although this can be a form of resistance to exploration and change, it can also be a manifestation of underlearning. The therapeutic approach taken should differ depending on whether resistance or underlearning is being encountered. Underlearning exists on three levels: cognitive and behavioral, affective, and core identity.

In summary, as a result of the wide range of influences that can affect a COSA's life, substance abuse must be put in perspective as only one of many sequelae stemming from being the offspring of an addict. The prevention of substance abuse in this population cannot be approached in isolation. It must be seen in the wider context of all the different ways that having a chemically dependent parent affects one's life.

PAST AND CURRENT PREVENTION STRATEGIES AND PROGRAMS

The development of substance abuse prevention strategies for the offspring of substance abusers is in its embryonic stages. Although it is well-established that people with substance abusing parents are at high risk for substance abuse problems themselves, little empirical research has focused on population-specific prevention strategies. Furthermore, the handful of studies that have appeared have all focused exclusively on offspring of alcoholics, without any assurance that their findings are generalizable to families in which other drugs are abused. Several factors give rise to this limited focus: greater numbers of alcoholics, and thus offspring of alcoholics; less social stigmatization associated with alcohol than with other drugs and therefore more acceptance, particularly in schools and among parents of school-aged children; existence of a very active popular literature and a blossoming professional literature addressing issues pertinent to offspring of alcoholics.

Of the several prevention programs specifically for COAs that have been reported in the literature (Morehouse, 1979, 1984; DiCicco et al.,

1984; Lehr & Schrock, 1987; Riccelli, 1987), only a few have reported follow-up data over any period of time. The disappointing long-term results emphasize the embryonic state of this field.

Primary Prevention

To begin at first principles, and at the risk of appearing facetious, we must point out that the prevention of parental substance abuse should be the ultimate goal of primary prevention efforts because it by definition eliminates the COSA population. No substance abusers, no offspring of substance abusers. There exists a voluminous literature on primary prevention of substance abuse for a general population. Evaluation and follow-up data abound. Even the most cursory review of this literature is beyond the scope of this chapter; we refer you to the excellent review by Moskowitz (1989) containing more than 300 references and the review on similar programs for children and adolescents by Tobler (1990).

Failing to eliminate the COSA population, there are two goals of primary prevention: the prevention of fetal alcohol syndrome and effects (FAS and FAE) and the prevention of substance abuse among COSAs themselves. A review of prenatal and neonatal effects and prevention efforts is contained in Chapter 16. Although it has been hypothesized that prenatal exposure to substance use and abuse constitutes a risk factor for the later development of chemical dependence, long-term studies have not adequately evaluated the vulnerability of these populations to developing substance abuse problems.

What does the literature tell us about whether, and how, the prevention of chemical dependence among COSAs can be achieved?

There is no unanimity on the question of whether prevention efforts for children should strive for the prevention of all use or the development of responsible use. Certainly it can be argued that, with an increased risk for the development of substance abuse in the COSA population, it is most sensible to strive for the prevention of all use in order to preclude any potential for abuse. Although the argument has

surface appeal, and political correctness during the Reagan and Bush administrations, the fact remains that alcohol and drug use is well-ingrained in our culture. Among adolescents and young adults, alcohol use is a rite of passage. Would a no-use approach ultimately result in less successful prevention efforts by failing to attract youth who may be amenable to responsible drinking but not to preemptive abstinence? Such decisions must always take into account the age of the target population. In general, an abstinence approach is both more feasible and appropriate with elementary school children.

The conceptualization and evaluation of primary prevention programs for COSAs is clearly warranted, given the fact that approximately 25% of COSAs develop substance abuse problems. Unfortunately, the number of potential variables leading to or mitigating against substance abuse is immense. Knowledge, attitudes, behavior, psychodynamics of the family, and the temperament and personality of a given child are all relevant to issues of vulnerability and resiliency. The basic framework for understanding chemical dependence (disease concept vs. behavioral habit vs. regulation of negative affect) held by researchers and prevention workers also influences the variables each emphasizes.

The studies that have investigated knowledge and attitudes have shown success at changing those variables, but virtually no success at producing a lasting change in drinking behavior (DiCicco et al., 1984; Mauss, Hopkins, Weisheit, & Kearney, 1988). Moskowitz (1989) states that, following changes in knowledge and attitude, "[i]ntentions explain little of the variance in subsequent use after controlling for prior use, suggesting that substance use is not necessarily a consciously planned behavior" (p. 68). He goes on to quote McGuire (1974): "Attitudes are perhaps a partial determinant of action. . . . However, drug use in young people is probably not the most rational area of human behavior. An individual's decision to use drugs in a given situation derives from many factors, not just his general belief system regarding drug usage" (pp. 23–24). These remarks suggest the importance of internal psychological processes (regulation of affect and interrelationships of self and object representations) in substance use and abuse. Understanding the function and meaning of substance use for the individual is key to understanding the natural history of the disorder and is one variable that prevention strategies must take into account in order to be successful.

Research on the psychological functioning of COAs is beginning to appear (Hibbard, 1989; Transceau & Eliot, 1990). However, this exploration is in its infancy and without a unifying umbrella. It is also plagued by the same problem as the majority of descriptive COA research: viewing COAs as a homogeneous group. Clinical experience, as well as common sense, suggests a wide range of functioning and pathology in the COA population. Studies are only beginning to delineate and explore the mediating and moderating variables among COSAs (Chassin et al., 1993; Driscoll, 1991; Roosa, Beals, Sandler, & Pillow, 1990; Roosa, Dumka, Tien, & Tweed, in review). It is quite reasonable to assume that different characteristics in different COAs play a role in determining which develop substance abuse problems and which do not.

In addition to the large number of potential variables to be assessed in conceptualizing and evaluating primary prevention programs for COSAs, research is further confounded by the lack of distinction between prevention and treatment in high-risk populations. Williams (1990) gives an example from a 1979 symposium on services for children of alcoholics that illustrates this lack of clarity as to what defines treatment and prevention. The symposium defined treatment as "the process of providing services needed by the child. It is not necessarily a formal therapy program, but it may include activities usually thought of as 'prevention.'. . . The problem assessment and definition stage of the treatment process have some unique aspects for the children of the alcoholic parent. . . . There may be no presenting problem, no visible symptoms, no accurate developmental history, or no history at all" (p. 188).

Treatment of predisposing vulnerabilities, whether it be attitudes, coping skills, or psychological functioning, constitutes a preventive strategy for substance abuse. A multipronged approach can only enhance the likelihood of successfully preventing substance abuse problems in the offspring of substance abusers. The eventual role of genetic counseling can only be speculated about at this point.

It is heartening to observe the rapid evolution of pilot prevention programs for COSAs since the early 1980s, although outcome research has been inconsistent in its methodological quality and findings.

The California Department of Education funded a pilot project using school nurses to develop a curriculum and support and referral programs for preschool, middle, and high school children (Lehr & Schrock, 1987). The goals were to develop and provide educational opportunities for staff and parents about the disease of alcoholism and its effects on other family members and to increase students' knowledge of same, with an emphasis on problem-solving and coping skills in the everyday life of a chemically dependent family. Lastly, the program sought to ensure that every site would have a trained person to make appropriate referrals for children, parents, and school staff members requesting help. Lehr and Schrock provide no data or specific results. They simply state that, based on positive evaluations, a program that began with two school nurses expanded to include forty nurses and other personnel, including teachers, counselors, and psychologists.

Riccelli (1987) reported a pilot program implemented on a college campus using a structured eight-session educational and therapy group format for COSAs. Student evaluations following the group stated that they felt more comfortable with and less critical of themselves. They also reported an increased awareness of different options as to how one might deal with familial alcohol problems. Although in this case sufficient information was supplied for replication, the results are highly questionable because only six of the original twelve students completed the group.

The first extensive report that included follow-up came from the Cambridge and Somerville Program for Alcohol Rehabilitation (CASPAR). Although primary prevention of substance abuse in children, and children of alcoholics in particular, is the overall goal, CASPAR champions the more modest goal of "helping the child *understand* what amounts to the *central fact* of his or her life—the alcoholism of a parent and its effect on the family" (Deutsch, DiCicco, & Mills, 1982; italics in original). The unique aspect of CASPAR is the use of teachers who receive special training, rather than guidance counselors or school nurses.

CASPAR sees five stages in their work with children of alcoholics: 1) pre-identification, 2) identification, 3) referral and intake, 4) intervention, and 5) follow-up and reinforcement. The pre-identification stage includes a carefully designed 10-session sequential curriculum. Recognizing the power of denial and the "no talk rule" in alcoholic families, discussion of alcoholism is confined to the last three sessions. This discussion is preceded by factual information on alcohol, attitudes about alcohol and drinking, and responsible decision making in drinking situations. This stage provides opportunities for identification of COAs by the teacher as well as self-identification by the students.

Another novel component of the CASPAR program is the use of trained and supervised peer leaders, themselves COAs, to lead the structured after-school groups. Weekly journal entries and attendance at an Alateen meeting with another group member are additional requirements of the group. There appears to be tremendous face validity to this program for breaking down isolation and building friendship and trust among children in dire need of someone to understand them. As we outline later, CASPAR developed many program components that other prevention workers have independently discovered.

Unfortunately, although the basic education groups have shown a steady rise in enrollment, a corresponding increase in participation in the CAF (children of alcoholic families) groups has not occurred. This finding indicates that an eagerness for information pertinent to personal and family problems does not necessarily lead to an openness to discuss these problems. This lack of openness may reflect the power of the alcoholic family norms of secrecy and isolation, or it may have more to do with the fact that only 50% of the children who choose to participate in the program have an alcoholic parent (Davis, Johnson, DiCicco, & Orenstein, 1985). It appears that aspects of the program other than alcohol-related information attract youngsters, perhaps the additional adult attention or the opportunity to discuss personal feelings or intrapersonal problems.

The data also reveal that boys more than girls, and older more than younger children, are reluctant to participate in the CAF groups (DiCicco, Davis, Travis, & Orenstein, 1984). This is not surprising in light of what we know about the socialization of boys and girls with respect to feelings (Chodorow, 1978) and is paralleled by the differing rates of use of psychotherapy by men and women.

Of particular importance is the fact that follow-up data demonstrate that although knowledge and attitude changes about alcohol persist, the decrease in drinking behavior that occurs while the children are in the groups does not continue after the cessation of the groups (DiCicco et al., 1984). The authors conclude, "It becomes evident that changing youthful drinking behavior is tantamount to changing a culture" (p. 168).

At the end of the 1980s, the dearth of evaluative studies and the laxity with which most were reported or carried out made it difficult to arrive at any significant conclusions other than that more rigorously conducted studies were needed.

Mauss, Hopkins, Weisheit, and Kearney (1988) state that "contemporary alcohol education programs are generally based on the assumptions that if an adolescent knows something about alcohol and alcoholism, holds attitudes tolerant of moderate use and abstinence but intolerant of excessive use, has high self-esteem and has well-developed skills in decision-making and coping, then the adolescent will be unlikely to abuse alcohol. . . . Although evaluative research *has not shown* even these more sophisticated programs to be particularly effective" (p. 51; italics ours).

The conundrum is this: Studies suggest that variables such as self-esteem and perceived well-being (Chassin, Presson, & Sherman, 1985; Hull & Young, 1983; Kleinot & Rogers, 1982) plus attitudes that reflect a distinction between responsible and irresponsible substance use (Gorsuch & Arno, 1979; Olmstead & Smith, 1980) are influential on drinking behavior. Therefore, Mauss noted, "it is not unreasonable for health educators to expect that enhancing self-esteem, attitudes and decision-making skills could have an important impact on problem drinking among youth" (Mauss, Hopkins, Weisheit, & Kearney, 1988, p. 52). Unfortunately, the reality is that evaluative studies repeatedly demonstrate virtually no lasting impact on drinking behavior despite how much time, effort, talent, and money was spent on the development and delivery of a curriculum with very good face validity.

Mauss, Hopkins, Weisheit, & Kearney (1988) concluded that parental, peer, and environmental factors are of such substantial influence that the type of classroom-based programs that have thus far been used are relatively impotent. Their closing comment is, "Surely any school-based program hoping to have any appreciable impact will have to be embedded in a comprehensive, community-wide prevention effort directed at all the major social influences and institutions that shape our youth" (p. 60). In effect, we must realize that schools are only one aspect of the social context affecting children. Unless the larger social context delivers the same prevention messages children encounter at school, the impact of the intervention will be slight. One is reminded of lack of impact carried by the adage "Do as I say, not as I do."

The second generation of prevention research for COAs is attempting painstaking efforts to ferret out some of the subtleties in constructs such as self-esteem and stress to refine their approach to the problem. New methods for recruiting target populations are being tested. Furthermore, community-based prevention efforts are being explored (St. Pierre, Kaltreider, Melvin, & Aikin, 1992) as well as the most ambitious project to date, a communitywide prevention program, the Midwestern Prevention Project (see Pentz, 1993, for a summary).

Emshoff (1990) reported on an 18-session program for children in grades 6 through 8 that combined didactic information and skill building, along with self-disclosure and discussion in a group process model. The focus in this program is more on hypothesized moderating or mediating variables than on alcohol information per se. The guiding philosophy stresses the importance of mental health beyond its relation to alcohol abuse. The author stated "the intervention was designed to do what parents normally do, that is to help children learn to live with themselves in their environments, to establish good relationships, to learn to make constructive decisions and follow them through, and to know where and how to seek help when needed" (p. 238). Results showed that following the intervention, participants experienced a greater sense of control and less loneliness and depression, had a more positive self-concept, and were able to establish stronger social relations.

As for the effect on alcohol use, participants reported low levels of use both before and after the program. Although these results are encouraging, a bevy of further questions must still be answered. Was there something about the recruitment procedure that resulted in this bias? Would the intervention have yielded the same results with youngsters having higher levels of use? Would the level of use have changed? Emshoff planned to collect follow-up data for at least two years, but those efforts have been suspended for lack of funding (Emshoff, personal communication, August 1993).

Probably the most significant aspect of this program, first described by Emshoff and Moeti (1989), is the recruitment procedure they used. They showed the entire school a film depicting scenes of an alcoholic family and the different responses of the three children to parental drinking. After the film came a brief discussion and an invitation to attend a longer discussion group later in the school day. Such a procedure allows students the opportunity to avoid embarrassment or stigmatization by using the excuse of avoiding class to attend the group discussion. This is a legitimate concern as stigmatization has been demonstrated in children labeled as having alcoholic parents (Burk & Sher, 1988).

The most thorough and methodologically sound research on primary prevention for COAs is underway at the Program for Prevention Research, Arizona State University. They conducted a series of studies designed to inform an empirically based prevention program for COAs. The results suggested that a stress process model was applicable to the intergenerational transmission of alcoholism. According to this model, high levels of environmental stress contribute to the risk of mental health problems, and this risk is either exacerbated or diminished by other environmental and personality factors. Family stress was implicated as a risk factor and the family members' self-esteem as a protective or moderating factor (Roosa et al., 1989).

Working from the premise that parental treatment and recovery are unlikely, the research team targeted the child's skills for coping with stress and bolstering his or her self-esteem and use of social supports. They developed an eight session curriculum focused on these targets. A pilot study was conducted with 26 children from grades 4–6 from three elementary schools. Another 55 children served as controls. All subjects responded to a film recruitment procedure similar to that described above. Measurements of self-esteem and emotional problems were given before and after the program. Although results were not overwhelmingly positive, they did show trends in the desired direction and supported further investigation of the program model. The most promising result of this project was the number of children who responded positively to the recruitment procedure.

Thus far, the Arizona group is focusing on characteristics of the recruitment, the interventions, the students, and their families with the

hope of developing a comprehensive and effective prevention program. No data have been analyzed to date on the impact of the pilot interventions on drinking attitudes or behavior. Current efforts are to incorporate a parent involvement component. There is no expectation that a single-shot intervention will have a significant impact on such a pervasive social problem (Roosa, personal communication, July 1993).

Another study (Gensheimer, Roosa, & Ayers, 1990) examined the impact of the recruitment procedure on children's self-selection into the prevention program. The good news in this study was that of 844 children from grades 4–6 who were shown the film, 37% attended a follow-up meeting and one-third of those obtained parental permission to participate in the program. However, there were a few peculiarities about this group that raise further questions. The group obtaining parental permission was overrepresented by females, fourth graders, and children whose parents had divorced. Furthermore, although the follow-up and permission groups showed greater concern over parental drinking than the no-interest group, as would be expected, one-third of those who reported no concern attended the follow-up meeting, and of those ultimately participating in the program, 60% showed no concern.

This raises the question of what the draw to an alcohol prevention program is for children who report no concern over parental drinking but also no difference in quantity or frequency of parental alcohol use from other children. Perhaps what they are drawn to is an opportunity to hear and express thoughts and feelings about family stress, parental conflict, and a child's isolation and loneliness. This possibility is supported by the fact that the follow-up group scored higher on depression than the no-interest group. So again, there is good news and bad news. On one hand, the procedure was effective in recruiting children who had a need for a safe, open environment in which to explore their feelings. On the other hand, the procedure was not effective in recruiting the target population. Before drawing conclusions, it is best to recall Cork's finding that the vast majority of COAs in her study were more concerned with their parents' arguing and fighting than their drinking.

This outcome also returns us to the question of the efficacy or economics of a program designed specifically for COAs, especially as there is a growing body of literature that suggests that it is aspects of the COAs experience other than parental drinking per se, such as trauma, significant loss or abuse, parent behavior, family system strength, (Driscoll, 1991; Fisher, Jenkins, Harrison, & Jesch, 1993; Roosa et al., 1993; Roosa, Dumka, Tein, & Tweed, in review; Williams & Corrigan, 1992), that give rise to emotional and behavioral problems. Additional support for this idea is developing in the field of sexual abuse, where research is beginning to suggest that it is the environmental (especially parental) response to the abuse that has the biggest impact on the child (Nash et al., 1993). Another thread that ties together these two areas of traumatic childhood experience comes from studies that demonstrate an impairment in object relations (more accurately, object representations) in COAs (Hibbard, 1989; O'Connell, 1990) and survivors of childhood sexual abuse (Leifer, Shapiro, Martone, & Kassem, 1991; Stovall & Craig, 1990). Object representations are the internal, unconscious images people have of themselves in relationship with others and the feelings connected with those relationships (Kernberg, 1975). These object representations develop early in a child's life by the internalization of his or her relationships with the significant others in the child's environment. This theoretical framework, which holds that the environment mediates a child's internal development, is the same conclusion being reached by research on the impact of growing up with an substance abusing or sexually abusive parent.

Secondary Prevention

Secondary prevention, the amelioration of effects, has in essence become the preferred method of primary prevention, as outlined above. Most primary prevention programs have gradually moved in the direction of attempting to improve self-esteem and teach coping skills, stress reduction, and conflict resolution as the primary means of preventing substance abuse. As a result, the literature on secondary prevention has essentially already been covered. There are no longitudinal long-term studies demonstrating whether mental health during adulthood has been improved by intervening on problems during childhood. Although this concept seems to have abundant face validity, we should be cautious in accepting it without question and further research.

Studies of resiliency have documented the profound importance of a child's ability to develop a close bond with at least one caregiver during the first year of life. Every principle of child development theory would support this finding. It is therefore of extraordinary importance to study programs such as the Georgia Perinatal Addiction Project that respond to identification of pregnant addicts and perinatal addiction by providing a full year of recovery support and parent effectiveness training. If the data show that enhanced support of the parental function during the first year of a child's life can increase resiliency, and if resiliency factors can be shown in other research to decrease the chances of offspring's eventually developing chemical dependence, we will finally have a rational approach to prevention.

Finally, although intervention and treatment of parental substance abuse has been demonstrated to have a trickle-down benefit for children (Moos & Billings, 1982), there is regrettably no confirmation that this has any impact on the subsequent rate of substance abuse among offspring. There have been several reviews of studies on family systems and the recovery process (Janzen, 1978; Kaufman, 1985; O'Shea & Phelps, 1985), but one variable that is consistently overlooked is the effect of parental treatment on the future development of substance abuse problems in the offspring.

Tertiary Prevention

The continuing care needed to arrest problems at their present state, the hallmark of tertiary prevention, has its most obvious role in the lifelong response required by FAS and FAE babies, as well as those who have incurred severe physical and mental damage as a result of complications of poor prenatal care, birth trauma, or neonatal complications of maternal and fetal addiction. The rapidly growing socio-medico-economic problems connected to these conditions are covered in Chapter 16.

PROPOSED PREVENTION OF SUBSTANCE ABUSE AMONG COSAS

The above review quickly confirms that the question of prevention programs for COSAs is quite complex, and there are no definitive answers regarding the most effective prevention strategies. This is true in part because research documents that changes of attitudes do not reliably translate into changes in behavior, and information is still missing, particularly regarding longitudinal studies. There is no substitute for following subjects for several decades after exposing them to specific prevention strategies. Clearly, COSAs have been identified too recently as a high-risk group to have been followed over sufficient time to draw conclusions regarding our prevention efforts.

The most significant point to be made in this final section is that the emotional component of the impact on children of parental substance abuse means that primary prevention cannot be separated from secondary prevention. In other words, one cannot hope to be effective in preventing substance abuse among COSAs who are already emotionally affected by their parents' alcohol or drug use without also addressing that emotional impact. If prevention efforts do not address the current source of pain in a child's life, the child will be justified in concluding that the people providing education about alcohol and drugs do not know the first thing of real importance, because the first thing of importance is that the child's heart has already been bruised. Unless this bruise is addressed, the education will be seen as irrelevant.

Possibly in response to the basic fact that COSAs must first and foremost have their experience validated, a recent publication from the COA Foundation (1993) notes that virtually every program has converged to essentially the same perspective. The 10 programs surveyed all operate from a family systems approach and believe that COSAs are at high risk, both physiologically and emotionally, for their own substance abuse. These programs also work to enhance COSAs' general coping, decision-making, problem-solving, and communication skills. Another key goal is to provide a safe and nurturing place for children to discuss and understand their feelings. A small group process (keeping children of similar ages together) is used by each, using unconditional acceptance, praise and support, and some personal disclosure by leaders. Most group meetings open with a check-in, and then use short presentations of factual material, continuation of the message through a structured activity, discussion, and a closing ritual. Whether these programs are consciously aware that chemical dependence has an increased rate of transmission in families that have lost their rituals (Wolin, Bennet, & Noonan, 1979), they have all found ways of importing rituals into their meetings.

Our survey of existing programs has led us to conclude that the most pragmatic, cost-effective way to reach children in large numbers has been pioneered by the student assistance movement. The essence of student assistance programs includes the following:

— Children are counseled with complete confidentiality.
— Counselors are separate from school grading and evaluation.
— Services are provided on the school grounds.

All three of these points are precisely parallel to the principles of effective employee assistance programs, with appropriate modifications for students.

A two-phase approach to students is necessary. Phase One includes a general approach to all students, with or without family histories of substance abuse. This initial approach should be primarily educational, including a component for educating parents as well, especially on how to talk to their children about alcohol and drug use. The goals of Phase One are twofold: All students receive basic alcohol and drug information and COSAs are encouraged to self-identify for Phase Two. In addition, it would be useful to promote attitudes among all students that support their COSA classmates.

This latter point deserves additional attention. The conclusion of some prevention workers that peer and social influences are of paramount importance in the decision to drink or use other drugs cannot be dismissed as idle wishes for an ideal world. Without concrete cultural changes, prevention efforts are struggling against an overwhelming current. Although many feel that such cultural changes are too grandiose ever to be accomplished, it is important to remember the transformation during the past two decades of our country's attitudes toward tobacco. Certainly, attitudes toward alcohol are more deeply ingrained than those toward tobacco, but the fact remains that attitudes that seemed insurmountable have been changed.

Fortunately, cultural attitudes can also be addressed within subcultures first. Each community, each school, and each classroom represents a subculture. The same prevention efforts that are doomed to failure when only a few scattered schools are targeted may succeed when a critical mass of schools are all targeted at the same time. Phase One should focus not only on transferring basic facts to a class of students, but should work toward stimulating empathy among non-COSAs for their classmates. Even slight improvements in the classroom atmosphere, leading to greater peer support (or lessened stigmatization) for COSAs who wish to self-identify and enter Phase Two could have a profound impact.

Phase Two is geared toward COSAs who self-identify, and approaches them on a more emotionally supportive level. Secondary prevention is the goal. How can children be helped today to reduce the impact of their parents' chemical dependence on their own lives? How can their sense of isolation be broken, their fears, pain, and anger validated, and their safety protected in the process? It is here that COSAs should be given a concerned and helping hand, while they are still in the middle of their experience with intoxicated parents. Once their current feelings are listened to and sorted out, it becomes far easier for children to take seriously the increased risk they may be running for their own chemical dependence.

During Phase Two, programs can be designed to incorporate protective factors that have been found to increase resiliency. The very act of self-identifying for Phase Two represents an act of pronounced autonomy (from the alcoholic family) and a strong social orientation (joining a group of other COSAs). Immediate and pervasive validation of these two strains, independence and the willingness to ask for help, should be provided. In fact, efforts should be made to provide activities that continue to reinforce the interdependence of these two, demonstrating that those who recognize their limits and make appropriate requests for assistance ultimately achieve the greatest independence.

Group activities that promote novel experiences, vigorous play, self-esteem, new hobbies, and creativity should be used to give COSAs the experience of potency, laughter, and solace in the middle of their family's tragedy. In particular, participants in Phase Two must be given practical guidelines for how they can best respond to their families, protecting their own interests without inflaming the situation. Perhaps the best avenue toward a sense of potency is to lead COSAs into activities that express age-appropriate levels of responsibility and helpfulness. Perhaps graduates of the program might be given leading roles in portions of the Phase One classes, sharing their experience and making it clear that peer support for COSAs self-identifying is of critical importance. Such a role adds meaning to an individual's experience by using that experience to begin transforming the culture and facilitating other COSAs in their search for help.

Follow-up data from programs that demonstrate the capability to alter youngsters' attitudes toward alcohol and other drugs have reported that these changes are not self-perpetuating. Given the present culture, they fade. The only antidote to this tendency of changed attitudes to revert would seem to be continuous reinforcement of the new attitudes. Prevention cannot be conceived as a single event. It must be developed as a consistent part of the COSA's life. Student Assistance Programs are likely to be effective only when they are continuously present and active from kindergarten through graduate school. Just as sobriety is a way of life for the recovering addict, not a one-time achievement, primary prevention for COSAs must be a way of life until it has been incorporated into the very fabric of our culture.

Incorporating primary prevention into the very culture surrounding a COSA should not be seen as an overwhelming task. It would require far less effort than transforming the culture in which adults live. Young people possess an altruism that leaves them horrified when one of their own has been physically or sexually abused. It is not out of the realm of possibility that being raised by an alcoholic or drug-addicted parent would be seen by most youngsters as an abusive situation, and that genuine empathy and support would naturally be extended toward classmates with the misfortune of being trapped in such a family. Children live in a powerful subculture, one that is capable of overwhelming the strongest efforts of adult culture to influence their offspring. The power of this subculture can be put to positive use, and not simply be the source of aggravation for adults. Although such a transformation could never be forced on youngsters by an adult world, it could be stimulated by exposing youngsters to the realities overtaking the lives of their friends, and then relying on the natural power of their altruism to take the situation seriously. Such exposure would occur during Phase One, particularly when the graduates of Phase Two speak honestly about their experience.

A final word must be said regarding the eventual role genetic research will play in our prevention efforts. When genetic counseling for substance abuse becomes a reality, all primary prevention programs will have to be adjusted to accommodate the central role it will occupy. Although the eventual role genetic testing and counseling will play cannot be determined at this time, it is never too early to begin pondering the social implications that will emanate from the technological progress expected. For example, who will guarantee protection of civil liberties and confidentiality once individual COSAs can be identified as being at the highest possible risk of chemical dependence? Will insurance companies and employers have access to this information? Will stigmatization reappear as people are classified as forming a "biologic underclass?"

These questions are not idle musings of aging liberals. Automobile insurance companies will want to know which 16-year-olds are genetically predisposed to substance abuse. Their industry-generated surveys will document that a significantly higher number of accidents occur in this group. Public revolt against already exorbitant insurance rates will lead insurance companies to "champion the rights of consumers" when they demand that each applicant take a simple blood test. Life insurance companies will feel justified in charging higher rates to genetically positive COSAs in order to protect the lower rates of the majority of their customers. The end result will be that no one will want to be tested. The risks are too high. Thus, we will lose the most valuable tool for targeting our prevention efforts on the group at highest risk.

If the above scenario appears fantastic, we need only turn our attention to attitudes recently taken toward "crack babies." Grade school teachers were terrified by the prospect of being inundated by hyperactive, aggressive, damaged students. The belief that this damage stems primarily from the direct effects of cocaine has yet to be clearly established to the degree that it is believed. Cocaine addicts make poor parents. Bonding can be disrupted from birth. We do not know which effects come from pharmacology and which come from lack of nurturing. The lesson here is that the clear definition of a high-risk group is a mixed blessing. Both good and harm can come from knowing who is at risk. The less surprised we are by the stigmatization that will occur when genetic markers for substance abuse are available, the more prepared we must be to put our technological advances to use for the good of COSAs.

HYPOTHESES TO GUIDE FUTURE RESEARCH

In conclusion, we are left with two hypotheses capable of generating research strategies. These hypotheses appear to be consistent with our clinical experience, accepted theoretical frameworks, and some available research data.

The first hypothesis, which we shall call the Resilience Hypothesis, combines support of parental function during the first year of life, the enhancement of resilience, and the potential efficacy of resilience in preventing chemical dependence. Although many links in this hypothesis are clearly speculative, it provides a framework for weaving several lines of research into an integrated approach to prevention without the immense commitment required to complete longitudinal studies over multiple generational cycles. The Resilience Hypothesis predicts that individuals will develop greater resilience if their infancy environment is stabilized, particularly in terms of consistent, nurturing parenting. The second facet of this hypothesis is the prediction that COSAs with high levels of resilience are less likely to become chemically dependent. If research on these two fronts proves positive, then a coherent approach to prevention can be undertaken in the first year of each COSA's life.

The second hypothesis, which we shall call the Validation–Education Hypothesis, combines supportive counseling (most often in the school setting) for children who are currently living in chemically dependent families with education about chemical dependence and their increased risk. It is probably essential that this support and education be present in age-appropriate ways from kindergarten throughout a student's education. Early exposure to a validating and educating environment, repeated exposure, and consistently age-appropriate approaches to COSAs should be the goal. The prediction is that continuous opportunities to express feelings, dispel loneliness, and receive validation for one's perceptions and worth could increase the impact of education about chemical dependence. This impact should be measured in several ways. First, we can look at an individual's decision to use alcohol and other drugs. Second, we can look at the incidence of abuse and dependence. Third, we should also determine whether those who become chemically dependent are less resistant to entering recovery. We must not forget that it would be an immense victory if we could substantially decrease the length of time individuals were actively chemically dependent before entering recovery, even if the rate of chemical dependence itself was not decreased.

Until we learn how to conduct prevention effectively, it is unlikely that our society will abandon its efforts to get it right. No matter how complex and difficult the problems involved in prevention may be, it is simply unacceptable to allow frustration to abort our commitment toward this goal. The population at risk is huge and continually growing. Any suffering we relieve is worth our efforts. In small increments, over generations, we will develop valuable expertise.

REFERENCES

Alcohol Alert, no. 9, PH 288, July, 1990.

Anderson, E., & Quast, W. (1983). Young children in alcoholic families: A mental health needs-assessment and an intervention/prevention strategy. *Journal of Primary Prevention, 3* (3), 174–187.

Begleiter, H. (1984). Event-related brain potentials in boys at risk for alcoholism. *Science, 225,* 1493–1496.

Bennett, L.A., Wolin, S. J., & Reiss, D. (1988). Cognitive, behavioral, and emotional problems among school-age children of alcoholic parents. *American Journal of Psychiatry, 145* (2), 85–190.

Burk, J. P., & Sher, K. J. (1988). The "forgotten children" revisited: Neglected areas of COA research. *Clinical Psychology Review, 8,* 285–302.

Cambridge and Somerville Program for Alcohol Rehabilitation (CASPAR).

Cermak, T. (1990, 1991). *Evaluating and treating adult children of alcoholics* (2 vols.). Minneapolis: Johnson Institute.

Chassin, L., Pillow, D. R., Curran, P. J., Molina, B.S.G., & Barrera, M. (1993). Relation of parental alcoholism to early adolescent substance use: A test of three mediating mechanisms. *Journal of Abnormal Psychology, 102,* 3–19.

Chassin, L.A., Presson, C. C., & Sherman, S. J. (1985). Stepping backward in order to step forward: An acquisition-oriented approach to primary prevention. *Journal of Consulting and Clinical Psychology, 53,* 612–622.

Chodorow, N. (1978). *The reproduction of mothering.* Berkeley. University of California Press.

Clair, D., & Genest, M. (1987). Variables associated with the adjustment of offspring of alcoholic fathers. *Journal of Studies on Alcohol, 48,* 345–355.

COA Foundation (1993). *Profiles: Ten prevention programs for children of alcoholics.* New York: COA Foundation.

Cork, M. (1969). *The forgotten children.* Ontario: Paperjacks.

Cotton, N. S. (1979). The familial incidence of alcoholism: A review. *Journal of Studies in Alcoholism, 40,* 89–116.

Davis, R. B., Johnson, P. D., DiCicco, L., & Orenstein, A. (1985). Helping children of alcoholic parents: An elementary school program. *The School Counselor, 32,* 357–363.

Deutsch, L., DiCicco, L., & Mills, D. J. (1982). In Roosa et al., U.S. Department of Health and Human Services (1989), *Prevention, intervention, and treatment: Concerns and models.* Publication no. ADM 83-1192, NIAAA Alcohol and Health Monograph no. 3. Washington, DC: USGPO, 147–174.

DiCicco, L., Davis, R. B., Hogan, J., MacLean, A., & Orenstein, A. (1984). Group experiences for children of alcoholics. *Alcohol Health and Research World, 8,* 20–24.

DiCicco, L., Davis, R. B., Travis, J., & Orenstein, A. (1984). Recruiting children from alcoholic families into a peer education program. *Alcohol Health and Research World, 8,* 28–34.

Driscoll, M. J. (1991). *Adult children of alcoholics and post-traumatic stress.* Unpublished doctoral dissertation. Alameda: California School of Professional Psychology.

Emshoff, J. G. (1990). A preventive intervention with children of alcoholics. *Prevention in Human Services, 7,* 225–253.

Emshoff, J. G., & Moeti, R. L. (1989). In *Family Relations, 38.*

Ervin, C. S., Little, R. E., Streissguth, A. P., & Beck, D.E. (1984). Alcoholic fathering and its relation to child's intellectual development: A pilot investigation. *Alcoholism: Clinical and Experimental Research, 8,* 362–365.

Fisher, G. L., Jenkins, S. J., Harrison, T. C., & Jesch, K. (1993). Personality characteristics of adult children of alcoholics, other adults from dysfunctional families, and adults from nondysfunctional families. *The International Journal of the Addictions, 28,* 477–485.

Fulton, A., & Yates, W. (1990). Adult children of alcoholics: A valid diagnostic group? *The Journal of Mental and Nervous Diseases, 178* (8), 505–508.

Gabrielli, W. F., Mednick, S. A., Volavka, J., Pollack, V. E., Schulsinger, F., & Itil, T. M. (1982). Electroencephalograms in children of alcoholic fathers. *Psychophysiology, 19,* 404–407.

Gensheimer, L. K., Roosa, M. W., & Ayers, T. S. (1990). Children's self-selection into prevention programs: Evaluation of an innovative recruitment strategy for children of alcoholics. *American Journal of Community Psychology, 18,* 707–723.

Goodwin, D. (1976). *Is alcoholism hereditary?* New York: Oxford University Press.

Gorsuch, R. L., & Arno, D. A. (1979). The relationship of children's attitudes toward alcohol to their value development. *Journal of Abnormal Child Psychology, 7,* 287–295.

Hibbard, S. (1989). Personality and object relational pathology in young adult children of alcoholics. *Psychotherapy, 26,* 504–509.

Hindman, M. (1975). Children of alcoholic parents. *Alcohol, Health and Research World, 6,* 2–6.

Hull, J. G., & Young, R. D. (1983). Self-consciousness, self-esteem, and success–failure as determinants of alcohol consumption in male social drinkers. *Journal of Personality and Social Psychology, 44,* 1097–1109.

Janzen, C. (1978). Family treatment for alcoholism: A review. *Social Work, 23,* 135–144.

Johnson, J. L., & Rolf, J. E. (1988). Cognitive functioning in children from alcoholic and non-alcoholic families. *British Journal of Addiction, 83,* 849–857.

Kaufman, E. (1985). Family systems and family therapy of substance abuse: An overview of two decades of research and clinical experiences. *International Journal of the Addictions, 20,* 897–916.

Kernberg, O. (1975). *Borderline conditions and pathological narcissism.* New York: Jason Aronson, Inc.

Kleinot, M. C., & Rogers, R. W. (1982). Identifying effective components of alcohol misuse prevention programs. *Journal of Studies on Alcohol, 20,* 897–916.

Knop, J., Teasdale, T. W., Schulsinger, F., & Goodwin, D. W. (1985). A prospective study of young men at high risk for alcoholism: School behavior and achievement. *Journal of Studies on Alcohol, 45* (4), 273–278.

Kohut, H. (1971). *The analysis of the self.* Madison, CT: International Universities Press, 27.

Lehr, K., & Schrock, M. M. (1987). A school program for children of alcoholics. *Journal of School Health, 57,* 344–345.

Leifer, M., Shapiro, J. P., Martone, M. W., & Kassem, L. (1991). Rorschach assessment of psychological functioning in sexually abused girls. *Journal of Personality Assessment, 56,* 12–28.

Li, T.-K. (1987). *Alcohol and alcoholism,* supplement 1, 91–96.

Li, T.-K., Lumeng, W., McBride, W. J., & Waller, M. B. (1979). Progress toward a voluntary oral consumption model of alcoholism. *Drug and Alcohol Dependence, 4* (1–2), 45–60.

Mauss, A. L., Hopkins, R. H., Weisheit, R. A., & Kearney, K. A. (1988). The problematic prospects for prevention in the classroom: Should alcohol education programs be expected to reduce drinking by youth? *Journal of Studies on Alcohol, 49,* 51–61.

McGuire, W. J. (1974). Communication-persuasion models for drug education. In M. Goodstadt (Ed.), *Research of methods and programs of drug education.* Toronto: Addiction Research Foundation.

Miller, D., & Jang, M. (1977). Children of alcoholics: A 20-year longitudinal study. *Social Work Research Abstracts, 13,* 23–29.

Millon, T. (1981). *Disorders of personality: DSM-III; Axis II.* New York: John Wiley & Sons.

Moos R. H., & Billings, A. G. (1982). Children of alcoholics during the recovery process: Alcoholic and matched control families. *Addict. Behavior, 7,* 155–163.

Morehouse, E. R. (1979). Working in the schools with children of alcoholic parents. *Health and Social Work, 4,* 145–162.

Morehouse, E. R. (1984). Working with alcohol-abusing children of alcoholics. *Alcohol Health and Research World, 8,* 14–18.

Moskowitz, J. M. (1989). The primary prevention of alcohol problems: A critical review of the research literature. *Journal of Studies on Alcohol, 50,* 54–88.

Nash, M. R., Hulsey, T. L., Sexton, M. C., Harralson, T. L., & Lambert, W. (1993). Perceived family environment, psychopathology and dissociation. *Journal of Consulting and Clinical Psychology, 61,* 276–283.

National Committee for the Prevention of Child Abuse Fact Sheet #14, 1989.

O'Connell, P. (1990). *Adult children of alcoholics: A Rorschach study.* Unpublished doctoral dissertation. Alameda: California School of Professional Psychology.

Olmstead, D. W., & Smith, D. L. (1980). The socialization of youth into the American mental health belief system. *Journal of Health and Social Behavior, 21,* 181–194.

O'Shea, M. D., & Phelps, R. (1985). Multiple family therapy: Current status and critical appraisal. *Family Process, 24,* 555–582.

Pentz, M. A. (1993). In J. S. Baer, G. A. Marlatt, & R. J. McMahon (Eds.), *Addictive behaviors across the life span: Prevention, treatment, and policy issues.* Newbury Park, CA: Sage Publications.

Prewett, M. J., Spence, R., & Chaknis, M. (1981). Attribution of causality by children with alcoholic parents. *International Journal of the Addictions, 16,* 367–370.

Riccelli, C. (1987). Adult children of alcoholics on campus: Programming for a population at risk. *Journal of American College of Health, 36,* 117–122.

Roosa, M. W., Beals, J., Sandler, I. N., & Pillow, D. R. (1990). The role of risk and protective factors in predicting symptomatology in adolescent self-identified children of alcoholic parents. *American Journal of Community Psychology, 18,* 725–741.

Roosa, M. W., Dumka, L., Tien, J. Y., & Tweed, S. (in review). *Parent problem drinking, stress, and other daily influences on child mental health.*

Roosa, M. W., Gensheimer, L. K., Short, J. L., Ayers, T. S., & Shell, R. (1989). A preventive intervention for children in alcoholic families: Results of a pilot study. *Family Relations, 38,* 295–300.

Roosa, M. W., Tein, J. Y., Groppenbacher, N., Michaels, M., & Dumka, L. (1993). Mother's parenting behavior and child mental health in families with a problem drinking parent. *Journal of Marriage and the Family, 55,* 107–118.

Schuckit, M. (1981). Twin studies on substance abuse: An overview. In L. Gedda, P. Parisi, & W. E. Nance, (Eds.), *Twin research: 3. Epidemiological and clinical studies.* New York: Alan R. Liss.

Schuckit, M. A. (1982). Anxiety and assertiveness in sons of alcoholics and controls. *Journal of Clinical Psychiatry, 43,* 238–239.

Schuckit, M. A. (1985a). Behavioral effects of alcohol in sons of alcoholics. In M. Galanter (Ed.), *Recent developments in alcohol,* vol. 3. New York: Plenum Press, 11–19.

Schuckit, M. (1985b). Genetics and the risk for alcoholism. *Journal of the American Medical Association, 254* (18), 2614–2617.

Steinglass, P. (1980). A life history model of the alcoholic family. *Family Process, 19,* 211–226.

Steinglass, P., Bennett, L., Wolin, S., & Reiss, D. (1987). *The alcoholic family.* New York: Basic Books.

Stovall, G., & Craig, R. J. (1990). Mental representations of physically and sexually abused latency-aged females. *Child Abuse and Neglect,* 233–242.

St. Pierre, T. L., Kaltreider, D. L., Melvin, M. M., & Aikin, K. J. (1992). Drug prevention in a community setting: A longitudinal study of the relative effectiveness of a three-year primary prevention program in boys' & girls' clubs across the nation. *American Journal of Community Psychology, 20,* 673–705.

Tobler, N. S. (1990). Meta-analysis of 143 adolescent drug prevention programs: Quantitative outcome results of program participants compared to a control or comparison group. *Journal of Drug Issues, 16,* 537–567.

Transceau, G., & Eliot, J. (1990). Individuation and adult children of alcoholics. *Psychological Reports, 67,* 137–142.

Werner, E. E. (1986). Resilient offspring of alcoholics: A longitudinal study from birth to age 18. *Journal of Studies on Alcohol, 47,* 1.

West, M. O., & Prinz, R. J. (1987). Parental alcoholism and childhood psychopathology. *Psychological Bulletin, 102* (2), 204–218.

Williams, C. N. (1990). Prevention and treatment approaches for children of alcoholics. In M. Windle & J. S. Searles (Eds.), *Children of alcoholics: critical perspectives.* New York: Guilford Press.

Williams, O. B., & Corrigan, P. W. (1992). The differential effects of parental alcoholism and mental illness on their adult children. *Journal of Clinical Psychology, 48,* 406–413.

Wolin, S. J., Bennet, L. A., & Noonan, D. L. (1979). Family rituals and the recurrence of alcoholism over generations. *American Journal of Psychiatry, 136,* 589–593.

Wolin, S., & Wolin, S. (1993). *The resilient self.* New York: Villard Books.

CHAPTER 18

ETHNIC MINORITIES

JOSEPH E. TRIMBLE

A long time ago we never had these drug problems in our villages. Now we do and they're killing our spirit and our children. Our healing ways of the grandfathers don't work on this problem. It's another one of those problems given to us by the waneentum *[white man]. The way I see it the* waneentum *can't stop the problem with their own kind. How do they expect us to stop a white man's problem in our villages when they can't stop it themselves?*

A Coast Salish elder speaking to
concerned tribal parents (1990)

The poignant and powerful words spoken by the American Indian elder on one cold, wet winter evening in the Pacific Northwest echo the sentiments of countless parents and concerned citizens in hundreds of ethnic minority communities across the country. Today, ethnic communities decry the intrusive influence of the drug and alcohol peddler. Numerous ethnic minority elders recall a time decades ago when drug use was not a concern—not even a remote one—in their villages, neighborhoods, and communities.[1] For most African Americans, American Indians and Alaska Natives, Asian Americans, Pacific Islanders, and Hispanic Americans, drug abuse was, indeed, a white man's problem. Now, and for the past few decades, drug use and abuse is everyone's problem as the pattern of use and abuse seems to consume all but a few American communities. Along with the frustration, pain, and senseless deaths that result from drug abuse, ethnic communities must struggle with treating and preventing a problem that doesn't fit within their own traditional healing systems. The anger and frustration engendered by the presence of psychoactive substances is intensified by the assumption that prevention and treatment strategies are not effective in general; because the strategies appear to be designed for use with the dominant culture, the prognosis for creating drug-free communities in diverse and culturally unique settings appears grim. The feelings and perceptions of ethnic minorities are not unfounded. Available evidence substantiates and validates their myriad concerns.

This chapter reviews research and commentary on the prevention of drug problems in America's ethnic minority populations. To set the scene, discussion focuses on the specification of ethnic minorities, a historical overview of ethnic minority drug use problems, and the sociocultural conditions that coexist with the presence of drugs. The chapter proceeds to examine the prevalence rates and provide a historical overview of prevention and treatment efforts. The chapter concludes with a critical summary of what is known and what can be promoted in the future to cut into the problem and its dreadful consequences.

SPECIFICATION OF ETHNIC MINORITY POPULATIONS

America's population consists of a complex mosaic of indigenous native groups and descendants

The author wishes to thank the Tri-Ethnic Center for Prevention Research at Colorado State University for providing support to prepare and write this chapter (NIDA grant P 50 DA07074).

of seemingly countless countries. Even the descendants come from immigrant stock who represent diverse ethnic and cultural traditions within their home countries. America's population also is a play of colors where practically every conceivable skin coloration is represented. For a variety of historical and socioeconomic reasons, ethnic groups with darker skin tones were and continue to be subjugated as oppressed minorities. The people who make up these groups are referred to as America's ethnic minority populations. In social and political terms, they are categorized as African Americans, Asian and Pacific Americans, American Indians and Alaska Natives, and Hispanic Americans. The four groups are not static, homogeneous entities and the use of a single label—an "ethnic gloss"—does not capture their broad and varied sociocultural characteristics (Trimble, 1991).

The ethnic composition and acculturative status of each of America's ethnic minority groups probably are as complex and diverse as the dominant culture. The marbling of each group can be seen in the way each group is described. African Americans are those who can trace their ancestry to various African countries. King, Moody, Thompson, and Bennett (1983) maintain that "blacks as a race is an illusion if one means by it a homogeneous group with common anatomical and psychological characteristics" (p. 6). The heterogeneity of African Americans can be understood if one considers the influences of social class, progeny from mixed marriages, and those who are descendants or are from the Caribbean basin and Central and South America. American Indians and Alaska Natives are extremely diverse groups representing more than 450 identifiable tribal units whose members reflect varying degrees of intermarriage, acculturative status, and personal identification (Trimble & Fleming, 1989). Wong (1982) asserts that at least 32 distinct groups make up the Asian-American and Pacific Island category. Moreover, Morishima et al. (1979) add that "given the diversity of languages, norms, mores and immigrant/American born [status], it is evident that to [label them

as Asian Americans and Pacific Islanders] implies a homogeneity which is lacking" (p. 3). On the Hispanic classification, Padilla and Salgado de Snyder (1985) assert that it "is a term used to designate those individuals who reside in the United States and whose cultural origins are in Mexico, Puerto Rico, Cuba, and other Latin American countries. As such the term Hispanic is not accepted by individuals, and it is not uncommon to find reference to Latinos, or La Raza, in place of Hispanic in some communities" (p. 158).

At one level of discourse, it makes sense to use the broad categories to refer to these groups. In each case, there is a common thread that binds the groups as a whole; American Indians and Alaska Natives are the indigenous aboriginal peoples of North America, African Americans can trace their origins to African countries, and Asian Americans can trace their roots to an array of different countries. At another level, however, to use the "ethnic gloss" as though the group members share a common understanding of their own ethnicity and nationalistic identification can be highly misleading. As one reads through the mounting literature about the groups, one gets the impression that they share some modal characteristic that sets them apart from other groups—we find constant references to studies comparing blacks with whites, American Indians with non-Indians, Asian Americans with other ethnic minority groups. The comparisons and the manner in which the groups are viewed lead the naïve reader to conclude that members of the respective groups must be alike in some manner.

Anthropologist Dwight Heath forcefully argues that "categories of people such as those compared under the rubric of 'ethnic groups' are often not really meaningful units in any sociocultural sense" (1978, p. 60). He goes on to point out "that the ways in which people define and maintain 'social boundaries' between or among self-identified categories are often far more important and revealing of sociocultural dynamics" (p. 60). Use of the categories for research purposes provides results that can be puzzling. In addition to the fact that ethnic comparative research results can reinforce stereotypes, they also can lead one to conclude that all members of the group in question act, react, respond, and behave in some generalized consistent manner. In fact, the labels belie the intrinsic importance culture and degree of ethnic identification play (Cheung, 1991). Most researchers fail to include measures of ethnic identity and cultural orientation; they presume that the labels and the respondents chosen to represent them are sufficient to tap cultural salience. Consequently, if researchers rely solely on the labels to capture culture vicissitudes, they stand to convey findings that are, at best, superficial; the results may well be meaningless because the labels bear little or no relation to the intrinsic cultural complexity of the groups (Heath, 1987, 1991). In reading ethnic and culture-specific comparative studies, the conclusions should be treated with caution and prudence—consider the proof provided by the researcher that the intricacies of ethnicity and culture have been sufficiently covered.

Emergence of Ethnic Minority Populations

America's dominant ethnic minority populations are increasing in size at a rate greater than the dominant population. Much of the accelerated growth is occurring in metropolitan areas, principally in East and West Coast areas. The rapid population increases of the ethnic groups present some interesting and potentially disturbing implications.

In 1988, the American Council on Education (ACE) released a carefully worded report describing the social and economic conditions of African Americans, Hispanics, and American Indians—three ethnic minority groups who make up about 90% of the total ethnic minority population in the United States. "In 1988," the authors of the report maintain, "we are seeing the emergence of another 'one-third of a nation' . . . who constitute our minority population—many of whom are afflicted by the ills of poverty and discrimination" (American Council on Education, 1988, p. 2). Most notably, the ACE-sponsored

document indicates that within the next decade, one-third of all school age children, 42% of all public school students, and 21.8 million of the 140.4 million projected to be in the labor force will be of ethnic minority background. The long history of oppression, racism, and discrimination experienced by these groups will no doubt accompany the rapid population and demographic growth. Along with the trends, we are likely to witness a continued use and abuse of psychoactive drugs unless an accelerated intense increase in appropriately designed research on epidemiological, treatment prevention, and intervention topics can be implemented.

According to the 1990 Bureau of Census reports, the demographic characteristics of ethnic minorities are unevenly distributed throughout the United States. Most nonwhites or ethnic minorities reside in concentrated regions of the United States. The population patterns indicate that Hispanics, especially those of Mexican origin, are concentrated in Texas, New Mexico, Arizona, and southern California, whereas Asian Americans and African Americans tend to be concentrated in metropolitan areas along the western and eastern coastal areas and American Indians and Alaska Natives reside in the western states and Alaska. The distribution patterns also reveal that all of the five groups can be found in some proportion in virtually every state—this is even true for American Indians, who number close to 1.9 million out of a general population rapidly approaching 260 million people. Given the population distribution of those who make up "one-third of the nation," it is safe to conclude that one can find varying levels of drug use and abuse among these groups in virtually every state along with the attendant problems of racism, poverty, and oppression.

Geographic Patterns of Drug Use

The use of psychoactive drugs occurs in all 50 of the United States. Because of population distribution patterns, use levels are higher in areas with dense populations; thus one finds drug use to be greater in America's metropolitan areas than in rural areas. Some metropolitan areas such as Detroit, Washington–Baltimore, New York City, and Miami tend to show greater drug use patterns among ethnic minorities (Johnson, Williams, Dei, & Sanabria, 1990). In these cities, ethnic minorities collectively are in the majority, so the finding is not an exaggeration. More than that, it does not support the notion that ethnic minorities have greater problems with drugs than the dominant culture.

Concentrations of ethnic minorities occur in rural and remote areas of the country, particularly for American Indians and Hispanics (more likely Mexican American). Drug use appears to be a problem in these settings, too. Segal (1992) points out that the drug use prevalence rates in certain Alaska Native villages are quite high and in a few instances reach epidemic-like levels. Beauvais, Oetting, Wolf, and Edwards (1989) found that American Indian youth in rural areas have higher drug use rates than non-Indian youth for nearly all drugs. Among Hispanic youth, Gilbert and Alcocer (1988) report high incidences of polydrug use; the authors emphasize that alcohol use quite often leads to a progressive use and abuse of hard drugs.

The distribution of ethnic minority drug use nationwide may give credence to the notion that they are inclined to use drugs more frequently than the dominant culture. Undoubtedly, cultural orientations do contribute to differential patterns in drug use rates and patterns (Heath, 1987; Trimble, 1994). Unfortunately, it appears that culture, and all that it implies, is not factored into descriptions of use rates among ethnic minorities. The notion tends to be reinforced by the generalized news media. It appears that the electronic and print media tend to focus their drug use stories on the problems that occur in America's inner-city communities. A cursory review of the drug use stories appearing in the weekly news magazines reveals the frequent use of photos of African-American and Hispanic drug users, crime statistics showing disproportionate numbers of ethnic minorities arrested for drug re-

lated crimes, and harrowing tales of drug abuse in public housing projects. What we rarely see in the magazines are stories and photos of drug use that occur in the affluent suburbs or predominantly nonminority communities and neighborhoods. Yet we know from the ongoing drug use studies of Johnston, O'Malley and Bachman (1989), and the National Institute on Drug Abuse (1991c) that drug use occurs among almost all groups. Both the accounts in the news media and research reports tend to emphasize inner-city drug problems and that, in itself, fosters the stereotypic notion that ethnic minorities, especially African Americans, are more likely to be addicts than whites and Anglos. There is no definitive evidence available to support this contention (Trimble, Padilla, & Bell, 1987; Tucker, 1985).

HISTORICAL OVERVIEW OF ETHNIC MINORITY DRUG USE

Few students of American history are unaware of the massive mid-nineteenth-century immigration of Chinese to the West Coast, brought in principally to work on railroads and related service industries. Along with their customs and traditions, the Chinese brought their proclivity for opium smoking. One could find an opium den in practically every Chinese-American community, especially in West Coast cities. The use and presence of opium increased and with the rise in usage came municipal legislation intended to outlaw and regulate its use. San Francisco and New York were the first municipalities to put through opium use regulations. By most accounts, many Chinese and Americans abused opium but there is no historical record of any attempt to treat and even prevent the addiction among the Chinese other than the use of interdiction (Segal, 1988; Inciardi, 1992). The laws and taxes imposed on opium were a deliberate attempt to regulate its use among the Chinese (Helmer, 1975; Morgan, Wallack, & Buchanan, 1989). It has been suggested that the laws and regulatory practices were deliberate and intended to control the Chinese, their employment patterns, and their interactions with other Americans (Banks, 1990; Helmer, 1975). Apart from the federal government's nineteenth-century effort to regulate alcohol use among American Indians, the opium statutes were the first set of laws set out to control drugs along with the habits and behavior of an ethnic group. The interdiction of alcohol use among American Indians and opium among Chinese was racially motivated. It was born out of the fear that somehow the effects of the alcohol and drug use presented a threat that the dominant culture couldn't control. Helmer (1975) points out that the "primary event that precipitated the campaign against the Chinese and against opium was the sudden onset of economic depression, the high unemployment levels, and the disintegration of working-class standards of living" (p. 32). He goes on to emphasize that "the ideological role of the anti-opium campaign was to get rid of the Chinese" (p. 32). Drug use and abuse was not the burning issue it seems to be today, but rather a means to control and further oppress an undesirable and underrepresented ethnic group. The divisive strategy masked as a stroke for promoting social welfare was used to control and regulate other ethnic groups, particularly African Americans and Mexican Americans.

At about the time the opium laws went into effect, concerns about the use of cocaine among southern United States African Americans began to surface. Banks (1990) cites several examples of newspaper accounts of "cocainized negroes," wild rampages, orgies, crime, and rape allegedly attributed to highly sensationalized accounts of cocaine use. "Historians question the validity of this 'epidemic,'" maintains Banks, "based on its thinly-veiled political intent and the fact that many of [the] stories were not substantiated" (p. 76). Fictional or not, the early twentieth-century accounts of African-American cocaine use added another pejorative to the already long list of negative stereotypes about the group (Helmer, 1975).

Early depictions of drug use among Chinese and African Americans proved to be a fertile ground for research; however, the research was quite biased and unsophisticated. Williams (1914)

was one of the first to study "hard" drug use among African Americans. After examining hospital and arrest records, he called southern blacks "dope fiends" and blamed an epidemic of cocaine use for their violent and aggressive lifestyles. However, Green (1914), after reviewing admissions records at the Georgia State Sanitarium between 1909 to 1914, found only three narcotic addiction cases among African Americans. The records also revealed that 142 white patients were diagnosed as having a "drug psychosis" problem. Several other "studies" attempted to support the notion that a "new menace" was created as cocaine made its way into African-American communities. Journalists helped to advance the stereotype of the "cocaine-crazed Negro." It was difficult for the cautious eye to separate fact from fiction during this period. It was not difficult, however, for certain segments of America's population to use the media fabrications to justify denying African Americans due process and access to equitable opportunities.

In the early 1920s, Mexicans and Mexican Americans were singled out as yet another population who required some form of control because of their alleged obsession with marijuana. Although it is difficult to isolate the cause of the so-called Mexican marijuana menace in the American West and Southwest, Bonnie and Whitebread (1974) believe that the Federal Bureau of Narcotics can shoulder most of the responsibility. During the 1930s, marijuana became known as the "killer weed" or "evil weed" and its protracted use led to an "incurable habit." In 1934, Harry J. Anslinger, director of the Federal Bureau of Narcotics, initiated a vigorous prolonged campaign to introduce marijuana laws in states with large Mexican-American populations. The laws apparently were motivated by allegations that the "marijuana menace" led to intense increases in "crime and deviant social behavior." Was marijuana a menace and was it used widely by Mexican Americans, as alleged by journalists of the 1930s?

Helmer (1975) identified and compiled the narcotic violation arrest rates for ethnic minorities between 1934 and 1941, the time period when the alleged "Mexican problem" reached its peak (Helmer, 1975). His compilations show that the Mexican arrest rates were lower than those of any other group, including whites. Clearly the Mexicans were singled out at that time for reasons other than their drug use. Morgan (1990) asserts that "the anti-Mexican crusade was engineered by the Federal Bureau of Narcotics (FBN) in the mid-1930s for reasons that had little to do with the Mexican population in the Southwest or marijuana for that matter" (p. 236). Helmer (1975) and Himmelstein (1983) incriminate the FBN for fabricating a problem based more on fictional accounts than on hard data.

Legal control of psychoactive drug use is a product of twentieth-century thought in the United States (Heath, 1992). Control efforts accelerated during the 1930s and reached their current levels during the late 1980s. Many of the drug laws were directed at the formulation and enactment of policies that promoted a common good. For the most part, Americans have viewed drug abuse as unhealthy and believed that prolonged use contributes to the social and moral decay of the nation. However, some of those who directed the nation's drug control and regulatory agencies used their positions to control certain populations, especially ethnic minority groups. "Control offered a means of protecting cherished values," maintains Walker (1981), "for a primarily white and putatively mobile society; it portended order in place of chaos" (p. 14). The early twentieth-century policies directed at the Chinese immigrants, southern African Americans, and Mexicans primarily living in California were racist; the policies may have been interpreted as a humanitarian gesture, but they were clearly coercive (Walker, 1981).

Drug laws and their corresponding campaigns typically produce policies imbued with political agendas (Morgan, Wallack, & Buchanan, 1989). The political agendas that include drug legislation more often than not are fueled by myths and exaggerations of drug use patterns. To a large extent, "the conflict over social justice (through social and political reform) is what the story of narcotics in America is about" (Helmer, 1975, p. 53). Chinese, Mexican Americans, and blacks were overrepresented in many drug reporting accounts between 1900 and the late 1930s; to an extent, these groups are still overrepresented in contemporary drug use reporting systems. The justice carried out against the disproportionate numbers of ethnic minority narcotic offenders created more than the usual outcomes. For the Chinese and Mexicans, the social reforms actually suppressed their potential participation in California's labor force (Helmer, 1975; Morgan, 1990). Therefore, Morgan (1990) asserts that "it is vital to understand that the importance of crusades against minorities lies not only in their victimization but also in the misrepresentation and falsification of their culture" (p. 250). Thus, the early history of drug use among ethnic minorities is understood best by examining the manner in which policy and drug laws were used for oppressive purposes and further social and class conflict. The story is not one where we learn about lifetime use patterns, addictive lifestyles, and straightforward humanitarian efforts to treat and prevent the effects of drug abuse.

CHARACTERISTICS OF ETHNIC MINORITY DRUG USE

Tallies of the numbers of ethnic minorities participating in alcohol and drug treatment programs and in drug-related emergency hospital admissions suggest that they may be overrepresented when compared with the dominant culture. Survey data maintained by the National Institute on Drug Abuse's (NIDA), Drug Abuse Warning Network (DAWN), and the Client-Oriented Data Acquisition Process (CODAP) systems show that ethnic minorities are heavily represented. Although a variety of explanations have been offered in an attempt to characterize the "overrepresentation effect" none appear to offer any promise. Few can effectively pin down causal reasons for the continued extensive and excessive drug use among the dominant ethnic groups. When the "effect" is added to the social and economic realities of the groups, a certainty emerges. Ethnic minorities have been and continue to be deeply affected by racism, discrimination, and poverty, along with the pain, despair, and hopelessness associated with oppressive lifestyles.

Literature Citations and Ethnic Minority Drug Abuse

Most drug-related epidemiological data files indicate that psychoactive drug use occurs with varying frequency among all of America's ethnic minority groups. Hence, Tucker (1985) observed that "there is no lack of commentary on the substance abuse problems faced by ethnic minorities in the United States" (p. 102). On reviewing the scant number of literature reviews on the topic, one finds that ethnic minorities have been the "objects" of a good deal of research, but little attention has been given to the cultural factors that influence their lifestyles (Cheung, 1991). For example, there are numerous studies comparing the epidemiology of drug use between ethnic groups but few etiological and within-group findings. Although Iiyama, Nishi, and Johnson (1976) point out that the literature up to the mid-1970s is quite comprehensive, Tucker (1985) also assures us that there "are no major substantive reviews of the empirical literature on ethnic minority drug use" (p. 1026). Trimble, Padilla, and Bell (1987) agree with Tucker and go on to add, "we lack even the basic and essential information necessary to understand the rate and extent of drug use among ethnic minority groups and individuals" (p. 1).

One of the first major and comprehensive summaries of ethnic minority drug abuse was sponsored by the National Institute on Drug Abuse (NIDA) (Austin, Johnson, Carroll, & Lettieri, 1977). The volume provides summary tables of 93 articles found in the literature dating back to the early 1950s. The NIDA-sponsored review does not provide an integrated comprehensive discussion of the findings. Instead, the basic components of each of the 93 articles are laid out in tables showing the authors, publication date, number of pages, number of references, sample sizes and types, age, ethnicity, geographic area, methodology and procedures, instrumentation, and dates when the study occurred. Complete reference citations also are included. The editors conclude the following: the dimensions of the problem are still not well understood, disagreement exists on the meaning of many of the findings, no clear picture exists on how the findings can influence and direct social policy, interpretations and theoretical generalizations are not convincing, and there is an absence of any theory to sufficiently explain the results.

In 1972, a National Conference on Drug Abuse was held in Washington, D.C. As a result of some background materials prepared for the meeting, an annotated bibliography of 245 citations was published, built largely on the interest and discussions generated by the conferees and sponsors (Iiyama, Nishi, and Johnson, 1976). In selecting the articles, the editors chose to include articles that focused on opiates, principally heroin—research on the abuse and use of marijuana, hallucinogens, amphetamines, barbiturates, and inhalants was omitted primarily because of the concern about the prevalence of heroin addiction in the represented ethnic populations. Oddly enough, most of the 28 Native-American citations dealt with the use of peyote, which is now classified as a psychedelic (along with LSD-25, mescaline, PCP, hashish, and marijuana). Presumably, the editors felt the need to include some citations about drug abuse among American Indians and assumed that peyote use was a problem among many of the tribal groups. In fact, this is an erroneous conclusion because the drug is highly controlled among many American Indians, particularly through the efforts of members of the Native American Church movement.

Iiyama, Nishi, and Johnson (1976) compiled an interesting and informative list of citations of which almost 80% focused on blacks and 23% on Puerto Ricans. Before the list of annotated bibliographic entries, the editors provided a 55-page summary of their findings complete with plausible interpretations and discussions. The editors tended to focus on the research results peppered with summaries of various strategies used by researchers. The summary review contains rich and enlightening speculations that prompt far more questions than answers, especially the meaning and implication of the findings and their relevance for shaping public attitudes and policy. Perhaps most compelling are the editors' bold and incisive conclusions. They contend "that although addiction among minorities is perceived by the public as a serious social problem, many facts indicate that the extent of the problem does not warrant the amount of public concern and attention given" (p. 53). The editors boldly conclude that it is society's response to narcotics addiction that is the major source of the problem. "The true problem," Iiyama, Nishi, and Johnson (1976) contend, "is the symbolic transformation of a relatively small public health concern into a gigantic moral problem" and that "minorities continue to be the focus of blame for drug addiction as well as the objects of social control efforts" (pp. 57–58).

In 1985 and 1987, two short literature reviews on ethnic minority drug abuse appeared in the literature. Tucker (1985) bases her review of 126 articles on her contention that "no comprehensive review of drug abuse *by* American ethnic minorities has ever been undertaken" (p. 1021; italics mine). She argues that the literature on the subject lacks a distinct ethnic focus and that "the literature tells us much about heroin addicts . . . but very little about drug addiction within Afro-American or Puerto Rican *culture*" (italics Tucker's; p. 1026). Using this point as her lead theme, Tucker builds her well-written review on the drug issues that "bind ethnic minorities; those that have distinctive relevance by virtue of the *sociopolitical status* of an ethnic minority" (p. 1024; italics in original). Tucker acknowledges the finding that more ethnic minorities are conducting research on their respective populations, especially during the 1970s, and therefore some of the culture-specific concerns are being

addressed. Like the other reviewers, Tucker points out that there are still limitations inherent in drug abuse research and the body of ethnic minority literature, including the following:

— There are no comprehensive reviews on empirical and clinical literature.
— There are no regular comprehensive drug abuse assessments.
— There are no etiological studies.
— Too many studies focus on comparisons between ethnic groups and too few studies focus on applying results for use in service delivery domains.
— Few theories account for the special circumstances of ethnic minorities.
— There is no literature to guide and direct the design, selection, and development of intervention and prevention programs.
— Little support exists to provide for the development of ethnic group-specific treatment and prevention programs.

These findings alone would provide for a comprehensive research and development agenda that could easily consume two decades of intensive effort.

In 1983, in response to growing national pressure applied by ethnic minorities concerning the seemingly growing problem of minority drug abuse, the National Institute on Drug Abuse convened a meeting of 13 researchers of ethnic minority background. Trimble, Padilla, and Bell (1987) edited and compiled the proceedings. By their own admission, some of the attendees at the NIDA-sponsored workshop were not drug abuse experts or even experts in the vicissitudes of their respective cultural and ethnic groups. However, they were of one voice in their recommendation that knowledge gaps existed in the ethnic minority drug abuse field and that a number of problems existed in the interpretation and implementation of some of the research findings. Like Tucker and Iiyama, Nishi, and Johnson, they put forth a call for research that distinguished "ethnic groups on the basis of values, norms, life conditions, history and heritage and adaptive problems" and stated "that the common division in drug and alcohol studies between 'white' and 'non-white' populations is grossly inadequate for examining drug abuse within a culture and each ethnic group needs to be studied in its own right" (p. 36).

Trimble (in press) identified 186 articles published between 1953 and 1988 that contained relevant information concerning research efforts and appropriate commentary concerning the topical field. Several criteria were used in the selection of the citations, including the frequency of the citation as it appeared in reference sections of publications and representativeness of the drug types. Studies on alcohol and peyote were excluded for logistic and practical reasons, hence the 186 citations included articles on sedative hypnotics, opiates, stimulants, psychedelics (because of the presence or absence of studies focusing on these psychoactive drug types, alternate drug categories were created to include opiates, marijuana, heroin, cocaine, methadone, and a generalized "other" category). Articles dealing with six ethnic minority social and political groups (American Indian and Alaska Native, Asian American and Pacific Islander, black, Hispanic/Mexican American, General, and Puerto Rican) were included. In this grouping he included articles that compared findings between ethnic groups and between Anglos and ethnic groups. The articles listed include detailed descriptions of methods and procedures, sample selection, instrumentation, and the general purpose of the study or article.

The counts show that almost twice as many articles were published in the 1980s than between 1950 and 1969 (4 in 1950, 41 in 1960, 72 in 1970, and 80 in 1980), revealing that the topic is receiving more attention. The geographic location in which the studies were conducted shows that 59.3% of the research was conducted in New York (24%), California (14.6%), and Kentucky (10.7%)—only 103 of 186 citations make reference to states, however. Studies conducted in the District of Columbia, Florida, Illinois, Texas, and Puerto Rico (four to six articles each), comprise 19.4% of the articles. Finally, 27 states did not show reported research on the topic during the period of the review.

Overall, the tabulations of the citations show that the majority of the studies are multiethnic comparative studies and focus primarily on adults concerning multiple drug and opiate topics. The findings also reveal that 29 studies compared Anglos with one or more of the ethnic groups, which is slightly less than *all* of the studies of the six ethnic groups combined. The number of citations for Asian Americans is the lowest for all other categories, with a total of 1,843 subjects who were included in three multidrug studies and one on opiates; Asians were included in a number of multiethnic studies, so more information is available on this group. The tabular results show that no studies on ethnic minorities and marijuana use were available for review and only one on methadone use was available. In general, the patterns show that researchers are somewhat driven by the desire to compare different types of drug use among different types of ethnic groups—the irony here is that significantly more detail is devoted to precisely describing drug types than to describing the subject populations.

Despite the presence of ethnic minorities in every state (and therefore every geographic region), Trimble's analysis shows that researchers tend to concentrate their work in a few areas of the country. The seven states of the Plains region (Iowa, Minnesota, Missouri, North and South Dakota, Nebraska, and Kansas) appear to generate the least amount of work, followed closely by the six New England states. The area with the largest concentration of studies is the Mid-Atlantic region, where most of the studies emanate out of New York City. A modest amount of work appears to have been performed in the South, but the tabulations are biased because the majority occur in Kentucky and Texas, principally in Lexington and Fort Worth.

Trimble's results offer a few summary conclusions. First, drug use researchers appear to be most interested in conducting and writing about ethnic comparative topics. All of the major groups are pooled in an effort to identify and describe between- and within-group drug use patterns. Research on African Americans received the most attention and Asian-Pacific Americans received the least. Most of the citations focus on adults. Second, much of what we know about ethnic minority drug use comes from survey research, where there appears to be a reliance on interview and questionnaire procedures. Third, treatment efficacy topics dominate the literature. Little attention is given to primary and secondary prevention topics. Consequently, we know something about the perceived effectiveness of treatment modalities but very little about prevention and epidemiological correlates among the major ethnic minority groups. We also know very little about the etiology of drug use and abuse among the groups. Finally, most of what we know about the subject was generated in certain regions of the United States. Because drug use occurs among ethnic groups in all 50 states, large information gaps do exist. When the results of the citation review are compared with earlier literature reviews, it is clear that the ethnic minority drug use field has not progressed in any significant manner. Even more disturbing is the possibility that many ethnic minority community and neighborhood prevention programs may be initiated in the absence of a strong research database—program planners may have little empirical evidence on which to build an intervention plan, which can increase the likelihood of program failure. Community drug intervention planners should have information about the efficacy of a strategy or model. Vicarious intervention plans, regardless of the intended audience, must not be implemented if the planners and organizers have no theoretical or data-based set of propositions. The present and future livelihood of many potential drug abusers is much too fragile to be subjected to untested whim and nonvalidated hunch.

Prevalence Rates Among Ethnic Minorities

The dearth of published articles focusing on ethnic minority drug abuse belies the ethnic minority drug use prevalence rates. Drug use surveys among ethnic groups are sparse and except for one or two groups, ongoing studies are sporadic

and limited to certain geographic areas. However, the results of some of the surveys indicate that use rates exceed those of the dominant populations on a per capita basis.

Maddahian, Newcomb, and Bentler (1985, 1986, 1988) conducted a five-year longitudinal study of three ethnic minority groups in the Los Angeles area; youth in the 7th, 8th, and 9th grades in 11 schools were given surveys designed to tap various notions about drug use. The researchers found differences between the ethnic groups in their use rates. However, they did not find differences between Asian, black, and Hispanic youth dropouts and continuing participants on drug use and intentions to use drugs. In a related finding, however, the researchers observed that there were differences between intention to use and actual future use rates across the groups. Although the sample sizes for the three ethnic groups were small and restricted to one metropolitan area, the nature of the work is precisely the kind that should be carried out nationwide.

Two recurring drug use surveys, the High School Seniors Survey (Johnston, O'Malley, & Bachman, 1988), and the National Household Survey on Drug Abuse (NIDA, 1991c) have been compiling drug patterns for nearly two decades. In the past, survey results from both projects downplayed drug use among ethnic minorities largely because of sampling and procedural matters.

The 1991 National Household Survey (NHS) compiled drug use rates from 32,594 respondents in four regions of the United States. African Americans and Hispanics were well-represented in the sample; other ethnic minority groups were involved, but their responses were grouped in a general "Other" category.

NHS results show that 39% of the African Americans and 31% of the Hispanics reported lifetime use of any illicit drug. Males in both groups used drugs more than females. Both groups reported heavy lifetime use of alcohol— 79% for African Americans and 77% for Hispanics. Slightly less than 50% of both groups reported using alcohol in the past month. Marijuana was the next most frequently used drug;

36% of the African Americans and 27% of the Hispanics reported use at some point in their lives. About 11% for each group reported use of cocaine. For all three drugs, a higher percentage of whites reported use than African Americans and Hispanics.

The National Institute on Drug Abuse collects national data annually through the Drug Abuse Warning Network (DAWN). In 1990, 503 sample hospitals with 533 separate emergency room facilities supplied the DAWN with patient drug abuse data. In 1990, multiple drug use was reported for 49% of emergency room episodes; 47% involved African Americans and 42% involved Hispanics (NIDA, 1991a). "Suicide was the drug use motive in 57% of episodes involving white patients; 35% of those involving Hispanic patients, and 24% of those involving African American patients" (p. 15).

The DAWN 1991 emergency room report shows that alcohol combined with other drugs, cocaine, and heroin/morphine were the three most frequently mentioned drugs. African Americans reported the highest use rates for all three drugs—34% for alcohol in combination, 49% for cocaine, and 6% for heroin/morphine. Twenty-two percent of the Hispanics mentioned use of cocaine as the motive for admission to the hospitals.

Again in 1990, 135 medical examiners from 27 metropolitan areas reported 5,830 drug-related deaths to DAWN (NIDA, 1991b). The report indicates that "decedents were white in 53 percent of the cases, Black in 29 percent, and Hispanic in 16 percent" (p. 7). Cocaine was reported 43% of the time for the deaths, followed by alcohol-in-combination and heroin/morphine. African-American deaths were more likely to be the result of cocaine than deaths of whites and Hispanics (66%, 27%, and 53%, respectively). Heroin/morphine use was reported in 34% of the cases; Hispanic deaths were higher than those of whites and African Americans (46%, 30%, and 35%, respectively).

Data generated by the DAWN and the National Household Survey are limited to African American and Hispanics and, therefore, tell us little about use rates among American Indians and Asian-Pacific Americans. Nonetheless, the reports contain rich information that can assist us in tracking drug use patterns over time and in different regions of the country.

With one exception, longitudinal and cross-section studies of drug use patterns among specific ethnic minority groups are nonexistent in the literature. The exception to this unfortunate finding is American Indians. Since 1974, Oetting, Edwards, and Beauvais (1989) at Colorado State University have been assessing drug use among samples of American Indian youth largely from reservation communities in the western states. The Colorado-based researchers found that drug use for Indian youth increased from 1975 through 1981, dropped off slightly for a few years, then gradually increased to the point where it has leveled off. Oetting, Edwards, and Beauvais compared their drug use with comparison date from the National Household Survey. Overall, the Indian use rates were much higher than those of other American youth. To account for some of their findings, the research team agree that much of "the anti-drug publicity has been aimed generally at the 'good kids' and it seems to have influenced them. But anti-drug efforts have apparently not been able to reach those young Indians who have a high potential for deviance" (p. 13). About 20% of the Indian youth reported in the Colorado State University studies are at highest risk—these are the youth who use drugs with some regularity.

Since 1988, researchers at the National American Indian and Alaska Native Mental Health Research Center in Denver, Colorado have been conducting a longitudinal study of Indian drug use in a boarding school (Dick, Manson, & Beals, 1993). Over the past three years, the researchers have found that more than 80% of the Indian youth report using alcohol. More than 20% reported using alcohol every weekend. About 70% reported using marijuana—close to one-fourth reported that they used it at least 10 times in the previous month. More than 40% reported using other drugs three or more times in the previous month (King, Beals, Manson, & Trimble, 1992). The Denver-based researchers indicate that use rates were declining slightly in 1992 (S. Manson, personal communication, February 11, 1992).

Data generated from the Colorado longitudinal surveys are consistent with other short-term studies on American Indian drug use. May (1982) summarized studies reporting alcohol and drug use patterns in a number of communities. The findings are somewhat dated, but they point to a disturbing pattern. May reports that between 56% and 89% of the youth from four Indian communities indicated that they drank alcohol.

In his analysis of marijuana use rates, May showed that between 22% and 78% of Indian youth indicated that they tried it at least once—in one study, 27% were shown to be heavy users of the drug. Inhalant use rates were reported to range between 4% and 62% in the studies included in May's review. Some 13% reported heavy use of inhalants in one area of the country. Overall, May's review of Indian drug use patterns reveals a good deal of variation from one community to the next. Despite the variation in the results, May demonstrates that Indian youth use rates exceed those of the general population. In a similar article, Weibel-Orlando (1984) reinforces May's conclusions and adds that "there is overwhelming evidence of the profound effects early drug socialization . . . has on individual drinking and drug use patterns" among American Indians (p. 329).

Studies conducted among Indians in the Pacific Northwest and Alaska Natives reveal somewhat similar use rates to those previously reported. Survey data generated from Indian youth in Washington show that at least 20% reported using marijuana, tobacco, and inhalants and that more than half of the youths tried alcohol (Gilchrist, Schinke, Trimble, & Cvetkovich, 1987). In Alaska, Segal (1989) conducted a comprehensive survey of drug use among a sample of more than 4,000 Alaskan youth. Alaska Natives and American Indians made up 23% of the sample. Native youth showed higher drug and al-

cohol use than the other ethnic groups, including whites. About 75% of the native sample indicated that they tried one or more drugs. About 71% of the Alaska Natives and 66% of the Indians tried marijuana, 40% reported using stimulants, 21% tried hallucinogens, and 33% used inhalants; 70% of the Alaska Natives and 53% of the Indians used "chew" or smokeless tobacco; and 88% of the Indians and 75% of the Alaska Natives tried alcohol.

The 1988 Alaska study was a follow-up of a similar survey conducted by Segal and his associates in 1983 (Segal, 1983). In both surveys, it is clear that drug use among Alaska Natives was fairly high. Drug use changes did occur between 1983 and 1988, but they were modest at best. Percent changes for the entire Alaskan sample of high school youth ranged between +18.4% to –1.1%; the former represents an increase in inhalant use and the latter a decrease in depressant use. These figures represent the youths' opportunity to try psychoactive substances. Segal (1988) summarizes his survey research with the point that "the changes within the [Alaskan] regions suggest that while there is *general consistency* across regions concerning use of some substances, there are also some patterns idiosyncratic to different locations" (p. 95; italics mine). Considering the geographic size and remoteness of most Alaskan communities, Segal's findings are alarming; the findings almost beg an answer to the question, "How do drugs find their way into small, remote communities?"

Although African Americans constitute the largest ethnic minority group in the United States, little published drug use studies have been dedicated to this group. Instead, what one finds in the literature are short-term site-specific surveys that often compare African-American drug use with that of other ethnic groups. Some of the studies focus exclusively on alcohol consumption. Fernandez-Pol, Bluestone, Missouri, Morales, and Mizruchi (1986) compared drinking rates between urban African Americans and Puerto Ricans and found that African-American women drink less than African-American and

Puerto Rican men. Womble and Bakeman (1986) also report similar findings. In addition, some limited survey findings suggest that African-American youth use alcohol less often than youth from other ethnic groups (Herd, 1988). However, African-American youth are more likely to engage in polydrug use than other American ethnic groups; they show higher use rates than those of young Hispanics and whites, especially for alcohol and heroin, alcohol and PCP, and cocaine and heroin (Schinke, Schilling, & Gilchrist, 1986). African-American adult males consume more alcohol than white males on a per capita basis; in fact, some data indicate that alcohol-related cirrhotic mortality rates among African Americans is twice that of whites (Herd, 1988). Because of the shortage of work in the area, Keil (1989), in a comparative overview of drug use among older ethnic minority women, points to the need for more comprehensive studies of this segment of the population.

The bulk of the African-American drug use survey findings emphasize urban and inner-city patterns. Nobles, Goddard, Cavill, and George (1987), in an effort to describe the culture of drug use among Oakland, California African-American youth, found that they were highly knowledgeable about drug distribution and use. More than 80% of the youth knew what specific drugs were being sold, slightly more than 70% knew someone who was on drugs, and about 90% witnessed drug use on a daily basis. Two-thirds of the youth felt that people like themselves were attracted to the drug lifestyle. Maton and Zimmerman (1992) surveyed 150 African-American male adolescents from Baltimore on two separate occasions. Most of the youth were school dropouts, which is a difficult population to identify and track. The researchers found that 61% tried alcohol, 39% used some marijuana, and 16% tried hard drugs (cocaine, "smack," and depressants). Results from their study suggest that lifestyle patterns are a moderate predictor of marijuana and hard drug use; leaving school also weighed heavily in predicting drug use patterns. Drug use among some African Americans and other ethnic groups often leads to violent lifestyles (Spunt, Goldstein, Bellucci, & Miller, 1990). Budd (1989), for example, found that the majority of homicide victims who tested positive for cocaine use were African-American males.

Literature on the psychosocial characteristics among America's homeless populations is increasing (Dennis, Buckner, Lipton, & Levine, 1991). According to Fischer and Breakey (1991) the "*new* homeless population is younger and more heterogeneous than the old skid row populations including a greater proportion of single women and an overrepresentation of minorities, particularly Blacks and Hispanics" (p. 1115). Milburn and Booth (1992) surveyed 414 homeless people in Washington, D.C. in the winter of 1988; 87% were African American. The two researchers found that 62% of the African-American adults reported using drugs at some point in their lives; 38% reported using drugs within the previous year. Twenty-six percent were using drugs at the time of the interview. Marijuana (17%) and cocaine (16%) were the two most frequently cited illicit drugs used by the respondents; 86% reported ever using alcohol, 74% used it within the past year, and 59% were currently using alcohol.

Milburn and Booth (1992) also compared illicit drugs among homeless and nonhomeless African Americans. Homeless African-American adults were more likely than their nonhomeless counterparts to use PCP, cocaine, and marijuana; this finding was true across all age categories. Older homeless African Americans were more likely to have used alcohol than the nonhomeless group. Homeless men were much more likely than women to use illicit drugs. The researchers conclude that drug abuse is more of a problem among homeless African-American adults living in shelters than for nonhomeless African Americans, but lifetime use rates vary with the duration of homelessness and the financial status of the individual.

A few researchers are studying drug use among African-American students in colleges and universities. Most notable and illuminative is the survey of students at a historically

African-American university carried out by Wilson and Taylor (1990). Using an extensive questionnaire, the research team surveyed more than 300 African-American undergraduates. Lifetime use rates were tabulated and the results show that 83% of males and 90% of females reported ever using alcohol; 58% reported using it in the previous month. For marijuana, 58% of males and 41% of females reported lifetime use. Cocaine use ranged from 9% for males to 4% for females; use of crack and heroin was reported by a few of the respondents. Respondents believed that drugs were easy to acquire, especially those who reported using them more frequently than other students.

How do the above drug use findings compare with a national sample of African Americans? In the 1985 National Household Survey, some attention was given to drug and alcohol use among three African-American age cohorts (18–25, 26–34, and 35+). Results show lifetime use rates are highest for alcohol; more than 80% indicated so for each cohort. Marijuana use was the second highest, with lifetime rates of 21% for the 35+ group and 50% for the 18–24 age group. The survey also found that stimulants, sedative hypnotics and tranquilizers, and cocaine yielded lifetime use rates of about 15% for the first two age cohorts and around 8% for the 35 and older group.

Drug use rates for African Americans are scattered among various segments of the population. Many of the findings are dated and limited to certain sections of the country. The results provide us with a snapshot view of the population, but they tell us little about longitudinal patterns of use. Therefore, there is an urgent need to generate more epidemiologic findings compiled from well-designed multiyear studies that include samples from all segments of the African-American population.

Drug use surveys among America's Hispanic populations are less prevalent than for African Americans; hence we know even less about the problem among America's fastest growing ethnic group. Gilbert (1989) reminds us "that much of the scant data that are available are limited in their generalizability, reliability and, most impor-

tantly, their usefulness to persons providing services targeted to Latino adolescents" (p. 36).

The most comprehensive review of Hispanic drug use to date can be found in the work by Chavez and Swaim (1992). The two researchers argue that the Hispanic drug use findings contain several contradictory findings. The inconsistent array of prevalence rate findings can be attributed to deficiencies in research design, the diversity and complexity of the Hispanic population, and variations in gender, Hispanic subgroups, socioeconomic status, community characteristics, educational attainment, and acculturation. Chavez and Swaim strongly emphasize that Hispanic drug use studies that do not account for the fluctuations in these characteristics and factors are likely to obscure differences among disaggregated samples. Given these concerns, the following summary of Hispanic drug use must be viewed with prudence and discretion.

The National Household Survey (NIDA, 1989) provided drug use comparative findings for Hispanic groups and whites. For all respondents between the ages of 12 to 35 and older, 87% of the Hispanic males and 72% of the females reported having ever tried alcohol; differences between the two sexes were also found for illicit drug use and these differences were greater for Hispanics than for whites. Cocaine and crack use also were found to be higher among Hispanics.

Perhaps the most comprehensive set of drug use findings was generated through the large-scale and comprehensive Hispanic Health and Nutrition Examination Survey (NIDA, 1987). Survey data were collected between 1982 and 1984 from slightly more than 8,000 Cuban Americans, Mexican Americans, and Puerto Ricans. For all three groups, males were more likely than females to have ever tried drugs; Cuban Americans collectively were less likely to use drugs than the other two groups. Lifetime use rates for marijuana were similar for Mexican Americans (42%) and Puerto Ricans (43%); they were lower for Cuban Americans (20%). Cocaine use was highest for Puerto Ricans (28% overall; 41% among males and 14% among females);

Mexican and Cuban American rates were almost half that of Puerto Ricans (11% and 9%, respectively). For all three groups, inhalant use rates were less than 5%.

Two large-scale drug use surveys were sponsored by the Texas Commission on Alcohol and Drug Abuse (Fredlund, Spence, & Maxwell, 1989). Results from both surveys show that Hispanic use rates were less than those of whites but higher than those of blacks. The highest rates for marijuana and cocaine use were found among Hispanic school-age youth.

Chavez and Swaim (1992) point out that Hispanic residential patterns yield quite different drug use results. For example, Chavez, Beauvais, and Oetting (1986) found overall use rates in a rural Southwest community to be considerably higher than those of the general population in the United States. They also found that alcohol and inhalant use were much higher in the community when compared with studies focusing on urban Hispanic use rates. These findings, however, contradict those reported by Schinke and colleagues (1992). The New York City–based researchers found not only that the ethnic and racial background factors were not strong predictors of substance abuse but that non-Hispanics reported higher lifetime drug use rates than Hispanics. Longshore, Hsieh, Anglin, and Annon (1992) also found similar results among blacks and Hispanics in the Los Angeles area.

In closing this brief section on ethnic minority drug use patterns, attention must be given to use rates among Asian and Pacific Americans. Earlier in this chapter, reference was made to the seemingly small number of articles devoted to drug use among Asian Pacific groups. Unfortunately, the number of published articles describing prevalence rates among this ethnic group are limited in scope and few in number. In general, the findings from the limited number of studies run counter to clinical and anecdotal testimony (Nakashima, 1986). Asian-Pacific drug use survey results tend to show that rates are much lower overall than those of other ethnic groups and of the general U.S. population. Clinical ad-

missions and "street talk" testimony portray another picture that suggests that use rates are much higher—even epidemic-like—than surveys report (Zane & Sasao, 1992). There is also a good deal of variation in the findings. Most survey samples are small and drawn from urban environments, primarily on the West Coast. Results are also compounded and perhaps confounded by intergenerational differences, culture-specific impressions concerning what constitutes "hard drugs," and differences within the Asian-Pacific population.

A summary of some of the findings can help to illustrate the nature and patterns and assist promote comparisons with the other ethnic groups. Zane and Sasao (1992) summarized two studies conducted in Los Angeles among 7th and 8th grade Asian youths. The results suggest that the lifetime use rates of cigarettes, marijuana, and alcohol were lower than those of African American, Hispanic, and white youth. Sasao (1989) surveyed about 125 residents of a Japanese community in southern California; 73% reported a lifetime use of alcohol and 55% of cigarettes. Yee and Thu (1987) surveyed some 840 Southeast Asian refugees living in Houston, Texas; 45% reported using alcohol or cigarettes. Finally, in a series of studies, Lubben, Chi, and Kitano (1989) interviewed almost 1,100 Asian Pacifics in the Los Angeles area. The research team found that alcohol use among the males was similar to that among same-age groups in the general population; Japanese and Filipino males reported the highest level of alcohol consumption (25% and 20%, respectively).

Zane and Sasao (1992) point out that drug use research on Asian Pacifics does not provide good estimates. Nonetheless, based on the limited number of surveys, they conclude that alcohol use has been underestimated; use of barbiturates, tranquilizers, and pain reduction drugs is evident among older Asian Pacifics; cultural differences influence use rates; and prevalence rates, as limited as they are, will soon be outdated.

In some respects, the words of Zane and Sasao stand as markers for the entire field of ethnic minority drug use surveys. Indeed, the data that exist are informative, even alarming at times. Soundly developed survey research on ethnic minority drug use is needed, especially if we hope to learn whether prevention and intervention strategies work. For the moment, however, we know that drug use is a problem in ethnic minority communities. The problem may be exaggerated; it may not be as great as we are led to believe by the media. Whatever the case, prevention and intervention programs are underway and hopefully are chipping away at the problem.

PREVENTION STRATEGIES AND PROGRAMS[2]

The literature shows that there are only a handful of articles describing drug use prevention programs intended specifically for ethnic minorities; these are limited to American Indian youth (Trimble, in press). Certainly, ethnic minorities may be involved in large-scale prevention efforts occurring in school and in ethnically mixed neighborhoods and communities. The literature findings are consistent with the observations of other researchers. King (1982) was unable to identify any studies describing prevention programs for African-American women; Womble (1990) reinforces this finding. Tucker (1985) is more direct when she points out that the state of "prevention activities directed toward minority concerns is very dismal" (p. 1037). She also cites the review of prevention programs conducted by Schaps et al. (1981)—the authors found that "only 3 of the 127 programs served populations that were more than 50% minority!" (p. 1037). Nathan (1983) concurs with the observation and adds that "we have chosen to concentrate our prevention efforts on the majority population in part because minorities do not avail themselves of treatment or prevention programs in numbers proportional to the problems they experience with alcohol" (p. 462).

A number of researchers have drawn attention to the need for developing and increasing prevention efforts intended for specific ethnic groups. Payton (1981) emphasized that "although

minority groups may not have an accurate count of drug use patterns as a result of missing or biased data their concern for preventing drug abuse is as great as that of the majority group" (p. 21). Taking a more direct stance, Brown (1985) lays the responsibility for promoting prevention right on the doorstep of federal government agencies. However, he reminds us, "for the minority community there appears to have been a particular ambivalence regarding federal drug abuse policy" (p. 213). Like many of his counterparts, Brown believes that the community of scholars, planners, and practitioners must mount an effort to construct culturally appropriate and effective treatment and prevention programs for minorities. Similar comments have been voiced for specific ethnic minority groups (Aron, Alger, & Gonzalez, 1974; Crisp, 1980; Harvey, 1985; May, 1982; Trimble, 1984; Willer & Vokes, 1989).

At-Risk Youth

A growing body of studies indicates that certain youth are more susceptible to drug use than others (Hawkins, Lishner, & Catalano, 1985; Kandel, Kessler, & Margulies, 1978; Johnson, Williams, Dei, & Sanabria, 1990, Benson & Donahue, 1989). The presence of crime, crowding, unemployment, homelessness, poor nutrition, and dysfunctional family life are known to increase the likelihood of drug use. Youth who are surrounded by these conditions are said to be at risk because the circumstances appear to be directly related to the presence of drugs in the neighborhoods and communities.

Other factors can influence youths' drug use. Family rearing practices, conflicts between parents, and the family's socioeconomic status, including poor living conditions, combine to increase the risk for delinquency, truancy from school, and drug use (Baumrind, 1985; Farrington, 1979; McCord, 1981; Needle et al., 1988; Nurco, Shaffer, & Crisin, 1984). School performance and commitment to education contribute somewhat to the high-risk conditions (Kandel, Kessler, & Margulies, 1978). The strongest pre-

dictor of drug use, however, is the peer group (Kandel, 1982; Oetting & Beauvais, 1986). Agnew (1991) points out that the nature of peer interaction, including closeness, attachment, time spent together, and pressure, influence the likelihood of delinquency and drug use. It is very likely that many ethnic minorities live in communities where the conditions fit the high-risk profile. Moreover, targeting prevention efforts at high-risk youth makes good pragmatic sense. The factors that contribute to risk merit serious attention and should be included in any comprehensive prevention program (Coie et al., 1993).

Federal Government Response

Currently, three federal agencies are responsible for stimulating and providing support for drug and alcohol treatment and prevention programs: the National Institute on Alcohol Abuse and Alcoholism (NIAAA), the National Institute on Drug Abuse, and the Center for Substance Abuse Prevention (CSAP). In the past decade or so, NIAAA and NIDA supported a handful of prevention efforts directed specifically at ethnic minority groups. CSAP, in its short history, has supported numerous drug and alcohol prevention and intervention projects in ethnic communities.

In 1986, the United States Congress legislated the Anti-Drug Abuse Act; a major portion of the act led to creation of CSAP. CSAP's major mission is to promote the concepts of no illicit drugs and no illegal or high-risk use of alcohol or other legal drugs; to accomplish this laudable and ambitious goal, CSAP emphasizes youth and families living in high-risk settings (CSAP, 1991). CSAP currently sponsors and promotes a variety of activities and programs toward this goal, including demonstration grants for the prevention of alcohol and other drug abuse among high-risk youth, model projects for pregnant and postpartum women and their infants, and community partnership grants. In addition, they sponsor communication programs that reach targeted populations with specific prevention messages and develop communication tools and ma-

terials that respond to the specific needs of certain audiences. Out of the communication effort, CSAP established the National Clearinghouse for Alcohol and Drug Information and the Regional Alcohol and Drug Awareness Resource Network. Clearly the CSAP, with the assistance of the U.S. Congress, formulated a variety of significant activities designed to reduce and possibly eliminate drug and alcohol use and abuse.

Projects funded through CSAP's Community Partnership Demonstration Program (CPP) shed a good deal of insight on the magnitude of the drug use problem in the United States. The CPP program is designed to demonstrate the effectiveness of using community resources to plan, coordinate, and implement prevention programs. To be eligible for an award, a community must establish a partnership with at least seven local organizations or agencies—examples include health clinics, social service agencies, schools, colleges and universities, private business and industry, religious organizations, law enforcement agencies, civic organizations, and professional organizations. Each applicant must submit a rigorously developed prevention model or plan including a thoroughly developed implementation and evaluation plan.

In 1990, CSAP awarded 252 community partnership grants; grant awards ranged from $98,000 to $1,040,000, with an average of $320,000. Many of the awards are for a five-year period. Twenty-six of the awards went to communities in California and 23 went to programs in Massachusetts; the remaining awards were distributed among communities in most of the other 50 states. Thirty-three percent of the grants focused on drug prevention programs targeted exclusively for whites, 5% were awarded to American Indian communities, 2% to Asian-Pacific and Hispanic communities, and 1% were awarded to African-American communities. Fifty-seven percent of the awards went to communities that proposed multiethnic-oriented projects. Thus, 10% of the awards went to communities that proposed an ethnic-specific prevention effort. The CPP is far and away CSAP's largest and most expensive program. Evaluation and outcome results from the large venture will be available sometime during the mid-1990s.

Beginning in 1987, CSAP supported and continues to support drug prevention demonstration grants targeted to high-risk youth. Many of the CSAP projects focus on ethnic minority youth. The overall objective of the CSAP program is to decrease the factors that protect and bolster the resiliency of vulnerable youth (CSAP, 1991). CSAP encourages communities, schools, and other nonprofit groups to develop prevention strategies that include the individual, the family, the school, the peer group, and the community— in a word, a multifaceted effort that includes elements that could contribute to decreasing youths' risks. Seventy percent of the CSAP-funded High-Risk Youth (HRY) projects are focused on the individual. Prevention strategies range from life skills training to cultural enrichment programs; 50% focus on family- and school-based risk factors and involve family life, parenting skills, and school and tutoring advocates and training.

The majority of the HRY projects use prevention and intervention strategies and approaches that have been tested in controlled research settings. Many of the programs strive to teach youths basic personal and social skills. Grounded in the fundamentals of social learning theory and persuasive communication theory, cognitive–behavioral strategies are developed to influence and build youths' social and personal competence (Bandura, 1977; McGuire, 1964). Out of the cognitive–behavioral tradition emerged drug use prevention strategies such as social assertiveness skills training (Pentz, 1983), cognitive–behavioral skills training (Schinke & Gilchrist, 1984), and life skills training (Botvin et al., 1984). Each of the intervention approaches guides youth through a process in which they develop and internalize communication, problem-solving, and decision-making skills, particularly in life situations where drug use may be involved (Bell & Battjes, 1987).

From 1987 to 1991, CSAP funded numerous HRY projects that focused on the five major high-risk groups. Projects that emphasized the individual and personal risk factors model focused on social and life skills training; individual or group therapy or counseling, tutoring and homework support, mentoring and role model encouragement, and alternative and modified individual level activities. Descriptions of two of the projects can enhance our understanding of the specific individual-level prevention strategies (CSAP, 1991).

Using a life skills training model, the Early Intervention with Substance Abusing Adolescents Program at the Philadelphia Psychiatric Center selected court-referred youth 13 to 19 years of age to participate in one of two activities. After the program, research findings showed that the youths' negative attitudes toward marijuana, alcohol, and cigarette use increased and getting in trouble with the police while drunk or drinking alcohol decreased.

In the New Orleans Alcohol and Drug Abuse Community Project, elementary school African-American youth were invited to participate in an after-school program. The intervention plan emphasized self-esteem building, supervised homework exercises, and free play. Evaluation results revealed that youth who participated in self-esteem activities showed significant improvement on standardized tests.

CSAP projects aimed at reducing family risk factors emphasized family therapy, family skills training, play therapy, parent training programs, and parent involvement programs. About 50% of the high-risk youth projects used some sort of parent skills training strategy in tandem with other activities. A summary description of one of the program follows: In Corpus Christi, Texas, the Parents Association for Drug Rehabilitation and Education (PADRES) chose to devote their prevention strategy to Hispanic youth and their parents. Parents were required to attend two counseling sessions. During the sessions and on other occasions, PADRES staff created opportunities for parents to become involved in program activities. A new community tradition emerged that led to greater communication between youth and the parents and the community as a whole.

As indicated earlier, peers appear to have a strong influence on youths' drug and alcohol use. Several of the CSAP high-risk youth projects emphasized peer-based activities that included positive peer clubs and groups, modifying peer group norms concerning alcohol and drug use, peer resistance and refusal skills training, providing positive peer models, and peer leadership development and counseling interventions. An example of one of our many interesting projects emphasizing this strategy occurred in Atlanta, Georgia. Through the use of peer resistance training, Super II Project was able to demonstrate a significant decrease in youths' alcohol and drug use. Parents and guardians were also included in the training program.

It is well-known that community norms can influence the use of drugs. Recognizing this finding as critical in preventing drug use, several CSAP projects chose to focus their efforts on cultural enhancement programs, orientations to the availability of community services, rites of passage, organizing positive drug-free youth groups, enhancing community service activities, conducting media education campaigns, and providing safe areas for youth to play. Examples of the community-based activities include the development and production of a cable television program by the Comprehensive Afro-American Adolescent Services Project at the University of Cincinnati, an Outward Bound type program developed by the Cherokee Challenge Early Intervention Project in Cherokee, North Carolina, and the community services project developed in Hartford and Bridgeport, Connecticut for African-American and Hispanic youth by the Targeted Primary Prevention Program.

Certainly, CSAP is responsible for supporting a wide range of drug prevention activities. In addition to this support, CSAP is keenly interested in compiling detailed information on the nature and effectiveness of the projects for specific ethnic minority and cultural groups. As part of that venture, CSAP asked several investigators to survey the project coordinators of the many ethnic-specific projects. Results compiled from a survey of projects targeted for American Indian and Alaska Native communities illustrate the depth and range of the activities. By 1988, CSAP awarded 18 grants that targeted communities with sizeable American Indian and Alaska Native populations; some 24 tribes and villages were represented in the prevention activities. Fleming and Manson (1990) conducted an extensive evaluation of the characteristics and effectiveness of the 18 programs. The results of their assessment produced some interesting insights concerning the importance and significance of substance abuse prevention and intervention efforts.

Ninety-four percent of the community-based programs emphasized primary prevention activities; primary prevention activities are developed for the purpose of preventing a health-related problem among those who may be at risk. Some of the primary activities involved the use of educational materials, promotion of Indian identity and self esteem through cultural events, and the use of self-help groups. Individual and group therapy and counseling were found in 88% of the projects; secondary and tertiary levels of prevention tend to emphasize the use of counseling and psychotherapy, so the activities are intended to prevent a problem from intensifying and to intervene in hope of alleviating the problem.

Because the 18 programs were based at the community level, the opinions of local staff were important in shaping the project's design to fit local needs and cultural perceptions. Sixty-one percent of the projects reported that the success of the activities centered on improving relationships with their clients' families; 56% felt that it was important to support and maintain open communications across all levels of the project's operation.

Fleming and Manson (1990) asked their respondents to identify factors that placed Indian youth at risk for using drugs and alcohol. Eighty-eight percent singled out poor self-esteem and parental abuse of alcohol as the greatest contributor to high risk. The respondents also identified additional contributing factors including peer and friends use of drugs; abuse, neglect and family conflict; sexual abuse and emotional and psychological difficulties; previous suicide threats or attempts; and alienation from the dominant culture's social values. The researchers also asked their respondents to identify factors that presumably prevented one from using and abusing drugs. Protective factors listed include a well-defined spiritual belief system, a positive sense of self-worth, ability to make good decisions about personal responsibilities, and the ability to act independent of others' influences. The respondents also believed that friends and peers who act in healthy and responsible ways can serve as models for at-risk youth.

Basically, Fleming and Manson were able to demonstrate that some Indian community members had a good sense of the social and psychological factors that contribute to drug use; they also seemed to recognize the factors that are essential to preventing the problems from occurring or getting worse. More to the point, many Indian communities appear to have keen insight into drug and alcohol abuse problems and the commitment and knowledge necessary to intervene. Communities may require technical and expert assistance in certain phases of prevention and intervention programs, but such assistance is not an absolute necessity.

Additional evidence demonstrates that many other American Indian communities are actively involved in preventing substance abuse. Owan, Palmer, and Quintana (1987) surveyed nearly 420 schools from Head Start to the secondary school level with large American Indian and Alaska Native enrollments and 225 different tribal groups that were receiving grant support for alcohol and drug abuse projects from the Indian Health Service. Both the school and community respondents indicated that alcohol and drug abuse education was a major priority, followed by a concern for building self-esteem and developing effective coping and decision-making skills. Owan, Palmer, and Quintana (1987) draw some important conclusions that emphasize the

need for "early intervention to combat alcohol and substance abuse among Indian youths" (p. 71). They also emphasize that Indian youth need strong families in order to promote positive self-esteem, identity, and values. "Weak families," they argue, "produce uprooted individuals susceptible to 'peer clusters' prone to alcohol and substance abuse" (p. 71).

A careful review of many of the drug and alcohol prevention programs operating in many Indian communities shows that a good deal of borrowing and exchange of conventional intervention and prevention approaches occurs. Indian program staff identified education, self-esteem, identity, value clarification, and family dynamics as major factors that need attention. Respondents mentioned the need to emphasize the use of counseling and psychotherapeutic techniques wherever possible in their programs. The survey results suggest, therefore, that Indian staff are borrowing certain intervention techniques and approaches and blending them with local cultural lifeways and thoughtways. This blend of approaches appears to be producing positive outcomes (Owan, Palmer, & Quintana, 1987).

Related Prevention Efforts

Over the past decade or so, several investigators developed and initiated drug abuse prevention and intervention programs in certain ethnic communities around the country. The number of efforts are scant and limited to certain geographic areas; the majority emphasize the use of primary prevention strategies. There is, however, a rich and growing literature on the use of tertiary forms of prevention that center on culturally efficacious and sensitive treatment approaches. The literature contains an abundance of articles emphasizing ethnic minority mental health issues—many of the topics include detailed discussion concerning the clinical treatment of drug and alcohol abuse. Currently, the cross-cultural clinical treatment literature is so vast that even a summary would not do justice to the topic; however, the reader is encouraged to consult the litera-

ture for more information (Santisteban & Szapoc-znik, 1982; Hubbard et al., 1986; Phillips & Phin, 1981; Smith-Peterson, 1983; Costello, 1987; Zitar, 1987; Hanson, 1985; Gorelick, 1992).

Given the high-risk vulnerability of many ethnic minority youth coupled with the drug use prevalence and use rates, it makes sense that a concerted and concentrated effort incorporating primary prevention strategies should be mounted. CSAP efforts appear to be moving rapidly in this arena. Before the implementation of the CSAP projects, however, concern was expressed by a few researchers about the general effectiveness of prevention programs. Goodstadt (1987) argues that the "evidence concerning the effectiveness of prevention strategies is scarce" and that the prevailing strategies "have had limited or no impact" (p. 31). Moreover, he argues that there is "no consistent evidence that (school-based programs) have positive effects" and "they may even have negative effects" (p. 31). Speaking specifically to the primary prevention of alcohol problems, Moskowitz (1989) not only concurs with Goodstadt's position but adds that "although such programs may influence knowledge, beliefs, or attitudes, they generally do not affect behaviors or problems" (p. 79). The criticisms and observations of these two researchers emerged from their critical review of prevention programs, the design of the intervention, data collection instruments and procedures, and the strategies themselves. Both also agree that primary prevention efforts should continue, but problems concerning effective diffusion should be resolved (Moskowitz, 1989).

One of the recurring problems found in the ethnic minority drug literature concerns the relationship between the community and the prevention-oriented strategies. Crisp (1980) found in his survey of Washington, D.C. program specialists that the community's interest, needs, and preferred prevention strategies differed from those of agencies. The perceptual differences derived from the culturally biased flavor and nature of the models and strategies. Crisp's observation is consistent with the findings of other researchers

concerned about the match between theory and practice and the cultural uniqueness and interests of ethnic enclaves. Maypole and Anderson (1987) remind us that there are just a few culturally specific prevention activities available, but the paucity of such efforts in no way reflects the concern for building relationships between the researcher and the community. "The black church," maintain Maypole and Anderson, "may be [a major support system]" because "it is deeply rooted in the cultural and traditions of blacks" (p. 136). This institution may be a most useful vehicle for developing and sustaining community prevention efforts.

Blending conventional prevention strategies with the interests, goals, and cultural lifeways should be the goal of any ethnic specific prevention. In addition, the prevention strategy should be flexible enough to accommodate cultural nuances; if it isn't, it will probably be rejected, especially given the heightened awareness of the importance of diversity and cultural concerns in contemporary life.

In the past decade, we have been exploring a blend of conventional psychological theory and local indigenous cultural lifeways and thought-ways in an effort to prevent Indian adolescent drug and alcohol use (Schinke et al., 1985; Schinke et al., 1988; Moncher et al., 1989). Because of the unique bicultural and sometimes multicultural demands placed on American Indian youth, prevention and intervention approaches must blend psychological theory and the unique cultural circumstances. As a consequence of the blend, Indian youth should learn biculturally effective competence skills that "blend the adaptive values and roles of both cultures in which [they] were raised and the cultural by which they are surrounded" (La Framboise, 1982, p. 12).

In our drug abuse prevention training and research, the methods and approaches are organized in such a way that they can be used by Indian youth and conducted by American Indian para-professionals, teachers, counselors, and parents. The methods center on providing information

intended to change knowledge and attitudes, assisting with problem solving, providing opportunities to formulate and use coping skills, improving interpersonal communication skills, and promoting the organizing of supportive peer clusters and social networks.

In the early 1980s a behavioral–cognitive skills enhancement program designed to prevent drug use among Indian adolescents was implemented under controlled conditions in the Pacific Northwest (Schinke et al., 1985; Gilchrist, Schinke, Trimble, & Cvetkovich, 1987). To assist in organizing and implementing the project and in designing the cultural components of the training curriculum, an Indian advisory committee was formed; the formation and use of an Indian advisory committee is an absolute must for any prevention or intervention effort. In keeping with local Coast Salish tradition in the Pacific Northwest, the project was named *La-quee biel* (to prevent) by a prominent Indian doctor (shaman) from one of the participating reservations. The intent of *La-quee-biel* was to determine the feasibility of blending social learning theory with local Indian cultural lifeways and thoughtways and assess the impact of the blended perspective.

The 12-member Indian advisory board met regularly to review, critique, change, and approve the implementation plans, curriculum, and intervention materials. The board also assisted in identifying communities where the intervention eventually took place. The board also monitored the pilot testing of the intervention materials. During the intervention phase of *La-quee-biel*, the board was provided with progress reports and summary analysis of the research findings.

Between the fall of 1984 and the spring of 1985, a total of 102 Indian youth participated in the prevention effort at three intervention sites (one urban and two rural). Numerous pieces of information were collected from the youth in an effort to assess the effectiveness of the intervention approach. Overall, the analysis of the measures modestly supports the potential for a bicultural competence skills intervention approach among American Indian youth. Gilchrist, Schinke, Trim-

ble, and Cvetkovich (1987) report that at a six-month follow-up, Indian adolescents who completed the skills-enhancement program had lower rates of alcohol, marijuana, and inhalant use than their peers who did not receive the skills training. Although the number of Indian youths who participated in the intervention approach was relatively small, the overall effort generated a good deal of enthusiasm from a number of constituent groups.

Did *La-quee-biel* work? Did our cognitive–behavioral prevention plan have an impact on the drug avoidance skills of the youth? The answers to both questions are affirmative. The group leaders and youth did learn something; analysis of our data collection tells us so (Gilchrist, Schinke, Trimble, & Cvetkovich, 1987; Schinke et al., 1988; Trimble, 1992). However, prevention and intervention methods must be approached with a degree of healthy skepticism. Part of our assessment plan involved a three- and six-month follow-up. In some instances, we painfully learned that some of our youth did engage in drug use at least at an experimental stage. One 12-year-old user told us, "I really liked the SODAS course. I learned a lot and I thought I could handle my friends. At home it's different. My mom drinks and smokes and so does my uncle. I see them drunk all the time and it hurts because it's my mom. And I say 'They do it so it must not be so bad.' I'm confused sometimes." Youths can learn and benefit from the program, but for the training to be effective, it must have home and community support. Teaching youths prevention skills in a community rife with drug and alcohol use is likely to create emotional tension for them, cause them to question what is normative, and erode respect and allegiance to kin. However, the point made by the 12-year-old may well reflect the fundamental problem with many prevention efforts. Emphasizing an individual's refusal skills, attitudes, and beliefs may produce short-term results. For any prevention effort to achieve even a modicum of success with youth, it must systematically involve peers, parents, community leaders, and related community institutions, all of whom work in concert to achieve the same goal.

RECOMMENDATIONS AND CONSIDERATIONS

Sprinkled throughout this chapter are suggestions and recommendations to improve our knowledge of ethnic minority drug use. The suggestions are contextual and flow from specific literature and research findings. There are additional considerations and recommendations that demand serious consideration. In some instances, if we delay research and development, the drug use and abuse problems in ethnic minority communities could reach epidemic levels, placing remedies, solutions, and interventions well into the future.

The following recommendations and considerations represent an integration and synthesis of concerns proffered by others who have written in the field. Where appropriate, references are provided for more in-depth study.

— The relationship between culture and ethnic orientations and drug use is based on the assumption that anything that is cultural is good and positive. What are the specific cultural and ethnic activities that have either a positive or negative impact on drug use? (See Fleming & Manson, 1990.)

— A good deal remains to be learned about the relationship between peer groups and their use and nonuse of psychoactive substances. Are there culture-specific lifeways that can be used to enhance the positive influence of peers? (See Fleming & Manson, 1990.)

— It is essential that future studies distinguish ethnic groups on the basis of values, norms, life conditions, history and heritage, and adaptive problems. The common division in drug and alcohol studies between white and nonwhite populations is grossly inadequate for examining drug abuse within a culture; each ethnic group must be studied in its own right (Tucker, 1985; Trimble, 1991; Cheung, 1991; Heath, 1992). On this point, Cheung (1991) accurately and appropriately points out that "it is important to recognize also the differences among members of the same ethnic group with respect to ethnic factors such as ethnic identification, cultural, and structure incorporation, generational status, age at immigration, adaptation problems, and ethnic community involvement" (p. 598).

— What psychological characteristics are associated with drug abuse? There is a need to determine the extent and the level of pathology, self-perception, social skills, experienced anxiety, guilt, rejection, and alienation from the surrounding community and one's own family.

— There is the need to examine alternative measures to assess the extent and kinds of abuse. Measures must be developed to reflect the varying differences accruing from cultural differences. Operationalizations of substance abuse must be behaviorally anchored. In conducting research investigations, attention should be given to the use of case-controlled retrospective studies between those who are and those who are not abusive and the use of cohort prospective designs that identify two groups on a common abuse-related characteristic and track them to see which develop drug abuse patterns.

— The efficacy of particular treatment and prevention strategies must be evaluated. Some that have been described include family effectiveness training, crisis intervention, bicultural education, and youth intervention programs. The question of their efficacy with regard to the target populations remains. For example, how effective are educational programs with youth in various settings? What is the efficacy of peer-support groups in drug-free and drug-supplemented programs? (See Lapge & Sherlock, 1991.)

— To what extent are available prevention techniques differentially effective among different age groups? How do prevention programs differ depending on age and generation of the target group?

— What treatment modalities (indigenous and traditional) are available to effectively deal with substance abuse and addictions? What expectancy variables define the treatment and therapeutic relationship? From the ethnic minority's point of view? From the therapist's viewpoint?

— According to Kumpfer, Moskowitz, Whiteside, and Klitzner (1985), programs that involve volunteers from all relevant community elements and institutions in a coordinated manner are likely to be successful. Prevention efforts should be coordinated with the community and strategies should reflect local norms, values, beliefs, and preferred practices.

— Kumpfer, Moskowitz, Whiteside, and Klitzner (1985) emphasize that prevention approaches should emphasize healthy lifestyles. Health consciousness efforts should include units dealing with cigarette and smokeless tobacco topics along with those central to drug and alcohol use. Youth should not be the sole recipients of these campaigns; adults and the elderly should be included in a health consciousness campaign that extends across the developmental lifespan.

— What are the natural support systems and culture-specific ways of strengthening them to promote the prevention of drug use and abuse? Along similar lines, what treatment modalities (indigenous and traditional) are available that may be included in prevention strategies? What are culture-specific expectations that define treatment models and therapeutic relationships? From the client's perspective? From the therapist's viewpoint? (See Trimble, 1984.)

There are probably many other considerations and recommendations that could be added to the list. For the moment, the recommendations included in this chapter provide enough for a lengthy research and development agenda. Moreover, it is possible that many of the points raised in this chapter may stimulate new ideas and strategies.

SUMMARY

We end where we started. Countless ethnic minority parents, community leaders, school personnel, and youth are concerned—even angry—about drug use among their kind. Voices of concern can be heard emanating from remote Alaskan villages, small Hawaiian villages, and inner-city ghettoes in large metropolitan areas. They all seem to be of one mind about the urgent need to prevent and eliminate a problem that tears up family life, holds people hostage, and imprisons the minds of youth. Many blame the federal government for not pouring more resources into interdiction efforts, treatment programs, and research ventures. Still others blame the *waneentum* (the outsiders or the whites). Others cast blame on the growing demoralization

of community values, beliefs, and sanctions. Some are truculent and are willing to wage war against drug pushers and drug lords; some are frustrated and hardened by the enormousness of the problem and feel hopeless. Moods vary, as do opinions about what recourse is open to those who desire to put an end to the problem.

Sadly, drug and alcohol use is endemic in the American way of life. Among ethnic minorities, it has a long and sordid history—alcohol and the first American, opium and the immigrant Chinese, marijuana and Mexican Americans, and cocaine and African Americans. Part of this chapter explores the source of ethnic groups' drug associations and points out that the association may be more fiction than fact—a contrivance sparked by certain government officials, fueled by the needs of business and industry, and fanned by the print media. Does this continue today? Consider the stereotypic images of the drunken Indian, the black heroin addict, and the Southeast Asian opium addict that run the circles of discussion in corners and pockets of this country.

Summaries of drug use and prevalence rates among ethnic minority youth are provided in the chapter. Use rates vary among and between groups and are irregular over time. Rates are alarmingly high among some groups and small among others. There appear to be more drug use surveys conducted among American Indians and Alaska Natives—America's smallest minority group—than among any other group. Why? Do researchers hope to squelch the harsh stereotype of the "drunken Indian?" Is it born out of a fascination with the vanquished "noble redman?" Or is the drug and alcohol problem real and at epidemic levels? Whatever the researcher's motive, we know that drug use among America's indigenous people is high and apparently not declining at any predictable rate. But what about the use rates among Asian-Pacific Americans, African Americans, and Hispanics? Why are there no large-scale longitudinal studies focusing on each of the specific groups—studies that tell us something meaningful within each of the cultural groups? (See Tucker, 1985.)

Following the discussion on prevalence and use rates, the chapter turns to discussion on the characteristics of youth likely to use drugs. It then turns to a discussion of federal government attempts to prevent substance abuse—a massive, expensive series of countermeasures and strategies sponsored by the Center for Substance Abuse Prevention. Examples of culture-specific programs are provided that are laid alongside prevention programs that emphasize the individual, the family, the parents, the school, and the community. Right now, about 300 communities with support from CSAP have formed partnerships with community agencies, institutions, and nonprofit organizations to orchestrate cultural and ethnic-specific prevention campaigns. A description of a cognitive–behavioral drug abuse prevention program is provided toward the end of the chapter. Researchers worked closely with American Indian tribal members to design and implement a prevention program with their youth. Results and follow-up investigations were encouraging. Moreover, the prevention effort demonstrated that one ethnic community can work with the research community to achieve mutual goals. The procedure should become policy, as it seems to be a most reasonable approach for sharing knowledge, skills, and wisdom.

Discussing the many sides of drug abuse among ethnic minorities can be depressing, especially if one reads or hears horrid stories about a teenager in Dallas, a family in San Francisco, or a young child in Boston. Perhaps the most alarming story was told to me by a colleague recently while we were driving across a snow-covered Colorado highway. The story may have been changed—even embellished—with the many times it has been told. Here is one version. A police officer wearing everyday casual clothes was sitting in the back of an elementary school classroom. It was a kindergarten class made up mostly of African-American youth. The teacher was talking about drugs and alcohol. On a subtle and unobtrusive cue from the teacher, the officer lit an incense cone that smelled a lot like marijuana. More than half of the class asked at one

point or another "Who is smoking a joint in here? Who has pot?" The school was located in a small rural community somewhere in the southern part of the United States. No more needs to be said.

NOTES

1. Many of the more commonly used psychoactive drugs have their origins principally in Southeast and Southwest Asia and South and Central America. Others, such as marijuana, peyote cactus, and the *Psilycybe Mexicana* mushroom are indigenous to Central and North America. The commonly used psychoactive drugs of today undoubtedly were used by those who resided in areas where the substances were prevalent. There is some ethnographic evidence that suggests that the use of certain psychoactive substances by aboriginal and indigenous peoples was not viewed as problematic; the drugs were used in religious, ceremonial, and socially controlled settings. For certain North American tribal groups, that is still the case. Now, unlike the past, the vast majority of psychoactive drugs are used in settings devoid of religious ceremonies and traditional sanctions and controls. For more details, see the works of Inciardi (1992) and Efron, Holmstedt, and Kline (1967).

2. The author wishes to apologize to the thousands of people who are actively involved in preventing drug abuse in ethnic minority communities. The material provided in this section was selected from government reports and the professional literature. Page limitations prevented me from including summaries of the many exciting programs throughout the country.

REFERENCES

Agnew, R. (1991). The interactive effect of peer variables on delinquency. *Criminology, 29,* 47–72.

American Council on Education (1988). *One-third of a nation.* Washington, DC: ACE.

Aron, W., Alger, N., & Gonzalez, R. (1974). Chicanoizing drug abuse programs. *Human Organization, 33,* 388–390.

Austin, G. A., Johnson, B. D., Carroll, E. E., & Lettieri, D. J. (Eds.). (1977). *Drugs and minorities* (Research Issues 21). Washington, DC: USGPO.

Bandura, A. (1977). *Social learning theory.* Englewood Cliffs, NJ: Prentice-Hall.

Banks, R. (1990). Living the legacy: Historical perspective on African-American drug abuse. In J. Debro & C. Bolek (Eds.), *Drug abuse research issues at historically black colleges and universities.* Atlanta: Clark Atlanta University, 56–110.

Baumrind, D. (1985). Familial antecedents of adolescent drug use: A developmental perspective. In C. L. Jones & R. J. Battjes (Eds.), *Etiology of drug abuse: Implications for prevention.* (NIDA Research Monograph 56). Rockville, MD: National Institute on Drug Abuse.

Beauvais, F., Oetting, E. R., Wolf, W., & Edwards, R. W. (1989). American Indian youth and drugs: 1975–1987—A continuing problem. *American Journal of Public Health, 79* (5), 634–636.

Bell, C. S., & Battjes, R. (1987). *Prevention research: Deterring drug abuse among children and adolescents.* NIDA Research Monograph 63 (ADM 87–1334). Washington, DC: USGPO.

Benson, P., & Donahue, M. (1989). Ten-year trends in at-risk behaviors: A national study of black adolescents. *Journal of Adolescent Research, 4* (2), 125–139.

Bonnie, R. J., & Whitebread, C. H. (1974). *The marijuana conviction: A history of marijuana prohibition in the United States.* Charlottesville: University Press of Virginia.

Botvin, G., Baker, E., Renick, N., Filazzola, A., & Botvin, E. (1984). A cognitive-behavioral approach to substance abuse prevention. *Addictive Behaviors, 9,* 137–147.

Brown, B. S. (1985). Federal drug abuse policy and minority group issues—reflections of a participant–observer. *The International Journal of the Addictions, 20* (1), 203–215.

Budd, R. D. (1989). Cocaine abuse and violent death. *American Journal of Drug and Alcohol Abuse, 15* (4), 375–382.

Center for Substance Abuse Prevention (1991). OSAP mobilizes to combat a national crisis. *The Fact is. . . .* Rockville, MD: National Clearinghouse for Alcohol and Drug Information.

Chavez, E., Beauvais, F., & Oetting, E. R. (1986). Drug use by small town Mexican-American youth: A pilot study. *Hispanic Journal of Behavioral Sciences, 8* (3), 243–258.

Chavez, E., & Swaim, R. (1992). Hispanic substance use: Problems in epidemiology. In J. Trimble, C. Bolek, & S. Niemcryk (Eds.), *Ethnic and multicultural drug abuse: Perspectives on current research.* Binghamton, NY: Haworth.

Cheung, Y. W. (1991). Ethnicity and alcohol/drug use revisited: A framework for future research. *The international Journal of the Addictions, 25* (5A & 6A), 581–605.

Coie, J., Watt, N., West, S., Hawkins, J., Asarrow, J., Markman, H., Ramey, S., Shure, M., & Long, B. (1993). The science of prevention: A conceptual framework and some directions for a national research program. *American Psychologist, 48* (10), 1013–1022.

Costello, R. M. (1987). Hispanic alcoholic treatment considerations. *Hispanic Journal of Behavioral Sciences, 9,* 83–89.

Crisp, A. D. (1980). Making substance abuse prevention relevant to low-income black neighborhoods. *Journal of Psychedelic Drugs, 12* (2), 139-156.

Dennis, D., Buckner, J., Lipton, F., & Levine, I. (1991). A decade of research and services for homeless mentally ill persons: Where do we stand? *American Psychologist, 46* (11), 1129-1138.

Dick, R., Manson, S., & Beals, J. (1993). Alcohol use among American Indian adolescents: Patterns and correlates of students drinking in a boarding school. *Journal of Studies on Alcohol, 54,* 172–177.

Efron, D. H., Holmstedt, B., & Kline, N. S. (1967). Ethnopharmacologic search for psychoactive drugs. *Proceedings of a symposium held in San Francisco, California* (no. 1645). Washington, DC: USGPO.

Farrington, D. P. (1979). Longitudinal research on crime and delinquency. In N. Morris, & M. Torry (Eds.), *Crime and justice: An annual review of research,* vol. 1. Chicago: University of Chicago Press, pp. 289–348.

Fernandez-Pol, B., Bluestone, H., Missouri, C., Morales, G., & Mizruchi, M. S. (1986). Drinking patterns of inner-city black Americans and Puerto Ricans. *Journal of Studies on Alcohol, 47* (2), 156–160.

Fischer, P. J., & Breakey, W. R. (1991). The epidemiology of alcohol, drug, and mental disorders among homeless persons. *American Psychologist, 46* (11), 1115–1128.

Fleming, C., & Manson, S. (1990). *Substance abuse prevention in American Indian and Alaska Native communities: A literature review and OSAP pro-*

gram survey. Rockville, MD: Office for Substance Abuse Prevention.

Fredlund, E. V., Spence, R. T., & Maxwell, J. C. (1989). *Substance use among students in Texas secondary schools—1988.* Austin: Texas Commission on Alcohol and Drug Use.

Gilbert, M. J. (1989). Alcohol use among Latino adolescents: What we know and what we need to know. *Drugs and Society, 3* (1/2), 35–53.

Gilbert, M. J., & Alcocer, A. M. (1988). Alcohol use and Hispanic youth: An overview. *Journal of Drug Issues, 18* (1), 33–48.

Gilchrist, L., Schinke, S., Trimble, J., & Cvetkovich, G. (1987). Skills enhancement to prevent substance abuse among American Indian adolescents. *International Journal of the Addictions, 22* (9), 869–879.

Goodstadt, M. S. (1987). Prevention strategies for drug abuse. *Issues in Science and Technology, 16,* 28–35.

Gorelick, D. (1992). Sociodemographic factors in drug abuse treatment. *Journal of Health Care for the Poor and Underserved, 3* (1), 49–58.

Green, E. M. (1914). Psychoses among Negroes: A comparative study. *Journal of Nervous and Mental Disease, 41,* 697–708.

Hanson, B. (1985). Drug treatment effectiveness: The case of facial and ethnic minorities in American—Some research questions and proposals. *The International Journal of the Addictions, 20* (1), 99–137.

Harvey, W. B. (1985). Alcohol abuse and the black community: A contemporary analysis. *Journal of Drug Issues,* 81–91.

Hawkins, J. D., Lishner, D. M., & Catalano, R. F., Jr. (1985). Childhood predictors and the prevention of adolescent substance abuse. In C. L. Jones & R. J. Battjes (Eds.), *Etiology of drug abuse: Implications for prevention.* (NIDA Research Monograph 56). Rockville, MD: National Institute on Drug Abuse.

Heath, D. (1978). The sociocultural model of alcohol use: Problems and prospects. *Journal of Operational Psychiatry, 9,* 55–66.

Heath, D. B. (1987). Anthropology & alcohol studies: Current issues. *Annual Review of Anthropology, 16,* 99–120.

Heath, D. B. (1991). Uses and misuses of the concept of ethnicity in alcohol studies: An essay on de-

construction. *The International Journal of the Addictions, 25* (5A & 6A), 607–627.

Heath, D. B. (1992). Political pharmacology: Thinking about drugs. *Daedalus: Journal of American Academy of Arts and Sciences, 121* (3), 269–291.

Helmer, J. (1975). *Drugs and minority oppression.* New York: Seabury Press.

Herd, D. (1988). Drinking by black and white women: Results from a national survey. *Social Problems, 35,* 493–505.

Himmelstein, J. (1983). *The strange career of marijuana.* Westport, CT: The Greenwood Press.

Hubbard, R., Schlenger, W., Rachael, J., Bray, R., Craddock, S., Cavanaugh, E., & Ginzberg, H. (1986). Patterns of alcohol and drug abuse in drug treatment clients from different ethnic backgrounds. *Annals of the New York Academy of Science, 472,* 60–74.

Iiyama, P., Nishi, S. M., & Johnson, B. D. (1976). *Drug use and abuse among U.S. minorities: An annotated bibliography.* New York: Praeger.

Inciardi, J. (1992). *The war on drugs II: The continuing epic of heroin, cocaine, crack, crime, AIDS, and public policy.* Mountain View, CA: Mayfield.

Johnson, B. D., Williams, T., Dei, K. A., & Sanabria, H. (1990). Drug abuse in the inner city: Impact on hard-drug users and the community. In M. Tonry & J. Q. Wilson (Eds.), *Drugs and crime. (Crime and Justice: A Review of Research,* Vol. 13). Chicago: University of Chicago Press.

Johnston, L. D., O'Malley, P. M., & Bachman, J. G. (1988). *Illicit drug use, smoking, and drinking by America's high school students, college students, and young adults: 1975–1987.* Washington, DC: USGPO.

Johnston, L. D., O'Malley, P. M., & Bachman, J. G. (1989). *Illicit drug use, smoking, and drinking by America's high school students, college students, and young adults.* DHHS no. 89-1602. Rockville, MD: National Institute on Drug Abuse.

Kandel, D. B. (1982). Epidemiological and psychosocial perspectives on adolescent drug use. *Journal of American Academic and Clinical Psychiatry, 21,* 328–347.

Kandel, D., Kessler, R., & Margulies, R. (1978). Antecedents of adolescent initiation into stages of drug use: A developmental analyses. In B. Kandel (Ed.), *Longitudinal research on drug use:*

Empirical finding & methodological issues. Washington, DC: Hemisphere Publishing Corp.

Keil, B. (1989). Drugs, gender, and ethnicity. Is the older minority woman at risk? *Journal of Drug Issues, 19* (2), 171–189.

King, L. (1982). *Alcoholism: Studies regarding black Americans. Alcohol and Health Monograph 4: Special Population Issues* (ADM, 82-1193). Washington, DC: USGPO.

King, J., Beals, J., Manson, S., & Trimble, J. (1992). A structural equation model of factors related to substance use among American Indian adolescents. In J. Trimble, C. Bolek, & S. Niemcryk (Eds.), *Ethnic and multicultural drug abuse: Perspectives on current research.* Binghamton, NY: Haworth.

King, L. M., Moody, S., Thompson, O., & Bennett, M. (1983). Black psychology reconsidered: Notes toward curriculum development. In J. Chunn, P. Dunston, & F. Ross-Sheriff (Eds.), *Mental health and people of color: Curriculum development and change.* Washington, DC: Howard University Press.

Kumpfer, K., Moskowitz, J., Whiteside, H., & Klitzner, M. (1985). Future issues and promising directions in the prevention of substance abuse among youth. *Journal of Children in Contemporary Society, 18* (1/2), 249–278.

La Framboise, T. D. (1982). *Assertion training with American Indians: Cultural/behavioral issues for trainers.* Las Cruces, NM: ERIC Clearinghouse on Rural Education and Small Schools.

Legge, C., & Sherlock, L. (1991). Perception of alcohol use and misuse in three ethnic communities: Implications for prevention programming. *The International Journal of the Addictions, 25* (5A & 6A), 629–653.

Longshore, D., Hsieh, S., Anglin, M., & Annon, T. (1992). Ethnic patterns in drug use treatment utilization. *Journal of Mental Health Administration, 19* (3), 268–277.

Lubben, J., Chi, I., & Kitano, H. (1989). The relative influence of selected social factors on Korean drinking behavior in Los Angeles. *Advances in Alcohol and Substance Abuse, 8* (1), 1–17.

Maddahian, E., Newcomb, M., & Bentler, P. (1985). Single and multiple patterns of adolescent substance use: Longitudinal comparisons of four ethnic groups. *Journal of Drug Education, 15,* 311–326.

Maddahian, E., Newcomb, M., & Bentler, P. (1986). Substance use and ethnicity: Differential impact of peer and adult models. *Journal of Psychology, 120,* 83–95.

Maddahian, E., Newcomb, M., & Bentler, P. (1988). Adolescent drug use and intention to use drugs: Concurrent and longitudinal analysis of four ethnic groups. *Addictive Behaviors, 13,* 191–195.

Maton, K. I., & Zimmerman, M. A. (1992). Psychosocial predictors of substance use among urban black male adolescents. In J. Trimble, C. Bolek, & S. Niemcryk (Eds.), *Ethnic and multicultural drug abuse: Perspectives on current research.* Binghamton, NY: Haworth.

May, P. A. (1982). Substance abuse and American Indians: Prevalence and susceptibility. *International Journal of the Addictions, 17* (7), 1185–1209.

Maypole, D., & Anderson, R. (1987). Culture-specific substance abuse prevention for blacks. *Community Mental Health Journal, 23* (2), 135–139.

McCord, J. (1981). Alcohol and criminality. *Journal of Studies on Alcohol, 42,* 739–348.

McGuire, W. J. (1964). Inducing resistance to persuasion. In L. Berkowitz (Ed.), *Advances in experimental social psychology, Volume 1.* New York: Academic Press.

Milburn, N. G., & Booth, J. A. (1992). Illicit drug and alcohol use among homeless black adults in shelters. In J. Trimble, C. Bolek, & S. Niemcryk (Eds.), *Ethnic and multicultural drug abuse: Perspectives on current research.* Binghamton, NY: Haworth.

Moncher, M., Parms, C., Orlandi, M., Schinke, S., Miller, S., Palleja, J., & Schinke, M. (1989). Microcomputer-based approaches for preventing drug and alcohol abuse among adolescents from ethnic/racial minority backgrounds. *Computers in Human Behavior, 5* (2), 79–93.

Morgan, P. A. (1990). The making of a public problem: Mexican labor in California and the Marijuana Law of 1937. In R. Glich & J. Moore (Eds.), *Drugs in Hispanic Communities,* New Brunswick: Rutgers University Press, 233–252.

Morgan, P. A., Wallack, L., & Buchanan, P. (1989). Waging drug wars: Prevention strategy or politics as usual. *Drugs & Society, 3* (1/2), 99–124.

Morishima, J., Sue, S., Teng, L., Zane, N., & Cram, J. (1979). *Handbook of Asian American/Pacific Islanders mental health research.* Rockville, MD: National Institute of Mental Health.

Moskowitz, J. M. (1989). The primary prevention of alcohol problems: A critical review of the research literature. *Journal of Studies on Alcohol, 50* (1), 54–88.

Nakashima, J. (1986). Substance abuse: The dark side of "Nikei Boulevard." *Rice Paper, 10,* 1–3.

Nathan, P. E. (1983). Failures in prevention: Why we can't prevent the devastating effect of alcoholism and drug abuse. *American Psychologist, 38,* 459–467.

National Institute on Drug Abuse (1985). *National household survey on drug abuse: Population estimates 1985* (ADM 87-1539). Washington, DC: USGPO.

National Institute on Drug Abuse (1987). *Use of selected drugs among Hispanics: Mexican Americans, Puerto Ricans and Cuban-Americans— Findings from the Hispanic health and nutrition examination survey* (HHANES) (ADM 87-1527). Washington, DC: USGPO.

National Institute on Drug Abuse (1989). *National household survey on drug abuse: Population estimates 1988* (ADM 89-1636). Washington, DC: USGPO.

National Institute on Drug Abuse (1991a). *Annual emergency room data, 1990* (ADM 91-1839). Rockville, MD: Division of Epidemiology and Prevention Research, National Institute on Drug Abuse.

National Institute on Drug Abuse (1991b). *Annual medical examiners data, 1991* (ADM 91-1840). Rockville, MD: Division of Epidemiology and Prevention Research, National Institute on Drug Abuse.

National Institute on Drug Abuse (1991c). *National household survey on drug abuse: Population estimates 1991* (ADM 92-1887). Rockville, MD: Division of Epidemiology and Prevention Research, National Institute on Drug Abuse.

Needle, R., Laver, Y., Su, S., Brown, P., & Doherty, W. (1988). Familial, interpersonal, and intrapersonal correlates of drug use: A longitudinal comparison of adolescents in treatment, not in treatment, and non-drug using adolescents. *The International Journal of the Addictions, 23,* 1211–1240.

Nobles, W., Goddard, L., Cavill, W., George, P. (1987). *The culture of drugs on the black community.* Oakland, CA: Black Family Institute.

Nurco, D. N., Shaffer, J. W., & Crisin, I. H. (1984). An ecological analysis of the interrelationships among drug abuse and other indices of social pathology. *The International Journal of the Addictions, 19* 441–451.

Oetting, E., & Beauvais, F. (1986). Peer cluster theory: Drugs and the adolescent. *Journal of Counseling and Development, 65* (1), 17–22.

Oetting, E. R., Edwards, R. W., & Beauvais, F. (1989). Drugs and Native-American Youth. *Drugs and Society, 3* (1/2), 1–34.

Owan, T., Palmer, I., & Quintana, M. (1987). *School/ community-based alcoholism/substance abuse prevention survey.* Rockville, MD: Indian Health Service, Office of Health Programs, Alcoholism/ Substance Abuse Program Branch.

Padilla, A., & Salgado de Snyder, N. (1985). Counseling Hispanics: Strategies for effective intervention. In P. Pedersen (Ed.), *Handbook of cross-cultural counseling and therapy.* Westport, CT: Greenwood, pp. 157–164).

Payton, C. R. (1981). Substance abuse and mental health: Special prevention strategies needed for ethnics of color. *Public Health Reports, 96* (1), 20–25.

Pentz, M. A. (1983). Prevention of adolescent substance abuse through social skills. In T. J. Glynn, C. G. Leukefeld, & J. P. Ludford (Eds.), *Preventing adolescent drug abuse: Intervention strategies,* NIDA Research Monograph 47 (ADM 83–1280). Washington, DC: USGPO.

Phillips, P., & Phin, J. (1981). The drug treatment process among minorities. In A. J. Schecter (Ed.), *Drug dependence and alcoholism, Vol. 2: Social and behavioral issues.* New York: Plenum.

Santisteban, D., & Szapocznik, J. (1982). *The Hispanic substance abuser: The search for prevention strategies.* New York: Grune and Stratton.

Sasao, T. (Aug. 1989). *Patterns of substance use and health practices among Japanese Americans in southern California.* Paper presented at third annual conference of the Asian American Psychological Association, New Orleans, LA.

Schaps, E., Di Bartolo, R., Moskowitz, J., Palley, C., & Churgin, S. (1981). A review of 127 drug abuse prevention program evaluations. *Journal of Drug Issues, 11,* 17–43.

Schinke, S., Botvin, G., Trimble, J., Orlandi, M., Gilchrist, L., & Locklear, V. (1988). Preventing substance abuse among American Indian adolescents: A bicultural competence skills approach. *Journal of Counseling Psychology, 35* (1), 87–90.

Schinke, S., & Gilchrist, L. (1984). *Life skills counseling with adolescents.* Baltimore, MD: University Park Press.

Schinke, S., Orlandi, M., Vaccaro, D., Espinoza, R., McAlester, A., & Botvin, G. (1992). Substance use among Hispanic and non-Hispanic adolescents. *Addictive Behaviors, 17* (2), 117–124.

Schinke, S. P., Schilling, R. F., & Gilchrist, L. D. (1986). Prevention of drug and alcohol abuse in American Indian youths. *Social Work Research and Abstracts, 16,* 18–19.

Schinke, S., Schilling, R., Gilchrist, L., Barth, R., Bobo, J., Trimble, J., & Cvetkovich, G. (1985). Preventing substance abuse with American Indian youth. *Social Casework: The Journal of Contemporary Social Work, 4* (66), 213–217.

Segal, B. (1983). *Patterns of drug use: Report of a statewide school survey.* Juneau, AK: Department of Health and Social Services.

Segal, B. (1988). *Drugs and behavior: Cause, effects, and treatment.* New York: Gardner.

Segal, B. (1989). Drug-taking behavior among school-aged youth: The Alaska experience and comparisons with lower-48 states. *Drugs and Society, 4* (1/2), 1–174.

Segal, B. (1992). Ethnicity and drug-taking behavior. In J. Trimble, C. Bolek, & S. Niemcryk (Eds.), *Ethnic and multicultural drug abuse: Perspectives on current research.* Binghamton, NY: Haworth, 269–312.

Smith-Peterson, C. (1983). Substance abuse treatment and cultural diversity. In B. Bennett, C. Vourakis, & D. Wolf (Eds.), *Substance abuse: Pharmacologic, developmental, and clinical perspectives.* New York: Wiley.

Spunt, B., Goldstein, P., Bellucci, P., & Miller, T. (1990). Race/ethnicity and gender differences in the drugs-violence relationship. *Journal of Psychoactive Drugs, 22* (3), 293–303.

Trimble, J. E. (1984). Drug abuse prevention research needs among American Indians and Alaska Natives. *White Cloud Journal of American Indian Mental Health, 3* (3), 22–34.

Trimble, J. E. (1991). Ethnic specification, validation prospects, and the future of drug use research. *The International Journal of the Addictions, 25* (2A), 149–170.

Trimble, J. E. (1992). A cognitive-behavioral approach to drug abuse prevention and intervention with American Indian youth. In L. A. Vargas & J. D. Koss-Chioino (Eds.), *Working with culture: Psychotherapeutic intervention with ethnic minority children and adolescents.* San Francisco: Jossey-Bass, 246–275.

Trimble, J. E. (1994). Cultural variations in use of alcohol and drug. In W. Lonner & R. Malpass (Eds.), *Psychology and culture.* Boston: Allyn and Bacon, 79–84.

Trimble, J., & Fleming, C. (1989). Providing counseling services for Native American Indians: Client, counselor, and community characteristics. In P. Pedersen, J. Draguns, W. Lonner, & J. Trimble (Eds.), *Counseling across cultures, third edition.* Honolulu: University Press of Hawaii, 177–204.

Trimble, J. E., Padilla, A., & Bell, C. (Eds.). (1987). *Drug abuse among ethnic minorities* (DHHS Publication no. ADM 87-1474). Rockville, MD: National Institute on Drug Abuse.

Tucker, M. B. (1985). U.S. ethnic minorities and drug abuse: An assessment of the science and practice. *The International Journal of the Addictions, 20* (6/7), 1021–1047.

Walker, W. O. (1981). *Drug control in the Americas.* Albuquerque: University of New Mexico Press.

Weibel-Orlando, J. C. (1984). Substance abuse among American Indian youth: A continuing crisis. *Journal of Drug Issues, 14,* 314–335.

Willer, B., & Vokes, D. (1989). *Prevention of chemical dependency among Native American families and youth.* Buffalo: State University of New York at Buffalo.

Williams, E. H. (1914). Negro cocaine "fiends" are a new southern menace. *New York Times, 12* (Feb. 8), 15.

Wilson, G. P., & Taylor, K. B. (1990). Substance use at an historically black university: An analysis of the results of two surveys. In J. Debro & C. Bolek (Eds.), *Drug abuse research issues at historically black colleges and universities.* Atlanta: Clark Atlanta University, 193–216.

Womble, M. (1990). Black women. In R. Engs (Ed.), *Women, alcohol and other drugs.* Dubuque, IA: Kendall/Hunt, 127–135.

Womble, M., & Bakeman, V. (1986). A comprehensive culturally specific approach to drunk driving for blacks. *Alcoholism Treatment Quarterly, 3* (2), 103–113.

Wong, H. (1982). Asian and Pacific Americans. In L. Snowden (Ed.), *Reaching the underserved: Mental health needs of neglected populations.* Beverly Hills, CA: Sage, 185–204.

Yee, B.E.K., & Thu, N. D. (1987). Correlates of drug use and abuse among Indochinese refugees: Mental health implications. *Journal of Psychoactive Drugs, 19* (1), 77–83.

Zane, N., & Sasao, T. (1992). Research on drug abuse among Asian-Pacific Americans. In J. Trimble, C. Bolek, & S. Niemcryk (Eds.), *Ethnic and multicultural drug abuse: Perspectives on current research.* Binghamton, NY: Haworth.

Zitar, M.L.P. (1987). Culturally sensitive treatment of black alcoholic families. *Social Work, 32,* 130–135.

CHAPTER 19

INNER-CITY YOUTH

AMADO M. PADILLA
DAVID DURAN
WADE W. NOBLES

Inner-city youth and young adults are at high risk for substance abuse, which further lessens their chances for educational and occupational advancement. The problem is so severe that drastic measures must be taken to enable inner-city youth to see alternatives to substance use. In this chapter, we will begin with an overview of the research literature on substance abuse with inner-city youth. Then we will discuss some current model prevention programs that have been established to serve the needs of young people in cities. Finally, we offer recommendations regarding prevention strategies based on our review and knowledge of the field.

Before reviewing the relevant literature, it is important to state an obvious fact regarding inner-city residents. Unfortunately, the majority of residents in our inner cities can be characterized as very poor, mostly from a minority background, likely to be from a single-parent home, exposed to alcohol and drug users, undereducated, unemployed or underemployed, homeless or near homeless, and in poor general health compared with suburban and small-city dwellers. For many of these individuals, their life chances may seem hopeless. It is no wonder that alcohol and drugs seem to provide at the least a temporary escape from the harsh realities of life in the inner city. However, there are alternatives for inner-city residents if mental health professionals, members of the community, the business sector, public service agencies, and policymakers offer the leadership required to pool resources to make a difference in our major urban areas.

The task is not impossible and some wonderful programs are beginning to emerge from the pulling together of many different individuals to make change happen in communities that have experienced near-epidemic rates of substance abuse in the past. The aim of this chapter is to contribute to the growing awareness that substance abuse is not endemic to inner cities and that we need not continue to lose generation after generation of our youth to the downward spiral of alcohol and drug abuse.

OVERVIEW OF LITERATURE

In an important series of studies, Richard Dembo and his colleagues have shown that different social groupings and drug use subcultures coexist among youths living in environments where there are different degrees of perceived risk. In this research, Dembo and his collaborators (Dembo et al., 1985; Dembo, Blount, Schmeidler, & Burgos, 1986) have reported that non-drug-using adolescents are less likely to be involved in street culture and give little status to drug-using peers who are involved with gangs.

Dembo, Farrow, Schmeidler, and Burgos (1979) have also reported that inner-city youth are sensitive to the influence of the perceived level of risk for the neighborhoods in which they live. Interestingly, nonusers saw themselves at high risk and reported that they felt very vulnerable to future drug involvement. Furthermore, nonusers who do not choose their friends on the basis of drug use are also more likely, because of exposure to drugs and peer pressure, to eventually become involved with drugs.

Obviously, to counter such exposure and peer pressure, primary prevention efforts must focus on teaching and rewarding non-drug-involved youth activities that emphasize the use of nondrug behaviors as critical variables in selecting friends and associates. In the past, many substance prevention programs, for example, placed an emphasis on the actual drugs and how their intrinsic properties resulted in the abasement of youth. In other programs, the belief was that factual knowledge (such as information on the damage done to vital organs) would increase resistance on the part of children and adolescents to substance abuse. In addition, these traditional approaches often focused on the way in which substance use in concert with a susceptible personality led to problems or on how certain cultural forces (such as machismo among Latino males) were conducive to excessive alcohol use.

Research findings (Dembo et al., 1985) suggest that professionals who implement intervention programs must be aware of the importance of environmental risk in the etiology of drug use and misuse and must consider this factor in the development of intervention strategies and programs. Furthermore, because drug users in inner-city, high-risk settings appear to be responding to social forces rather than acting out disturbed personality problems, intervention personnel should be trained to use ethnographically informed group dynamic techniques in an attempt to devalue the status associated with, and to alter the norms reinforcing, heavy drug use (Dembo et al., 1985).

In particular, drug availability and the perceived status of drug-using and gang-involved youth are seen to bear a direct relationship to friends' use of various drugs. According to Dembo et al. (1985), contrary to theoretical expectations, judged availability of drugs in the neighborhood and at the school were not directly related to drug involvement in any of the settings. The environmental experiences of the youths studied, especially their relationship to elements of the drug use subcultures existing in their neighborhoods, were critical factors in understanding their drug use.

The relationship between neighborhood setting and drug use appears to be drug-specific. For alcohol and tobacco, familiarity with peer use was highly predictive of personal use, independent of how tough or drug-involved the neighborhood was thought to be, but quite dependent on neighborhood perceptions for personal marijuana use. Further, the relationship became more predictive as the neighborhood was perceived by the youth as tougher and more drug-involved.

Sociocultural views of nonmedical drug use among inner-city youths argue that this behavior is learned, motivated, peer-oriented, and adaptive, reflecting a commitment to a lifestyle that is socially and culturally valued.

Youths who perceive their neighborhood to be tough and drug-oriented are much more likely to report marijuana use for both themselves and their peers than those who do not perceive their neighborhood as tough. This relationship is different for alcohol use. Here the person is likely to report alcohol use for him- or herself and peers regardless of "toughness" perceptions of the neighborhood.

In sum, it is not physical environment per se that is so important, but how the youth interacts with the people in it and how he or she perceives those people in relation to him- or herself. Hence, users and nonusers coexist in the same physical space (Blount & Dembo, 1984).

Youngsters may gain access to particular drugs either in their neighborhood or at their school. These two distribution sources are differentially emphasized by the boys and girls studied by Blount and Dembo (1984). These researchers found that drug availability in the neighborhood was more important in understanding the drug use of the boys. Furthermore, ease of access to various substances in the neighborhood or at school was not directly related to personal drug involvement. The influence of drug availability on the youths' drug-taking occurred through a complex relationship of availability and friends' use of alcohol and marijuana (Dembo, Farrow,

Schmeidler, & Burgos, 1979). Again, whether a young person turns to alcohol or drug use is related to peer use and *then* on environmental factors such as a ready supply of drugs or alcohol.

Some professionals and many parents believe that an effective deterrent to youth substance abuse is to make the young person afraid to experiment with alcohol or drugs. Another reason why the fear strategy prevails in some school systems is one of expediency. An already-full curriculum necessitates that alcohol and drug education be covered as part of a life skills class along with nutrition and sexuality. As a result, alcohol and drugs get only limited coverage rather than comprehensive treatment that enables students to learn effective strategies for decision-making around friendship selection and staying drug-free, especially in environments where drugs are readily available.

This strategy of fear inducement emphasizes the cognitive domain and includes as its main assumption the belief that knowledge is an effective deterrent to substance abuse. However, there is no evidence that knowledge leads to attitude and behavior change. Knowledge has a short-term effect and it seldom translates into action. The efficacy of the cognitive approach has been questioned, especially in relation to long-term behavior control or change. Information is an essential part of any approach, but it cannot be the only component of a prevention program, especially where inner-city poor and minority youngsters are concerned.

Facts related to the harmful effects of alcohol and drugs are secondary to strategies that enhance psychosocial skills in the areas of stress reduction, values awareness, decision-making, and behavioral alternatives (Moskowitz, 1983). In his study, Moskowitz (1983) found that drinking was associated with low self-esteem, inadequate interpersonal and social skills, poor family relationships, a lack of refusal skills, and an absence of a sense of power. More interesting was the fact that social and economic conditions not only correlated strongly with these characteristics, but they possibly perpetuated them. Thus, a

prevention strategy that addresses many of the personal and social deficiencies related to minority status may be more effective than the factual or cognitive approach that emphasizes negative consequences of substance abuse only. Social competency and assertiveness training that are designed to empower the person may also indirectly influence the process, resulting in alcohol and drug abstinence or reduction. An important point to be made here is that this prevention approach suffers from the same shortcoming that plagues the entire substance abuse prevention field, namely the lack of an evaluation component that validates the effectiveness of the program (Moskowitz, 1983).

Prevention programs for these inner-city populations should be more in tune with the whole life situation than with just problem drinking or drug use, which is usually a symptom of personal and cultural disjunctions exacerbated by minority status. For this reason, some prevention specialists have advocated a developmental approach. The value of such an approach is that it focuses on modifying and strengthening the negative personality derivatives of minority status. However, a sociopsychological approach may be best for minority youth because such an approach incorporates both social and cultural considerations within a developmental framework and this serves as a heuristic model for prevention among minority groups. Contrary to popular belief, there is a strong abstinence sentiment in minority communities, especially among women and youth, which must be taken into account in planning and implementing prevention programs. This is why it makes sense to embed substance education and prevention into regular activities engaged in by inner-city youth.

According to Globetti (1988), another critical component in prevention programs involves incorporating peer leaders in out-of-school leisure and sports groups. Ideally, prevention strategies should include every facet of life in the community, especially the family, the school, and the informal social groups in which youth participate. Several workshops on such varied topics as dance, drama, and crafts were infused with units on alcohol education (Globetti, 1988).

Some preventive measures affect the supply of alcohol and drugs and the places in which they are used. Another category of preventive measures focuses on drinking practices of people once access to alcohol has been obtained; it consists of various forms of alcohol education as a means of shaping drinking attitudes and practices, especially among young people. The idea here is to make drinking practices safer, even if people don't change their drinking behavior. For African Americans, the lack of awareness has created a lack of commitment in taking action to eliminate alcohol problems. The implication for alcoholism prevention among African-American youth is that there is a need for a massive and comprehensive educational campaign targeted not only toward black youth, but also toward their parents and other adults to increase awareness of the severe impact of alcoholism on blacks.

Another internal factor that may to some extent be under the control of African Americans themselves is the location of alcohol outlets in and near black residential areas. The most important external factor to consider in establishing alcoholism prevention measures is the manner in which alcohol problems have been historically compounded by institutional racism.

Recent evidence indicates that the level of racial consciousness among African Americans is associated with attitudes toward the use of alcohol and other substances. There is no significant difference between black and white teenagers in terms of involvement in drinking. Dawkins (1988) maintains that primary prevention of alcoholism among black youth requires involvement of all of the major institutions in the black community, including families, churches, schools, political organizations, the business community, and social and civic groups. In addition, holistic approaches to chemical dependency treatment based on culturally sensitive practice modalities are gainir.g wide acceptance within the broader black community (Thompson & Simmons-Cooper, 1988).

Not much information exists on substance use patterns of African-American youth who do not come to public attention through the criminal justice or mental health system (Gary & Berry, 1985). The most striking finding reported by Gary and Berry was that racial consciousness was of central importance in determining the substance use attitudes of their study sample. Individuals with strong African-American racial identity were less likely to be involved in heavy substance use.

Gary and Berry argue that it is vitally important to have a clear and definable target population in any prevention strategy. Individuals and their cultures plus the social group or organization, the community, and the interaction of all these factors must be considered in designing substance abuse prevention strategies.

Finally, a critical element to emerge from the Gary and Berry study was the central role played by the black church in preventing substance abuse. Accordingly, a recommendation that emerged for mental health planners and practitioners was that any effort to provide prevention and intervention programs for African-American communities needed to incorporate the black church. These specific aspects of prevention programs for African-American youth will be discussed in the context of an Afrocentric approach to prevention.

Youths not involved in drug or alcohol use appear to be good candidates for drug abuse prevention efforts. Dembo et al. (1983) report data that confirm that drug-free youths responded rather well to programs that involved such traditional prevention agents as staff members of a drug program, a physician, or a school-based drug educator. However, the situation was different for the users of marijuana and other drugs, particularly those living in high-drug-use neighborhoods, where Dembo et al. reported findings that suggest that the influence of drug use subculture was greatest. Using respected neighborhood residents as role models, particularly residents who had overcome their personal abuse of drugs, appeared to be the most effective strategy for intervening in current drug use.

Alcohol consumption for white youth was consistently higher than for blacks and Asian Americans, and Hispanics reported greater use than blacks. For marijuana use, there was also a significant overall difference by ethnicity. White students consumed significantly more alcohol than other ethnic groups, followed by Hispanics. The lowest level of alcohol use was found among black adolescents. White students also had the highest marijuana use, followed by Hispanic students.

In terms of hard drugs, white adolescents again showed the highest level of use, followed by Hispanics. The lowest level of hard drug use was among black students (Maddahian, Newcomb, & Bentler, 1986).

SUBSTANCE ABUSE AMONG HOMELESS YOUTH

In a review of the literature on alcohol, drug abuse, and mental health problems among the homeless, Fischer (1991) concluded that research on the homeless population conducted over the past decade has been largely descriptive, with the result that much is known about the sociodemographic characteristics of homeless populations. Recent studies portray the "new homeless" as younger and more heterogeneous than the old skid-row populations. The homeless are also composed of greater proportions of women and minorities (particularly African Americans and Hispanics), an alarming number of families with young children, and increasing numbers of people with mental illness and histories of drug abuse.

According to Weinreb and Bassuk (1990), only very recently have incidental findings of substantial rates of substance abuse among homeless families—especially single mothers—reawakened interest in the epidemiology of alcohol-related problems and raised questions concerning the role of drug abuse in the life history of the homeless. Weinreb and Bassuk (1990) discuss the plight of drug-addicted mothers and their children and the absence of adequate drug intervention services for these mothers. As a consequence, homeless children are at great risk to

eventually become addicts themselves. Accordingly, homeless children and adolescents constitute a special population in our review of prevention programs for inner-city youth.

When turning specifically to the question of homeless children and adolescents, very little is known other than anecdotally. For instance, Reverend Ritter (1989), the founder of Covenant House, estimates that there may be between 200,000 and 300,000 homeless children and adolescents living in our cities. He believes that this is a conservative estimate and points out that according to U.S. Census procedures, the homeless are not counted until they reach 21 years of age. According to Ritter, the family profile of the average Covenant House youngster is "almost invariably, that of a single-parent family, a child of divorced parents or of no marriage at all. These youngsters, mostly adolescents and teenagers, are almost always a product of the child welfare system and repeated placements, have long histories of involvement with the police and of failure in school, and long histories at home of physical and sexual abuse, alcoholism, and drug abuse" (p. 156).

Furthermore, a great number of the chronically homeless teenagers engage in polydrug use and commercial sex. As further evidence of the severity of the problems of homeless youth, Ritter estimates that as many as 25% of the boys have either attempted or contemplated suicide.

In her review of literature, Fischer (1991) identified only two studies that dealt specifically with homeless adolescents. In the first study by Robertson (see Fischer, 1991), drug abuse was found in two-fifths and alcohol abuse in about half of the Hollywood homeless teenagers sampled. In the second study carried out by Shaffer and Caton (see Fischer, 1991), approximately 90% of the homeless adolescents sampled in New York City had mental health problems.

In sum, homeless youth as a group appear to have fallen through the cracks in prevention efforts directed at inner-city youngsters. Two actions are called for: research on the number of homeless youth and their substance abuse involvement, and strategies for incorporating these

TABLE 19.1   Critical Elements of Successful Approaches Used in Model Prevention Programs

COMPREHENSIVE APPROACHES	EXAMPLE
Addressing multiple dimensions of youths' lives	Individual Family Peer group School Community
Addressing multiple public-health domains	Agent (drugs) Host (the individual) Environment
Use of a variety of services	Self-esteem enhancement activities General skills training Information and awareness enhancement Refusal skills training Youth leadership training Education or training of parents Counseling

INDIRECT APPROACHES	EXAMPLE
Use of program names that will omit any reference to drug use or prevention services	Soaring Eagles American Variety Theatre Company Peer Consultants in Training Adventure Alternatives
Use of activities as enticements	Sports, dance, music, drama, food, games, movies, family outings, day camps, field trips, wilderness activities
Use of indirect prevention techniques	Sports and creative arts Themes of dramatic productions Cultural identity development Leadership development Experiential games

(continued)

youth into community prevention efforts that include some form of residential stability, education, and employment.

COMMON FEATURES OF ADOLESCENT DRUG USE PREVENTION

In an extensive survey of 138 adolescent drug use prevention programs and a case study analysis of 10 programs (U.S. General Accounting Office, 1992), a framework of key ideas for prevention programs is presented. This framework is important and deserves serious consideration by any agency planning to provide prevention services for adolescents. The following are the key features of seemingly effective prevention programs identified in the GAO report: a comprehensive prevention strategy, an indirect approach

TABLE 19.1   Critical Elements of Successful Approaches Used in Model Prevention Programs   *continued*

EMPOWERMENT APPROACHES	EXAMPLE
Use of role models	Recruitment of male staff Recruitment of role models from the community
Development of leadership skills	Public speaking training Question/answer sessions with adults Community service activities Peer leadership training
Development of general skills	Academic assistance Parenting education and training Values clarification workshops Communication skills training Problem-solving/coping skills training Vocation preparation

Source: Adapted from the 1992 U.S. General Accounting Office Report on Adolescent Drug Use Prevention (Tables 1–3).

to substance abuse prevention, a goal of empowering participating youth, an active participatory approach, a culturally sensitive orientation, and organization around highly structured activities.

The framework is an invaluable guide to any agency or community group planning a prevention program for youth. The critical elements of several components of the framework are depicted in Table 19.1. As indicated in Table 19.1, the first element involves comprehensive approaches to prevention services. This must of necessity involve not only the young person, but also the family, school, peers, and community. This involvement can be achieved through the coordination and collaboration of multiple service agencies, as noted in the table. The more comprehensive the prevention program, the greater the chance for success because the entire ecosystem of the young person is involved in one way or another in the decision to resist drugs.

The second component shown in Table 19.1 is an indirect approach to prevention; that is, programs that engage inner-city children and adolescents in activities such as sports, dance, and field trips that also communicate positive messages about remaining drug-free. According to the GAO report, the service providers associated with these programs saw it as essential that the name of the agency or service omit any reference to drug use or prevention services. Youth who become engaged as active participants in such programs are very likely to resist drugs in their environment because the programs offered them an alternative to drugs.

Another critical component is the empowerment skills young people learn as part of their participation in these indirect drug prevention activities. Central to the empowerment approaches are appropriate role models for the participants, especially drug-free adult males from the community who can guide inner-city youth away from drugs. As shown in Table 19.1, the empowerment skills include leadership training, communication skill development, and community service activities. Collectively, the intent is to see change in academic achievement, problem-solving behavior, and vocational preparation.

The GAO report points out that very few of the 138 prevention programs surveyed have adequate evaluation plans and data collection strategies for assessing program impact. Thus, at this stage it is still difficult to know with certainty which program features have the greatest effect on enabling inner-city youth to remain drug free. Furthermore, there may be no single set of best features; they may vary depending on the targeted individuals, their family, peers, school, and community.

The report also stresses several concerns that all programs seem to experience as they attempt to provide services in the inner city. These concerns are maintaining continuity with program participants, coordinating and integrating the various service components, providing accessible services to all youth in need, obtaining funds to maintain long-term continuity, and attracting and keeping leaders and staff for the program. However, the case studies in the GAO report indicate that these problems can be surmounted and high-quality programs can be instituted for children and adolescents in the inner city.

PARTNERSHIP FOR A DRUG-FREE AMERICA

In existence since the 1980s, the Partnership for a Drug-Free America is a nonprofit organization representing the nation's advertising and communications industries. It uses its knowledge of print and electronic media to communicate directly to youth that drugs are not cool. In 1992, the partnership launched a highly specialized antidrug public service advertising program for inner-city children (Dnistrian, 1992).

As a part of its focus on inner-city youth, the Partnership carried out a study involving interviews with a total of 7,288 students. The students were in grades 2 through 6 and from both public and parochial schools in the five boroughs of New York City. In the study, public schools in which 74.5% or more of the students were below the poverty level were designated as below-

poverty schools. The poverty-level designation for parochial schools, which have much lower numbers of poor students, was set at 50% of students below poverty. In all, 68% of the children interviewed fell below the poverty line established by the researchers.

Based on these interviews, the Partnership study arrived at five major conclusions regarding the children living below the poverty line and their attitudes and vulnerabilities to drug use. Each of these conclusions is presented in detail here because of their importance in prevention program planning and implementation.

Conclusion 1: Poor, urban children are effectively reached by media messages, which help them learn about the risks of drugs. This is an important general conclusion because it supports the idea of the Partnership that children can learn about drugs from a variety of sources, including television. An overwhelming number of children interviewed learned about the risks of drug use from Partnership media messages aimed at the general population over the preceding five years. In support of this conclusion, the following was learned:

- Nine out of ten children learn about drugs from TV commercials, and two out of three learn "a lot" about drugs from TV. This source of information reinforces what the children learn at home and in school about the harmful consequences of drugs.
- The specific drug messages that have appeared have been learned at very high levels. Specifically, nine out of ten students believe that a person should never take crack, cocaine, or marijuana; 95% or more of children in grades 4–6 say that a person will die, get sick, or have a messed-up brain if he or she uses drugs; nine out of ten in grades 4–6 fear getting hooked or being in danger from using drugs.
- Interestingly, it was found that children could repeat, verbatim, the antidrug messages that they had heard on TV.

Conclusion 2: The findings also showed that the children interviewed were extremely vulnerable to drug use. The children needed and wanted help from adults in protecting them from drugs. These children were scared of external pressures in the environment and internal temptations to try drugs. Specifically, the interviews showed the following:

— At least 67% of the children reported that they feared that someone would make them take drugs and 31% of the children in grades 4–6 were afraid they could be tempted to try drugs.
— Importantly, children felt isolated in their fear. Fully 75% of the children in grades 4–6 believed that they were different in how they felt about drugs, despite the fact that the great majority of children their own age were drug-free and expressed the same fears regarding drugs.
— Drugs are more the norm in the neighborhoods of poor, urban children. This is illustrated by the fact that 14% of children in grades 4–6 say that some friends use marijuana, compared to 10% of children their age in the general U.S. population; 10% say some friends use crack, compared to 5% in the general U.S. population.
— In all, 25% of children in grades 4–6 in New York City's poor areas have friends who are using illegal drugs; for younger children in grades 2–3, it's approximately 10%.
— In focus interview sessions with selected children, it was learned that children felt funny about both the idea of trying drugs and about saying no to drugs. Children wondered how others their own age felt about similar problems.

Conclusion 3: Inner-city children need encouragement and support to resist drugs. In addition, they need the skills to be able to resist the temptation to engage in drug experimentation. Specifically, these children were not confident about their ability to resist the pressures to try drugs and needed assurance that it was possible to resist without being isolated from their peers or risking social disapproval. Among children in grades 4–6, the findings showed the following:

— 70% found it hard to say no to drugs, compared to 44% of the same age group in the general population.
— 60% indicated that everyone tries drugs (any kind) sometime, and 75% felt that everyone tries marijuana.

— 75% said they were afraid that they would not know how to say no, and more than one out of five said that they would not know what to do if offered drugs.

These findings show clearly why children need training in how to resist drugs. Such training entails self-esteem, assertiveness, and the willingness to meet social disapproval from peers. The benefits of such a decision for the young person must outweigh the social disapproval of resisting drugs. This is one of the major challenges in drug prevention programs.

Conclusion 4: Importantly, positive peer influences do exist in inner-city neighborhoods to help protect children from drug use. Although children believe that they are alone in their antidrug efforts, the opposite is true. Media messages such as those produced by the partnership attempt to communicate that children are not alone and that there are adults around to help them resist drugs. For instance:

— 76% of children in grades 4–6 and 88% in grades 2–3 reported that none of their friends used illegal drugs.
— 90% of children in grades 4–6 interviewed do not believe that a person is more cool or popular if he or she uses drugs.
— 90% of all children do not believe that drug users have more fun.
— 90% of the respondents in grades 4–6 do not believe that using drugs helps the user to get a boyfriend or girlfriend.
— 90% in grades 4–6 believe that users of marijuana stand to lose their friends.
— 90% in grades 2–3 believe that marijuana use can mess up your life.

In essence, these findings show that young inner-city children can be influenced positively about the harmful consequences of substance abuse before they are seriously challenged to use drugs. Building on this strength, prevention programs must be directed at developing the necessary skills to continue resisting drugs.

Conclusion 5: The family plays an important and crucial role in helping to inform and motivate inner-city children to resist drugs and cannot be excluded from any prevention effort.

- Among the survey respondents, 66% of the children in grades 2–3 and 55% of the children in grades 4–6 lived with both a mother and a father present in the home.
- Importantly, the vast majority of the children (90% of children in grades 2–3 and 97% grades 4–6) were afraid of using drugs because it would make their parents sad.
- The most important life goal for children in grades 4–6 was making their parents proud of them.
- Nearly all of the respondents, 93%, learned about drugs from their parents as well as from other sources.
- Nearly 75% of the students in grades 4–6 were not aware that their own drug use could influence a younger sibling to also use drugs.

In summary, the findings of the partnership study are very important because they show that the problem of drugs in the inner city is not hopeless. In fact, the findings reveal that the vast majority of inner-city elementary school-age children are defiantly antidrug. However, the findings also show that the youngsters are afraid of pressure to use and sell drugs. This is exactly why organizations such as the Partnership for a Drug-Free America are so vital in the effort to curtail drug use in the inner city. Their ability to produce antidrug TV ads targeted for inner-city youth has proven critical, but this is not sufficient. Other prevention programs in the community must be available for children and adolescents. Among other goals, these programs must show youth that they are not alone and that they can learn the empowering skills to resist drugs.

An important question related to the partnership's antidrug ads is whether the media have any influence on adolescent drug use. Some information that bears on this research question comes from the National High School Senior Survey, which annually assesses drug use among the nation's high school seniors (Partnership for a Drug-Free America, 1992). In recent years, there has been some decline in the rate of drug use among high school seniors. According to

Lloyd Johnston, one of the three investigators who administered the senior survey, two factors driving the decline of illicit drug use among teenagers are: an increasing perception of risk associated with drugs and drug use and increasing social disapproval among youth of drugs and drug use. The information gathered as part of the survey showed that "the Partnership's national campaign has effectively delivered the message of drug risk and social disapproval to teenagers. The survey found that students have a 'very high level of recall' of Partnership messages; that, in students' opinions, the messages held 'a high degree of credibility' and had 'an impact on their drug-using behaviors and attitudes" (Partnership for a Drug-Free America, 1992, p. 1).

To give the reader some idea of the ads prepared by the partnership, one of the best-known ads shows a frying skillet and an egg. The voice-over to the ad says, "This is your brain," referring to the egg, and the egg is cracked and dropped into the skillet and begins to fry noisily. After a short pause, the voice-over says, "This is your brain on drugs." After another short pause, the voice-over asks, "Any questions?"

In conclusion, the inner-city program supported by the partnership emphasizes five distinct but interrelated strategies using the media to educate youth about drugs. These strategies are as follows:

- Reinforce young people's self-esteem to enable them to avoid the dangers of drugs
- Encourage resistance and demonstrate how to respond when confronted with an offer of drugs
- Suggest positive alternatives to drug use and recognize through celebration how ordinary children have resisted drugs
- Encourage the participation of family members and friends in drug prevention
- Show the strong social stigma surrounding drug use and those who prey on children by giving or selling them drugs

These themes are all communicated in one way or the other to young persons in the approximately 375 antidrug ads that have been created to date (Partnership for a Drug Free America, 1992).

The success of the ads is illustrated by the fact that as recently as 1986, only one-third of high school seniors were willing or able to acknowledge the risks associated with cocaine use. This figure rose rapidly after 1986, reaching nearly two-thirds of high school seniors who by 1991 could identify the risks of cocaine use. Whereas from 1979 to 1986 about 12% of seniors used cocaine during the preceding year, that figure dropped to 3.5% by 1991.

AMERICA'S PRIDE: AN INTERNATIONAL DRUG PREVENTION PROGRAM

America's PRIDE is a drug prevention program for high school youth that has been very active in the inner city. Using a team approach, PRIDE encourages students to reach out to their friends, younger students, and the community with an assertive antidrug message. The major goal of the organization is to support drug-free activities in the school and in the community. The guiding principles of PRIDE are as follows:

- All youth deserve the opportunity to reach their full potential in an alcohol- and drug-free environment.
- Youth are capable and responsible individuals who, with proper guidance and direction, can become tomorrow's leaders.
- The best agents of primary and secondary prevention are peers who can effectively reduce the use of alcohol and other drugs.
- The prevention of alcohol and other drug use is the responsibility of everyone in the community.

The PRIDE youth program is composed of three age-appropriate programs (elementary, middle, and high school) that all have the same objectives: no drug use, an overall healthy lifestyle, a focus on positive prevention techniques, and the involvement of youth as resources (Michael Basket, personal communication, 1993).

In addition, PRIDE is careful to monitor the research findings regarding youth and substance abuse. It makes these research findings available via its newsletter, brochures, press releases, and conferences. PRIDE also carried out a national study of drug use among students during the 1992–1993 school year.

The PRIDE findings were based on the responses of 236,745 students in seven grade levels in 40 states. Questions about 10 types of drugs were asked in each of the seven grade levels, for a total of 70 instances. Drug types studied were cigarettes, beer, wine coolers, liquor, marijuana, cocaine, uppers, downers, inhalants, and hallucinogens. Some of the findings reported by PRIDE in a press release (PRIDE, 1993) were as follows:

- On the basis of annual use (at least once in the past year), 56 of the 70 instances (80%) showed significant increases or no change and 14 involved decreases.
- On the basis of monthly use, 54 instances (77%) showed significant increases or no change and 16 involved decreases.
- Marijuana posted significant increases in all seven grade levels for both annual and monthly use, the only drug to do so.
- For middle school (grades 6–8), significant increases were detected in annual use of marijuana and hallucinogens. There were no significant decreases for any drug.
- For senior high (grades 9–12), significant increases were found in annual use of cigarettes, marijuana, and hallucinogens. There were, however, significant decreases in beer, wine coolers, liquor, uppers, and downers. The use of cocaine (including crack) and inhalants remained unchanged.
- The most startling change in drug use patterns was the increase in marijuana use by African-American students in all grade levels. Among African Americans in middle school, annual use of marijuana rose 71% among males and 100% among females. Overall, African-American students continue to use less marijuana than white students, but the difference is smaller than in previous years.
- Use of hallucinogens, including LSD and PCP, rose significantly on an annual basis in the eighth grade (2.4% to 2.7%), eleventh grade (5.6% to 6.4%), and twelfth grade (7.1% to 8%). There was no significant decrease in hallucinogen use for annual or monthly usage.

The nature of polydrug use among America's youth indicates to the PRIDE leadership that prevention efforts should not be directed at any single drug. Focus should be on the early sequence of drugs that young people are first likely to try and on the conditions that lead them into experimentation and use. In addition, the important thing to learn from the PRIDE survey findings is that youth-oriented substance abuse prevention efforts must be continuous.

Thus far, we have discussed several national efforts that have targeted inner-city youth for substance abuse prevention. Although these programs incorporate many cultural aspects of the minority groups being served, they are not specifically designed as culture-specific models of prevention. There are such model programs, however, that are an important part of any serious efforts at prevention for minority youth in the inner city. The next section discusses an Afrocentric approach to prevention that has been successfully implemented with African-American youngsters.

AN AFROCENTRIC APPROACH TO PREVENTION

Optimal Afrocentric prevention planning should include a culturally consistent service delivery process that reflects the belief that all African-American youth can lead a drug-free life; a process wherein knowing and knowledge are connected directly to the youths; programmatic techniques and practices characterized by cooperation and mutuality; the blending of individual achievement with collective advancement; the desire to continually guide youths to a higher level of understanding and functioning; the underlying goal of personally contributing to one's own as well as others' fulfillment; training and learning that is linked to the students' and community's well-being and welfare; and a process wherein cooperative effort is used to continually develop and expand the natural resiliencies of youths.

If the prevention program is to be effective with African-American inner-city youths, it must be consistent with the cultural substance of the population to whom it is targeted. In terms of program activities, it is believed that the prevention plan should have the following characteristics.

In its objectives, the Afrocentric prevention plan should aim at the development of sense of consciousness, confidence, competence, commitment, and character in African-American adolescents, to make them contributing members of their families, communities, and society. The program activities must enable African-American adolescents to believe and experience the feeling that there are positive things that they can do well and that benefit the family or the community. By providing the youths with opportunities to experience success, the program would help to develop a sense of confidence. Additionally, the program would develop competencies in youths by providing them with opportunities to acquire new skills, knowledge, and practices. Finally, the program activities would develop a sense of consciousness in the adolescents by providing them with an understanding of their position in world history. If African-American adolescents understand the critical contributions African Americans have made to world civilization, then pride, awareness, and commitment to self, family, and community would become possible. The essential task of the service delivery process is to create the conditions wherein youths can acquire the essential information about the African and African-American contributions to world civilization. By knowing what was in the past, youths can conceive of an alternate reality to what is known at present.

In its purpose, the Afrocentric prevention plan should require and reflect a systematic and intentional process of enculturation and immersion in African cultural traditions that provide the basis for the insulation and inoculation of African-American adolescents from the contemporary pressures to engage in self-destructive behavior. These cultural traditions provide the basis for the development and expansion of the natural resiliency factors that exist within youths and that have traditionally enabled African Americans to overcome some of the worst excesses of racism. It should be clear to all participants in the programmatic activities that there is a cultural basis of the program and that it is rooted in African and African-American traditional cultural precepts.

In its content, the Afrocentric prevention planning should be based on, and reflect, an emphasis on spirituality. The emphasis on spirituality is designed to enable youths to perceive and understand such principles as reciprocity, responsibility, restraint, and respect. The content of the program should serve to develop a consciousness and awareness of a supreme being and the intimate relationship that exists between human beings and the supreme being and other human beings. The language used in the program should be simple and direct, yet challenging to the target population. In their activities, the service providers should make use of symbolic imagery (such as proverbs, analogies, and folktales) as a primary mechanism for the transference of information. The use of proverbs represents an important teaching process of traditional African and African-American communities that allows the learner to engage in abstract thinking of applying general principles (the proverb) to a specific situation (the event). It is through this process of synthesis and induction that the learner comes to acquire knowledge of more complex problems. The prevention specialist, in fact, is the bridge. It is the prevention specialist's job to make the inoculation strategy come alive. The prevention specialist must carry the complex and technical information supporting human growth and development to the life and minds of African-American adolescents. The prevention component of the program should provide experiences and applications that African-American adolescents can use and understand.

The Afrocentric model of prevention has as its basis a holistic, humanistic, and naturalistic orientation. The Afrocentric prevention plan should reflect a holistic orientation that deals with the totality of the individual existence. It should address the social, physical, spiritual, and mental aspects of the youths. It cannot just be a substance abuse prevention program. It must go beyond the prevention activities and begin to address issues of development in the broader context. Thus, the content of the Afrocentric model should provide youths with psychosocial skills and attributes that increase their capacity to resist negative environmental influences.

Accordingly, substance abuse prevention must respect and reflect the geopolitical and psychocultural reality of the client. In this regard, prevention practitioners who work with at-risk African-American youths must do so from an Afrocentric perspective. In effect, optimal prevention activity for African-American youths can be achieved only when it is designed to promote culturally consistent growth and development for African-American youths. The optimal can be achieved only when the prevention activities, objectives, interests, and goals are defined and driven by the cultural values, precepts, and axioms of the clients' culture. As such, optimal substance abuse prevention is a culturally consistent health promotion for at-risk African American youths.

A STATE RESPONSE TO PREVENTION EDUCATION

In an interesting publication, *Not Schools Alone,* the California State Department of Education (1990) issued a set of guidelines for schools and communities regarding prevention of use of tobacco, alcohol, and other drugs among children and youth. According to this report, early attempts to prevent alcohol and drug use by students have been largely ineffective because there were many misconceptions about the problem of substance abuse. Initially, it was believed that drug use could be diagnosed like any other physical, emotional, or skill deficiency and that it was due to a lack of information, willpower, or moral character. Naturally, the response of schools around the country from the late sixties to the mid-1970s was focused on teaching students drug information, communication skills, and the physical and legal consequences of drug use. The assumption that information leads to attitude change and then to behavior change was proven to be incorrect and misleading.

Whether a student is inclined to smoke, drink, or use drugs is largely determined by the influence groups, or systems, that define his or her daily environment—that is, family, school, friends, and community. Each of these key influence groups has either a positive or negative impact on a young person's development, learning, and behavior (California State Department of Education, 1990).

Alcohol abuse and alcoholism is the number-one health problem in the black community (Prevention Pipeline, 1993b). Although African Americans are still less likely than whites to drink, those who do are more likely to suffer alcohol-related problems such as drunkenness and esophageal cancer, especially if they are low-income males. However, most Americans hear far more about the dangers of illegal drugs in ghettos—particularly crack cocaine—than they ever hear about alcohol. For example, the health department in Los Angeles County reported that four times as many African Americans died in 1990 from alcohol-related causes as from cocaine use. Two out of every three accidental drug deaths in the county were alcohol-related (just 5% were due to cocaine), and hospital emergency rooms admitted more patients who had overdosed on alcohol in combination with other drugs than just from cocaine (Prevention Pipeline, 1993b)

— Nearly two-thirds of all high school students have tried illicit drugs before graduation. Today's youth start using tobacco, alcohol, and other drugs on average at age 12.
— More than $2 billion is spent each year on confinement in public and private juvenile facilities for delinquents.
— Roughly 51% of African-American children, 45% of Hispanic children, and 17% of white children have been characterized by a leading expert as at risk.

Studies have shown that access to information and services alone may not have much impact on changing the behavior of adolescents at risk. What does reduce risk-taking behavior among adolescents is the focus of intense investigation. A review of 100 successful prevention programs found two common themes: individual attention and multicomponent, multiagency, communitywide programs. Other common components include early intervention, basic skills training, healthy school climate, parent involvement, peer involvement, connection to the working world, social and life-skills training, and attention to staff training and supervision.

The review also found that successful programs tended to focus primarily on the antecedents of high-risk behavior rather than the presenting behavior itself. Greater relative emphasis to the protective factors of adult attention and communitywide support is urged. Early intervention is key. The programs and services must work with children, families, and communities from the outset. In-school programs offering comprehensive health and social services are important and in greater need in our inner-city schools.

In prevention program planning and implementation, it is important to remember that young people are inherently strong, vigorous, creative, dynamic, and resourceful (Prevention Pipeline, 1993a). These are the attributes that make it possible for the majority of inner-city adolescents to negotiate one of life's most difficult passages and move successfully into adulthood. These are precisely the qualities that must be nurtured and reinforced in prevention programs for adolescents living in unhealthy, risky environments if these youngsters are to succeed (Prevention Pipeline, 1993a).

RECOMMENDATIONS

In developing programs to address the problems of alcohol and drug abuse in the inner city, it is important to have specific attainable goals and guidelines for achieving such goals. The goals should take into account the particular concerns of the community. No longer can we rely on the drug-prevention messages from schools or the media. In working to prevent initial drug use and stop drug use among those already using drugs and alcohol, it is essential to develop strategies that focus on the unique characteristics of each population. In addition, because of the different ethnic compositions of our inner cities, what works in one urban area may not work in another. Issues of language, culture, and relation to the predominant culture all must be addressed when developing and assessing programs. There is no single right program for the inner city; the challenge that faces professionals today is in reaching the largest number of youth with the most comprehensive plan that can be developed. It is important to consider the changing demographics of our nation and the fact that all recommendations must be dynamic in their conceptualization and flexible in their application. A major obstacle faced in the examination of programs is the lack of proper evaluation and assessment procedures for programs that were identified as effective with inner city residents. If the work of these programs is to be replicated, it is important to be able to look at the effectiveness of these programs against some form of evaluation.

In reviewing successful programs, themes that addressed the population served became apparent. Among the themes we find especially important are individual attention to clients, multi-agency support, parent training, and community-wide involvement. Additional features include a comprehensive strategy, an indirect approach to prevention services, a program that emphasizes a participatory approach, and cultural sensitivity to inner-city youth.

When delivering primary prevention services, it is important to include a strong abstinence component for children. Furthermore, the involvement of parents is crucial in developing a strong antidrug theme. The strong emphasis on raising self-esteem has also been shown to be critical in primary prevention. Self-esteem provides the individual with the inner strength necessary to resist drug use and to make effective personal decisions regarding conduct. Social competency training has also been seen as an effective deterrent in preventing future drug and alcohol use by increasing the child's sense of self and decreasing risk factors that may lead the young person to feelings of self-doubt and that mask assertive refusal skills. Central to this prevention program is the use of the community in sponsoring and supporting recreational activities such as dance, drama, and sports. The role of peers, parents, and teachers is crucial to the success of such programs. The young person needs to learn that support exists for these activities. Lastly, the ready availability of drugs and alcohol in the inner city needs specific attention. For many inner-city children, the easy availability of drugs and alcohol is difficult to escape. Parents should work with their city councils and police departments to develop plans for supporting businesses other than liquor stores in their communities. It is important for communities and police departments to create drug free lanes to schools in order to provide safe passage to and from school.

In the development of secondary prevention programs, what is needed is an emphasis on attitudes toward drinking and drug use. The use of respected community leaders and peers has been found to be effective in preventing future use. In addition, because of the many sociological forces associated with drug use in the inner city, it is important to focus on devaluing the status of drug use. Successful programs focus on getting children involved in the development of the program with highly structured activities that provided a chance for the young person to see alternatives to drug use. The influence of peers and parents is still important at this phase and can be influential in providing alternatives to drug use. The role of recognizable role models is also important.

Programs addressing the needs of inner-city youth who are regular drug users face even more difficult challenges. The emphasis of these programs is to help the individual reintegrate into society through job training, educational support, and a drug-free environment. These individuals are perhaps best reached by individuals of similar backgrounds who have gone through similar drug use experience and who are now living drug-free. The recovering drug user or addict can provide a model of life without drugs. These young people have many obstacles facing them, but with support and encouragement, programs can be designed to foster a life free from drugs. The development of basic living skills, job training, and support for abstinence from drug usage is vital. The involvement of parents is also important in the recovery process.

In developing any of these types of programs, it is important to recognize that there are many realistic problems that make implementation very difficult. These problems include obtaining funding, providing accessible services, coordinating with the many service agencies, maintaining contact and interest of the participants, attracting and retaining qualified staff, and, most importantly, finding methods of evaluating the effectiveness of the program for implementation elsewhere. The goal of all professionals should be to incorporate the best elements of the effective programs while attempting to address the specific issues that face the communities they serve.

REFERENCES

Blount, W. R., & Dembo, R. (1984). The effect of perceived neighborhood setting on self-reported tobacco, alcohol, and marijuana use among inner-city minority junior high school youth. *The International Journal of the Addictions, 19* (2), 175–198.

California State Department of Education (1990). *Not schools alone: Guidelines for schools and communities to prevent the use of tobacco, alcohol and other drugs among children and youth.* Sacramento: California State Department of Education.

Dawkins, M. P. (1988). Alcoholism prevention and black youth. *The Journal of Drug Issues, 18,* 15–20.

Dembo, R., Allen, N., Farrow, D., Schmeidler, J., & Burgos, W. (1985). A causal analysis of early drug involvement in three inner-city neighborhood settings. *The International Journal of the Addictions, 20,* 1213–1237.

Dembo, R., Blount, W. R., Schmeidler, J., & Burgos, W. (1986). Perceived environmental drug use risk and the correlates of early drug use or nonuse among inner-city youths: The motivated actor. *The International Journal of the Addictions, 21,* 977–1000.

Dembo, R., Farrow, D., Schmeidler, J., & Burgos, W. (1979). Testing a causal model of environmental influences on the early drug involvement of inner city junior high school youths. *American Journal of Drug & Alcohol Abuse, 6,* 313–336.

Dembo, R., Schmeidler, J., Taylor, R. W., Agresti, D., & Burgos, W. (1983). Preferred resources for help with a drug problem among youths living in different inner city neighborhood settings. *Advances in Alcohol and Substance Abuse, 2* (1), 57–75.

Dnistrian, S. (1992). Partnership messages target urban kids. *Partnership Newsletter, 6 (#2 Winter Supplement),* 1–2.

Fischer, P. J. (1991). *Alcohol, drug abuse and mental health problems among homeless persons: A review of the literature, 1980–1990.* Rockville, MD: Alcohol, Drug Abuse, and Mental Health Administration.

Gary, L. E., & Berry, G. L. (1985). Predicting attitudes toward substance use in a black community: Implications for prevention. *Community Mental Health Journal, 21,* 42–51.

Globetti, G. (1988). Alcohol education programs and minority youth. *The Journal of Drug Issues, 18,* 115–129.

Maddahian, E., Newcomb, M. D., & Bentler, P. M. (1986). Adolescents' substance use: Impact of ethnicity, income, and availability. *Advances in Alcohol and Substance Abuse, 5* (3), 63–78.

Moskowitz, J. (1983). Preventing adolescent substance abuse through drug education. In T. Glynn, C. Leukefeld, & J. Ludfard (Eds.), *Preventing adolescent drug abuse: Intervention strategies.* Research monograph 47. Rockville, MD: National Institute on Drug Abuse, pp. 233–249.

Partnership for a Drug-Free America (Sept. 1992). *The influence of media on adolescent drug use: Can kids be influenced by what they see on TV and in other media?* New York: Unpublished document.

Prevention Pipeline (1993a). Interventions for adolescents at risk. *Prevention Pipeline, 6* (3), 87–89.

Prevention Pipeline (1993b). A potent brew: Booze and crime. *Prevention Pipeline, 6* (5), 87-89.

PRIDE (1993). *After a decade of progress, students return to drug use: Increases in marijuana and hallucinogens cited* (press release). Atlanta: PRIDE.

Ritter, B. (1989). Abuse of the adolescent. *New York State Journal of Medicine* (March), 156–158.

Thompson, T., & Simmons-Cooper, C. (1988). Chemical dependency treatment and black adolescents. Special issue: Alcohol problems and minority youth. *Journal of Drug Issues, 18* (1), 21–31.

United States General Accounting Office (1992). *Adolescent drug use prevention: Common features of promising community programs.* Report to the Chairman, Subcommittee on Select Education, Committee on Education and Labor, House of Representatives. Washington, DC: Superintendent of Documents.

Weinreb, L. F., & Bassuk, E. L. (1990). Substance abuse: A growing problem among homeless families. *Family and Community Health, 13* (1), 55–64.

CHAPTER 20

THE ELDERLY

MEYER D. GLANTZ
ZILI SLOBODA

When talking or writing about the elderly, it seems obligatory to begin by saying that older Americans constitute more than 12% of the United States population and by noting that of all age groups, they are the most sharply increasing in number. It is almost as if we need to be reminded that the elderly are a significant part of the American population. As of 1990, approximately one in every eight Americans is 65 years of age or older; if adults 60 years or older are included instead of age 65 and up, then older adults constitute approximately 17% of the population (U.S. Senate Special Committee on Aging et al., 1991). Due to the aging of the large baby boom generation, by the year 2030, 20% of the U.S. population will be 65 years of age or older.

Perceptions of the elderly are often determined more by stereotypes than by data. The elderly are a very diverse group—in fact, the most heterogeneous of any age group. This diversity extends to all dimensions, ranging from health and functionality to psychological, social, and economic status. Partially in an attempt to cope with this diversity, many gerontological researchers distinguish the "young" elderly (65 to 75 years of age) from the "frail" elderly (76 years and older). Among the more common stereotypes of the elderly are those that assume that the young elderly have relatively the same characteristics and problems as the frail elderly.

In fact, the young elderly are quite different and, as a group, they are generally functioning well.

Another widely held stereotype is that there are no drug abuse problems among the elderly. The public, policymakers, and even healthcare professionals generally do not associate substance use problems with the elderly. The inaccuracy of this belief grows every year. Elderly substance abusers are not now and will not in the future be limited to a few skid-row alcoholics and aging, burned-out heroin addicts. Furthermore, there is reason to believe that elderly substance abuse will escalate over the next several decades. A number of articles have reviewed the literature on substance-related problems and the elderly and the conclusions of the research are summarized here. Although the substance abuse research literature is sparse, some findings appear to be well-founded.

ILLICIT DRUG USE

There does not *now* appear to be a significant abuse problem related to illicit drugs among the elderly; in fact, only a few percent of the currently elderly population has ever had a single illegal drug experience. This low prevalence of current involvement is due in part to a cohort/cultural lack of drug involvement and acceptability, to the reduced survivorship of abusers, and to

The views expressed in this chapter are those of the authors and do not necessarily represent the opinions or policies of the National Institute on Drug Abuse, the U.S. Department of Health and Human Services, or the federal government.

the maturing-out phenomenon, which reflects the observation that abusers tend to decrease involvement with illicit drugs as they age past 26 years of age.

The particular causes of the low prevalence of elderly drug involvement today are very significant because neither they nor their dampening effects on elderly drug abuse may be as constant over time and across groups and cohorts as has been believed. First, the maturing-out phenomenon appears to be less common than was previously hypothesized, with more abusers extending their career of drug involvement, often by changing the drugs and methods of obtaining them. Second, the increased availability of methadone clinics and other factors are facilitating the survival probability of abusers, meaning greater longevity for a greater number. Third, although cohort, cultural, and historical factors mitigate against the current elderly population having illegal drug involvement, these factors are increasingly less relevant to future elderly cohorts. With the aging of the baby-boom cohort, an age group notorious for their illegal drug experimentation and involvement, the age-related risk distribution may change. By the time the boomers reach their senior years, the elderly may become one of the higher-risk groups for drug abuse. (For a more extensive discussion of elderly illicit drug abuse, see Glantz & Backenheimer, 1988; Glantz, 1981).

Indications of a shift in drug acceptability among older adults can be seen in a trend analyses of data from the National Household Survey on Drug Abuse (NHSDA) conducted by the National Institute on Drug Abuse. The NHSDA was initiated in 1971 to monitor the level of drug abuse behaviors in the general population. Conducted bi- and tri-annually until 1989, when it began being conducted annually, the survey has used a consistent methodology for data collection and serves as the best measurement of drug use among a national probability sample of U.S. households. In 1991, the survey was expanded from a sample size of approximately 8,000 to 31,000. The expansion of the sample size has enabled more detailed analyses of special population groups ordinarily underrepresented in prior surveys.

Although the NHSDA is a cross-sectional survey, examination of the trends of drug use by age group provides insights into differences in age cohorts. In the past, the age group showing the highest rates of drug use was the 18–25 age group, with markedly lower rates for those 26 and older. In 1979, almost 70% of those surveyed in the 18–25 age group reported they had used an illicit drug sometime in their lives and the annual prevalence rate for this group in that same year was close to 50% (NIDA, 1991a).

As subsequent birth cohorts have entered this peak-use age range (as captured in more recent surveys), the drug use prevalence rates for 18- to 25-year-olds have decreased to the current levels of just over 50% lifetime prevalence and 29% annual prevalence. However, the survey has shown that as the baby boomers have aged, their drug use has not changed dramatically. Indeed, trend analyses of these data indicate that the most significant U.S. population changes noted in drug-using behaviors over the past six years have been increases for those aged 35 and older (NIDA, 1991b). The findings not only support the hypothesis that drug use is a cohort-related phenomenon, but demonstrate that because they are a more drug-tolerant and drug-involved cohort, baby boomers are not maturing out but are aging with drug involvement not substantially curtailed. If these trends continue, the baby boomers may well become an elderly cohort with a significant number of active drug abusers.

Other surveys support this observation. Data from the 1992 NHSDA show that rates and prevalence of illicit drug use have dropped steadily since 1979 for 12- to 34-year-olds but not for those 35 and older (SAMHSA/OAS, 1993b). The authors of the NHSDA report state that the trend for the over-35 group is determined by the "aging of the heavy drug using cohorts of the 1970s, [i.e. the baby boomers], which has resulted in an overall shift in the age distribution of illicit drug users." In 1979, only 10% of illicit drug users were age 35 and older; according to the 1992 NHSDA

data, 23% of the illicit drug users are over 35. Corroboration can also be found in data from the Drug Abuse Warning Network (DAWN).

DAWN collects information on drug abuse-related hospital emergency room episodes from a representative sample of nonfederal short-stay hospitals located throughout the coterminous United States, including 21 oversampled metropolitan areas. The 1992 DAWN data estimates show a continuation of the general upward trend in emergency room drug mentions that began in 1990. However, the percentage of increase for both heroin- and cocaine-related episodes among the 35 and older age group exceeded the general rate of increase (SAMHSA/OAS, 1993a).

Also somewhat reflective of changes in levels of tolerance of drug-using behaviors are perceptions of drug-related physical and psychological harmful effects held by those surveyed. The relationship between drug use and negative perceptions of drug use, as measured by physical and psychological harm and feelings of social disapproval of drug use, has been best discussed by Bachman, Johnston, O'Malley, and Humphrey (1988). Prevention programming (both school- and community-based) has moved since the 1970s to include components to affect social norms of children and youth. The beneficial consequences of these efforts are reflected in the NHSDA and in the survey of high school seniors, Monitoring the Future, conducted by the University of Michigan. Both of these surveys have documented the downward trends in drug use among youth and the association of the downward trends with increased negative perceptions of drug use. However, we should not be too sanguine about these trends, as we have not been able to significantly affect those who report heavier and more frequent drug use and those whose lives have become more involved with drugs. More efforts are needed to address the more vulnerable populations. These may increasingly include the elderly.

Decreases in these perceptions of drug-related harm and disapproval have been noted over time in cohorts aged 35 and older. Statisti-cally significant decreases in perception of harmful effects associated with cocaine, heroin, and occasional use of marijuana were noted for this age group between the 1988 and 1990 surveys (NIDA, 1991b). This means that compared to previous 35-and-older cohorts, currently middle-aged and older adults do not view drug involvement as being as harmful, and thus as aversive. This further supports the hypothesized trend that with the aging of the baby boomers, drug use is becoming more acceptable and therefore more common among older adults.

Epidemiological research on drug-abusing behaviors has identified factors associated with the initiation of illicit drug use through either cross-sectional or longitudinal studies. These studies implicate biological, genetic, familial, psychological, physiological, and environmental variables with the initiation of illicit drug use. Very few studies have been able to specify factors or processes associated with the maintenance or progression of these behaviors. All of the studies focus on children and youth; few have included young adults or the elderly.

Information about risk factors associated with drug use problems among the elderly is derived from the literature on compliance to medication regimens. Other than demographics such as age and gender (the younger elderly and women being at greater risk for drug problems), marital status, living arrangements, educational status, reading ability, memory capacity, health beliefs and attitudes, and availability of social support systems have been explored in relation to low compliance and drug misuse (Kail & Litwak, 1989; German & Burton, 1989; Hulka, Cassel, Burdette, 1976; Brown & Chiang, 1983–1984). It is known that misuse is much more likely to occur if the older person is taking a psychoactive drug; significantly, drug interactions (particularly including the use of alcohol in combination) are the most common misuse in these cases (Gold-stein, Folkman, & Lazarus, 1989). This study found that misuse increases with the number of drugs taken. Risk factors or predisposition (vulnerability) to use of illicit drugs or pur-

misuse of drugs for psychological effects have not been studied among the elderly.

Epidemiological information that is needed for prevention programming for the elderly should address the following questions:

- What are the nature and common patterns of inappropriate drug use in older people?
- What is the extent of elderly drug-using behaviors, including initiation of drug use and progression to drug abuse and dependence? What role do alcohol and prescribed psychoactive drugs play?
- What are the characteristics of elderly people who misuse and abuse drugs? What markers make these individuals identifiable?
- What are the drug-using trends over time, how do cohorts differ on their attitudes, behaviors, and vulnerabilities, and what impact do the characteristics of older drug users and drug use patterns at any time have on these trends?
- What factors predispose or make an older individual vulnerable to the use of drugs and influence the onset of drug-using behaviors and progression to abuse and dependence?
- What factors can protect the older vulnerable individual from inappropriate drug use?
- What are the social, biomedical, psychological, psychiatric, and economic effects of inappropriate drug-using behaviors?
- How can elderly substance misuse and abuse be detected and diagnosed as easily and as early as possible? What instruments and interview techniques are best suited for these assessments? If no adequate assessments are identified, how can existing instruments be modified for this population?
- Are patterns of substance involvement different for elderly men than for elderly women? Are there differing patterns or special factors that must be taken into account when considering elderly substance misuse and abuse among minorities and special populations?

ALCOHOL USE/ABUSE

More common today and (at least within the last five years) more commonly recognized is alcohol abuse among the elderly. There have been many comprehensive reviews of the literature on the epidemiology of alcohol abuse among the elderly (Gomberg, 1990; Liberto et al, 1992; Glantz & Backenheimer, 1988; Abrams & Alexopoulos, 1991; Smart & Adlaf, 1988). Research suggests that the elderly in general, as well as elderly problem drinkers, consume less alcohol than their younger counterparts. There has been some controversy over whether this phenomenon is limited only to previous elderly cohorts, but it appears that this is not just a cohort effect; alcohol consumption does tend to decrease with age, particularly among heavier drinkers. There is, however, a cohort effect indicating that successive cohorts have fewer abstainers, and there are some indications that the finding of a decrease in alcohol consumption with age may be less the case for younger cohorts. Some decrease in alcohol use with age may be related to the elderly's greater biological sensitivity to the effects of alcohol; they experience more intense reactions and therefore potentially more disruptive behavioral effects. Some of the tapering of use with age may be related to psychological factors. Nevertheless, alcohol problems are probably underrecognized and underreported among the elderly.

Certain elderly subgroups are heavier users of alcohol; for example, elderly men are greater alcohol consumers than women (Schuckit, Morrissey, & O'Leary, 1978). Similarly, certain groups, such as hospitalized and outpatient elderly, have been found to have much higher rates of alcohol abuse than their age peers in the general community; rates may range above 20% (Liberto, Oslin, & Ruskin, 1992). Estimates of alcohol problems in community-dwelling elderly vary enormously. Research reports are inconsistent on the general population rate of elderly alcohol abuse and dependence, although these rates are certainly less than those of younger adults; part of the variation in rates is probably attributable to the variations of the assessments and diagnostic criteria for abuse used in different studies. The Epidemiologic Catchment Area study, using DSM-III diagnostic criteria, found in a combined sample analysis of 4,600 elderly residents of three large cities that the six-month prevalence of alcohol abuse ranged between

1.9% and 4.6% for men and between 0.1% and 0.7% for women (Holzer et al., 1984). Although authoritative, this is probably a somewhat conservative estimate given the survey characteristics, the limited and strict assessment methodology of the study, and the diagnostic criteria, which are only somewhat applicable to the diagnosis of patterns of alcohol involvement in the elderly.

One of the greatest barriers to the timely intervention of elderly drug and alcohol use problems is the difficulty of recognition and correct identification of the problem by physicians, caretakers, family and even the elderly themselves. Several reports substantiate the difficulties involved and the all-too-frequent failures to identify cases of drug dependence (Miller, Whitcup, Sacks, & Lynch, 1985; Whitcup & Miller, 1987), failure to recognize drug abuse within a group of elderly alcoholics (Finlayson, Hurt, Davis, & Morse, 1988), and the problems associated with identifying alcohol inappropriately used in combination with other drugs (Glantz, 1985; Glantz & Backenheimer, 1988).

Behavioral and psychological symptoms that in a younger population would typically lead family members or health professionals to be concerned and possibly to suspect drug or alcohol use problems are often, when an elderly person is the sufferer, attributed to disease or the "normal" concomitants of old age. Additionally, for a variety of reasons, many elderly drinkers conceal their use of alcohol. Because many elderly alcohol abusers are more likely to follow a more low-level drinking pattern (often a higher-frequency "maintenance" drinking pattern), extremes of behavior are less evident and the alcohol problem less detectable. For all of these reasons, many cases of elderly alcohol abuse are not recognized. Also of concern are anecdotal reports of some family and health care providers who suspect an older person of higher levels of drinking but who take no action, believing that old age is so painful and filled with fears and losses that drinking while you "fall apart and wait to die" is reasonable. There are even reports of family members and caretakers encouraging or facilitating drinking among their elderly charges. Lastly, many people will not acknowledge that an elderly person might have an alcohol problem; for a variety of reasons, they do not want to see the problem, so they do not see the evidence of it.

There is good reason to believe that some cases of "senility" are unsuspected drug or alcohol use- or abuse-related problems. There have been many anecdotal reports of this type of misidentification problem and empirical confirmation is beginning to appear in the literature. In a study of 200 outpatients with suspected dementias, 5% suffered dementias due to previously unidentified drug-related problems and toxicities and 4% suffered from alcohol-related dementias (Larson et al., 1985). Even the elderly sufferers themselves may make the same misattribution, assuming that the some of the problems they are experiencing are related to age or infirmity. Some may try to hide the problem as a means of coping and they may even drink more as a means of coping with their anxiety about their dysfunctions.

Patterns of Elderly Problem Drinking Onset and Continuation

Many researchers and clinicians distinguish between different patterns of drinking onset. Glatt and Rosin (1964; see also Rosin & Glatt, 1971) contrasted early-onset elderly drinkers who developed their alcoholism earlier in their lives and continued it into old age with late-onset elderly alcohol abusers who began drinking late in life. Glatt and Rosin believed that early-onset elderly drinkers were more likely to have more characterological psychopathologies and personality dysfunctions than late-onset drinkers who used alcohol as a coping mechanism to adapt to the stresses of old age. This taxonomy has been accepted by many researchers and clinicians and several studies have looked at the prevalence of the two onset patterns (Atkinson, Tolson, & Turner, 1990). It is estimated that of all elderly with alcohol problems, between one-third and one-half developed the problems later in life.

An alternative taxonomy has been proposed by Carruth, Williams, Mysak, and Boudreauz (1975), who described three groups of older problem drinkers. In the first observed pattern, the elderly late-onset drinkers had no history of problem drinking until old age; those in the second pattern, the late-onset exacerbation drinkers, had intermittent alcohol problems until old age, when they developed a more severe or persistent problem; those described by the third pattern, the early-onset drinkers, had a substantial history of alcoholism, which they continued into old age. Gomberg (1980) hypothesized a similar distinction between "reactive problem drinkers," whose problem drinking began late in life, "intermittent problem drinkers," whose periodic intervals of drinking include old age, and "survivors," whose long history of drinking extends into old age.

We believe that the three-category onset classification is more descriptive and useful. Late-onset alcoholism appears to more often be reactive and therefore to have a better prognosis. Although the majority of late-onset alcohol abusers do demonstrate some concomitant anxiety or depression, the affective pathology is often also of more recent origin and therefore more tractable.

Early-onset alcoholism typically seems to involve greater comorbid psychopathology and dysfunction and a much more extensive lack of resources and support. Therefore, it is much more difficult to successfully treat early-onset alcoholism, as psychotherapy requires not only intervention directed at the foci identified for the late-onset drinker but must also deal with the comorbid psychopathology, the other areas of impairment, and the long-compounded history of problems (Blow et al., 1992).

The majority of all alcoholics are probably intermittent drinkers; most have had periods of sobriety and controlled limited drinking, and this is also true for intermittent elderly alcoholics. The importance of distinguishing and identifying these intermittent elderly drinkers lies in their greater vulnerability to use alcohol as a coping mechanism and their much greater vulnerability to rapidly escalate their drinking and relapse once they have reinitiated an old pattern. This group often demonstrates some psychopathology, and is often more fatalistic and difficult to treat that late-onset drinkers, but less so than early onset alcoholics. Both prevention and treatment must be tailored differently for the intermittent drinker than for the late-onset drinker.

The National Institute of Alcohol Abuse and Alcoholism has sharply increased its efforts over the last seven years to increase awareness and assistance for older problem drinkers. However, these efforts have still been relatively limited and the public's awareness of and concern about elderly drinking has not substantially changed. In addition, most physicians and other "gateway" healthcare and service providers are neither sensitized to nor trained in detecting alcohol problems among the elderly; most alcohol abuse treatment professionals have little or no training in treating elderly alcoholics and most treatment facilities do not have programs targeting the elderly. Most prevention efforts continue to be directed toward younger populations.

Obviously, prevention and treatment interventions must be different for elderly individuals, following the different onset patterns. Discussion of some of these issues is included in a later section of this chapter, but must be limited to preventive interventions.

The importance of onset and continuation patterns is not limited to alcohol abuse. This descriptive categorization might be helpful in conceptualizing elderly drug abuse, particularly in the near future as the younger, more drug-involved cohorts age. A taxonomy of late-onset abusers, intermittent users, and survivors seems to be a good classification for the illicit-drug-involved elderly, and the characteristics of these groups identified for elderly alcohol abusers probably also apply to elderly drug abusers. The classification and its implications may also apply to elderly abusers of licit drugs.

LICIT DRUG USE, MISUSE, AND ABUSE

Older adults account for approximately 35% of the use of licit prescriptions and a similar percentage of the use of general over-the-counter

(OTC) medications. Although the elderly's use of licit prescribed and OTC drugs is greatly disproportionate to their numbers, this level is not necessarily inappropriate because the elderly have a disproportionately large number of medical problems. This high level of use may lead to polypharmacy, side effects, and drug interaction problems. Often these are problems of physician-perpetrated misuse, such as suboptimal but unintentional drug prescribing, and they can be ameliorated or at least minimized with care, attention, and the dissemination of timely, accurate information. Elderly patients are sometimes unintentionally noncompliant, which also leads to licit drug use problems. Patient and physician education and patient self-advocacy programs are increasingly supported and available and these efforts can be enormously successful in reducing these unintended iatrogenic problems. Given the obvious and significant benefits of such programs, it is clear that they should be increased. More education-based programs are needed to ensure that prescribing physicians obtain a complete medical and prescription and OTC drug use history and a current comprehensive assessment of function before prescribing additional drugs.

This is especially important as elderly adults are more susceptible to drug interactions, drug side effects, and idiosyncratic drug reactions because of the age-related changes in drug metabolism. Therefore, even greater care in prescribing, monitoring, and management is necessary with the elderly than with most other groups, and this level of care should be a standard. Many serious and even life-threatening misuse problems can be avoided by ensuring that the prescribing physician has a complete and up-to-date medical history for each patient, a complete list of all the prescribed and OTC medications they take, and information about their nutrition, alcohol use, and other lifestyle factors. Patients' drug regimens must be evaluated for side effects and interactions, directions and warnings must be made clear (preferably in easy-to-read printed form), and all of a patient's questions must be answered. Many elderly people prepare lists of questions to ask the physician and have the physician write infor-

mation and instructions, bring a tape recorder, or ask a companion to listen to the information. Ensuring that pharmacological interventions are prescribed by or at least reviewed by physicians specializing in the specific medical problem area can also be very beneficial. Patient self-advocacy, in which elderly patients or their families make sure that the use of any treatment or medication, its intended effects, and its potential side effects and problems are clearly explained and discussed with the patient provides perhaps the greatest benefit. Programs must be initiated to encourage and instruct the elderly to be their own advocates and ensure that drug use regimens are optimally planned and implemented.

Misuse may also be perpetrated by the elderly themselves or by those who care for the elderly. In some cases, the misuse is unintentional, so programs that assist the elderly in becoming knowledgeable about and organizing their medication can be helpful in avoiding these problems. Mechanical aides can be very helpful, such as calendar pill boxes in which the patient loads the compartments of the box according to which pills they take at which times. Several excellent books and programs are available and the elderly and their caretakers should be encouraged to use them. Examples include the *Elder-Ed: Using Your Medications Wisely* program, sponsored by the National Institute on Drug Abuse (1979), and publications such as those by Wolfe and Hope (1993), and Silverstone and Hyman (1982). There are also several health newsletters that include discussions of drug use relevant to the elderly.

A few types of misuse may be perpetrated more knowingly but with no intention for abuse and no awareness of possible harm. Currently, the most common misuse problems among the elderly are likely to be underuse, unintentional failure to follow prescription directions, drug interactions, side effects, inadvertent over- or underuse of PRN medications due to uncertainty about proper use, and inappropriate combination or use with other drugs, foods, or alcohol. Information, education, patient advocacy, and health-care benefit plans that cover medication costs are the remedies for these types of misuse.

Some elderly people perpetrate more active forms of misuse, such as intentionally not taking their medications; modifying their drug regimen on their own; self-medicating with old prescriptions, prescriptions intended for other patients, or OTC drugs; taking alcohol in combination with their drugs; and not providing complete information to their physicians.

When the intent of these modifications is the creation of a psychoactive effect, then drug abuse is occurring. There is no evidence at this time that this form of drug abuse among the elderly is common, although this may change in the future. However, other types of abusive drug problems are currently widespread.

The differentiation of misuse from abuse is not a mere semantic issue. The implications and corrective actions for each are very different. Misuse is inappropriate drug use that is unintentional and not desired by the perpetrator. Misuse is a mistake that the perpetrator would willingly correct if he or she had the appropriate information, resources, and ability. Abuse implies that the inappropriate use is knowingly committed with an intended pharmacological consequence and that the perpetrator would not willingly correct the drug use simply as a result of receiving accurate information (for a more extensive discussion of this issue, see Glantz, 1985).

The elderly comprise one of the few groups that may be involved in drug abuse without being the perpetrators themselves. In cases where the perpetrator is improperly or inappropriately prescribed drugs in a negligent, uninformed, inexpert fashion inconsistent with informed medical standards, then this must be considered abuse. This is particularly true when a psychoactive drug is prescribed. Sufficient geropharmacological information and training is available to healthcare providers that it is no longer reasonable to excuse inappropriate prescribing to the elderly because of a purported lack of drug use information or geropharmacological educational opportunities.

We know that there is considerable general mismedication among the elderly (Kusserow, 1989) and that this may involve common psychoactive drugs (Closser, 1991). Falls, hip fractures, and other accidents have been associated with presumably problematic psychoactive drug prescriptions (Ray et al., 1987; Ray, Griffin, & Downey, 1989; Skegg, Richards, & Doll, 1979). Evidence exists that overdrugging in institutions ("chemical straitjacketing") of the elderly occurs all too often (Beers et al., 1988; Burns & Kamerow, 1988; Buck, 1988). Exacerbated rather than resolved sleep difficulties (Schneider-Helmert, 1988) and cognitive impairments (Larson, Kukull, Buchner, & Reifler, 1987; Scharf, Fletcher, & Graham, 1988; Scharf, Saskin, & Fletcher, 1987) have been reported as other serious consequences of psychoactive drug-prescribing practices for the elderly. Physicians, family members, caretakers, and the elderly must be extremely vigilant in recognizing the possibly problematic sequelae of the use of any drugs, particularly psychoactive drugs. At this time, the greatest drug-abuse-related problem in the elderly is the inappropriate use of prescription psychoactive drugs. Although they are participants and the victims, the elderly are not the primary perpetrators.

Elderly adults currently account for more than 35% of the prescribed psychoactive drugs. This is highly disproportionate in terms of their numbers. However, unlike the situation with general prescribed medications, this disproportionate level is not justifiable on the assumption that the elderly suffer disproportionately from conditions that warrant such medications. In fact, compared with other adult age groups, the ECA study found that the elderly have the same or (in most cases) lower prevalence of all mental disorders, with the exception of organically related cognitive impairments (Myers et al., 1984). Nor can the inappropriately high level of psychoactive drug prescribing be attributed to the hypochondriasis of the elderly, as they have been shown to be less hypochondriacal than younger people. Compounding this finding, research shows that the elderly are more likely to be long-term rather than short-term users of drugs such as anxiolytics (for reviews of the relevant literature, see Glantz & Backenheimer, 1988).

Overuse of prescription psychoactives by the elderly is of particular concern because the elderly experience the most side effects (including mental impairments) and the most adverse drug reactions (including death) of any adult age group. They are also the most vulnerable to drug interactions, idiosyncratic responses, accumulations, and other drug use problems. They are more problematic psychotherapeutic drug treatment candidates than younger adults. Therefore, when an elderly person presents with a mental health problem, careful diagnosis by a gerontologically trained mental health professional should be the first step in determining appropriate treatment. Ironically, the elderly are the least likely group to be diagnosed and treated by mental health professionals and, despite their problematic responses to many psychopharmacological treatments, they are the least likely to receive psychotherapy. Of those elderly who do receive some type of outpatient mental health service, 88.6% are treated in the general medical sector rather than in the mental health sector. General medical sector physicians frequently serve as gatekeepers to the mental health sector. These physicians and the elderly themselves often think of older adults as being inappropriate and unsuccessful psychotherapy candidates. They often think of the elderly's psychological problems as "natural" or expected because of the many losses, stresses, and physical problems associated with old age. Some think that these psychological problems are "just part of getting old."

These stereotypes, as well as common misconceptions about psychotherapy, encourage the belief that the elderly's psychological problems are most appropriately treated by medication. Generally speaking, the psychiatric problems of most elderly adults are treated by healthcare providers who are not experts in psychiatric diagnosis or treatment. It is not surprising that this often leads to inappropriate overuse of psychoactive medications; this must be considered a form of other-perpetrated drug abuse. (For more extensive discussions of this issue and the relevant literature, see Glantz, 1985, and Glantz & Backen-

heimer, 1988). The only current preventive intervention programs addressing any of these problems are information-oriented. As discussed, these are relevant to misuse rather than abuse problems.

The elderly are at least as appropriate and at least as responsive to psychotherapy as any other age group. As an example, cognitive therapy is increasingly being used successfully with a variety of populations, including the elderly. Although some modifications and attention to special issues are necessary, research and experience show that cognitive therapy can be a highly appropriate and a very effective intervention for the elderly suffering from a diverse range of psychiatric problems (Glantz, 1989, 1994).

DEVELOPMENTAL CYCLE

Glantz (1992) presents a comprehensive developmental psychopathology model of drug abuse etiology that is descriptive and explanatory for many patterns of drug abuse that develop before and during adolescence. He points out in his conclusion, "there is the clear implication in this model that effective preventive and early treatment intervention is possible." The focus of the model is on the individual and his or her psychiatric and biobehavioral characteristics and on the interaction of these characteristics with the environment and with interpersonal relationships, societal groups, and institutions such as the family, peers, and schools.

If we extend this model to examine the continuing adult developmental process, particularly focusing on social roles and transitions, and the influence of each developmental phase on subsequent phases, we begin to understand that prevention of drug abuse must be ongoing and multidimensional throughout the lifespan. Not only must prevention and treatment efforts be directed toward the elderly, but they must also be specifically designed to accommodate the characteristics, cohort experiences, and circumstances of the target group. The resulting programs may need to be very different to be effective for different target groups. Currently, our prevention and early intervention programs are targeted to and designed for children and youth. We must extend these at both ends to include infants, preschoolers, young adults, and older populations.

Several promising general models of prevention have evolved to include components that not only affect knowledge and attitudes about drugs but also provide life skills and drug-resistance skills and create or enhance antidrug social norms in the macro- and microcommunities. Although these models are designed to meet the needs of "troubled" youth, they appear to be effective for the general population and could be modified to suit the special needs of both young and older adults. Other prevention models proving to be effective address specific high-risk behaviors such as family dynamics and bonding, academic achievement, and social behaviors. These interventions address some of the psychopathology and social factors mentioned in Glantz's model.

Essential to this developmental approach are validated age-appropriate instruments to identify high-risk individuals as well as specific interventions to prevent problem substance abuse later in life. Prevention and early intervention programs targeting the elderly must consider the aspects specified by Glantz's developmental model as well as its extension, and incorporate them into intervention components. (Discussion of some of the specific factors that must be taken into account when designing intervention programs for the elderly can be found in Glantz, 1989, 1994).

Prevention must become an ongoing effort that targets critical life points. Multiple messages and channels for prevention are needed to saturate communities, groups, and individuals to create a comprehensive antidrug environment and mindset. Some specific prevention actions are also clearly indicated.

PREVENTION RECOMMENDATIONS

Following from the unrealistic but prevalent societal attitudes and beliefs about drinking and drug use in the elderly, it is not surprising that few programs intended to prevent these problems have been developed, disseminated, or supported. Those that have been employed are typically based on the assumption that substance abuse problems in the elderly are limited to medication use and are almost always results of misinformation and (accidental) misuse that are correctable through information dissemination programs and more careful monitoring of medicines. This is not true now, and unless prevention efforts are increased, it is likely to be even less the case over the next several decades.

The issue of inappropriate drug use among the elderly is not a new one. Although concerns about alcohol and drug abuse among the elderly are more recent, concern about the misuse of drugs (one form of inappropriate drug use) has existed for more than 30 years. However, despite these concerns, prevention efforts, even for the more accepted and noncontroversial misuse, have focused on two types of intervention strategies: information dissemination and prescription-monitoring procedures. In these strategies, compliance or adherence to drug regimen are the outcomes of interest. A review of the literature has not produced a favorable assessment of either of these approaches (Levy & Glanz, 1981).

This chapter has emphasized the need to view drug abuse among the elderly from a developmental perspective. Any assessment of the factors associated with these behaviors must include such a perspective. Prevention for the elderly should therefore incorporate "back to the future" strategies, dealing with past developmental experiences within the context of current lifestyle and functioning. Prevention strategies that target children and youth today must establish objectives to prepare them for their own personal futures as adults and seniors in this society. Strategies targeting the elderly must incorporate knowledge regarding beliefs, attitudes, and practices relative to drug-using behaviors from their childhood, youth, and adulthood. In other words, the strategies must be culture-specific. Furthermore, separate strategies must be developed and implemented for misuse as opposed to abuse, for self- versus other-perpetrated misuse and abuse patterns, and for patterns involving illicit versus legal drugs.

Prevention of drug-abusing behaviors is a complex activity and prevention strategies must be sensitive not only to the level of abuse (initial use to dependence) and etiology but also to the developmental and cultural paths of the target group. Despite agreement in the field regarding available information on drug-abusing behaviors among the elderly and the need for effective prevention and early interventions, there is a dearth of research in this area. Given the current focus of American society on youth, research in this area will not be augmented in the immediate future. We fear that until the current drug abusers and potential future abusers now in their 30s and 40s reach their 60s and become burdens on the healthcare system, such research will not receive the support it needs. For other types of health problems, the prevention emphasis has been on the healthcare providers and on personal beliefs, attitudes, and knowledge regarding the problem of interest. The premise of this approach is to make the healthcare provider aware of the problem, enable diagnosis and assessment of the problem, and teach the requisite skills needed to recognize and treat the problem through appropriate medication, monitoring, proper referral, and, when appropriate, counseling or psychotherapy. This is a beginning, but prevention efforts must also focus on the individual or group at risk. This is particularly true when healthcare providers have been involved as perpetrators of misuse and abuse.

Available models that explain health behavior are in their infancy. Social learning, skills development, the health belief model, cognitive theory, and the theory of reasoned action have not been well tested in older populations. These models must be modified to incorporate the complexities of physical, psychological, and social aging. This approach is particularly important when the target behavior is drug abuse.

Certainly, given the state of drug abuse prevention in the United States, the field is moving in the direction of more theory-based and more comprehensive approaches. This movement currently focuses on youth, including multiple-problem youth, but has failed to address issues of aging, even into early adulthood. If we wait until substance abuse is common among the elderly, prevention efforts will undoubtedly be too little and too late.

RECOMMENDATIONS FOR AN OPTIMAL PREVENTION STRATEGY

We have identified potential etiologies and models for substance abuse behaviors and suggested intervention points and strategies to prevent these problem behaviors. These can be depicted in the paradigm shown in Table 20.1.

Following are some general considerations and recommendations and some more specific ideas for implementation.

Effective prevention of substance abuse problems among the elderly requires action, resources, and changes in societal attitudes and behaviors, not merely corrective or educational information. An important first step is a national initiative to correct the inaccurate stereotypes and widespread discriminatory and denigrating attitudes toward the elderly. This includes the general societal reconceptualization of the problems of the elderly as not necessarily being medical or having primarily medical or pharmacological solutions; a "pill for every problem" orientation creates more problems than it solves.

Although the elderly have had at least some success in advocating for themselves as a group, they often do not advocate for and protect themselves as individuals. This is particularly true in the case of medical psychiatric and psychological problems and issues of quality of life. There is a need to support institutional and organizational advocacy for the elderly and to encourage and support the elderly (and their families) to be assertive in seeking the best possible quality of life and to be active in understanding and obtaining the assistance and interventions they need. This includes defining a good quality of life for the elderly as involving not only financial and

TABLE 20.1   Intervention Strategies

ETIOLOGY	INTERVENTION STRATEGIES
Misinformation	Develop elderly-specific drug use standards and use guides for wide dissemination to professionals, with particular attention to psychoactive drugs and drugs with psychoactive side effects.
	Direct patient education and drug use monitoring provided by prescribing physicians and other health-care professionals; printed "elderly user friendly" drug use guides provided by prescribing or pharmacy.
	Indirect education through user-friendly drug packaging information inserts, mass media, and brochures.
	Mass-media patient education to develop self-advocacy and self- and familial responsibility for drug prescription and use. Indirect tracking of potential problems through pharmacy monitoring.
Iatrogenic	Develop elderly-specific drug use standards and prescription guides for wide dissemination, with particular attention to psychoactive drugs and drugs with psychoactive side effects. Develop elderly-specific suspicion and detection protocols and guides for the early detection of inappropriate or problematic drug use; detection facilitation materials for drug interactions, side effects, and toxicities should be included.
	Provider education in appropriate prescription of drugs for elderly, detection and diagnosis of substance use problems, referral for dependency treatment, and methods to provide medication information to patients.
	Monitoring of prescribing patterns of health providers. Increased monitoring of prescribing patterns in care and custodial facilities.
	Strict enforcement of prescribing standards.

(continued)

medical well-being but also the personal and interpersonal qualities of life and experience expected by younger adults.

To assist the elderly in advocating for themselves, readily usable programs and guidelines must be developed and widely disseminated. General guidelines discussing how to be an active advocate for one's own care as well as more specific guidelines discussing norms and problems and reviewing and recommending interventions, including considerations of possible problems, are necessary. These more specific guidelines might cover such topics as psychoactive drug use, drug side effects and interactions, psy-

TABLE 20.1 Intervention Strategies *continued*

ETIOLOGY	INTERVENTION STRATEGIES
Psychopathology	Provide education in diagnosis and referral as well as appropriate pharmacological and psychotherapeutic treatment of elderly.
	Public and provider education to inform about effectiveness and appropriateness of psychotherapy and other non-pharmacological interventions.
	Caretaker education in detection and help-seeking procedures.
	Increase number of trained geropsychologists, geropsychiatrists, and other geriatrically trained mental healthcare providers; increase availability of geriatric mental health diagnosis and treatment services and access and financial support for services.
Physical and psychological dependence	Provider and caretaker education in detection, diagnosis, and help-seeking and referral procedures
	Expansion of treatment of elderly alcohol abuse as elderly drug abuse is likely to increasingly include patterns in which alcohol is abused in combination with other drugs.
	Develop elderly-specific protocols for treatment of drug abuse and dependence.
	Develop and disseminate elderly-oriented services and programs for the treatment of drug abuse and dependence.

chotherapy, sleep and sleep-related problems, depression, anxiety, intellect and memory functioning, and chronic and episodic pain management. The creation and dissemination of such materials will probably require the collaboration of government agencies with national and local elderly advocacy and consumer groups. Media campaigns could also play an important role. Most of the few existing programs and publications must be updated and expanded.

It would also be helpful if self-administrable and scorable assessments for the identification of drug or alcohol problems, including misuse and abuse, were developed for and disseminated to the elderly. A simple symptom checklist, followed by a discussion of the checklist's possible indications and the appropriate actions to take, would probably be accepted and used. Perhaps more than any other age group, the elderly are likely to use and be responsive to such warning or suspicion indices. Warning signs indices and advocacy programs for family members of elderly people would also be helpful. As part of routine medical and psychiatric history taking, healthcare professionals should inquire about lifetime histories of drug and alcohol use to identify intermittent abusers who may reinitiate substance abuse. If a patient is identified as a potential intermittent abuser, increased attention to the possible signs of current substance abuse are called for and prescriptions of abusable drugs must be made more conservatively and with greater monitoring.

In addition to the interventions involving healthcare professionals described above, more elderly-specific substance abuse training and continuing education for treatment and diagnosis should be required of professionals who provide services for older adults. Programs that support drug development should be required to assess medications for effects on older adults and efforts should be made to identify and develop drugs and use regimens that are optimally suited for the elderly. Standardized computer pharmacy databases linked by networks across all pharmacies in an area and containing registers of prescription drug use should be developed and their information made available to patients, who can easily arrange for comprehensive printouts to be sent to their physicians or themselves. This would greatly facilitate the identification of many misuse and some abuse problems. Education programs and guidelines should be developed and widely disseminated to encourage healthcare professionals to not provide services outside of their specialties and to encourage the elderly to seek psychological, psychiatric, and psychopharmacological diagnosis and treatment only from professionals with expertise and credentials in these specialty areas.

Better support for the treatment of psychiatric conditions comorbid to elderly substance abuse is necessary. Relatedly, early-onset drug and alcohol abuse survivors should not be ignored or written off regardless of their resistance to treatment or the seeming intractability of their problems. Programs should be developed and attempts should be made to help these long-term abusers. Considerable practical and financial support may also be needed.

Lastly, it is important to reiterate that the baby boomer cohort, now in its 30s and 40s, is aging. There is every indication that this cohort will be at risk for substance abuse in their elder years. Although the exact forms of abuse and the involved substances cannot be predicted at this time, this cohort's vulnerability to abuse is known. Using the principles and ideas described above, programs must be developed now to prevent the future substance abuse in this group. In addition, law enforcement agencies must be prepared to attend to the elderly as a potential market in the future for illegal drugs.

REFERENCES

Abrams, R., & Alexopoulos, G. (1991). Geriatric addictions. In R. Frances & S. Miller (Eds.), *Clinical textbook of affective disorders.* New York: Guilford Press.

Atkinson, R., Tolson, R., & Turner, J. (1990). Late versus early onset problem drinking in older men. *Alcoholism: Clinical and Experimental Research, 14,* 574–579.

Bachman, J., Johnston, L., O'Malley, P., & Humphrey, R. (1988). Explaining the recent decline in marijuana use: Differentiating the effects of perceived risks, disapproval, and general lifestyle factors. *Journal of Health and Social Behavior, 29,* 92–112.

Beers, M., Avorn, J., Soumerai, S., Everitt, D., Sherman, D., & Salem, S. (1988). Psychoactive medication use in intermediate-care facility residents. *Journal of the American Medical Association, 260,* 3016–3054.

Bernstein, L., Folkman, S., & Lazarus, R. (1989). Characterization of the use and misuse of medications by an elderly, ambulatory population. *Medical Care, 27,* 654–663.

Blow, F., Cook, C., Booth, B., Falcon, S., & Friedman, M. (1992). Age-related psychiatric comorbidities and level of functioning in alcoholic veterans seeking outpatient treatment. *Hospital and Community Psychiatry, 43,* 990–995.

Brown, B. B., & Chiang, C. (1983–84). Drug and alcohol abuse among the elderly: Is being alone the key? *International Journal of Aging and Human Development, 18* (1), 1–12.

Buck, J. (1988). Psychotropic drug practice in nursing homes. *Journal of the American Geriatric Society, 36,* 409–418.

Burns, B., & Kamerow, D. (1988). Psychotropic drug prescriptions for nursing home residents. *Journal of Family Practice, 26,* 155–160.

Carruth, B., Williams, E., Mysak, P., & Boudreauz, L. (1975). Community care providers and older problem drinkers. *Grassroots* (July supplement), 1–5.

Closser, M. (1991). Benzodiazepines and the elderly: A review of potential problems. *Journal of Substance Abuse Treatment, 8,* 35–41.

Finlayson, R., Hurt, R., Davis, L., & Morse, R. (1988). Alcoholism in elderly persons: A study of the psychiatric and psychosocial features of 216 inpatients. *Mayo Clinic Proceedings, 63,* 761–768.

German, P., & Burton, L. C. (1989). Clinicians, the elderly and drugs. *Journal of Drug Issues, 19* (2), 221–243.

Glantz, M. D. (1981). The prediction of elderly drug abuse. *Journal of Psychoactive Drugs, 13,* 117–126. Reprinted in D. Petersen & F. Whittington (Eds.), *Drugs, alcohol, and aging.* Dubuque, IA: Kendall Hunt Publishing, 1982.

Glantz, M. D. (1985). The detection, identification and differentiation of elderly drug misuse and abuse in a research survey. In E. Gottheil, K. Druley, T. Skoloda, & H. Waxman (Eds.), *Alcohol, drug abuse and the aging.* Springfield, IL: Charles Thomas.

Glantz, M. D. (1989). Cognitive therapy with the elderly. In A. Freeman, K. Simon, L. Beutler, & H. Arkowitz (Eds.), *A comprehensive handbook of cognitive therapy.* New York: Plenum.

Glantz, M. D. (1992). A developmental psychopathology model of drug abuse vulnerability. In M. Glantz & R. Pickens, (Eds.), *Vulnerability to drug abuse.* Washington, DC: American Psychological Association.

Glantz, M. D. (1994). Cognitive therapy with elderly alcoholics. In T. Beresford & E. Gomberg (Eds.), *Alcohol and aging.* New York: Oxford University Press.

Glantz, M. D., & Backenheimer, M. (1988). Substance abuse among elderly women. *Clinical Gerontologist, 8,* 3–26.

Glatt, M., & Rosin, A. (1964). Aspects of alcoholism in the elderly. *Lancet, 2,* 472–473.

Gomberg, E. (1990). Drugs, alcohol, and aging. In L. T. Kozlowski et al. (Eds.), *Research advances in alcohol and drug problems,* vol. 10. New York: Plenum, pp. 171–213.

Holzer, C., Robins, L., Myers, J., Weissman, M., Tischler, G., Leaf, P., Anthony, J., & Bednarski, P. (1984). Antecedents and correlates of alcohol abuse and dependence in the elderly. In G. Maddox, L. Robins, & N. Rosenberg (Eds.), *Nature and extent of alcohol problems among the elderly.* Washington, DC: National Institute on Alcohol Abuse and Alcoholism, USGPO.

Hulka, B., Cassel, L. K., & Burdette, J. (1976). Communication, compliance and concordance between physicians and patients with prescribed medications. *American Journal of Public Health, 66* (9), 847–853.

Kail, B., & Litwak, E. (1989). Family, friends and neighbors: The role of primary groups in preventing the misuse of drugs. *Journal of Drug Issues, 19* (2), 261–281.

Kusserow, R. (1989). *Medicare drug utilization review.* Washington, DC: Office of the Inspector General, Department of Health and Human Services.

Larson, E., Kukull, W., Buchner, D., & Reifler, B. (1987). Adverse drug reactions associated with global cognitive impairment in elderly persons. *Annals of Internal Medicine, 107,* 169–173.

Larson, E., Reifler, B., Sumi, S. Canfield, C. & Chinn, N. (1985). Diagnostic evaluation of 200 elderly outpatients with suspected dementia. *Journal of Gerontology, 40* (5), 536–543.

Levy, M. R., & Glanz, K. (1981). Drug misuse among the elderly: An educational challenge for health professionals. *Journal of Drug Education, 11* (1), 61–75.

Liberto, J., Oslin, D., & Ruskin, P. (1992). Alcoholism in older persons: A review of the literature. *Hospital and Community Psychiatry, 43,* 975–984.

Maddox, G., Robins, L., & Rosenberg, N. (Eds.) (1984). *Nature and extent of alcohol problems among the elderly.* Washington, DC: National Institute on Alcohol Abuse and Alcoholism, USGPO.

Miller, F., Whitcup, S., Sacks, M., & Lynch, P. (1985). Unrecognized drug dependence and withdrawal in the elderly. *Drug and Alcohol Dependence, 15,* 177–179.

Myers, J., Weissman, M., Tischer, G., Holzer, C., Leaf, P., Orvaschel, H., Anthony, J., Boyd, J., Burke, J., Kramer, M., & Stoltzman, R. (1984). Six-month prevalence of psychiatric disorders in three communities; 1980–1982. *Archives of General Psychiatry, 41,* 959–967.

National Institute on Drug Abuse (1979). *Elder ed: Using your medications wisely: A guide for the elderly.* Washington, DC: DHHS Publication no. (ADM) 82-705.

National Institute on Drug Abuse (1991a). *The National Household Survey on Drug Abuse: Main findings, 1990.* Washington, DC: DHHS Publication no. (ADM) 91-1788.

National Institute on Drug Abuse (1991b). *The National Household Survey on Drug Abuse: Preliminary findings.* DHHS Publication press release, December.

Ray, W., Griffin, M., & Downey, W. (1989). Benzodiazepines of long and short elimination half-life and the risk of hip fracture. *Journal of the American Medical Association, 262,* 3303–3307.

Ray, W., Griffin, M., Schaffner, W., Baugh, D., & Melton, L. (1987). Psychotropic drug use and the risk of hip fracture. *New England Journal of Medicine, 316,* 363–369.

Rosin, A., & Glatt, M. (1971). Alcohol excess in the elderly. *Quarterly Journal of Studies on Alcohol, 32,* 53–59.

Scharf, M., Fletcher, K., & Graham, J. (1988). Comparative amnestic effects of benzodiazepine hypnotic agents. *Journal of Clinical Psychiatry, 49,* 134–137.

Scharf, M., Saskin, P., & Fletcher, K. (1987). Benzodiazepine-induced amnesia: Clinical and laboratory findings. *Journal of Clinical Psychiatry Monographs, 5,* 14–17.

Schneider-Helmert, D. (1988). Why low-dose benzodiazepine-dependence insomniacs can't escape their sleeping pills. *Acta Psychiatrica Scandinavica, 78,* 706–711.

Schuckit, M. A., Morrissey, E. M., & O'Leary, M. R. (1978). Alcohol problems in elderly men and women. *Addictive Diseases, 3,* 405–416.

Silverstone, B., & Hyman, H. (1982). *You and your aging parent: A guide to understanding emotional, physical, and financial needs.* Mount Vernon, NY: Consumers Union.

Skegg, D., Richards, S., & Doll, R. (1979). Minor tranquilizers and road accidents. *British Medical Journal, 1,* 917–919.

Smart, R., & Adlaf, E. (1988). Alcohol and drug use among the elderly: Trends in use and characteristics of users. *Canadian Journal of Public Health, 79,* 236–242.

Substance Abuse and Mental Health Services Administration, Office of Applied Studies (1993a). *Estimates from the Drug Abuse Warning Network; 1992 estimates of drug-related emergency room episodes. Advance report #4.* Rockville, MD: Department of Health and Human Services.

Substance Abuse and Mental Health Services Administration, Office of Applied Studies (1993b). *Preliminary estimates from the 1992 National Household Survey on Drug Abuse. Advance report #3.* Rockville, MD: Department of Health and Human Services.

U.S. Senate Special Committee on Aging, American Association of Retired Persons, Federal Council on Aging, & U.S. Administration on Aging (1991). *Aging America: Trends and projections, 1991 edition.* Washington, DC: DHHS Publication no. (FCoA) 91-28001.

Whitcup, S., & Miller, F. (1987). Unrecognized drug dependence in psychiatrically hospitalized elderly patients. *Journal of the American Geriatric Society, 35,* 297–301.

Wolfe, S., & Hope, R. (1993). *Worst pills, best pills II: The older adults' guide to avoiding drug-induced death or illness; second edition.* Washington, DC: Public Citizen Health Research Group.

CHAPTER 21

PSYCHIATRIC PATIENTS

DOUGLAS M. ZIEDONIS

Substance abuse prevention strategies must target high-risk groups; both children and adults with preexisting psychiatric disorders are at clear risk for developing substance abuse problems. Substance abuse is common among psychiatric patients and complicates the presentation, course, and treatment.

This chapter addresses the unique tasks of primary prevention of a secondary disorder (the psychiatric disorder occurred first and is the primary disorder) and the use of prevention efforts within a treatment setting. The wide variety of psychiatric disorders, settings, and age groups forces prevention efforts for this population to be individualized to match the unique needs of each subtype. Children and adolescents can develop unique psychiatric disorders that put them at especially high risk for future substance abuse. Prevention efforts targeted at adults must consider the unique aspects of different disorders and the mental health system. Although substance abuse disorders are classified as psychiatric disorders, there has been a historical split dividing substance abuse and other psychiatric services and research. Although mental health clinicians are experienced at secondary and tertiary prevention strategies for psychiatric illness, they have only recently recognized the importance of substance abuse prevention and treatment. On a hopeful note, important changes are beginning to occur in mental health settings because of the increased awareness of dual-diagnosis patients (those with both a psychiatric and a substance use disorder).

This chapter reviews the epidemiology of substance abuse among psychiatric patients, including prevalence rates and possible etiological considerations. Specific child and adult psychiatric disorders are reviewed for common presentation, comorbidity rates, causality issues, impact on course, and prevention implications. A review of the mental health system precedes general systems and policy recommendations. The chapter concludes with specific recommendations for primary, secondary, and tertiary substance abuse prevention among psychiatric patients.

DUAL DIAGNOSIS RATES AND RISK FACTORS FOR SUBSTANCE ABUSE

Psychiatric disorders and substance use disorders are common in the general population, as determined by the National Institute of Mental Health's (NIMH's) Epidemiological Catchment Area (ECA) Study (Robins & Regier, 1991). This study, performed in the early 1980s, estimated that 22.5% of the population has met criteria for a psychiatric disorder during their lifetime (lifetime rate) and 13% currently meet criteria for a psychiatric disorder (current rates). The careful reader will note whether reports specify lifetime or current rates of disorders. There are more than 200 psychiatric diagnoses in the *Diagnostic and Statistical Manual of Mental Disorders, Fourth Edition (DSM-IV),* which provides the accepted diagnostic classification system for psychiatric disorders in the United States (American Psychiatric Association, 1994). Psychiatric disorders encompass wide ranges of impairment, severity, and chronicity.

The ECA study also found that 16.7% of the population have a lifetime substance use disorder and 3.8% have a current substance use disorder (Regier et al., 1990). This study also found that substance use disorders are very common among psychiatric patients, with 29% having a lifetime substance use disorder and 20% having a current substance use disorder (Regier et al., 1990). The most common psychiatric disorders associated with substance use disorders are depression, anxiety, schizophrenia, and antisocial personality disorders. The rates of substance use disorders are significantly higher among psychiatric patients than among the general population. Researchers analyzing the ECA study asserted that "these data provide clear and persuasive evidence that mental disorders must be addressed as a central part of substance abuse prevention efforts in this country" (Regier et al., 1990, p. 2517).

Another recent study, The National Comorbidity Survey (NCS), was specifically mandated by the U.S. Congress to assess the comorbidity of substance use disorders and nonsubstance psychiatric disorders (Kessler et al., 1994). Between September 1990 and February 1992, 8,098 people were interviewed to assess rates and risk factors for substance use and other psychiatric disorders. This study used the Composite International Diagnostic Interview (CIDI) instrument to determine DSM-III-R diagnoses. Risk factors evaluated included family history of psychiatric disorders, adverse childhood experiences, social networks and support, and stressful life events. This study found that the prevalence of psychiatric disorders was even greater than the results of the ECA study, which had taken place ten years before. The NCS found that 48% of the population had a psychiatric disorder in their lifetime and 26% a substance use disorder. Of note, 14% of the population had three or more comorbid disorders, which accounted for 50% of the number of diagnoses. This high comorbidity is far more concentrated than had been known previously.[1]

Individuals with both a substance use and psychiatric disorder have been labeled dual-diagnosis patients. Dual-diagnosis patients may present with a variety of combinations of psychiatric and substance abuse disorders (such as schizophrenic cocaine abusers or depressed alcoholics). The primary disorder is the disorder that occurred first; however, the nature of the relationship between psychopathology and substance abuse is more complex. Individuals with a substance use disorder can also develop psychiatric symptoms or a psychiatric disorder from chronic drug abuse. Meyer believes that individuals who abuse drugs eventually connect their drug use behaviors with their psychiatric symptoms in a way that becomes meaningful to them (Meyer, 1986).

RISK FACTORS

Both substance abuse and other psychiatric disorders are complex behavioral disorders with uncertain etiologies that are influenced by many biological, psychological, and social factors. The stress/vulnerability model suggests that biological and genetic vulnerabilities can be intensified by psychosocial stress or reduced by psychosocial protective factors.

BIOLOGICAL FACTORS

A number of interesting biological hypotheses have been made based on linking brain changes that are found in a psychiatric disorder with similar brain changes caused by a specific drug. An example is the recent biological explanation for high rates of nicotine addiction among individuals with schizophrenia. These disorders may be linked through a common specific brain chemical (dopamine) that is important for both schizophrenia and addictive disorders. Nicotine can both directly and indirectly influence the release of dopamine in specific brain regions that are less active in individuals with schizophrenia. Therefore, nicotine may be especially reinforcing in individuals with schizophrenia through the combined mechanism of stimulating the brain reward center and correcting the defective brain functioning. The neurobiological vulnerability caused by a psychiatric disorder may account for the fact that psychiatric patients often have greater drug withdrawal symptoms than do nonpsychiatric patients. Increased symptoms are associated with lower likelihood of achieving drug abstinence and an increased likelihood of progressing from substance use to abuse. Several studies have shown that nicotine withdrawal can provoke depression in those with a history of depression, and that those with a history of anxiety or depression are less likely to succeed in smoking cessation (Glassman, 1993). Cocaine abusers with major depression also appear to have a more severe withdrawal syndrome than those without depression (Gawin & Kleber, 1986). Also, the route of administration and the frequency of use of specific drug types may result in different drug abuse susceptibilities for individuals with different psychiatric disorders.

Genetic predisposition may be an important factor in substance abuse comorbidity among psychiatric patients. A review of family history data reveals a strong familial relationship between alcohol dependence and both anxiety and depressive disorders (Schuckit, 1986; Merikangas, Leckman, et al., 1985). Also, family history accounts for an increased association between heroin dependence and depression disorders (Rounsaville, Kosten, et al., 1991; Mirin, Weiss, & Michael, 1986). Individuals with schizoaffective disorder (who have prominent symptoms of both schizophrenia and mood disorders) are likely to pass on to their children a genetic vulnerability to both disorders (Coryell & Zimmerman, 1987). Individuals with schizophrenia and an addiction disorder (perhaps a "schizoaddictive" disorder) appear to pass on a genetic vulnerability (Ziedonis & Fisher, 1994). A study of twins found that genetic factors contribute to the expression of alcohol abuse in schizophrenia (Kendler, 1985). Gender differences may be important in understanding the relationship between substance abuse and other psychiatric disorders (Weiss, 1991; Ziedonis, Rayford, Bryant, & Rounsaville, 1994). For example, women tend to develop psychiatric disorders before alcohol dependence, whereas men often develop alcohol dependence before psychiatric disorders (Hesselbrock, 1986).

Two biological theories have suggested that substance abuse can precipitate a psychiatric disorder: the brain poison theory and the kindling theory (Westermeyer, 1992). The brain poison theory suggests that specific types of drugs can cause a psychiatric disorder in individuals who do not have a genetic vulnerability or predisposition for a psychiatric disorder. For example, Andreasson studied a large Swedish data set and found higher rates of a history of cannabis use in patients who later developed schizophrenia (Andreasson, Allebeck, Engstrom, & Rydberg, 1987). The kindling theory links the brain poison and genetic vulnerability theories and suggests that exposure to a specific type of drug will precipitate a psychiatric disorder in individuals with a genetic vulnerability. Some epidemiological and family studies on the role of drugs that can induce psychotic symptoms (stimulants, hallucinogens, cannabis, and PCP) in genetically vulnerable individuals tend to support this theory (Westermeyer, 1992; Abraham, 1986).

PSYCHOLOGICAL FACTORS

In addition to biological factors, psychosocial factors may have an important etiological role in the development of substance abuse among psychiatric patients. In the context of genetic vulnerability, children who live with their mentally ill parents (including substance abusers) often undergo severe environmental stressors and psychological experiences that affect their development. The unpredictable behaviors and poor parenting skills of their parents can provoke anxiety and depression and result in neglect, missed opportunities for healthy growth, and increased efforts to bond with negative peer groups. These children are often victims of domestic violence. All these problems increase the odds of developing a substance abuse problem among children of the mentally ill. However, despite these risks, many of these children do not develop substance abuse disorders and appear to build coping skills or connect with positive forces that protect them from a negative environment. These resiliency factors are being studied in children of alcoholics and drug addicts, and further study may provide clues in learning about the causes of substance abuse and in designing prevention programs (Rutter, 1985; Wolin & Bennett, 1984).

Psychiatric patients may discover that specific types of drugs are reinforcing because of their ability to reduce psychiatric symptoms (Weiss, 1991). The self-medication theory (Khantzian, 1985) suggests that patients may self-medicate with alcohol or other drugs in an attempt to reduce or eliminate persistent psychiatric symptoms or even the side effects of their medications.

Some psychiatric patients with prolonged mental illness may actually prefer the label of being an alcoholic or drug addict to that of being mentally ill. In addition to a new identity, some are attracted to a drug-abusing subculture that acquaints them with a new peer group that appears to have clear behavioral expectations and norms (Weiss, 1991). Although both disorders are stigmatized, many famous individuals have admitted their substance abuse problem in an attempt to show others that this illness is treatable and preventable.

SOCIAL FACTORS

Social factors influence the high rates of substance abuse among psychiatric patients. Alcohol and other drugs are perceived as a mechanism to improve social interactions and decrease social alienation (Drake et al., 1991; Lieberman & Bowers, 1990).

The symptoms of a psychiatric disorder often counteract the positive influence of social factors such as marriage, family, work, and community that oppose the development of substance abuse. In fact, many individuals with prolonged mental illness are often unable to maintain a positive relationship in any of these social areas.

As a social factor, the mental health system may have either a positive or negative influence on patients. By designing substance abuse prevention programs within mental health settings, the system is taking the first step toward sending a clear antidrug message to patients. Unfortunately, the system has also sent mixed messages. For example, psychiatric treatment programs have a long history of permissiveness about and perpetuation of nicotine addiction. Not only is nicotine an addictive drug, it is often a gateway drug to other types of substance abuse. Mental health staff have not been given the clear message that substance abuse among psychiatric patients is their responsibility, and this leads to a neglect of substance abuse and its separation from all other aspects of psychiatric care.

Substance abuse among psychiatric patients increased with deinstitutionalization (when long-term psychiatric patients were discharged from state hospitals to community residential and treatment programs). Also, deinstitutionalization began in the 1960s, when a dramatic increase in entitlements and permissiveness toward drug experimentation also took place. Unfortunately, community programs were unprepared for deinstitutionalization and had severe funding and staff limitations. Once in the community, patients suddenly were not supervised and were unprepared to plan their own recreational activities. Entitlement programs provided patients with the resources to purchase alcohol and other drugs.

CHILD PSYCHIATRIC DISORDERS

Specific child psychiatric disorders are linked with the later development of substance abuse, including conduct, attention deficit, learning, and depressive disorders. Children with these disorders often have several childhood psychiatric disorders.

Conduct disorder is common among children. About 5% of school age children have the disorder, and it is four times as common among males as among females (Kaplan & Sadock, 1985). Conduct disorder is a pattern of disruptive behavior that lasts more than six months and includes antisocial activities that go beyond simple pranks. For example, these children repeatedly run away from home, lie, set fires, are cruel to animals and other people, are truant from school, or deliberately steal from others (American Psychiatric Association, 1994). These symptoms tend to alienate them from positive social forces, such as family and school, that oppose drug abuse. Children with severe conduct disorder often develop substance abuse and antisocial personality disorders (Robins, 1966; Robins & Price, 1991).

Attention deficit disorder (ADD) accounts for one-third to one-half of child psychiatry outpatients. The core of symptoms in ADD is the triad of impulsiveness, hyperactivity, and poor attention span. The incidence of ADD is estimated at about 5% to 10% percent of grade school children, with boys at three to four times the risk as girls. Parents of children with ADD have a high incidence of antisocial personality, depression, alcoholism, and their own history of attention deficit disorder (Beiderman et al., 1986).

Many children with ADD are also aggressive and defiant. Symptoms may interfere with developing important relationships within the family, school, and community, social forces that reduce the likelihood of drug involvement. These children often have subtle neurological impairments and may also meet criteria for conduct and mood disorders. Studies have linked ADD and later development of substance abuse (Mannuzza et al., 1991; Cantwell, 1988).

ADD can continue into adulthood and has features similar to personality disorders, including increased distractibility, impulsiveness, restlessness, and quick temper (Gittelman, Mannuzza, Shenker, & Bonagura, 1985). Several researchers have noted an association between ADD and cocaine addiction (Khantzian, Gawin, Riordan, & Kleber, 1984; Rounsaville, Anton, et al., 1991). They have speculated that adults with residual ADD take cocaine as a way to self-medicate and that the use of medications that treat childhood ADD may also help these adults. In a study of 299 treatment-seeking cocaine addicts, childhood conduct disorder was diagnosed in 54% of the male cocaine addicts and 47% of the female addicts, and ADD was diagnosed in 39% of males and 25% of females (Ziedonis, Rayford, Bryant, & Rounsaville, 1994). Alcoholics have also been subtyped according to a history of inattention, hyperactivity, and impulsiveness (Tarter, McBride, Baumpane, & Schelde, 1977).

Learning disorders also appear to be linked with substance abuse (Rutter, Tizard, & Whitmore, 1970). About 5% to 10% of children have a learning disorder, categorized according to the specific area of development affected, including problems with arithmetic, expressive writing, reading, articulation, language, and coordination. A diagnosis is made when the child has poor skills in a specific category and the performance level is markedly below intellectual capacity. Poor school performance may be linked to a demoralization syndrome of low self-esteem and acting out by children with a conduct disorder, learning disorder, or ADD. Impaired cognition may be an important risk factor for substance abuse (Tarter et al., 1984; Ervin, Little, Streissguth, & Beck, 1984).

Childhood depressive disorders occur in about 2% of children and 5% of adolescents. Unlike among adults, where women are twice as likely to have a depressive disorder than men, depression is more common among boys during childhood and equally common by gender during adolescence. A major depressive episode is manifested by specific symptoms that occur most of the day and nearly every day. The symptoms include depressed mood, decreased interests in doing things, psychomotor agitation or retardation, fatigue, feelings of worthlessness, and difficulty concentrating (American Psychiatric Association, 1994). About 20% of depressed children also have a conduct disorder, and this combination often predicts alcohol dependence and depression in adulthood (Harrington et al., 1991; Deykin, Levy, & Wells, 1987).

Among depressed adolescents, suicidal ideation and behavior are often associated with the use of alcohol and other drugs (Crumley, 1990). The typical adolescent at risk for suicide is a white male who is intoxicated and has access to a firearm. Suicide is associated with stressful precipitating events and underlying psychiatric disorders such as depression and conduct and personality disorders. Suicide is a leading cause of death among adolescents and young adults, with the incidence rate peaking at age 23 (Hollinger, 1987). Unfortunately, adolescents who abuse substances and attempt suicide are more likely to complete .suicide than those who do not abuse substances (Kaminer, 1992). The relationship between suicide, aggression, and alcohol abuse has been explored in genetic and neurochemical research that differentiates types of alcoholics (Cloninger, Reich, & Witzel, 1979). Preventing teenage suicide is a critical area for treatment and research initiatives, and substance abuse prevention efforts could have an important role in such efforts (Shaffer et al., 1988).

CHILDHOOD TRAITS OF AGGRESSION AND SHYNESS

Specific personality traits found in child psychiatric disorders have been linked to later substance abuse, including impulsiveness, aggression, shyness, social nonconformity, and novelty seeking (Tarter, Alterman, & Edwards, 1985; Kellam, Brown, Rubin, & Ensminger, 1983). Kellam and associates are conducting two prospective longitudinal studies of children that may help us better understand the causal link between child psychiatric disorders and later substance abuse and may suggest an effective prevention program for children with psychiatric disorders. These studies found that concurrent aggression and shyness in first grade predicted later substance abuse.

The first study, the Woodlawn Longitudinal Study in Chicago, closely evaluated 1,242 first graders and their parents, teachers, and peers, and then reevaluated these individuals 10 years later (1975–1976) and 25 years later (1992–1993). At the 10-year follow-up, 705 children were reeval-

uated and significant differences were found according to gender and behavioral traits. For males, first grade learning problems predicted teenage psychiatric symptoms and aggression predicted later substance use. Shyness appeared to inhibit later drug use, and none of these associations was significant for women. However, concurrent shyness and aggressiveness was associated with the highest likelihood of later substance abuse for both genders. Males and females who reported a positive connection to school were the least likely to be involved with substances at follow-up. Strong peer bonding increased drug abuse for males, and family bonding decreased drug abuse for females (Kellam et al., 1991; Kellam & Rebok, 1992).

Twenty-five years later, 950 of the original children were reevaluated as adults, and adult cocaine use was twice as common among those who had concurrent aggression and shyness during first grade (17%) compared to individuals with either shyness or aggression alone (about 10%). Analysis of the data links concurrent shyness and aggression in first grade with negative engagement in school in adolescence (low bonding), and the low school bonding is important in predicting later drug use (Ensminger & Slusarcick, 1992).

The second study by Kellam and associates, the Baltimore School District Study, attempted to see whether aggression and shyness among children could be changed and affect the outcome of later substance abuse (Kellam, Rebok, Ialongo, & Mayer, 1994). In this intervention study, children were randomly assigned to different classrooms in which half the children played a "good behavior game" on a regular basis and the other children did not. In the game, children in the classroom were assigned to one of three teams. Teams were positively rewarded if each child cooperated in completing a task. The use of positive peer pressure normalized working together. After six years, children in the "good behavior game" group had significant improvements over the control group in reducing shy and aggressive behavior, and delaying the onset of use of tobacco. This study may be an effective approach to peer-focused prevention programs for children with conduct and attention deficit disorders.

NICOTINE: A GATEWAY DRUG

Psychiatry is only beginning to awaken to the seriousness of nicotine addiction. Nicotine dependence is the most common comorbidity for adolescents and adults with psychiatric disorders and is associated with other substance use disorders (Kandel, Kessler, & Margulies, 1978). Historically, mental health settings have had a very permissive attitude toward tobacco use and have even used cigarettes as a behavioral reward in treatment. Some staff may smoke with patients as a way to improve communication and remove barriers (Feldman, 1984), but nicotine is a potent addictive drug that alters brain functioning and psychiatric symptoms. Also, cigarette smoking changes medication metabolism, side effects, and effectiveness.

Of all psychiatric patients in treatment, 50 to 85% are nicotine dependent, and individuals with depression, anxiety, alcohol dependence, and schizophrenia are particularly vulnerable to nicotine addiction. The rate of nicotine dependence among psychiatric patients is significantly higher than the general population rate of about 26%, even when age, sex, marital status, alcohol use, caffeine use, and socioeconomic status are controlled (Resnick, 1993; Hughes, Hatsukami, Mitchell, & Dahlgren, 1986; Glassman, 1993; Ziedonis, Kosten, Glazer, & Frances, 1994).

Studies suggest that there is an important relationship between depression and nicotine dependence that may be causal or result from common predisposing factors. Depression predicts a more difficult withdrawal from nicotine, and abstinence from nicotine increases the risk for a depressive relapse in those with a history of depression. The Epidemiological Catchment Area (ECA) study found that depression was more than twice as common among smokers than among nonsmokers, and smokers without a lifetime history of depression were twice as likely to stop smoking than were smokers with a history of depression (Glassman, 1993). The strong association of nicotine dependence and depression may be linked through genetic factors that increase the vulnerability for both disorders (Kendler et al., 1993; Glassman, 1993; Breslau, Kilbey, & Andreski, 1993). Nicotine dependence is twice as common among individuals with an anxiety disorder than in the general population; however, anxiety disorders are not associated with increased difficulty in smoking cessation (Breslau, Kilbey, & Andreski, 1991).

The rate of nicotine dependence among individuals with schizophrenia is between 50% and 90%. Smoking influences the course of schizophrenia. Compared with nonsmokers with schizophrenia, smokers with schizophrenia are more likely to have an earlier onset of schizophrenia and demonstrate more psychotic symptoms, increased medication side effects, and less social inhibition and greater inattentiveness. As with other psychiatric patients, smokers have higher rates of alcohol abuse and drug abuse than nonsmokers (Ziedonis, Kosten, Glazer, & Frances, 1994).

The strong association between nicotine dependence and other psychiatric disorders is influenced by biological, psychological, and social risk factors. Genetic vulnerability and possible dopamine and opioid neurotransmitter system linkages have been implicated as important biological factors. The psychological factor of self-medication may increase the use of nicotine because nicotine causes behavioral arousal and relaxation, including feeling more alert and less anxious, angry, and depressed. For schizophrenics, self-medication may also include attempting to improve concentration and alleviate feelings of boredom and social inhibition. Social factors supporting nicotine use include the lack of alternative recreational activities and permissiveness or even positive reinforcement for nicotine use while in psychiatric residences or treatment settings. Only recently have smoke-free units been enforced in psychiatric settings. The reasons why smoking has been ignored by mental health professionals may have important implications for treatment and prevention of nicotine dependence among psychiatric patients. Nicotine addiction should be a top priority in substance abuse prevention and treatment efforts among psychiatric patients, and more research is needed.

ADULT PSYCHIATRIC DISORDERS

The time period between the onset of the primary psychiatric disorder and the onset of the secondary substance abuse disorder provides a window of opportunity in which to perform primary substance abuse prevention efforts in mental health settings. Substance abuse prevention efforts targeting adult patients with a new psychiatric disorder should prove cost-effective and reduce the overall incidence rate of substance use disorders.

ANXIETY DISORDERS

There are several types of anxiety disorders, including phobia, panic, obsessive-compulsive, post-traumatic stress, and generalized anxiety disorders. Anxiety disorders are common in the general population, and the lifetime prevalence rate is about 15 to 25% and the current rate is about 7% (Regier et al., 1990; Kessler et al., 1994). In the ECA study, individuals with an anxiety disorder were almost twice as likely to have a substance use disorder, although there was a wide range according to specific anxiety disorder subtypes.

Controlled studies have explored the relationship of alcohol use and anxiety symptoms. Initially, alcohol use by anxious individuals has a relaxing effect, but long-term use can result in increased anxiety. Many individuals report that their anxiety disorder preceded their substance use disorder; however, they also report more severe anxiety symptoms after the onset of substance abuse (Stockwell & Bolderston, 1987). High school students report that they use drugs to reduce tension and anxiety (Johnston & O'Malley, 1986). Post-traumatic stress disorder (PTSD) can occur at any age after a traumatic event, and substance use can progress to abuse as a poor coping technique to deal with the painful memories of the trauma.

Treatment for anxiety disorders usually includes medication and psychotherapy. Common and effective medications include benzodiazepines (such as Valium or Xanax), but this type of medication can cause physical and psychological dependence.

MOOD DISORDERS

Mood disorders are common in the general population, with a lifetime prevalence of about 8% to 19% and current prevalence of 5% (Regier et al., 1990; Kessler et al., 1994). Women are twice as likely as men to develop a depression disorder. Depression is associated with low energy, anhedonia, and impaired social and work functioning, which increases the vulnerability to drug abuse through biopsychosocial mechanisms. Thirty-two percent of individuals with depression have a substance use disorder at some time in their lifetime, as do 64% of those with bipolar disorder (both mania and depression) (Dunner, Hensel, & Fieve, 1979). Women are more likely than men to have a primary depression and secondary alcohol use disorder (Hesselbrock, 1986).

Depression symptoms may be more severe with concurrent substance abuse because of reduced psychiatric treatment compliance or because drugs independently increase the severity of psychiatric symptoms. Although some depressed patients report using cocaine to help overcome feelings of boredom, emptiness, and fatigue, they often report a negative paradoxical reaction to cocaine use that includes tearfulness, extreme mood lability, and increased risk for suicide (Post, Kotkin, & Goodwin, 1974). Some depressed patients report self-medicating with alcohol to reduce symptoms of anxiety, insomnia, or depression. Often alcohol and other sedating drugs are abused in an initial attempt to reduce sleep problems. Alcohol and other sedatives can have an initial effect of reducing anxiety, but chronic use can actually increase the intensity and lability of the anxiety and depression. Depressed adults who abuse substances are at a much higher risk of suicide (Roy et al., 1990).

SCHIZOPHRENIA DISORDER

In the ECA study, lifetime substance use disorders were diagnosed in 47% of those with schizophrenia, including 34% with alcohol use disorder and 28% with a drug use disorder. These data support previous studies in psychiatric treatment settings that report current substance abuse in 25–50% of patients. A review of these clinical studies indicates that individuals with schizophrenia abuse more amphetamines, cocaine, marijuana, and nicotine than other psychiatric patients and the general population (Schneier & Siris, 1987).

Schizophrenia occurs in about 1–2% of the population and is characterized by a cycle of exacerbations and remissions. During exacerbations, patients experience psychotic symptoms and have impaired reality testing. The psychotic symptoms include hearing voices, severe language and communication disturbances, delusional beliefs, and bizarre behaviors. Antipsychotic medication is most helpful in reducing these symptoms. During remissions, patients are usually not psychotic and have improved reality testing. However, they continue to suffer from other difficulties that affect their ability to organize themselves and maintain the resources necessary for an unassisted adjustment in the community. Schizophrenics have underlying attention and arousal deficits, communication problems, and problems with regulating affect.

Substance abuse worsens the course of schizophrenia. Substance abuse causes individuals with schizophrenia to have increased symptoms of hallucinations, paranoia, depression, anxiety, violent behavior, and suicide attempts. Substance-abusing schizophrenics often have poor nutritional habits, engage in criminal activities, have financial problems, and become and remain homeless. These individuals require frequent psychiatric hospitalizations because they often do not comply with treatment and because other drugs decrease the effectiveness of medication and increase medication side effects (Westermeyer, 1992).

Ironically, compared with individuals with schizophrenia who do not abuse drugs, those who do abuse drugs often have a less severe schizophrenia disorder when not using drugs. Their baseline symptoms are less socially inappropriate, and they have a better prognosis (Dixon et al., 1991; Brady et al., 1990; Ziedonis, Kosten, & Glazer, 1993). The explanation for this apparent contradiction is not fully understood, although the stress-vulnerability model suggests that the impact of drugs (stress) on individual vulnerability is dramatic. It is conceivable that these higher-functioning individuals with schizophrenia might not have developed schizophrenia without the effect of drugs (as suggested in the earlier discussion on the brain poison and kindling theories). Among individuals with schizophrenia, a primary substance use disorder is associated with an earlier age of onset of schizophrenia. Another possibility is that higher-functioning individuals with schizophrenia are better able to relate to nonpsychiatric peers with whom they engage in drug experimentation. They may endure stress better, which may have helped them to better tolerate initial drug experimentation and maintain longer periods of drug use without complete psychiatric decompensation.

PERSONALITY DISORDERS

Psychiatric patients with personality disorders demonstrate chronic and pervasive maladaptive patterns of behavior that result in long-term difficulties in most spheres of their lives (American Psychiatric Association, 1994). Although about 5–10% of the population have a personality disorder, individuals with the disorder often do not seek psychiatric treatment unless they also have severe symptoms of depression or anxiety. The personality disorders most frequently associated with substance use disorders are the histrionic, narcissistic, antisocial, and borderline personality disorders. Individuals with these personality disorders are often very dramatic, unpredictable, and impulsive. They have symptoms similar to substance abusers, including using denial, excuse making, blaming, lying, minimizing, victim role-playing, grandiosity, and engaging in antisocial activities while obtaining drugs.

Most of the literature on personality disorders and substance abuse focuses on antisocial personality (ASP) disorder (Gerstley, Alterman, McLellan, & Woody, 1990; Grande, Wolf, & Schubert, 1984). Although only 4% of the population have an ASP diagnosis in their lifetime, the ECA study estimated that 84% of those with ASP had a comorbid substance use disorder in their lifetime. ASP is a poor prognostic factor in treatment, and is associated with increased risk for exposure to the HIV virus through needle sharing and high-risk sexual behaviors (Brooner et al., 1990). ASP is often associated with psychiatric patients who have already developed a substance use disorder, and clinicians should consider antisocial activities as a screening clue for early detection of substance abuse and a factor in treatment matching.

PSYCHIATRIC SYSTEMS ISSUES

The mental health system could be an important social factor in reducing the likelihood of psychiatric patients progressing from substance use to abuse. The adult and child mental health treatment systems have multiple levels of treatment, including inpatient, outpatient, consultation-liaison, emergency, partial hospitalization, outreach, and residential services. These services occur in a variety of private and public settings, and they maintain important linkages with other community agencies within supportive housing, criminal justice, vocational, child protection, general medical, and substance abuse treatment systems.

In addition, many individuals with mental health problems are treated outside the mental health system in primary medical care settings and religious settings. Medical professionals and clergy are often the first to be contacted by an individual seeking mental health assistance. Therefore, improving the linkages with these community resources may increase earlier access for psychiatric treatment and for primary substance abuse prevention efforts.

Another important historical development in the mental health system was the separation of substance abuse and mental illness agencies at the federal, state, and local levels. For example, almost 50% of the states still have separate mental health and substance abuse agencies with different treatment service systems, administrations, policies and procedures, funding sources, and entitlement programs (Davidson, Simsarian, & Marcus, 1993; Ridgely, Goldman, & Willenbring, 1990). This division occurs throughout the health care system. The federal research agencies are divided into the National Institute of Mental Health (NIMH), the National Institute on Drug Abuse (NIDA), and the National Institute of Alcohol and Alcohol Abuse (NIAAA).

Unfortunately, these divisions have formed access barriers for the dually diagnosed, who have had to seek separate treatment for each disorder: the substance abuse treatment took place within the substance abuse system, and the psychiatric treatment within the mental health system. Unfortunately, both systems ignored or rejected the dual-diagnosis patient, and numerous barriers limited access and the development of services directed at their special needs. Treatment occurred either sequentially (for example, first substance abuse and then psychiatric treatment or vice versa) or in parallel (separate treatment but during the same time period). Patients were often rejected from one system and referred to the other because both systems felt that the other system should assume primary responsibility for the patient's care.

Initial attempts to integrate mental health and substance abuse treatment services within either treatment setting often have been unsuccessful because of the boundaries between agencies, the limitations on target populations, the separation of funding sources, differing training and educational priorities, and differing treatment philosophies. For example, substance abuse treatment emphasizes the patient's personal responsibility for change, the therapist's confrontation of a patient's denial or minimization of the problem, the use of 12-step self-help involvement (such as Alcoholics Anonymous), and total abstinence from drug usage. Mental health treatment emphasizes the use of medications to help reduce symptoms, being supportive and helping a patient develop healthier coping skills before confronting ineffective defense mechanisms, and outreach into the community (Group for the Advancement of Psychiatry, 1991; Davidson, Simsarian, & Marcus, 1993; Ridgely, Goldman, & Willenbring, 1990).

Substance Abuse Prevention for Psychiatric Patients

This chapter will now summarize and propose specific recommendations for primary, secondary, and tertiary substance abuse prevention for child and adult psychiatric patients. Unfortunately, very little has been published on primary substance abuse prevention efforts for psychiatric patients. There is, however, an expanding literature on secondary and tertiary substance abuse prevention efforts.

Primary Prevention of Substance Abuse as a Secondary Disorder

Primary prevention aims to delay or eliminate an individual's initial involvement with alcohol and other drugs. Prevention efforts for psychiatric patients should focus on the unique aspects of the specific dual diagnosis combination. Tarter (1992) has suggested that prevention interventions should be individualized for each high-risk group.

Individual Focus

Primary prevention efforts attempt to help the individual develop social skills, problem solving

abilities, self-esteem, and ways to anticipate and manage transitional life events. Early access and appropriate psychiatric treatment also help reduce psychiatric symptoms that weaken the linkage to positive social supports of marriage, family, work, and community. Psychiatric treatment tends to focus on the individual and use specific biological, psychological, and social interventions. These interventions reduce the need for patients to self-medicate emotional problems with drugs. An increased understanding of the biological underpinning of dual diagnoses may lead to specific pharmacological interventions that treat the psychiatric disorder and prevent the progression from substance use to abuse. In addition, psychosocial prevention efforts are consistent with existing psychiatric treatment efforts to develop healthier coping and interpersonal skills. Specific psychosocial programs focus on helping the individual develop better problem-solving abilities, communication skills, and mood management. Patients often benefit from practical guidance on money management, which could be used to increase ability to purchase alcohol and other drugs. Psychiatric patients benefit from help in developing alternative highs that can replace the sensation-seeking aspects of substance abuse. This often occurs through planned vocational, social, and leisure activities. Psychiatric patients often have strong feelings of isolation and loneliness, and need help in arranging meaningful social activities. Helping to empower patients to organize these activities on their own or to seek out existing community resources may be an effective substance abuse prevention technique.

The ways in which specific psychiatric disorders increase an individual's vulnerability to substance abuse are an important area of future research. In the active phase of a psychiatric disorder, patients appear to be at increased risk of progressing from substance use to abuse. Psychiatric clinicians could focus prevention efforts on these time periods and reinforce these efforts when the psychiatric illness is in remission. Education on the stress-vulnerability aspects of psychiatric disorders could include information on effective and ineffective coping skills, such as self-medicating uncomfortable feelings. This education could be reinforced with action-oriented activities within treatment settings and reinforced in the patient's natural setting.

The specific characteristics of adult and child psychiatric disorders should be considered in developing prevention programs. Each specific psychiatric disorder requires a specific psychiatric treatment, and improved access to psychiatric treatment through increased screening, early diagnosis, referral, and treatment may reduce the likelihood of developing a substance use disorder.

CHILDREN WITH PSYCHIATRIC DISORDERS

Primary substance abuse prevention programs should target children with a psychiatric illness, especially those with conduct, attention deficit, learning, and depressive disorders. Successful prevention interventions have targeted the primary symptoms of these psychiatric disorders, which include aggression, inattention, impulsiveness, impatience, poor academic success, and low self-esteem. Reducing these symptoms may help the child connect to healthy support systems, including family, school, and community.

More information is needed on what factors build resiliency in children with psychiatric disorders. Helping children to develop these resiliency traits might provide important prevention strategies. Some children are able to endure the stress and deprivation of chronic family problems by developing their own sense of autonomy, social orientation, vigorous and spontaneous play, curiosity, self-reliance, ability to ask for help, involvement in hobbies and creative activities, and bonds with a positive primary caregiver (Werner, 1984; Wolin & Bennett, 1984). Werner believes that effective prevention programs reinforce the natural social bond between young and old.

Helping children develop alternative highs might delay the onset of substance use and could target the gateway drugs of alcohol and nicotine. These types of activities should be developmentally and age-appropriate. Adolescents may benefit from one-on-one relationship programs, job skills training, and organized physical adventures (Tobler, 1986). Adult prevention efforts might include some of these approaches as well.

ADULTS WITH PSYCHIATRIC DISORDERS

Adults with a psychiatric disorder are also at risk for developing a substance abuse problem, and the specific type of psychiatric disorder may suggest specific prevention efforts. Effective prevention among adults might target the window of opportunity between the onset of the primary specific psychiatric disorder and the onset of the secondary disorder. For example, social skills training for non-substance-abusing schizophrenic patients focus on helping patients with problem-solving and communication skills, mood management, assertiveness training, asking others for help, and make healthy living choices. With minor modification, existing approaches could reinforce non-drug-using activities and include drug resistance training.

Another strategy to reduce the likelihood of progression from use to abuse is to increase the amount of rewarding and structured activities. Many chronic psychiatric patients also need help managing disposable income from disability payments (such as Social Security Disability Insurance and Veterans Administration benefits). Westermeyer (1992) has suggested linking entitlements to healthy activities by allowing funds to be released only after participation in structured activities that benefit the patient or society (such as a day program, sheltered workshop, or public works).

Family Focus

The family could be an important resource and target for primary prevention efforts for both child and adult psychiatric patients, although some families may actually interact in a dysfunctional manner that increases family stress. Family members may benefit from family therapy and family education approaches.

Family support groups do exist for families with a member who is mentally ill. The National Alliance for the Mentally Ill (NAMI) is concerned with improving treatment and research efforts for the mentally ill and providing families with support, information, and advocacy.[2]

Prevention efforts might consider the needs of the other family members of psychiatric patients, such as siblings, children, spouses, and parents. Family therapy can decrease high-intensity expressed emotion (which occurs in families that are overinvolved and are very critical of the patient).

CHILDREN OF PSYCHIATRIC PATIENTS, INCLUDING THE DUALLY DIAGNOSED

Children of the dually diagnosed, psychiatric patients, or substance abusers are all at increased risk for substance use disorders and psychiatric disorders. The early identification of psychiatrically ill or substance-abusing parents might result in more immediate family interventions. Chapter 17 of this volume reviews several possible approaches and includes parent training, prenatal care, and support groups for children. Unfortunately, few treatment programs have considered or instituted this approach.

Parenting skills programs for dually diagnosed parents are being developed and evaluated (Ziedonis, Tanagho, & Ziedonis, n.d.; Perk-Hoff, 1991). Strengthening the parenting abilities of the dually diagnosed may be an effective tertiary prevention approach for parents and primary prevention approach for their children. Encouraging patients' identity as a parent may reduce their identity as a career substance abuser. These programs focus on developing parent skills and decreasing marital discord. Parents are taught how to solve problems, to become active in their children's school, and to help their children express themselves. Parents are taught the importance of resolving conflicts between themselves and disciplining their children in nonaggressive ways.

Peer Group Focus

Another important prevention approach might target the patient's peer group. In treatment and community programs, there are opportunities to encourage healthy peer group activities. Much of psychiatric treatment occurs in group therapy settings. For example, social skills training for the chronically mentally ill includes developing communication skills and receiving peer feedback and advice. Within this kind of program, patients could discuss peer pressure to use alcohol and other drugs and practice drug resistance exercises.

Community Focus

Treatment and community program settings provide another opportunity to reinforce antidrug messages by maintaining no-drug campus policies. Most community-based programs do attempt to reduce the availability of and access to drugs. The social climate can be influenced by the use of posters and wellness newsletters that reinforce antidrug messages. Policies on how drug usage will be dealt with are also needed. Consequences could be nonpunitive initially, but increasingly severe negative consequences and treatment requirements should be instituted if use continues. Programs that help patients make a positive contribution to the community strengthen positive social bonds. Community service programs might include volunteer work for programs with the elderly and youth and vocational training.

COMMUNITY PROGRAMS

Efforts to reinforce antidrug messages include having a range of housing based on the tolerance of alcohol or other drugs. Some residential programs have created "wet," "dry," and "damp" alternatives. In dry houses, alcohol and other drugs are not permitted on the premises. Although clients are not immediately extruded for use, there are consequences. Prevention efforts for psychiatric patients could be designed to integrate with general substance prevention efforts within public housing complexes and homeless shelters.

Prevention and treatment of nicotine dependence may serve a primary substance abuse prevention function for other types of substances. The literature clearly links cigarette smoking with other types of substance abuse. Nicotine addiction is commonly overlooked in community programs as well as treatment programs.

MENTAL HEALTH SYSTEM

Although primary prevention is recognized as a goal of community mental health centers, this goal is typically unrelated to clinicians' actual roles or previous training. However, prevention of comorbidity should be an important consideration in treating any psychiatric disorder. This clinical wisdom has been reinforced by a finding of high comorbidity in 14% of individuals interviewed in the National Comorbidity Study. The mental health system must assume responsibility for providing comprehensive services for patients who are dually diagnosed.

PREVENTING PRESCRIPTION DRUG DEPENDENCE

Prescription drugs have had a profoundly positive effect on the treatment of most psychiatric disorders. However, some of these medications can be misused and can cause prescription drug dependence. Primary substance abuse prevention efforts must target this problem and help ensure the careful and appropriate prescribing of medications, including stimulants such as ritalin, sedatives such as benzodiazepines (Fraser & Ingram, 1985), and antiparkinsonian drugs such as cogentin (Westermeyer, 1992). Prescription drug abuse can occur when physicians overprescribe because of a lack of knowledge and patient pres-

sure, when patients have several physicians, or when careless prescription writing is easily altered (for example, 10 pills becomes 100).

NATIONAL HEALTHCARE SYSTEM

The current U.S. healthcare system is considering enormous changes in priorities, access, administration, delivery, and funding of healthcare services. Now there is an opportunity to rethink the relationship between prevention and treatment.

Competition for limited resources has been a barrier to integration, and this issue will require compromise. Prevention efforts for psychiatric patients should reduce morbidity and mortality, which would offset other costs to the mental health system and the community. In addition, reimbursement for prevention services has been minimal, and ways to provide incentives to treatment settings to integrate these services should be considered. Prevention becomes more important as healthcare changes toward more managed care, market system forces, cost consciousness, and capitation systems.

Innovative ways to increase clinicians' awareness of substance abuse are needed. For example, the Partnership for a Drug-Free America (see Chapter 11 of this volume) sent a primary and secondary prevention media message to psychiatrists through the use of advertisement space in psychiatric professional journals. Their full-page advertisement included a Rorschach picture with a patient's cocaine-influenced description of this picture as "Death. A headless woman with black wings, reaching out to kill me." The ad provided information about the specific psychiatric symptoms of cocaine use and exhorted "First, rule out drug abuse" and "Your patients need *your* perspective, not cocaine's" (Partnership for a Drug-Free America, 1994).

SECONDARY SUBSTANCE ABUSE PREVENTION FOR PSYCHIATRIC PATIENTS

Secondary substance abuse prevention focuses on the early detection of substance abuse and the prompt initiation of substance abuse treatment. Common secondary prevention approaches include routine screening for substance use and related problems, immediate evaluation at triage locations, crisis intervention, networking with community resources, and rapid referral for immediate treatment (Kaplan & Sadok, 1985). How can secondary prevention efforts be improved in mental health settings, and how should they differ for psychiatric patients?

Several studies have demonstrated that simple, traditional substance abuse screening instruments can be used effectively in detecting substance abuse problems among psychiatric patients. As in many other healthcare settings, psychiatric patients will usually deny or minimize their substance use and related problems. Therefore, an effective screening approach must include assessments other than the patient's self-report. Community awareness and support could also be encouraged through highly publicized substance abuse awareness activities, such as "problem drinking awareness day," "smoking awareness day," "drug abuse awareness day," or "healthy living day" (which would address diet and sleep habits). Similar kinds of "awareness days" have been effective in medical care settings in screening for hypertension and depression. Second, future research must evaluate whether the standard diagnostic concepts and criteria used for psychiatric patients should be modified to include a broader spectrum of substance users and substance-related problems. The transition from use to abuse is a gray area that needs further definition, especially among psychiatric patients.

SCREENING

Mental health clinicians should integrate substance abuse screening techniques into every adult and adolescent psychiatric assessment. Clinicians should ask directly both the patient and significant others about alcohol and other types of drug use, including nicotine, caffeine, and prescription drugs. Patients should be questioned about past and current use, specific amounts, frequency, and last use. Although patients often report that they used a substance "in the past," they may exaggerate how far in the past. Patients are not likely to minimize their nicotine smoking patterns, however, and positive findings regarding nicotine suggest the need for a careful evaluation for other types of substance abuse. Smoking is associated with high rates of other types of substance abuse among both the general population and psychiatric patients (Ziedonis, Kosten, Glazer, & Frances, 1994).

Screening instruments can be helpful tools for the clinician if they are simple, valid, and accepted by patients. Some examples of commonly used tools include the CAGE (Mayfield, McLeod, & Hall, 1974), MAST (Michigan Alcohol Screening Test; Seltzer, 1971), DAST (Drug Abuse Screening Test; Skinner, 1982), Trauma Scale (Skinner et al., 1984), and urine drug toxicology and alcohol breathalyzer. Most of these instruments have been tested in several dual-diagnosis subtypes and found to have good specificity and sensitivity (Kofoed, 1991).

For example, the CAGE, a short and inexpensive tool, requires asking four simple questions:

- Have you ever felt the need to cut down on your drinking?
- Have you ever been annoyed by criticism of your drinking?
- Have you ever felt guilty about your drinking?
- Have you ever had an eye opener first thing in the morning?

If two or more of these questions are answered affirmatively, it is highly probable that an alcohol use disorder exists (the specificity and sensitivity are about 80%). CAGE is readily accepted by patients, minimizes defensiveness by being nonjudgmental, focuses on the issue of controlling use, and can provide information that helps present a diagnosis to the patient. CAGE questions can be adapted to other drug use by replacing drinking references with other drugs (Kofoed, 1991; Clark, Dube, & Lewis, 1992).

Urine toxicology and alcohol breathalyzer tests must be used routinely in all psychiatric settings.

Several studies have documented the substantial problem of denial in drug-abusing psychiatric patients. For example, a study at the University of California at Los Angeles found that one-third of the individuals with schizophrenia who came to the emergency room were recent cocaine abusers. Of this group, 50% denied their cocaine use; only urine drug test results provided information about current cocaine use (Shaner et al., 1993). Although a positive urine test result does not unequivocally indicate the presence of a substance use disorder, it can provide a major clue.

Clinicians should be aware of other clinical clues from reviewing a patient's current psychiatric symptoms and general well-being. For example, schizophrenics who abuse substances often use verbal threats, are resistant to psychiatric treatment, have increased psychiatric emergency room and inpatient visits, have periods of homelessness or malnourishment, and have a recent history of trauma. For other dual diagnosis combinations, patients who abuse substances have an increased severity or frequency in psychiatric symptoms, have crisis-filled lives, and have peers in treatment who are known substance users. One of the difficult aspects of early diagnosis is that the transition from substance use to abuse can be vague and not well-defined.

THE FULL SPECTRUM OF SUBSTANCE USE

More attention must be given to the full spectrum of substance use among psychiatric patients. This information may have important implications for specific interventions within primary, secondary, and tertiary substance abuse prevention. For example, what kinds of consequences result from what amount of alcohol use among individuals with a preexisting psychiatric disorder? Is any amount too much? Can some level of alcohol or other drug usage be helpful? Does the type of diagnosis and the type of substance used matter? There may be a need to broaden our definitions of alcohol and drug problems and interventions (Skinner, 1990).

For adolescents, there has been some effort to define levels of substance use. Simkin (1994) has summarized the literature into four levels based on the work of Schaeffer (1987) and Nowinski (1990). In the first level, adolescents use substances for experimentation, curiosity, thrill-seeking, and acceptance by peers. In this level of substance use, the individual learns the effect of drugs on moods. In the second level, the adolescent is actually seeking the mood swing that the drug causes. Often this mood swing is a pleasurable experience, and it may help the individual deal with difficult but ordinary feelings, such as anger, sadness, or boredom. Level three is consistent with the definition of substance abuse, and level four with substance dependence, including continued use despite adverse consequences, preoccupation with use, and loss of control. An improved understanding of the levels of use may help improve prevention.

ESTABLISHING THE DIAGNOSIS

In establishing a substance abuse diagnosis, the mental health clinician must consider all available information from the patient, significant others, case managers, and other clinicians. Some clinicians may benefit from using structured diagnostic instruments such as the Structured Clinical Interview for DSM-III-R (SCID; Spitzer & Williams, 1985), which uses DSM criteria. In addition, the clinician should draw a time line indicating the relative age of onset of substance abuse as compared to other psychiatric disorders and consider the possible impact the disorders had on one another. The evaluation should determine the substance abuse family history, severity of the substance use disorder, and patient's motivation for substance abuse treatment.

MOTIVATIONAL LEVEL

Assessing the level of motivation for substance abuse treatment is an important aid to treatment planning. Motivation is a state, not a trait, and it can be improved with the appropriate intervention. Prochaska, DiClemente, and Norcross (1992) have defined five stages of a patient's readiness for changing substance abuse behaviors: 1) precontemplation or denial (a patient is unaware of the need to change), 2) contemplation (a patient is aware of the need to change but is not yet ready to try to change); 3) preparation (patient tries to change on own but is unsuccessful); 4) action (patient comes to treatment desiring to change the behavior); and 5) maintenance (patient has been able to consistently change the behavior for more than three to six months). These stages of change can be assessed using the Change Assessment Scale and the Processes of Change Assessment Inventory (Rosenblum, 1991). The level of motivation should be linked to the specific types of interventions in substance abuse treatment (Miller & Rollnick, 1991). Using a simple five-point scale, the patient's level of motivation has been found to predict early sobriety among some dual diagnosis patients (Ries & Ellingson, 1990). A patient's motivation may increase when continued substance abuse threatens his or her housing, psychiatric treatment, vocational rehabilitation, family, marriage, and freedom from jail.

IMMEDIATE REFERRAL

Mental health organizations should first attempt to develop and integrate substance abuse treatment within their own settings, especially for those with prolonged mental illness. Typically, some of the initial barriers to treatment have been waiting lists and strict admission criteria that exclude either substance abuse or psychiatric disorders. Detoxification programs should occur in a variety of settings, including outpatient and residential settings. Current inpatient psychiatric units provide detoxification services only if symptoms include severe and disabling psychosis or suicidal thoughts. Detoxification is a critical time for some psychiatric patients because of increased psychiatric symptomatology. An increase in symptoms may result in worse initial treatment outcomes for psychiatric patients as compared to nonpsychiatric patients (for example, depressed smokers versus depressed cocaine addicts). Also, there is a need to increase outreach efforts into the community for both psychiatric and substance abuse problems.

Because the vast majority of addicted psychiatric patients will be in denial or just contemplating treatment, and not in the action stage, mental health staff must be taught substance abuse treatment motivational enhancement techniques. Mental health systems might develop specialized dual diagnosis consultation services to assist general psychiatric units in integrating substance abuse treatment. For example, the Connecticut Mental Health Center in New Haven, Connecticut has successfully used this approach and has developed a specialized team that attends psychiatric staff meetings and provides consultation on diagnostic issues, motivational enhancement, treatment planning, action-oriented treatment, and community resources (Ziedonis & Fisher, 1994).

TERTIARY SUBSTANCE ABUSE PREVENTION FOR THE DUALLY DIAGNOSED

This concluding section of the chapter reviews treatment matching, phases of dual-diagnosis treatment, and changes that must occur within the mental health system to integrate substance abuse treatment into the ongoing treatment of the dually diagnosed.

Treatment Matching

The core of substance abuse treatment for psychiatric patients is treatment matching. After a comprehensive patient assessment, a treatment plan is developed that outlines specific treatment interventions to address specific patient needs, characteristics, and diagnoses. Usually the psychiatric diagnosis dictates the emphasis of either an addiction or psychiatric treatment model. However, new dual-diagnosis treatment models are being developed.

In addition, patients differ in their motivation for treatment, previous number of treatment efforts, and amount of support from family and friends. All these factors are considered in deciding the appropriate level of treatment. Levels vary according to the intensity of the treatment and the setting (inpatient, outpatient, or day hospital) (Ziedonis & Fisher, 1994).

Phases of Treatment

The engagement phase of treatment includes assertive outreach by mental health network providers to gain the confidence and trust of individuals with mental illness. This process provides patients with assistance in practical problems in the community. The persuasion phase often occurs within mental health treatment settings during individual or group therapy. The goals of this phase are to increase the patient's awareness of how drugs affect their lives. In the mental health setting, patients are given information on healthy living habits (including the negative effects of alcohol, nicotine, and other drugs). In addition, group therapy provides a setting for peer support and confrontation. Ultimately, the goal is to increase the patient's commitment to substance abuse treatment.

In the active treatment phase, the patient is motivated to abstain from drugs and is interested in obtaining the skills to help reduce the likelihood of using drugs. Specific skills are developed, including problem-solving, communication, and mood management skills. Behavioral and cognitive approaches are used, and there is ongoing urine toxicology monitoring. In the maintenance phase, the patient has achieved three to six months of continuous abstinence and desires to focus on relapse prevention skills and improving vocational and social activities. For long-term maintenance, some dually diagnosed patients become further involved in 12-step groups in the community (such as Alcoholics Anonymous). All four of these phases of treatment are considered in service development.

Substance Abuse Treatment System for the Dually Diagnosed

Mental health and substance abuse treatment systems are currently considering whether dual-diagnosis treatment should be part of their primary responsibility. The overall trend, however, is to provide integrated treatment in one program.

Concurrent Treatment

The concurrent (but separate) treatment approach requires mental health and substance abuse treatment systems and clinicians to coordinate activities and work together to improve patient care. Because dual-diagnosis patients often require intensive clinical efforts and varied community resources, each system might expect that the other system will assume primary responsibility for treatment. If responsibilities are unclear, treatment is adversely affected.

As awareness of the dual-diagnosis problem increases, most agencies are adapting by developing new services for at least some specific dual-diagnosis combinations. For example, many traditional substance abuse treatment programs are now able to provide dual-diagnosis treatment services for individuals with comorbid anxiety, depression, or personality disorders.

Addiction Treatment Integrated into the Mental Health System

The departments of mental health in several states have taken the leadership role in efforts to develop an integrated and comprehensive service system for the dually diagnosed (Drake et al., 1991; Davidson, Simsarian, & Marcus, 1993). For example, the Connecticut Department of Mental Health took "responsibility for providing comprehensive services for those adults who are working to recover both from a prolonged mental illness and a substance use disorder" (Davidson, Simsarian, & Marcus, 1993, p. 1).

Coordination of Services

Currently, substance abuse services for the dually diagnosed are poorly coordinated and lack authorized leadership. Drake and colleagues (1993) have successfully improved coordination of substance abuse services for the dually diagnosed by developing continuous treatment teams. These multidisciplinary teams serve as the primary clinician for a relatively small number of patients, and are involved in the patient's treatment in all settings. The teams are outpatient-oriented and execute intensive case management within the patient's natural environment.

Treatment Principles

The first step toward integrating substance abuse treatment within a mental health system is to develop overarching treatment values and principles that articulate a unified philosophy and approach to care. Successful programs have an active outreach component into the community that increases patient awareness and motivation for treatment, an integrated mental health and substance abuse approach, broad-based and comprehensive services, and flexibility to meet individuals' needs. Providers are optimistic and convey a conviction that improvement and recovery are possible (Drake et al., 1993; Davidson, Simsarian, & Marcus, 1993).

Program structures that provide psychological and social interventions include individual therapy, group therapy, family services, and self-help groups. A comprehensive dual-diagnosis group therapy program should include groups that are oriented to the different levels of motivation for treatment. These include persuasion groups, relapse prevention groups, and maintenance groups. Persuasion groups are designed for patients who minimize their substance abuse. These groups provide support and education in a nonconfrontational manner and attempt to increase awareness of the substance abuse problem and the patient's commitment to active treatment. Relapse prevention groups are for patients who are committed to the goal of abstinence and ready to take active steps in making changes in their lives. Patients are provided with information about both their psychiatric and substance use disorders and the potential for a relapse with either. Patients learn the triggers for their drug use and they develop strategies to resist the triggers. The patient's cognitive beliefs and distortions can be explored to better understand their expectations about avoiding future substance

abuse. Also, therapy can help patients improve their mood management, problem-solving abilities, and communication skills. Maintenance groups are designed for those who have three to six months of continuous abstinence and want to move to the next level of substance abuse treatment by working on long-term lifestyle issues such as greater involvement in vocational rehabilitation. Increased involvement in 12-step programs in the community also occurs during this stage.

Self-help groups can provide a non-drug-using peer group and aid in the development of a healthy value system to guide patients through the steps in recovery. These meetings provide a setting for patients to share their own experience, strength, and hope. Another important aspect of treatment is family education and therapy. Interventions in this area strengthen an important social structure that may oppose a drug-abusing lifestyle.

The emphasis on medications differs between substance abuse and psychiatric treatment programs. Psychiatric staff must be aware of the cautious attitude of 12 step members and substance abuse treatment staff to the use of medications. Unfortunately, lack of information and the stigmatization of mental illness has resulted in poor advice to stop psychiatric medications. Staff must develop medication monitoring systems and review the psychology of prescribing medications. For example, patients should be warned against using nonaddictive medication in an addictive manner. Staff must be aware of how they and the patient perceive the use of medication, and the message should be clear that medications are only one tool in the toolbox and are not magic bullets. Staff and patients can review the Alcoholics Anonymous publication *The A.A. Member: Medications and Other Drugs* (1984; Ziedonis & Kosten, 1991).

A medical management component is important because patients are at risk for multiple medical problems including infectious diseases such as HIV, sexually transmitted diseases, and injuries such as head trauma. The spread of HIV is a growing problem for many of the dually diagnosed.

The mental health treatment system must coordinate with community agencies to provide safe, stable housing. These agencies can often develop and maintain evening and weekend activities as well. Case managers provide an important link for patients to community programs through conservatorship, money management, outreach, leisure activities, and vocational services.

Administrators are considering how to use existing social mechanisms to link the receipt of disability payments (entitlement) to participation in structured recovery programs, work adjustment programs, or subsidized employment opportunities (Westermeyer, 1992). This kind of arrangement might provide an important lever for keeping a patient engaged in treatment.

There is a need for program evaluation in all clinical settings. These efforts could provide a rich source of data and improve clinical services. One effective mechanism has been to bring computers into community mental health clinics.

Integrating Substance Abuse and Psychiatric Techniques

Psychiatric and substance abuse techniques can and should be integrated and modified within specific system components. For example, the dual diagnosis relapse prevention (DDRP) psychotherapy approach was developed for psychiatric patients with cocaine abuse and schizophrenia who are motivated for substance abuse treatment (Ziedonis, 1992; Ziedonis et al., 1992). This action-oriented therapy approach modifies and integrates traditional substance abuse relapse prevention and traditional psychiatric social skills training of medication management and psychiatric symptom management (Marlatt & Gordon, 1985; Carroll, Rounsaville, & Keller, 1991; Liberman, DeRisi, & Meuser, 1989). These traditional approaches share a common cognitive–behavioral approach and use behavioral learning techniques including role-playing, coaching, homework, and positive feedback. Patients are taught relapse prevention strategies for both psychotic symptoms and substance use.

CONCLUSION

Child and adult psychiatric patients are at risk for developing a substance abuse disorder. Prevention strategies targeted at this population may decrease the incidence and prevalence of substance abuse disorders. In addition, these efforts should improve the morbidity and mortality of the primary psychiatric disorder.

NOTES

1. Unfortunately, only initial reports from this study were available when this book went to press, and more information on this study can be obtained from the NCS Study Coordinator, Room 1006, Institute for Social Research, University of Michigan, Box 1248, Ann Arbor, MI 48106.
2. NAMI's national office is located in Virginia (Help line 1-800-950-NAMI; address: NAMI, 2101 Wilson Boulevard, Suite 302, Arlington, VA 22201).

REFERENCES

Abraham, H. D. (1986). Do psychostimulants kindle panic disorder? (letter). *American Journal of Psychiatry, 143,* 1627.

Alcohol, Drug Abuse, and Mental Health Administration (1991). *Comorbidity of substance abuse disorders and other psychiatric disorders.* Washington, DC: ADAMHA.

Alcoholics Anonymous (1984). *The A.A. member: Medications and other drugs.* New York: Alcoholics Anonymous World Services.

American Psychiatric Association (1994). *Diagnostic and statistical manual of mental disorders* (4th ed.). Washington, DC: APA.

Andreasson, S., Allebeck, P., Engstrom, A., & Rydberg, U. (1987). Cannabis and schizophrenia. *The Lancet,* 1483–1486.

Beiderman, J., Munir, K., Knee, D., Habelow, W., Armentano, M. (1986). A family study of patients with attention deficit disorder and normal controls. *Journal of Psychiatric Research, 20,* 263–274.

Botvin, G. J. (1983). Prevention of adolescent substance abuse through the development of personal and social competence. In T. J. Glynn, C. G. Leukefeld, & J. P. Ludford (Eds.), *NIDA Research*

Monograph 47. Washington, DC: U.S. Department of Health and Human Services, 115–140.

Brady, K., Anton, Ballenger, J. C., Lydiard, B., Adinoff, B., & Selander, J. (1990). Cocaine abuse among schizophrenic patients. *American Journal of Psychiatry, 147,* 1164–1167.

Breslau, N., Kilbey, M. M., & Andreski, P. (1991). Nicotine dependence, major depression, and anxiety in young adults. *Archives of General Psychiatry, 48,* 1009–1074.

Breslau, N., Kilbey, M. M., & Andreski, P. (1993). Nicotine dependence, major depression, and anxiety in young adults. *Archives of General Psychiatry, 50,* 23–36.

Brooner, R. K., Bigelow, G. E., Greenfield, L., Strain, E. C., & Schmidt, C. W. (1990). Intravenous drug abusers with antisocial personality disorder: High rate of HIV-1 infection. In L. Harris (Ed.), *Problems of drug dependence, 1990: Proceedings of the 52nd annual scientific meeting of the Committee on Problems of Drug Dependence.* National Institute on Drug Abuse Research Monograph No. 105, DHHS Pub. no. ADM 91-1753. Washington, DC: USGPO, 488–489.

Cantwell, D. P. (1988). Families with attention deficit disordered children and others at risk. In R. H. Coombs (Ed.), *The family context of adolescent drug use.* New York: Haworth Press, 163–186.

Carroll, K. M., Rounsaville, B. J., & Keller, D. S. (1991). Relapse prevention strategies for the treatment of cocaine abuse. *American Journal of Drug and Alcohol Abuse, 7,* 249–265.

Clark, W., Dube, C. E., & Lewis, D. C. (1992). *Screening for alcohol and other drug problems* (Project ADEPT). Providence: Brown University.

Cloninger, C. R., Reich, T., & Witzel, R. (1979). Alcoholism and affective disorders: Familial associations and genetic models. In D. W. Goodwin & C. K. Erickson (Eds.), *Alcoholism and affective disorders: Clinical genetic and biochemical studies.* New York: SP Medical and Scientific Books.

Coryell, W., & Zimmerman, M. (1987). The heritability of schizophrenia and schizoaffective disorder: a family study. *Archives of General Psychiatry, 45,* 323–327.

Crumley, F. E. (1990). Substance abuse and adolescent suicidal behavior. *JAMA, 263,* 3051–3056.

Davidson, L., Simsarian, J., Marcus, K. (Oct. 1993). Providing services to persons dually diagnosed with prolonged mental illness and substance abuse: A report. White paper prepared for the Connecticut Department of Mental Health.

Deykin, E. Y., Levy, J. C., & Wells, V. (1987). Adolescent depression, alcohol and drug abuse. *American Journal of Public Health, 76,* 525–531.

Dixon, L., Haas, G., Weiden, P. J., Sweeney, J., & Frances, A. J. (1991). Drug abuse in schizophrenic patients: clinical observations and reasons for use. *American Journal of Psychiatry, 148,* 224–230.

Drake, R. E., Antosca, L. M., Noordsy, D. L., Bartels, S. B., & Osher, F. C. (1991). New Hampshire's specialized services for the dually diagnosed. In K. Minkoff & R. E. Drake (Eds.), *Dual diagnosis of major mental illness and substance disorder.* New Directions for Mental Health Services, no. 50. San Francisco: Jossey-Bass, 3–12.

Drake, R. E., Bartels, S. J., Teague, G. B., Noordsy, D. L., & Clark, R. E. (1993). Treatment of substance abuse in severely mentally ill patients. *Journal of Nervous and Mental Disease, 181,* 606–601.

Dunner, D. L., Hensel, B. M., & Fieve, R. R. (1979). Bipolar illness: Factors in drinking behavior. *American Journal of Psychiatry, 136,* 583–585.

Ensminger, M. E., & Slusarcick, A. L. (1992). Paths to high school graduation or dropout: A longitudinal study of a first-grade cohort. *Sociology of Education, 65,* 95–113.

Ervin, C. S., Little, R. E., Streissguth, A. P., & Beck, D. E. (1984). Alcoholic fathering and its relation to child's intellectual development: A pilot investigation. *Alcoholism, 8,* 362–365.

Feldman, R. (1984). Smoking and the psychiatric nurse. *Journal of Psychosocial Nurse Mental Health Service, 22,* 13–16.

Fraser, A. A., & Ingram, I. M. (1985). Lorazepam dependence and chronic psychosis. *British Journal of Psychiatry, 147,* 211.

Gawin, F. H., & Kleber, H. D. (1986). Abstinence symptomatology and psychiatric diagnosis in cocaine abusers. *Archives of General Psychiatry, 43,* 107–113.

Gerstley, L. J., Alterman, A. I., McLellan, A. T., & Woody, G. E. (1990). Antisocial personality disorder in patients with substance abuse disorders: A problematic diagnosis? *American Journal of Psychiatry, 147* (2), 173–178.

Gittelman, R., Mannuzza, S., Shenker, R., & Bonagura, N. (1985). Hyperactive boys almost grown up. I. Psychiatric status. *Archives of General Psychiatry, 42,* 937–947.

Glassman, A. H. (1993). Cigarette smoking: Implications for psychiatric illness. *American Journal of Psychiatry, 150,* 456–553.

Grande, T. P., Wolf, A. W., & Schubert, D. S. (1984). Associations among alcoholism, drug abuse, and antisocial personality: A review of literature. *Psychological Reports, 55,* 455–474.

Group for the Advancement of Psychiatry (GAP) Committee on Alcoholism and the Addictions (1991). Substance abuse disorders: A psychiatric priority. *American Journal of Psychiatry, 148,* 1291–1299.

Harrington, R. C., Fudge, H., Rutter, M., Pickles, A., & Hill, J. (1991). Adult outcomes of childhood and adolescent depression: II. Links with antisocial disorders. *Journal of the American Academy of Child and Adolescent Psychiatry, 30* (3), 434–439.

Hesselbrock, V. M. (1986). Family history of psychopathology in alcoholics: A review and issues. In R. Meyer (Ed.), *Psychopathology and addictive disorders.* New York: Guilford Press.

Hollinger, P. C. (1987). *Violent deaths in the U.S.: An epidemiologic study of suicide, homicide, and accidents.* New York: Guilford.

Hughes, J. R., Hatsukami, D. K., Mitchell, J. E., & Dahlgren, L. A. (1986). Prevalence of smoking among psychiatric outpatients. *American Journal of Psychiatry, 143,* 993–997.

Johnston, L. D., & O'Malley, P. M. (1986). Why do the nation's students use drugs and alcohol? Self-reported reasons from nine national surveys. *Journal of Drug Issues, 16,* 29–66.

Kaminer, Y. (1992). Psychoactive substance abuse and dependence as a risk factor in adolescent attempted and completed suicide. *The American Journal on Addictions, 1,* 21–29.

Kandel, D. B., Kessler, R. C., & Margulies, R. Z. (1978). Antecedents of adolescent initiation into stages of drug use: A developmental analysis. In D. B. Kandel (Ed.), *Longitudinal research in drug use: Empirical findings and methodological issues.* Washington, DC: Hemisphere.

Kaplan, H. I., & Sadok, B. J. (1985). *Comprehensive textbook of psychiatry.* Baltimore: Williams & Wilkins.

Kellam, S. G., Brown, C. H., Rubin, B. R., & Ensminger, M. E. (1983). Paths leading to teenage psychiatric symptoms and substance use: Developmental epidemiological studies in Woodlawn. In S. B. Guze, F. J. Earls, & J. E. Barrett (Eds.),

Childhood psychopathology and development. New York: Raven Press.

Kellam, S. G., & Rebok, G. W. (1992). Building etiological theory through developmental epidemiologically based preventive intervention trials. In J. McCord & R. E. Tremblay (Eds.), *Preventing deviant behavior: Experimental approaches from birth to adolescence.* New York: Guilford Press.

Kellam, S. G., Rebok, G. W., Ialongo, N., & Mayer, L. S. (1994). The course and malleability of aggressive behavior from early first grade into middle school: Results of a developmental epidemiologically based preventive trial. *Journal of Child Psychology and Psychiatry and Allied Disciplines, 35,* 259–281.

Kellam, S. G., Werthamer-Larsson, L., Dolan, L., Brown, C. H., Mayer, L., Rebok, G., Anthony, J. C., Laudolff, J., Edelsohn, G., Wheeler, L. (1991). Developmental epidemiologically based preventive trials: Baseline modeling of early target behaviors and depressive symptoms. *American Journal of Community Psychology, 19,* 563–584.

Kendler, K. S. (1985). A twin study of individuals with both schizophrenia and alcoholism. *British Journal of Psychiatry, 147,* 48–53.

Kendler, K. S., Neale, M. C., Maclean, C. L., Heath, A. C., Eaves, J. L., & Kessler, R. C. (1993). Smoking and major depression: A causal analysis. *Archives of General Psychiatry, 50,* 36–43.

Kessler, R. C., McGonagle, K. A., Shanyang, Z., Nelson, C. B., Hughes, M., Eshleman, S., Wittchen, H., & Kendler, K. S. (1994). Lifetime and 12-month prevalence of DSM-III-R psychiatric disorders in the United States: Results from the National Comorbidity Survey. *Archives of General Psychiatry, 51,* 8–18.

Khantzian, E. J. (1985). The self-medication hypothesis of addictive disorders: Focus on heroin and cocaine dependence. *American Journal of Psychiatry, 142,* 1259–1264.

Khantzian, E. J., Gawin, F. H., Riordan, C., & Kleber, H. D. (1984). Methylphenidate treatment of cocaine dependence: A preliminary report. *Journal of Substance Abuse Issues, 1,* 107–112.

Kofoed, L. (1991). Assessment of comorbid psychiatric illness and substance disorders. In K. Minkoff & R. E. Drake (Eds.), *Dual diagnosis of major mental illness and substance disorder.* New

Directions for Mental Health Services, no. 50. San Francisco: Jossey-Bass, 43–55.

Liberman, R. P., DeRisi, W. J., & Meuser, K. T. (1989). *Social skills training for psychiatric patients.* Elmsford, NY: Pergamon.

Lieberman, J. A., & Bowers, M. (1990). Substance abuse comorbidity in schizophrenia. *Schizophrenia Bulletin, 16,* 29–30.

Mannuzza, S., Klein, R. G., Bonagura, N., Malloy, P., Giampino, T. L., & Addalli, K. A. (1991). Hyperactive boys almost grown up: V. Replication of psychiatric status. *Archives of General Psychiatry, 48,* 77–83.

Marlatt, G. A., & Gordon, J. K., Eds. (1985). *Relapse prevention: Maintenance strategies in the treatment of addictive behaviors.* New York: Guilford.

Mayfield, D., McLeod, G., & Hall, P. (1974). The CAGE questionnaire: Validation of a new alcoholism screening instrument. *American Journal of Psychiatry, 131,* 1121–1123.

Merikangas, K. R., Leckman, J. F., Prusoff, B. A., Pauls D. L., & Weissman, M. M. (1985). Familial transmission of depression and alcoholism. *Archives of General Psychiatry, 42,* 367–372.

Merikangas, K. R., Weissman, M. M., Prusoff, B. A., Pauls, D. L., & Weissman, M. M. (1985). Depressives with secondary alcoholism: Psychiatric disorders in offspring. *Journal of Studies on Alcohol, 46,* 199–204.

Meyer, R. E. (1986) *Psychopathological and addictive disorder.* New York: Guilford.

Miller, W. R., & Rollnick, S. (1991). *Motivational interviewing: Preparing people to change addictive behavior.* New York: Guilford.

Mirin, S. M., Weiss, R. D., & Michael, J. (1986). Family pedigree of psychopathology in substance abusers. In R. E. Meyer (Ed.), *Psychopathology and addictive disorders.* New York: Guilford, 57–77.

Nowinski, J. (1990). *Substance abuse in adolescents and young adults: A guide to treatment.* New York: W.W. Norton.

Partnership for a Drug-Free America (1994). First, rule out drug abuse (advertisement). *Psychiatric Annals, 24,* 68.

Perk-Hoff, S. (1991). *The kid's connection,* 4th ed. Dallas: Rainbow Days.

Post, R. M., Kotkin, J., Goodwin, F. R. (1974). The effects of cocaine on depressed patients. *American Journal of Psychiatry, 131,* 551–517.

Prochaska, J. O., DiClemente, C. C., & Norcross, J. C. (1992). In search of how people change: Applications to addictive behaviors. *American Psychologist, 47,* 1102–1114.

Regier, D. A., Farmer, M. E., Rae, D. S., Locke, B. Z., Keith, S. J., Judd, L. L., Goodwin, F. K. (1990). Comorbidity of mental disorders with alcohol and other drug abuse. *Journal of the American Medical Association, 264,* 2511–2518.

Resnick, M. P. (1993). Treating nicotine addiction in patients with psychiatric co-morbidity. In C. T. Orleans & J. Slade (Eds.), *Nicotine addiction: Principles and management.* New York: Oxford University Press.

Ridgely, S. M., Goldman, H. H., & Willenbring, M. (1990). Barriers to the care of persons with dual diagnoses: Organizational and financing issues. *Schizophrenia Bulletin, 16,* 123–132.

Ries, R. K., & Ellingson, T. (1990). A pilot assessment at one month of seventeen dual diagnosis patients. *Hospital and Community Psychiatry, 127,* 89–94.

Robins, L. N. (1966). *Deviant children grown up: A social and psychiatric study of sociopathic personality.* Baltimore: William & Wilkins.

Robins, L. N., & Price, R. K. (1991). Adult disorders predicted by childhood conduct problems: Results from the NIMH Epidemiologic Catchment Area project. *Psychiatry, 54 (2),* 116–132.

Robins, L. N., & Regier, D. A. (1991). *Psychiatric disorders in America.* Free Press.

Rosenblum, D. (1991). *A transtheoretical analysis of change among cocaine users* (unpublished doctoral dissertation). Kingston: University of Rhode Island.

Rounsaville, D. J., Anton, S. F., Carroll, K., Budde, D., Prusoff, B., & Gawin, F. (1991). Psychiatric diagnosis of treatment-seeking cocaine abusers. *Archives of General Psychiatry, 48,* 43–51.

Rounsaville, B. J., Kosten, T. R., Weissman, M. M., Prusoff, B., Pauls, D., Anton, S. F., & Merikangas, K. (1991). Psychiatric disorders in relatives of probands with opiate addiction. *Archives of General Psychiatry, 48,* 33–42.

Roy, A., Lamparski, D., DeJong, J., Moore, V., & Linnoila, M. (1990). Characteristics of alcoholics who attempt suicide. *American Journal of Psychiatry, 147,* 761–765.

Rutter, M. (1985). Resilience in the face of adversity: Protective factors and resistance to psychiatric disorder. *British Journal of Psychiatry, 147,* 598–611.

Rutter, M., Tizard, J., & Whitmore, K. (1970). *Education, health, and behavior.* London: Longman.

Schaeffer, D. (1987). *Choices and consequences.* Minneapolis: Johnson Institute Books.

Schneier, F. R., & Siris, S. G. (1987). A review of psychoactive substance use and abuse in schizophrenics: Patterns of drug choice. *Journal of Nervous and Mental Disease, 175,* 641–652.

Schuckit, M. A. (1986). Genetic and clinical implications of alcoholism and affective disorder. *American Journal of Psychiatry, 143* (2), 140–147.

Seltzer, M. L. (1971). The Michigan Alcoholism Screening Test: The quest for a new diagnostic instrument. *American Journal of Psychiatry, 127,* 89–94.

Shaffer, D., Garland, A., Gould, M., Fisher, P., & Trautman, P. (1988). Preventing teenage suicide: A critical review. *Journal of the American Academy of Child and Adolescent Psychiatry, 27,* 675–687.

Shaner, A., Khalsa, M. E., Roberts, L., et al. (1993). Unrecognized cocaine use among schizophrenic patients. *American Journal of Psychiatry, 150,* 758–752.

Simkin, D. R. (1994). Levels of use in adolescents. *Newsletter of the American Academy of Psychiatrists in Alcoholism and Addictions,* (Spring).

Skinner, H. A. (1982). The Drug Abuse Screening Test. *Addictive Behaviors, 7,* 363–371.

Skinner, H. A. (1990). Spectrum of drinkers and intervention opportunities. *Canadian Medical Association Journal, 143,* 1054–1059.

Skinner, H. A., Holt, S., Schuller, R., Roy, J., & Israel, Y. (1984). Identification of alcohol abuse using laboratory tests and a history of trauma. *Annals of Internal Medicine, 101,* 847–851.

Spitzer, R. L., & Williams, J. B. W. (1985). *Structured clinical interview for DSM-III-R.* New York: Biometrics Research Department, New York State Psychiatric Institute.

Stockwell, T., & Bolderston, H. (1987). Alcohol and phobias. *British Journal of Addictions, 82,* 1178–1182.

Tarter, R. E. (1992). Prevention of drug abuse. *The American Journal on Addictions, 1,* 2–20.

Tarter, R. E., Alterman, A., & Edwards, K. (1985). Vulnerability to alcoholism in men: A behavior-genetic perspective. *Journal of Studies on Alcohol, 46,* 329–356.

Tarter, R. E., Hegedus, A., Goldstein, G., Shelly, C., & Alterman, A. I. (1984). Adolescent sons of alcoholics: neurospsychological and personality characteristics. *Alcoholism, 8,* 216–222.

Tarter, R. E., McBride, N., Baonpane, N., & Scheider, D. U. (1977). Differentiation of alcoholics: Children with history of minimal brain dysfunction, family history, and drinking pattern. *Archives of General Psychiatry, 34,* 761–768.

Thacker, W., & Tremaine, L. (1989). Systems issues in serving the mentally ill substance abuser: Virginia's experience. *Hospital and Community Psychiatry, 40,* 1046–1049.

Tobler, N. S. (1986). Meta-analysis of 143 adolescent drug prevention programs: Quantitative outcome results of program participants compared to a control or comparison group. *Journal of Drug Issues, 16,* 537–567.

Weiss, R. D. (1991). The role of psychopathology in the transition from drug use to abuse to dependence. In M. Glantz & R. Pickens (Eds.), *Vulnerability to drug abuse.* Washington, DC: American Psychological Press.

Werner, E. (1984). Resilient children. *Young Children, 40.*

Westermeyer, J. (1992). Schizophrenia and substance abuse. In A. Tasman & M. B. Riba (Eds.), *American Psychiatric Press review of psychiatry, 11.* Washington, DC: American Psychiatric Press, 379–401.

Wolin, S. J., & Bennett, L. A. (1984). Family rituals. *Family Process, 23,* 401–420.

Ziedonis, D. M. (1992). Comorbid psychopathology and cocaine addiction. In T. R. Kosten & H. D. Kleber (Eds.), *Clinician's guide to cocaine addiction: Theory, research and treatment.* New York: Guilford, pp. 337–360.

Ziedonis, D. M., & Fisher W. (1994). Assessment and treatment of comorbid substance abuse in individuals with schizophrenia. *Psychiatric Annals, 24,* 477–483.

Ziedonis, D. M., & Kosten, T. R. (1991). Pharmacotherapy improves treatment outcome in depressed cocaine addicts. *Journal of Psychoactive Drugs, 23,* 417–425.

Ziedonis, D. M., Kosten, T. R., & Glazer, W. (1993). The impact of drug abuse on psychopathology and movement disorders in chronic psychotic outpatients. In L. Harris (Ed.), *Problems of drug dependence 1992.* NIDA Research Monograph 153.

Ziedonis, D. M., Kosten, T. R., Glazer, W. M., & Frances, R. J. (1994). Nicotine dependence and schizophrenia. *Hospital and Community Psychiatry, 45,* 204–206.

Ziedonis, D. M., Rayford, B. S., Bryant, K., & Rounsaville, B. J. (1994). Psychiatric comorbidity in white and African-American cocaine addicts seeking substance abuse treatment. *Hospital and Community Psychiatry, 45,* 43–49.

Ziedonis, D. M., Richardson, R., Lee, E., Petrakis, I., & Kosten, T. (1992). Adjunctive desipramine in the treatment of cocaine abusing schizophrenics. *Psychopharmacology Bulletin, 28* (3), 309–314.

Ziedonis, D. M., Tanagho, A., & Ziedonis, P. X. (n.d.). *Parenting program for families in which a parent has both a psychiatric and substance abuse disorder: therapist's manual* (unpublished manuscript).

PART FOUR

CONTROVERSIAL PREVENTION ISSUES

CHAPTER 22

DRUG TESTING

DEBORAH L. ACKERMAN

The first task of prevention is to define the problem to be prevented and the goal of the intervention. Is drug abuse defined as regular use, or any use, of psychoactive substances? Is the desired outcome to prevent the use of particular drugs or categories of drugs, or to prevent or control the consequences of use? The definition of drug abuse and the degree to which it is tolerated vary considerably from culture to culture and within the same culture from time to time. Currently in our society, compulsive or irresponsible drug use that endangers drug users' lives or others' lives and property is not tolerated. The government has declared war on this type of drug use, and has strengthened its efforts to limit the availability of drugs by increased surveillance and harsher penalties for the manufacture, possession, and distribution of illicit substances. In addition, governmental and private employers have begun to require drug testing of potential and existing employees in an effort to eliminate drug use and abuse from the workplace.

The testing of employees for substance abuse is one of the most controversial issues in the current war against drug abuse. Advocates consider it an important weapon, capable of reducing on-the-job substance use and thereby restoring economic productivity. Critics have called it an invasion of employees' privacy, one with technical limitations and harmful consequences. Various drug testing programs have been challenged in the courts on the basis of a number of constitutional

and state protections. However, the courts have generally sanctioned drug testing when they were satisfied that the health and safety of other employees or the public were at stake and that such action by employers would substantially protect or benefit society (West & Ackerman, 1993).

A BRIEF HISTORY OF TESTING[1]

The purposes and methods of drug detection programs have changed considerably since they were first introduced more than 50 years ago. In clinical settings, various observational techniques have long been used to assist in diagnosing new patients. However, in the past half century, advances in the science of laboratory analysis have made it possible to screen urine for sugar, blood cells, abnormal metabolites, and ingested substances. Urine testing for drug use is now a routine procedure, especially in emergencies when drug intake is suspected, or to evaluate new patients on admission. In sports, drug testing has been used for decades to ensure a chemically fair contest. Currently, it also serves to promote a drug-free society by allowing "clean" athletes to set a good example and inspire today's youth to avoid drugs. Urine screening to detect drug use among military personnel and workers was introduced nearly 20 years ago to ensure operational readiness and on-the-job safety. More recent concerns about the rising costs associated with drug and alcohol abuse by employees have contributed

---

[1] A more detailed account by the author can be found in *Drug testing: Issues and options,* edited by R. H. Coombs & L. J. West, New York: Oxford Press, 1991, pp. 3–21.

to the rapidly growing extension of drug testing programs of the mass screening type into the workplace. Following is a summary of developments leading up to the various drug testing programs currently in place in our society.

In Medicine

Early methods to diagnose certain physical conditions relied on observational techniques such as examining the urine of diabetics to detect sugar. The only method to determine surreptitious drug use was to observe individuals' behavior. In the 1950s, an observational test for narcotic drug use, the nalorphine pupil test, was developed for use in hospitals and prisons. By the mid 1970s, after subsequent advances in analytic chemistry made it possible to detect drugs and their metabolites in urine, drug screening was introduced on hospitalization and as an aid to proper diagnosis of psychiatric outpatients. Urine testing is now seen as the simplest and most efficient tool for the diagnosis of substance abuse. As drug abuse has increased, more and more outpatient and inpatient drug rehabilitation programs use drug screening routinely to monitor drug-dependent individuals.

In Sports

Drug testing in athletics began in the 1930s with the mouse tail flick test to determine whether race horses had been given morphine, a widely used stimulant and performance enhancer. The method involved injecting horse's saliva under the skin of a mouse. If the mouse's tail became rigid, the test was positive and the horse was withdrawn from the race. By the 1950s, developments in analytic chemistry made it possible to screen the animal's saliva for a variety of substances, mostly performance enhancers and analgesics, simultaneously. A sample of saliva was taken after the race from the winner and from each horse that placed, came in last, or was the favorite. Today, further technological advances have made it possible to conduct pre-race testing

in both dogs and horses on blood or urine samples drawn before the race (Clarke, 1969).

In the late 1960s, the International Olympic Committee (IOC) began to screen the urine of competitors for performance-enhancing drugs to remove any unfair advantage that athletes who use such drugs might have. This reason was especially valid for CNS stimulants and (later) anabolic steroids, two groups of drugs that can improve physical performance and endurance. Analgesics were also banned in an effort to protect athletes from potentially dangerous side effects: Analgesics mask the pain of an injury and thereby may lead to more serious injury. Currently, the IOC bans substances in five categories: psychomotor stimulants, sympathomimetic amines, miscellaneous CNS stimulants, narcotic analgesics, and anabolic steroids. In addition, blood doping (withdrawing blood from an individual, freezing the red blood cells, and returning the thawed cells after the body has replenished the lost blood just before a competition) and the use of growth hormone are prohibited.

In January 1986, the National Collegiate Athletic Association (NCAA) initiated its drug testing program so that, according to its policy statement, no one participant might be pressured to use chemical substances in order to remain competitive. The NCAA's banned drug list is similar to the IOC's, except that it bans recreational drugs such as marijuana. The NCAA's legislation requires that all student athletes sign a consent form annually before participating in any sport. The use of several drugs prescribed for the treatment of asthma must be declared before competition, and corticosteroid use must be declared at NCAA championships or certified football games. Current testing is mandatory, but random unannounced testing has not been adopted.

Today in the United States, drug testing, combined with education to change athletes' attitudes about drugs, serves as a primary intervention to discourage children and adolescents from using street drugs. Athletes also serve as role models: "Clean" athletes will deter today's youth from becoming tomorrow's addicts. This is especially true in professional sports, although professional organizations have been somewhat slower to follow the lead of amateur athletic organizations (due largely to the influence of players' unions). Most allow testing as part of an annual preseason medical evaluation, and do not allow mandatory random drug testing. One aspect unique to professional sports is the employee assistance program, which allows the impaired athlete to receive treatment while continuing to play and receive a salary (Wagner, 1987).

In the Military, Law Enforcement, and the Workplace

Since the passage in 1914 of the Harrison Narcotics Act, American drug policy has been dominated by efforts to control the supply, demand, and distribution of illicit drugs. The earliest approach to reduce demand was the introduction of state and federal laws mandating criminal or civil commitment for narcotics addicts. Addicts were sentenced, on the basis of physical evidence and clinical criteria, to periods of involuntary confinement at the national hospitals operated by the U.S. Public Health Service. These hospitals were eventually taken over by the Federal Bureau of Prisons, which installed specialized addiction treatment units within most prisons. All of these operations used drug testing procedures to monitor the condition of inmates and parolees.

The first drug detection method to affect the public and protect public safety was the breath test for alcohol. In the 1930s, noninvasive breath analyzers, marketed under such names as the Drunkometer, Intoximeter, and Alcometer, were introduced to test drivers involved in accidents or otherwise suspected of driving while intoxicated. However, breath tests did not achieve widespread support until growing concerns about highway safety led to the passage in 1966 of the National Highway Safety Act. That legislation carried provisions for enforcement procedures regarding alcohol testing. By 1969, testing was performed for cause on drivers suspected of driving while intoxicated. In the 1970s and 1980s, random testing of motorists was introduced by means of roadblocks set up for such purposes, at first to gather data about the incidence and typology of alcohol use among drivers (Wolfe, 1974) but later to apprehend drunk drivers and remove them from the roadways. Vehicle stops that are purely at the discretion of the officer have been disallowed by the Supreme Court as being too subjective and possibly discriminatory. Stops must be truly random, or follow an objective pattern (such as stopping every nth car that approaches a checkpoint). Because of uncertainties about their constitutionality, sobriety stops have not been widely adopted. However, in as many as 21 states they have been applied with strict procedural controls. Similar measures were instituted in Australia, Great Britain, and several other countries at about the same time.

In the 1960s and 1970s, heroin addiction was seen as the greatest threat to the health and safety of American soldiers and workers. The military first instituted urine testing at that time to identify heroin users returning from Vietnam. By the early 1970s, the screening program was extended to detect other drugs among soldiers reporting for active duty. At the same time, some industries began to require urine drug tests of job applicants to identify heroin addicts and users of other psychoactive drugs before they were hired, and thereby to prevent the problems of increased illness and injury caused by addicted employees.

In the early 1980s, the first mass screening program was introduced by the U.S. Navy. The program was initiated after a 1980 Pentagon survey, conducted through anonymous questionnaires among 20,000 military personnel, showed that 27% of the under-25 population in the Navy were using drugs. Another impetus was the May 1981 crash of a Marine Corps aircraft aboard the aircraft carrier Nimitz in the Atlantic. Six of the 10 deck crew who died were found to have used illegal drugs within the preceding 30 days. Today, the Navy screens for amphetamines, barbiturates, cocaine, marijuana, opiates, and PCP. Drug programs in the other branches of the military are similar, but less extensive. All branches employ mass screening of all enlisted personnel; most also screen civilian employees in sensitive positions.

Most recently, concerns among U.S. government and private employers about the rising costs associated with drug and alcohol abuse by employees have led to the extension of mass screening programs into the workplace. In 1986, the National Institute on Drug Abuse estimated that the cost of employee drug and alcohol abuse was $100 billion per year in accident-related loss of life and property and reduced productivity. In 1988, that estimate had reached $135 billion per year. Two-thirds of the total is attributable to alcohol use alone. Based on anticipated population growth, the maturation of the baby boom generation, and growth and productivity in the workforce, these costs are expected to increase 2% per year. This means that by 1995, the total cost of drug and alcohol abuse will approach $160 billion (Hawks & Chiang, 1986; U.S. Department of Health and Human Services, 1990).

Workplace testing for drug use has increased dramatically in the past decade. Between 1982 and 1988, the portion of the nation's largest companies that test employees rose from 5% to 28%. The National Institute on Drug Abuse now estimates that the number has risen to 40%. Federal agencies also have developed plans to deal with problems of safety and drug abuse by employees. In 1985, the Federal Railroad Administration drafted guidelines to test employees in response to the startling findings that between 1972 and 1983 drug- or alcohol-related train accidents killed 42 people, injured 61, and cost $19 million in property damage. The program required the testing of applicants for sensitive positions, and of employees for reasonable suspicion or after accidents. By the mid-1980s, the U.S. Secret Service was testing applicants and probationary officers and the Department of Defense was screening civilian employees. A few other federal agencies also started or established guidelines for their own screening programs. However, widespread testing of employees in the public sector did not begin until 1986, when president Ronald Reagan provided the legal basis.

In March 1986, the President's Commission on Organized Crime issued its final report. Among its more than 50 recommendations were the following: The president should direct all federal agencies to formulate clear policy statements, implement guidelines, and include suitable drug testing programs; state and local governments and leaders in the private sector should support unequivocally a similar policy that any use of drugs in the workplace is unacceptable; and government and private sector employees who do not already require testing of job applicants and current employees should consider the appropriateness of such a testing program. On September 15, 1986, executive order 12,564 signed by then-president Reagan mandated a drug-free workplace and the passage of the Anti-Drug Abuse Act. In June 1987, Public Law 100-71, Section 503, Title V, was enacted to permit the administration to proceed with programs to test federal employees.

The *Mandatory Guidelines for Federal Workplace Drug Testing Programs: Final Guidelines,* prepared by the U.S. Department of Health and Human Services (1988) in response to the president's order, applies to all federal agencies and serves as a model for private industry. It requires all federal testing programs to test urine for marijuana and cocaine and authorizes testing for opiates, amphetamines, and phencyclidine. Tests for other substances may be done with written authorization from the secretary of the Department of Health and Human Services. Despite the well-documented heavy burden of morbidity and mortality caused by alcohol, the order mandating a drug-free federal workplace applies only to drugs listed in Schedules I and II of the Controlled Substances Act, and not to alcohol.

Today, there are three basic types of drug testing programs: pre-employment screening, testing for cause, and random testing. The majority of workplace programs involve pre-employment screening of job applicants. They may also require drug testing of current employees who wish to transfer to more sensitive positions. These tests are usually done with the applicant's or employee's full prior knowledge. Testing for cause is based on reasonable suspicion about an individual's current drug use or after he or she has been involved in an on-the-job accident. Random testing involves the selection of a sample from a pool of all employees, or of those in sensitive positions, and may be either announced or unannounced.

Urine screening programs in the military, the workplace, and the criminal justice system generally test for the most common drugs of abuse: amphetamines (stimulants), cocaine (also a stimulant), barbiturates (sedatives), benzodiazepines (tranquilizers), cannabis (marijuana, hashish), opiates (morphine, codeine, heroin), methadone (a synthetic opiate), phencyclidine (PCP or angel dust), and methaqualone (Quaalude). The usual procedure includes initial screening of urine samples by an immunoassay test, followed by more specific tests to confirm positive findings. A few private companies and federal agencies also test for alcohol after accidents and in other probable cause situations. However, a single urine specimen may not reflect accurately the degree of alcohol consumed because of the time elapsed since drinking, the stage of absorption, the quantity of urine in the bladder, the frequency of urination, and other variables. Unless tests for alcohol are performed on blood samples or by breath tests, the results must be interpreted with caution (Winek & Esposito, 1987).

EVIDENCE OF PROGRAM EFFECTIVENESS

The major rationale for urine drug screening is that it identifies drug users. A secondary rationale is that screening programs may deter drug abuse. In clinical settings, drug testing is for the good of the patient. It assists the clinician in making an accurate diagnosis and in instituting appropriate treatment. The testing of athletes is supposed to benefit both the sport and the player, and to act as a deterrent to drug use within society as a whole. In the criminal justice system, the traditional arena in which the war on drugs has been fought, drug detection helps to monitor patterns of drug

use and control the illegal activity of drug-dependent individuals. One of the reasons for detecting drug use among military personnel and employees is to identify and then to rehabilitate or remove the drug abuser from the workplace so that overall productivity and on-the-job safety will increase while on-the-job accidents and impairment-related medical expenses will decrease. In each of these arenas, the effectiveness of drug testing in meeting its goals has been studied. The following is an overview of those findings.

In Medicine

Drug testing in clinical settings is generally accepted as a necessary medical procedure. A routine toxicology screen is regularly ordered in the emergency room if a patient is unconscious and there are no witnesses to help determine the cause of coma and to aid in selecting proper treatment. Urine testing is also a simple and efficient technique to help in the prompt evaluation and ongoing clinical management of chemical dependency disorders and for the diagnosis of intoxication of any kind.

Several studies have evaluated the role of drug testing to monitor the progress of clients in drug rehabilitation programs and have found it to have variable degrees of usefulness. Kaistha and Tadrus (1978) found mandatory urine testing to have several important uses. It provides an objective indicator of clients' progress, it provides a tool for client confrontation, it exposes the real behavior of the client and thus helps generate an honest relationship with the clinician, it may help the client in certain legal situations, it can provide data for statistical evaluations of treatment plans, it can help in therapeutic communities, and it can assist in methadone treatment programs as a deterrent against diversions.

Singh, Singh, and Miller (1972) used urine testing to verify the reported drug use of addicts on a methadone substitution program. Test results from 100 addicts who were tested on days 15, 30, 45, and 60 of the program demonstrated that morphine and its metabolites along with quinine were present in 30% of the samples, despite patients' denials that they were taking these other drugs. The authors recommend that urine testing be used as a surveillance measure and that efforts should be made to gain the trust of addicts so that they will be more amenable to counseling.

In contrast, Milby et al. (1979) found drug testing to be marginally effective in the rehabilitation process. The authors compared outpatient psychotherapy among drug abusers with and without drug testing. At the end of three months, the subjects who were tested had decreased their barbiturate use and their association with drug-using friends; however, narcotic use did not decline in either group. The authors concluded that surveillance was only somewhat useful as an adjunct to psychotherapy.

DeAngelis, McCaslin, & Ungerleider (1978) discovered another purpose for testing during drug rehabilitation: to predict treatment success or treatment failure. They observed that time in treatment was significantly related to results of urinalysis during the first three months; clients who remained in treatment for longer periods were those whose average opiate use during the first three months was lowest.

In Sports

One of the most effective applications of drug testing may be in sports. The antidoping campaign was instituted to uphold the ethics of sports, protect athletes' health, and preserve fair competition. Since the institution of drug testing, the numbers of positive tests at competitions have been substantially reduced. Several sports policy-makers attribute the success of preventive efforts to those directed at the enhancement of athlete education, the development of strict policies dealing with athletes who use banned substances, and refinement of drug testing procedures (Puffer, 1986). However, problems still exist as some athletes successfully evade the process. Short-acting steroids can be taken throughout the training period and discontinued in time for a competition where testing will be performed.

In Norway, where random unannounced testing is performed, the program may be more effective. Oseid (1984) described the preventive (antidoping) measures that have been carried out there since 1976. Between 1977 and 1982, the percentage of positive tests was low, but the author attributed that to the large denominator—testing was done on all athletes in all sports, not just "loaded" sports (such as power and weight lifting and throwing events in track and field). In 1983, tests were refocused on those "loaded" sports and more tests were done at random. These changes netted four times as many positives as in the previous year.

One recent survey of college athletes in the United States indicates that drug testing may be having an effect opposite to the one intended. Coombs and Ryan (1990) surveyed 500 college athletes who were subjected to mandatory testing as part of their preseason medical evaluation. When compared with a group of 124 athletes exempt from testing, the tested athletes had fewer positive tests. Although most reported that they had reduced their use of drugs, 15% said that their drug use had increased. Among drug-using athletes, some claimed that they used drugs to celebrate having passed a drug test.

In the Military

When the military first instituted urine testing to identify heroin users returning from Vietnam, the screening method that was used could detect only morphine (the major metabolite of heroin excreted in urine). Consequently, to avoid detection, many returnees who knew the approximate dates of their debarkation were able to pass the test by temporarily switching to methadone, barbiturates, or tranquilizers to help them get through heroin withdrawal. Now that screening for multiple substances is possible, such problems do not exist.

There have been reports that the military's drug testing program has significantly reduced the prevalence of drug abuse. A report on mandatory screening in the Army and Air Force showed that the percentage of positive urine tests dropped from more than 20% in January 1983 to less than 1% in December 1987 (Goldsmith, 1988). The Navy's random, unannounced testing program lowered the number of specimens positive for marijuana from 48% in 1982 to 2% in 1988 (Mulloy, 1991). In addition, a survey of Navy personnel demonstrated that drug testing has been a deterrent to drug use. Eighty-three percent of young sailors considered the Navy's drug testing program to be the primary deterrent to drug abuse; 26% said that they would probably resume if the drug testing program were dropped (Mulloy, 1989).

A longitudinal study was conducted more than a decade ago by Rothberg and Chloupek (1978) to evaluate the subsequent military performance of soldiers who were identified by the Army's urine screening program as having used drugs when they reported for active duty. The study compared outcome measures from the medical and personnel files of more than 1,600 urine-positive and more than 2,400 urine-negative males. They found that urine-positive individuals were more likely not to complete their tour of duty and were more likely to be hospitalized and have more bed-days per hospitalization than their urine-negative counterparts. However, a separate analysis failed to demonstrate any benefit to the Army as a whole from drug testing. The authors constructed a drug-free cohort by deleting data on all those who had tested positive, and compared the outcomes of that group with those of a similarly sized random cohort that contained an estimated 2% urine-positive (the then current prevalence). Because the prevalence of drug use was so low in the random cohort, there was little difference between the two cohorts with regard to subsequent military performance.

A recent investigation has also found that test results may be useful in predicting the subsequent performance of individuals in the military. Blank and Fenton (1989) compared the service records of nearly 500 Navy recruits who tested positive for THC (tetrahydrocannabinol) with a control group who tested negative. After 2.5 years, 81% of the THC-negative and 57% of the THC-positive group were still in the Navy. Fourteen percent of the drug-positive group and 1% of the drug-negative group left the service for drug or alcohol problems. Twenty-one percent of the positives and 8% of the negatives were discharged for other behavioral or performance reasons. However, these comparisons did not attempt to control for differences between the groups that may have contributed to the difference in attrition, such as education, intelligence, and race. They did find significant differences in high school education; more of the THC-negatives had finished high school (94% vs. 87% of the THC-positives). In addition, a significantly higher percentage of the THC-positive group was black. Also, THC-positives as a group scored significantly lower than THC-negatives on the Armed Forces Qualification Test, a test that correlates highly with standardized measures of intelligence.

In Law Enforcement

McGlothlin (1980) described the success of the first year of a heroin control program in Singapore that combined urine surveillance with strict law enforcement. In 1975, Singapore experienced a sudden heroin epidemic that within two years involved an estimated 3% of the 15- to 24-year-old males. In 1977, the government responded with a comprehensive enforcement strategy to reduce the demand for heroin through large-scale arrests of suspected users and the immediate commitment of those with positive urines to drug rehabilitation centers. The primary rehabilitation emphasis was on instilling discipline, social responsibility, and sound work habits. Releases were placed on two years of compulsory supervision and were required to report at five-day intervals for urine testing. Within the first year of supervision, 63% showed no detected drug use. Supply reduction efforts were equally strong and although they were not immediately successful in limiting availability, heroin became very scarce and expensive. There was some evidence that addicts were substituting cannabis, psychotropic drugs, and alcohol, but the number of new heroin cases was minimal. McGlothlin concluded that, overall, the epidemic appeared to have been controlled.

In the United States today, drug testing of people who have been arrested or who are under the supervision of the criminal justice system serves several purposes. Drug testing of probationers and parolees is a method of monitoring drug use and verifying abstinence, which is often a condition of release. Because of the known association between drug abuse and criminal activity, individuals who are identified as drug-dependent can be referred to drug abuse treatment programs and regularly monitored for drug use, which is supposed to reduce both drug abuse and crime. Also, the testing of arrestees can help to identify individuals with health problems known to be associated with drug use, especially intravenous drug use, such as hepatitis and AIDS. Furthermore, urine testing of arrestees continues to serve as a surveillance tool and a data source, providing information on community drug use trends and patterns of drug availability.

In the Workplace

A few studies have examined the effectiveness of preemployment screening in identifying drug users, with contradictory results. One early study by Dupong (1971) reported on the usefulness of pre-employment screening in two New York City medical units of NY Telephone. During an 11-month period in 1970–1971, 10,841 male job applicants were examined and 1,023 specimens were found positive for one or more drugs. Applicants who tested positive were reinterviewed by an experienced physician, and their employment and medical histories were reevaluated. Three hundred forty-seven (3.2%) were later classified as too high a risk for employment because of drug involvement. The authors considered the program a success, even though a few problems were found, such as the use by a few

applicants of tranquilizers and sedatives to calm them for the interview process, and the legitimate use of some drugs for medical conditions that applicants neglected to report on their medical history forms.

In contrast, Hilker, Asma, Daghestani, and Ross (1975) described a different experience with pre-employment screening at the Illinois Bell Telephone company. In 1971, 488 applicants were tested. Thirty-two tests (6.6%) were positive for various drugs. Only three (0.6%) were positive on retest. One of these failed to show up for a third time; one was referred to a drug clinic, then hired when pronounced clean; the other was disqualified because of a medical condition. At the same time, another utility company in Chicago tested approximately 500 applicants and had similar results. In both companies, the positives were mainly for heroin. The authors concluded that the drug problem was not of sufficient magnitude in the population seeking employment to warrant screening every applicant. Screening was subsequently used only selectively on clinical indication.

More recently, Lewy (1983) reported on the lack of utility of pre-employment urine screening on prospective hospital employees in New York in 1981. Thirty-three (6.6%) examinations were positive for one or more of either Valium, barbiturates, amphetamines, phencyclidine, or opiates. Only 13 (2.6%) were confirmed to be positive. Of those with confirmed positive results, only one applicant was denied employment, and that case would have been suspected during the clinical preemployment examination.

The first case in which the Supreme Court upheld the government's right to require urine tests for Customs Service employees seeking drug-enforcement jobs was *National Treasury Employees' Union vs. Von Raab,* 86-1879 (1988). An attorney for the National Treasury Employees Union argued that in the two years since Customs Service employees had been required to provide a urine sample in a supervised setting and to test negative for drugs in order to obtain a promotion, only five employees out of a total of about 3,600 tested (0.1%) had positive results. The Customs Service already had many other tools to investigate employee drug abuse, including an aggressive internal affairs division. Nevertheless, the court upheld the government's right to require drug testing.

One study that compared the results of preemployment screening with subsequent job performance failed to support the assumptions that rehabilitating or removing the drug abuser from the workplace would result in increased productivity and decreased on-the-job accidents and impairment-related medical expenses. Parish (1989) used data from all employees hired over a six-month period at a large hospital in an urban area. Results of the screening were kept confidential. After a year of employment, the personnel folders of all employees studied were reviewed. Twenty-two of 180 employees (12%) had tested positive for drug use. Comparison of job performance variables, job retention, supervisor evaluations, and reasons for termination showed no significant differences between drug-positive and drug-negative employees. Drug-negative employees received better performance evaluations than did drug-positive employees, but the difference wasn't statistically significant. Eleven of the 158 (7%) drug-negative employees were fired during the study; none of the 22 drug-positive employees were fired. Because the groups were so small, valid statistical comparisons could not be made. Parish recommended that further studies of this kind are needed. If impairment in job performance is found to be associated with drug use, techniques to identify drug users should be supported. If no relation between job performance can be found, the money being spent on drug testing programs should go to other programs.

A recent report supports the assumption that job performance is related to drug use. Normand and Salyards (1989) described an ongoing evaluation of preemployment drug testing in the U.S. Postal Service. The study involves all 5,465 applicants (of whom 4,375 were hired) for permanent positions in 21 participating sites during the study period. Urine testing for amphetamines,

barbiturates, benzodiazepines, cannabinoids, cocaine, methadone, opiates, and phencyclidine was part of the preemployment medical evaluation. The results were not released to Postal Service personnel and therefore did not influence the decision to hire or any other personnel action. Two outcome measures, absenteeism and turnover (termination), were evaluated to determine whether they were related to drug test results and, if so, to describe the degree of association. The findings demonstrated that the drug-positive employees' odds of being fired were approximately 1.5 times the odds of drug-negative employees. Those who tested positive for cocaine were twice as likely to be terminated than those who tested negative. The frequency of absenteeism was also related to drug test results. Employees who tested positive for any drug were more than 1.75 times as likely to be absent as those who tested negative; those who tested positive for marijuana were twice as likely to take a moderate amount of leave; and those who tested positive for cocaine were more than three times as likely to take a large amount of leave.

In a separate study of postal workers in Boston by Zwerling, Ryan, and Orav (1990), in which test results did not influence hiring and the outcome measures were absenteeism and accidents, applicants who tested positive for marijuana or cocaine were found to have 78–128% more absences and 55–85% more industrial accidents than other employees. The authors compared these figures with previous estimates that workers who use drugs are involved in 200–300% more accidents, sustain 400% more compensable injuries, and use 1500% more sick leave than do workers who do not use drugs. They concluded that the risk in hiring drug users, though significant, may be lower than previously estimated.

Drug testing is expensive. The initial immunoassay screen may cost $15–$35 per urine sample, and up to $100–$200 for each confirmation test. Employers may be reluctant to pay to test all employees for drug use when so few are found to be positive or when no economic benefit has been realized.

A recent evaluation by Crouch and colleagues (1989) of the effectiveness of the drug testing program of the Utah Power and Light Company included a cost–benefit analysis. The UP&L's program includes pre-employment, before promotion, after accident, performance-related, voluntary, and rehabilitation screens. The authors compared two study groups (a drug-positive group and a voluntary rehabilitation group) with two control groups that were frequency matched by age, sex, job classification, years of service, and geographical area. The results of Student's t-tests that compared each study group with its control group demonstrated significantly more absenteeism in both the drug-positive and the drug rehabilitation groups than the control groups. Although there was no clear pattern related to drug-using groups in expenditures for medical benefits, medical injury accidents were reduced after the introduction of drug testing. The greatest costs to UP&L associated with drug-abusing employees were unexcused absences, the use of sick days, and employee turnover. The greatest savings was estimated to result from pre-employment screening because it eliminated employees at high risk for being terminated for drug abuse or for leaving voluntarily. The authors concluded that the initial startup costs and operating expenses for drug testing were more than made up by eliminating drug-positive employees at pre-employment screening.

Random selection may be more cost-effective because only a sample of eligible employees are actually tested. The Department of Transportation's random drug testing program went into effect in December 1989. Its testing programs affect 3,000,000 long-distance truckers; 538,000 aviation employees, pilots, flight attendants, and mechanics; and 200,000 merchant seamen and other mariners. The Transportation Department estimated that its program will cost more than $2.1 billion in the first 10 years but will save $8.7 billion in increased productivity, accident reductions, and medical savings. However, a recent study of one Department of Transportation testing laboratory found shortcomings that could limit the anticipated financial benefits. Wick, Brawley, and Berger (1992) compared pre-placement testing by a DOT laboratory with testing by an American Airlines laboratory of applicants for positions with that company. The authors found that the DOT laboratory was less sensitive to marijuana and cocaine, which represented the bulk of illicit drug use. The company's laboratory also detected barbiturates and benzodiazepines, two classes of drugs not tested for by the DOT laboratory that could have major safety—and economic—implications in the aviation industry.

As yet there are no published reports to prove the benefits of random testing. However, there have been a number of studies evaluating an analogous random testing procedure: sobriety checkpoints, or roadblocks, to detect drunk drivers. A number of studies are relevant with respect to the success of such random testing procedures to prevent alcohol-related traffic accidents. The majority demonstrate that the effectiveness of sobriety checkpoints is short-term and depends on the amount and type of related publicity, which increases a driver's belief in his or her risk of being stopped while driving drunk and his or her fear of punishment.

Under usual circumstances, a driver's risk of being stopped is very low. Beitel, Sharp, and Glauz (1975) computed the probability of arrest in Kansas City in 1972 given a particular blood alcohol level (BAL). They estimated the unconditional probability of being arrested by a skilled officer for driving while intoxicated (DWI) and the probability that a driver who has not been arrested was DWI. By using Bayes' theorem, they constructed a table of probabilities of arrest given a particular BAL. They determined that the probability of being arrested with a BAL greater than or equal to 0.10% was .005 (1 in 200).

Anda, Remington, and Williamson (1986) computed a still lower risk. They calculated the probability of being arrested while driving intoxicated in Michigan in 1982. Their data included information about the prevalence of driving while intoxicated within the previous four weeks obtained from a random telephone survey of 1,492 Michigan adults. The authors projected that 500,000 of the 6.3 million adults in Michigan had driven while impaired in the previous month. Using their estimates and police data on drunk-driving arrests in 1982, they estimated that the risk of being arrested during an episode of alcohol-impaired driving is 4 in 1,000, or .004. They also estimated the cost of each drunk-driving arrest in terms of police time, each arrest costing two to six hours of officer time. To arrest all drunk drivers would require at least 1 million police-hours per month, which would be equivalent to 6,250 officers working full-time to manage the paperwork and other logistic problems following drunk-driving arrests.

Christoffel (1984) evaluated the efforts that had been made in other countries and in some U.S. states to reduce drunk driving. In the 1970s in England, the "Cheshire Blitz" was instituted to routinely administer breath tests to all drivers involved in accidents or committing traffic violations between 10 P.M. and 2 A.M. In New Zealand, cars were stopped for equipment checks as a preliminary to breath tests. The most effective deterrence occurred in Australia, Canada, and the United States where roadblocks were used. Because the perceived likelihood of being arrested based on an officer's observing erratic driving behavior is low, roadblocks were most effective if well-publicized and if the punishment for drunk driving was swift and severe. Similarly, Homel (1983) found that the number of fatal accidents fell significantly in the first three months after random breath testing was introduced in New South Wales, Australia in December 1982. After surveying 400 drivers, the author concluded that the effects of random breath testing were maximized by both strict law enforcement and vigorous publicity. When drivers think that their chances of being stopped and tested are high, they will not drink and drive; however, as the threat of being stopped seems less likely, their prudence diminishes.

Ross (1985) analyzed data on injury accidents in Delaware between December 1982 and August 1983, when checkpoints were in use. During that period, there was a 10% decrease in injury accidents and a 32% decrease in alcohol-related injury accidents compared with a previous control period. One Maryland county had a 75% decline in deaths from alcohol-related accidents during a checkpoint period between July 1982 and July 1983. A survey of residents revealed that people in counties that frequently used checkpoints believed that they had a greater chance of being arrested, even though their reported drinking and driving behavior was similar to that of residents in other counties. The author suggested that more checkpoint activity might be required to attain a notable deterrent effect. Of possible deterrents, the author concluded, the most effective in the short term are those that affect the drivers' perceptions of the certainty of punishment.

CONTROVERSIES OVER TESTING

The current controversy over drug testing spans several arenas and generates ongoing debates within the medical, scientific, legal, and lay communities (West & Ackerman, 1993). One issue concerns the polarity between the right of the individual to privacy on one hand and the right (or need, or demand, or employment precondition) of others to know—the prerogatives of society— on the other. Other issues concern the relative effectiveness of urinalysis in providing accurate information about drug use and personal impairment. The technology of drug testing is not infallible. False positives and false negatives do occur. Furthermore, opponents of workplace drug testing have questioned the validity of testing, which should be to detect physical or mental *impairment* caused by drugs, rather than merely to detect the *presence* of drugs.

The most frequent legal argument against drug testing refers to protections guaranteed by the Constitution and the Bill of Rights. The Fourth Amendment guarantees the right of citizens to be "secure in their persons, houses, papers, and effects against unreasonable searches and seizures." The Fifth Amendment protects citizens against self-incrimination. Most people agree that forcing a worker to submit to a urine test does constitute a search under the Fourth Amendment; however, the principal controversy is whether drug testing represents an unreasonable search. The courts must balance the degree to which the search represents an intrusion on the individual's Fourth Amendment right and the degree to which the search reflects a legitimate government interest.

Drug testing has also been challenged because it violates an individual's right to privacy. Although the Constitution contains no specific provision guaranteeing such a right, it may be inferred from several provisions taken together along with the Fourth and Fifth Amendments. The right to privacy generally refers to an individual's self-interest in avoiding disclosure of personal information and in protecting his or her independence in making certain kinds of personal decisions. By requiring employees to reveal specific information about their persons, drug testing procedures may be an invasion of privacy. The right to privacy has also been invoked against the practice of directly observing urination to ensure that an individual does not substitute or tamper with the specimen.

An additional challenge to mandatory drug testing is based on the requirement of the Fourth and Fifth Amendments that the government provide an individual with due process before depriving him or her of life, liberty, or property. Although due process is not specifically defined in the Constitution, court decisions in drug testing cases have generally interpreted due process as a requirement that urine specimens be properly handled and that positive samples be accurately confirmed. Due process also applies to the procedures for termination of employment if a worker is to be discharged after a positive drug test has been confirmed.

The courts have generally sanctioned the use of drug testing when evidence has been presented that the health and safety of other employees or the public are at stake. They have also upheld testing if there is reasonable suspicion of a need to test. Testing programs are more likely to be sanctioned if employees who test positive are given a chance to be rehabilitated rather than fired.

Although private employers generally are not bound by constitutional restrictions because the company, rather than the state, is taking the action, the distinction between public and private employer is not always clear. For example, a public utility that is regulated by the federal government may be subject to constitutional restraints even if it is privately owned. A company doing business by contract with the government may be subject to the same standards as a public employer. Also, when the government requires private employers to conduct employee drug testing programs (in the transportation industry, for example), such a requirement may represent sufficient public involvement as to make it subject to constitutional guarantees. Furthermore, state constitutions may extend their protections to employees in private industry or state-regulated industries and limit the power of employers in ways that the federal constitution does not.

Another area of controversy pertains to the relative effectiveness of urinalysis in providing accurate information about drug use. Current technology makes it possible to test urine, blood, saliva, breath, and hair for the presence of alcohol, steroids, stimulants, sedatives, opiates, hallucinogens, and other chemicals. However, this technology is not infallible. Legal challenges have been made concerning the reliability of test results, especially the possibility of false-positive findings in pre-employment drug screening and in criminal proceedings. False negatives are more likely to be cited in arguments against the cost-effectiveness of drug testing programs.

Accuracy depends on the prevalence of drug use within the tested population. Screening methods are less accurate when tests are routinely administered to a population in which the overall prevalence of drug use is quite low. Both the sensitivity (ability to accurately detect) and specificity (ability to accurately reject) are impaired. When the sensitivity of a test is reduced, the number of false negatives is increased. This means that samples that do contain the screened-for substance are not identified. Conversely, when the specificity of a test is reduced, the number of false positives increases. Thus, samples are incorrectly identified as containing the screened-for substance. The consequences of each error depend on the purpose of the screening. A false positive may be more damaging to the employee, whereas false negatives undermine the entire drug testing program (Goldsmith, 1988).

Accuracy also depends on whether the proper procedures are followed for collecting, handling, and analyzing the urine. Even before a specimen reaches the testing laboratory, a number of problems can occur to invalidate the results. Deliberate tampering, dilution, or the adding of adulterants can invalidate the tests. Accidental contaminants or mislabeling may occur. It is therefore necessary to ensure a proper chain of custody during the collection, preparation, and analysis of each sample.

Montagne, Pugh, and Fink (1988a) advised that the reliability of the laboratory that performs the analysis must be considered. Unfortunately, in 1972 when Lundberg first called drug testing "chemical McCarthyism," the existing technology was so imperfect that the performance of even the best toxicology laboratories was grossly defective, with error rates on unknown samples commonly as high as 20–70%. However, the results of such screenings were responsible for an employee's getting and keeping his job, an addict's freedom, and a soldier's future employability (Lundberg, 1972).

A study by Frings, White, and Battaglia (1987) demonstrated that the accuracy of drug detection by laboratories has improved. All laboratories that participated in the study were currently performing urine drug testing for preemployment or continuing employment purposes. The laboratories were challenged to detect drugs in eight specimens at the concentrations at which they normally accept business. Of the 47 laboratories, 36 accurately identified all drugs present, 8 performed at 97.5% accuracy, and 3 performed

with more than 95% accuracy. The overall accuracy was better than 95%. The overall false-negative rate was 0.76% (14 of 1,832 trials) and the false-positive rate was 0.05% (1 of 1,847). The authors suggested that in previous studies of this kind, the laboratories may have been scored inaccurately because they used technology designed to detect higher concentrations of the drugs than were weighed into the study specimens. This points up the need for laboratories and clients to be specific about the threshold concentrations used to report positives and policies for reporting positives detected below those concentrations.

The validity of test results is another area of controversy. Although current screening methods can reveal whether a certain substance is present in the urine, they can't distinguish between legitimate and illicit use of prescription drugs or between certain street drugs and common foods and over-the-counter medications that have the same metabolites, and they can't determine how much, how often, or how recently a drug was taken (Willette, 1991). Related to these are concerns about the relationship between the pharmacodynamic (dose and response) and the pharmacokinetic (drug metabolism, distribution, and clearance) profiles of each individual (Goldsmith, 1988).

Perhaps most importantly, there is considerable debate over whether ingestion of a certain amount of a drug will without question impair a given individual's performance at certain tasks. Currently, although there is a statistically *relative* relationship between drug levels and degrees of impairment, there is no *absolute* correlation of the degree of behavioral impairment with the measured level of a detected drug in a given person. Morgan (1984) argued that cost estimates of drug abuse are based on the questionable assumptions that dysfunctional work (or life) and a history of use or the presence of a drug are causally related, and that people who use drugs will inevitably malfunction in a fashion similar to the drug abusers seen in treatment programs. He questioned these assumptions because there is no proven correlation between a positive urine test for drugs and observed or assessed human behavior. After reexamining the issue of drug screening 14 years after his initial commentary, Lundberg (1986) wrote that under no circumstances could impairment be diagnosed or even presumed from a urine test result. Similarly, Montagne, Pugh, and Fink (1988b) cautioned that test results are meaningful only if they are correlated with a clinical state.

The American Medical Association has called for the development of tests to detect impairment caused by drug and alcohol use rather than to detect drug use. In 1984, the AMA supported the testing program proposed by the Federal Railroad Administration that called for testing after accidents, before employment, and for reasonable cause, and the establishment of employee assistance programs to treat employees who have a drug or alcohol problem. However, it recommended to the FAA that a more effective approach would be to develop a method of detecting mental and physical impairments that may result from alcohol and drug abuse or dependence rather than a chemical method of detecting alcohol or drug use. Later, the House of Delegates adopted a report by the Council on Scientific Affairs that concluded that drug testing does not provide any information about mental or physical impairments that may be caused by drug use or about patterns of abuse (AMA Council of Scientific Affairs, 1987).

RECOMMENDATIONS AND CONCLUSIONS

The AMA Council on Scientific Affairs (1987) recommends that drug and alcohol testing of employees should be limited to pre-employment examination of people whose jobs affect the safety and health of others, situations in which there is reasonable suspicion that an employee's job performance is impaired by alcohol or drug use, and monitoring of patients in comprehensive programs of treatment or rehabilitation for alcohol and drug abuse or dependence. Lundberg (1986) argues that because functional impairment can-

not be diagnosed or even presumed from a urine test result, the principal purpose of urine screening is legal, not medical. He declares that if society feels that the problems of drug abuse are so great as to justify the threat to individual freedom through mandatory random urine drug screening, then the decision should be made by the electorate, probably through state-by-state referenda.

Because drug testing is expensive, the program that detects the greatest proportion of positives should be the most cost-effective. Cost can be minimized by applying screening programs to populations known to have a high prevalence of drug use and by conducting random testing. Although random testing is probably the most controversial, it may be the most effective both in reducing costs of drug abuse and in deterring drug use. By testing only a fraction of the target population, the expense of testing is kept low. In addition, the perceived risk and uncertainty involved in being selected and tested discourages drug use.

One additional consideration is the expense of defending drug testing programs in the courts. Most current programs can be legally challenged in one way or another. The determination in each case will depend on the nature of the search; who is searched, why, and when; and what is done with the results. The courts have generally sanctioned the use of drug testing when evidence has been presented that the health and safety of other employees or of the public are at stake. They have also upheld testing if there is reasonable suspicion of a need to test. Workplace testing programs are more likely to be sanctioned if employees who test positive are given a chance to be rehabilitated rather than fired. Within the context of current policies, Lubran and Jasper (1988) advise that drug testing programs require careful planning. They should include a written policy that specifies which drugs will be screened, who will be tested, the frequency and mode of testing, and what will be the sanctions if tests are positive; determination of a chain of custody for the urine specimen and maintenance of confidentiality; careful selection of the drug testing laboratory; establishment of what concentrations of each drug constitute a positive test; and interpretation of positive results by an expert.

When the damage to society is evaluated in economic measures, the rationale for drug testing programs is expressed in terms of money saved by the prevention of accident-related loss of life and property and reduced productivity. However, the majority of screening programs have not been set up to detect the costliest drug of abuse—alcohol. Alcohol abuse and alcoholism account for two-thirds of the total cost of alcohol and drug abuse. However, the majority of drug-testing programs analyze urine specimens, and urinalysis is not the most effective way to assess alcohol intoxication. Blood and breath are the specimens of choice for determining alcohol levels, with breath-testing being the less invasive procedure. Therefore, to maximize the effectiveness of detecting chemically impaired workers while minimizing the intrusion, drug testing programs should probably include breath tests for alcohol. It is highly probable that if Zwerling, Ryan, and Orav (1990) had tested applicants of the Boston Postal Service for alcohol use and included alcohol-positive subjects in their analysis, the costs due to accidents and absenteeism would have been substantially more, approaching the cited higher estimates of financial losses due to employee substance abuse.

As one weapon in the government's "war on drugs," drug testing has had some success. It has enabled employers to detect drug use among employees and applicants. When combined with drug treatment programs, it has contributed to the rehabilitation of the drug user. When applied to job applicants, it has identified drug users before they were hired. From the employer's perspective, therefore, drug testing has helped to prevent the consequences of drug abuse. However, to the individual drug user denied a job because of a positive urine test, and to the society on which he or she must remain (unemployed and) dependent, drug testing may compound the problems caused by drug addiction. Except within certain populations, such as the military where close surveillance is possible and toler-

ated, drug testing alone does not appear to prevent drug abuse and addiction. It must be a part of a concerted effort to educate and rehabilitate.

REFERENCES

AMA Council on Scientific Affairs (1987). Issues in employee drug testing. *Journal of the American Medical Association, 257* (22), 3110-3114.

Anda, R. F., Remington, P. L., & Williamson, D. F. (1986). A sobering perspective on a lower blood alcohol limit [letter]. *Journal of the American Medical Association, 256* (23), 3213.

Beitel, G. A., Sharp, M. C., & Glauz, W. D. (1975). Probability of arrest while driving under the influence of alcohol. *Journal of Studies on Alcohol, 36* (1), 109–116.

Blank, D. L. & Fenton, J. W. (1989). Early employment testing for marijuana: Demographic and employee retention patterns. In S. W. Gust & J. M. Walsh (Eds.), *Drugs in the workplace: Research and evaluation data.* NIDA Research Monograph 91. Washington, DC: ADAMHA, 139–150.

Christoffel, T. (1984). Using roadblocks to reduce drunk driving: Public health or law and order. *American Journal of Public Health, 74* (9), 1028–1030.

Clarke, E.G.C. (1969). Dope and doping. *Medicine, Science, and the Law, 9* (4), 218–223.

Coombs, R. H., & Ryan, F. J. (1990). Drug testing effectiveness in identifying and preventing drug use. *The American Journal of Drug and Alcohol Abuse, 16* (3–4), 173–184.

Crouch, D. J., Webb, D. O., Peterson, L. V., Buller, P. F., & Rollins, D. E. (1989). A critical evaluation of the Utah Power and Light Company's substance abuse management program: Absenteeism, accidents and costs. In S. W. Gust & J. M. Walsh (Eds.), *Drugs in the workplace: Research and evaluation data.* NIDA Research Monograph 91. Washington, DC: ADAMHA, p. 169–194.

DeAngelis, G. G., McCaslin, F. C., & Ungerleider, J. T. (1978). Drug use and employment patterns before and during treatment. *The International Journal of the Addictions, 13* (8), 1183–1205.

Dupong, W. G. (1971). Urine chromatography in testing for drugs in applicants for work. *Journal of Occupational Medicine, 13* (10), 459–464.

Frings, C. S., White, R. M., & Battaglia, D. J. (1987). Status of drugs-of-abuse testing in urine:

An AACC study. *Clinical Chemistry, 33* (9), 1683–1686.

Goldsmith, M. F. (1988). Drug testing upheld, decried physicians asked to help decide [news]. *Journal of the American Medical Association, 259* (16), 2341–2342.

Hawks, R. L., & Chiang, C. N. (1986). *Urine testing for drugs of abuse.* NIDA Research Monograph no. 73. Washington, DC: ADAMHA.

Hilker, R. R., Asma, F. E., Daghestani, A. N., & Ross, R. L. (1975). A drug abuse rehabilitation program. *Journal of Occupational Medicine, 17* (6), 351–354.

Homel, R. (1983). The impact of random breath testing in New South Wales, December 1982 to February 1983. *Medical Journal of Australia, 1,* 616–619.

Kaistha, K. K. & Tadrus, R. (1978). Need for urine drug testing. *Journal of Pharmaceutical Sciences, 67* (01–06), iv.

Lewy, R. (1983). Preemployment qualitative urine toxicology screening. *Journal of Occupational Medicine, 25* (8), 579–580.

Lubran, M. M. & Jasper, K. T. (1988). Drug abuse in the workplace. *Annals of Clinical Laboratory Science, 18* (1), 6–12.

Lundberg, G. D. (1972). Urine drug screening: Chemical McCarthyism. *The New England Journal of Medicine, 287* (14), 723–724.

Lundberg, G. D. (1986). Mandatory unindicated urine drug screening: Still chemical McCarthyism. *Journal of the American Medical Association, 256* (21), 3003–3005.

McGlothlin, W. H. (1980). The Singapore heroin control programme. *Bulletin on Narcotics, 32* (1), 1–14.

Milby, J. B., Toro, C., Thronton, S., Rickert, D., & Clarke, C. (1979). Some urine surveillance effects on drug abusers in psychotherapy. *British Journal of Addiction, 74,* 199–200.

Montagne, M., Pugh, C. B., & Fink III, J. L. (1988a). Testing for drug use, Part 1: Analytical methods. *American Journal of Hospital Pharmacology, 45* (6), 1297–1305.

Montagne, M., Pugh, C. B., & Fink III, J. L. (1988b). Testing for drug use, Part 2: Legal, social, and ethical concerns. *American Journal of Hospital Pharmacology, 45* (7), 1509–1522.

Morgan, J. P. (1984). Problems of mass urine screening for misused drugs. *Journal of Psychoactive Drugs, 16* (4), 305–317.

Mulloy, P. (1989). Yeas, nays of drug testing. *News Chronicle,* Thousand Oaks, CA, Jan. 8.

Mulloy, P. (1991). Winning the war on drugs in the military. In R. H. Coombs & L. J. West (Eds.), *Drug testing: Issues and options.* New York: Oxford University Press, 92–112.

Normand, J., & Salyards, S. (1989). A empirical evaluation of preemployment drug testing in the United States Postal Service: Interim report of findings. In S. W. Gust & J. M. Walsh (Eds.), *Drugs in the workplace: Research and evaluation data.* NIDA Research Monograph 91. Washington, DC: ADAMHA, pp. 111–138.

Oseid, S. (1984). Doping and athletes—Prevention and counseling. *Journal of Allergy and Clinical Immunology, 73,* 735–744.

Parish, D. C. (1989). Relation of the pre-employment drug testing result to employment status: A one-year follow-up. *Journal of General Internal Medicine, 4* (1), 44–47.

Puffer, J. C. (1986). The use of drugs in swimming. *Clinic in Sports Medicine, 5* (1), 77–89.

Ross, H. L. (1985). Deterring drunken driving: An analysis of current efforts. *Journal of Studies on Alcohol,* Suppl. 10, 122–128.

Rothberg, J. M., & Chloupek, R. J. (1978). A longitudinal study of military performance subsequent to civilian drug use. *American Journal of Public Health, 68* (8), 743–747.

Singh, J. M., Singh, M. D., & Miller, L. H. (1972). Behavior patterns of addicts on a methadone substitution program as indicated by urine analysis. In J. M. Singh, L. H. Miller, & H. Lal (Eds.), *International symposium on drug tolerance, addiction, abuse, and methadone treatment, 1971, Xavier University of Louisiana College of Pharmacy.* Mount Kisco, NY: Futura, 183–186.

U.S. Department of Health and Human Services (1988). *Mandatory guidelines for federal workplace drug testing programs: Final guidelines.* Washington, DC: Superintendent of Documents, USGPO.

U.S. Department of Health and Human Services (1990). *Seventh special report to the U.S. Congress on alcohol and health.* DHHS Pub. no. (ADM)87-1519. Washington, DC: Superintendent of Documents, USGPO.

Wagner, J. C. (1987). Substance-abuse policies and guidelines in amateur and professional athletics. *American Journal of Hospital Pharmacology, 44* (2), 305–310.

West, L. J. & Ackerman, D. L. (1993). The drug-testing controversy. *Journal of Drug Issues, 23,* 579–595.

Wick, R. L., Brawley, W. L., & Berger, B. T. (1992). A survey of pre-placement urinalysis drug findings. *Aviation, Space, and Environmental Medicine, 63,* 56–59.

Willette, R. E. (1991). Techniques of reliable drug testing. In R. H. Coombs & L. J. West (Eds.), *Drug testing: Issues and options.* New York: Oxford University Press, 67–91.

Winek, C. L., & Esposito, F. M. (1987). The validity of urine alcohol analysis in drunk drivers. *Legal Medicine,* 97–106.

Wolfe, A. C. (1974). *1973 U.S. national roadside breathtesting survey: Procedures and results. Interim report.* Prepared for the National Highway Safety Administration. Washington, DC: Superintendent of Documents, USGPO.

Zwerling, C., Ryan, J., & Orav, E. J. (1990). The efficacy of preemployment drug screening for marijuana and cocaine in predicting employment outcome. *Journal of the American Medical Association, 264* (20), 2639–2643.

CHAPTER 23

USER ACCOUNTABILITY

JOHN R. HEPBURN

The principal focus of U.S. drug control policy has been to interrupt the supply of illicit drugs. Government agencies attempt to prevent the growth and harvest of plants both here and abroad, to interdict efforts to import illegal drugs to the United States, and to arrest, prosecute, and confine those who manufacture, transport, distribute, and sell illegal drugs. In the terminology of classical economics, these law enforcement efforts are designed to curb the supply side of the exchange in this illegal market.

More recently, the demand side of the drug market has received increased attention. Users and potential users have been the focus of a variety of rather traditional educational and treatment programs that aim to reduce the level of demand for illegal drugs. In addition, there has been a surge of support for user accountability as a demand reduction strategy. In its simplest form, user accountability calls for policies that hold drug users legally accountable for their behavior.

The inclusion of user accountability as a strategy of demand reduction represents a major shift in social definitions, assumptions regarding human behavior, and social policy. This chapter reviews the development of the concept of user accountability as a demand reduction strategy, outlines a prototypical user accountability program, and assesses the problems and prospects of user accountability as a drug control policy.

CONCEPTUAL DEVELOPMENT OF USER ACCOUNTABILITY

To some degree, demand reduction has long been a part of the official response to "the drug problem"

in the United States. Government-sponsored pamphlets, films, speakers, and other forms of mass communication have sought to educate and inform the public of the dangers of drug use for more than 50 years. These efforts often sensationalized the effects of drug use and presented incomplete or inaccurate information, yet they were an integral part of the effort to reduce the demand for drugs. Not coincidentally, these efforts also legitimized legal action against drug users. For the most part, drug addicts—and not casual drug users—were subject to criminal sanctions, but drug control policies have changed substantially since 1988.

Demand Reduction as a Means of Drug Control

A wide variety of drug education and prevention programs were in operation during the first half of the 1980s, but the focus of most of these programs was on schools. In Texas' War on Drugs program, begun in 1979, school drug policies and youth groups were the basis of an educational approach to the prevention of drug use by young people (Barron, 1988). The Los Angeles Police Department initiated the Drug Abuse Resistance Education (DARE) program in 1983, assigning uniformed officers to teach school children how to "just say no" to drugs (Gates, 1986). In 1984, the Federal Bureau of Investigation (FBI) and the Drug Enforcement Administration (DEA) combined efforts to form the Sports Drug Awareness Program, which provided school athletic coaches with literature and training on drug abuse prevention (Webster, 1986). During this same period, Omaha, Nebraska initiated a comprehensive program to develop drug awareness in all public and private schools and to solicit public denouncement of drug abuse by local sports celebrities (Wadman & Crowley, 1986).

These and other prevention programs were, in effect, programs to reduce the demand for drugs. However, it was not until 1986 that demand reduction became an official strategy in the U.S. war on drugs. Both FBI Director William Webster (1986) and DEA Administrator John C. Lawn (1986) outlined the importance of demand reduction and called for more public education and prevention programs like their own Sports Drug Awareness Program. Also in 1986, drug abuse was declared Public Enemy Number One by the Board of Officers of the International Association of Chiefs of Police. After pointing out the futility of focusing all attention on only the supply side, the board resolved that "The only rational response left to the problem by the people of the United States will be found in the launching of an all-out, concentrated campaign with an additional strategy to include a major national effort to reduce demand for these illegal substances" (IACP Board of Officers, 1986, p. 2).

Federal funds to support increased public education and treatment programs were made available when the 1986 Anti-Drug Abuse Act formally established a demand reduction agenda and earmarked millions of dollars to support such programs. That same year, Lawn created a Demand Reduction Section within the DEA "to direct the agency's efforts in the area of drug abuse prevention and education," proclaiming that "the ultimate answer in solving the problem lies in reducing the demand. Until we can convince our citizens—particularly our young people—of what drug abuse is doing to their minds and bodies, the demand for drugs will always be there. And until the demand is reduced substantially, the supply will be available" ("DEA sets up new section," 1986, p. 4).

In 1987, the National Drug Policy Board was established by the Reagan administration to highlight a national concern with the drug problem (Koven, 1989). The board formed two coordinating groups—an enforcement group to address the issues of drug supply and a drug abuse prevention and health group to propose demand reduction strategies. Demand reduction was viewed as a means of reducing the supply of drugs, and demand was to be reduced by using education and treatment to define drugs as socially undesirable. That same year, the nation's major advertising agencies formed the Partnership for a Drug-Free America and began a sustained campaign of public service announcements designed to create a public consensus of intolerance toward drugs.

User Accountability and Demand Reduction

These early efforts to call attention to the need for demand reduction emphasized education, prevention, and treatment, especially among young people. Law enforcement was not a part of demand reduction, and anyone urging the arrest of drug users was criticized for wanting to redirect police activities away from those who were profiting from the crime—the drug trafficker and seller. Soon, however, law enforcement and punishment, which had been the exclusive province of the supply-side effort, became a part of the strategy to reduce demand. User accountability took on a special meaning as it was used to publicize and promote this new rationale for arresting users. As greater attention focused on demand reduction generally, the strategy of user accountability gained momentum and legitimacy.

In 1985, Charles Blau, head of the Organized Crime/Drug Enforcement Task Force (first formed by President Reagan in 1982), reported that drug users should be arrested and prosecuted because they are as much a part of a "conspiracy chain" as those who distribute it. At the same time, Attorney General Edwin Meese stated that "there is no such thing as a harmless recreational drug" and that he wanted "the individual drug users . . . to understand the moral responsibility that they bear" ("IDL update," 1985, p. 7). Early the next year, the President's Commission on Organized Crime recommended both the repeal of state laws that had decriminalized marijuana possession and the prosecution of drug users ("Justice Department to begin arresting," 1988).

In 1987, Donald Ian MacDonald, director of the White House Office of Drug Abuse Policy, stated publicly that the president had agreed to a plan to arrest drug users. In testimony before the House Select Committee on Narcotics Abuse and Control, MacDonald identified three general categories of people with regard to drug use. One category consisted of those who do not use drugs, and the White House policy was to educate these people against future drug use with drug prevention programs. A second category was made up of people already addicted to drugs, who needed treatment. Recreational drug users formed the third group, and White House policy called for legal sanctions against these occasional users to reduce demand. This policy was clarified by the testimony of Frank Keating, assistant secretary of the Treasury for enforcement: "We, as a law enforcement community, wish to make drug use painful. We wish to make sure that anyone who uses drugs, and who traffics in drugs, suffers" (O'Connell, 1987, p. 10).

By 1988, the use of criminal sanctions against drug users was gaining momentum. The nature of this impetus for user accountability is evident in the 1988 position paper of the International Association of Chiefs of Police, which also illustrates just how far the IACP had broadened its range of demand reduction activities since its 1986 resolution. IACP executive director Gerald Vaughn (1988, p. 18) wrote:

While demand reduction strategies primarily focus on prevention and education, it would prove to be more effective if used in conjunction with a carefully designed and prudent deterrence-oriented strategy that reinforces each citizen's right and responsibility to live, work, and be educated in a drug-free environment by holding those accountable who choose to consume illicit drugs. User accountability programs focus on a punitive
approach that seeks to deter drug abuse through criminal and/or social sanctions that send a powerful message that drug use will not be tolerated.

Although the way was prepared by MacDonald, Vaughn, Lawn, and others, a national policy of user accountability was not established until the passage of the Anti-Drug Abuse Act of 1988 (Koven, 1989). Among the Act's landmark provisions was the creation of a Cabinet-level director of drug policy (a "drug czar") to oversee the many activities and provisions authorized by the Act. It called for strict drug enforcement and a policy of zero tolerance and it increased the arsenal of weapons available in the war against the supply of drugs, including the death penalty for drug kingpins. The 1988 Act also laid out a comprehensive demand reduction strategy that included a user accountability provision. Drug users could be denied specific federal benefits, including grants, loans, contracts, or licenses provided by any agency of the federal government. People possessing even small amounts of illegal drugs could be fined up to $10,000 by the U.S. attorney general. The secretary of Housing and Urban Development was authorized to evict tenants engaged in any criminal acts, including use of drugs. Federal contractors were required to make good faith efforts to maintain a drug-free workplace or risk suspension, termination, or debarment from contracts. Furthermore, driver's license applicants in a four-state pilot program were to be tested for illegal drug use, and those who tested positive could be denied driving privileges for at least one year.

In 1989, the Drug Enforcement Administration's position on user accountability was articulated by DEA administrator John Lawn. The attention to drug users is warranted, Lawn argued, because "[u]ser accountability attacks the idea that there can be any such thing as a casual or recreational user of drugs" (1989, p. 49). To address this problem, Lawn proposed increased public education about the dangers of drug use, greater attention to establishing a drug-free workplace, and appropriate actions to increase the certainty and severity of punishment for illegal drug users.

User Accountability and a National Drug Control Strategy

By the end of the decade, the transformation was complete. The Office of National Drug Control Policy (ONDCP), directed by "drug czar" William Bennett, issued its first national strategy in 1989, highlighting the central importance of user accountability in future drug control policies.

> There are two ways to influence whether an individual decides to use drugs. One is to make him not want to use them. Information and moral persuasion obviously help shape an individual's preferences, attitudes, and desires. The other approach is to make an individual fear the consequences and penalties that society will impose for drug use by making it clear that the costs will outweigh whatever temporary benefits drugs can provide (Office of National Drug Control Policy, 1989, p. 47).

After noting that drug use should have a price, the 1989 *National Drug Control Strategy* urged a broad-based range of sanctions against users. Military-style boot camps and halfway houses were called for, as were legal fines, property forfeiture, and denial of federal contracts and benefits. Furthermore, the ONDCP advocated a variety of less formal sanctions, especially for first offenders and occasional users: suspended driver's license, notification of employer, identification in local newspapers, overnight or weekend detention, and forfeiture of cars driven during purchase or use of drugs. For juveniles, accountability could be achieved by notification of parents, suspension from school, community service activities on weekends, and suspension of (or delay in application for) driver's licenses.

Originally designed to harass and punish drug suppliers, asset forfeiture laws also became an important weapon in the war against drug users. The 1970 Comprehensive Drug Abuse Prevention and Control Act declared that all controlled substances and all materials and equipment used to manufacture or distribute controlled substances were subject to civil forfeiture. Subsequent modifications by Congress permit the forfeiture of all real property used in any manner to facilitate a violation of drug laws, including monetary instruments, homes, businesses, tracts of land, and vehicles. These state and federal laws have raised serious questions about the applicable rules of evidence and the placement of the burden of proof in these civil proceedings (Stahl, 1992). Further controversy surrounds the disposition of the seized assets and whether the availability of these assets to law enforcement agencies leads to profit-oriented police activities. When applied to casual users, asset forfeiture raises the added question of whether the punishment is disproportionate to the crime.

What has emerged, in summary, is a national policy designed to bring legal and social sanctions against drug users generally, but the specific target is the recreational or occasional drug user. Many states have enacted laws requiring stiff penalties against casual drug users (Knapp, 1989). For example, Indiana legislated court fees of $100–$400, with the funds to be used to support undercover police units and prosecutors. In New Jersey, people convicted of any drug offense automatically lose their driving privilege for six months to two years. In Rhode Island, anyone driving under the influence of drugs must pay a $400 fine, an amount that supports the offender's treatment. In Florida, driving under the influence of alcohol or drugs results in a suspended license, and all drivers' license applicants must complete a drug education course.

The most widely adopted approach to date is the reverse sting. Undercover police make controlled buys from drug sellers working the street, arrest the sellers, and then substitute their own undercover officers as sellers. People who buy (or attempt to buy) illegal drugs from these officers are arrested immediately after the transaction. Operation Sting was begun in Miami, Florida in 1986, and during its first year the program produced 927 felony arrests, 2,147 misdemeanor arrests, seizure of 1,000 vehicles, and forfeiture of $73,577 (Dickson, 1988). Reverse stings have been used with varying success elsewhere, including Nashville, Tennessee (Drug Enforcement Administration, n.d.), Inglewood, California (Carter & Knowles, 1987), and Washington, D.C. ("Justice Department to begin arresting," 1988). A variation of this approach has been used by the Los Angeles County Sheriff's Office, which watched known sellers to identify users and then arrested the users a short distance away (DEA, n.d.).

USER ACCOUNTABILITY IN OPERATION: THE MARICOPA COUNTY DEMAND REDUCTION PROGRAM

The Maricopa County, Arizona Demand Reduction Program has received high acclaim and national visibility. Begun in March 1989, it was heralded as a success only six months later by DEA Administrator John Lawn (1989). In September 1989, President Bush was asked how to fight a successful war against the casual drug user; he replied: "Go to Phoenix, folks. Take a look at what they're doing there." Soon thereafter, the program was profiled on national television network programs, including CBS's *48 Hours* and *Morning News,* ABC's *Primetime Live,* and NBC's *Today Show,* and in the *Wall Street Journal* and other newspapers from around the country. Legislators, prosecutors, and police administrators have visited Phoenix to see for themselves the inner workings of this program, which has captured the national spotlight.

A consortium of municipal, county, state, and federal law enforcement agencies located in Maricopa County, Arizona initiated the program. A task force made up of the heads of the 26 participating agencies proposed ways to address the problem of illegal drug use in the City of Phoenix and surrounding metropolitan area, with a combined population exceeding 2 million.

A formal structure of an executive committee and subcommittees developed (see Figure 23.1) and specific goals were identified. According to the executive committee, the mission of the Demand Reduction Program was as follows:

- To promote a wide, community-based commitment toward accomplishing the goal of a drug-free county
- To increase public awareness of the consequences of illicit drug use
- To assist public and private sector leaders in backing their commitment to a drug-free workplace with effective action
- To assist in the development and incorporation of educational programs
- To participate in coordinated programs to identify and target illegal drug users for concentrated enforcement efforts
- To provide low-cost counseling and treatment opportunities for drug users

The first four objectives strive to educate the general population and private sector employers to the fact that drug use is harmful and that those who use drugs will be held legally accountable. The goal is to create a communitywide awareness of the severity of the problem—to develop a moral consensus—and to alert drug users to the increased risk of legal sanctions. If effective, these demand reduction activities will prevent or deter drug use.

The final two objectives focus on the arrest, prosecution, and possible diversionary treatment of drug offenders. Here, the emphasis is on increased and coordinated law enforcement activities directed against individual offenders and on special treatment programs in lieu of prosecution. Together, they enlist the criminal justice system to achieve demand reduction via user accountability.

Do Drugs. Do Time

In Maricopa County, the message that users are subject to criminal penalty has been widely disseminated through the public campaign slogan "Do Drugs. Do Time." Depending wholly on private sector contributions of time, expertise, money, and equipment, a major advertising campaign informs the public that casual drug users

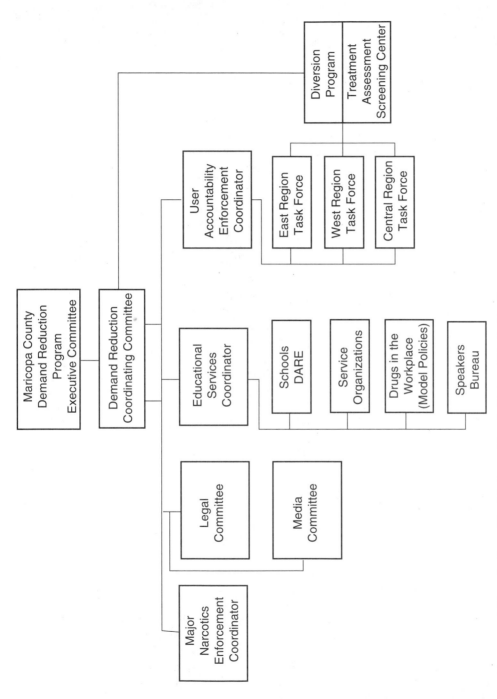

FIGURE 23.1. Organization of the Maricopa County Demand Reduction Program
Participating agencies include the Arizona Department of Public Safety, the Drug Enforcement Administration, the Federal Bureau of Investigation, the United States Attorney's Office, the Maricopa County Sheriff's Office, and the local law enforcement agencies of Arizona State University, the City of Phoenix, and each of the 17 other municipal police agencies in suburban Phoenix.

are the target of stepped-up law enforcement efforts. Placards on city buses, billboards above major streets and highways, and televised public service announcements proclaim that those who do drugs can expect to do time. As the examples in Figures 23.2 and 23.3 illustrate, this deterrent message is directed at stereotypical casual or recreational users: white, young adults with a high level of education and a comfortable style of living.

The promise of the "Do Drugs. Do Time." warning may be fulfilled in several ways. At minimum, people arrested for drug use will spend at least a few hours in the county jail while they are booked and await an initial hearing. It is hoped that the prospect of arrest, formal booking, and short confinement in a holding cell will be a sufficient sanction to deter many of the middle-class casual users targeted by this program. Because possession and use of even the smallest amount of illegal drugs are felonies in Arizona, "Do Drugs. Do Time." also implies that a period of incarceration awaits convicted users. Finally, even offenders who are diverted to a treatment program can be seen as "doing time" during the 6–24 months they are under the supervision and surveillance of the treatment program.

Arrest and Prosecution or Diversion to Treatment

The user accountability program consists of four separate components, as illustrated in Figure 23.4. Two of these components are heightened law enforcement efforts, the third is increased prosecution, and the fourth is diversion to treatment via the Adult Deferred Prosecution Drug Program. Increased enforcement by uniformed patrol officers is expected to result in increased arrests for drug use, as are the coordinated enforcement activities of the task force. These arrests, in turn, are backed by greater prosecution efforts by the county attorney. To minimize the added burden on the county attorney's office and on the courts, however, eligible offenders may be diverted from prosecution to a drug-specific treatment program.

Task Force Operations

A unique feature of this program is the formation of the Maricopa County Task Force, a committee representing the many law enforcement agencies in Maricopa County. Each agency has one or more representatives on the task force, but the size is made more manageable by dividing the county and its many agencies into three regions: east, central, and west. Each region has its own task force commander, and these commanders work with the task force coordinator to obtain the necessary assistance in personnel and equipment to carry out specific operations anywhere in the county.

The task force coordinates and conducts two types of operations. One is the reverse sting, used in an area of curbside drug sales. Drug sellers are arrested and replaced by undercover officers, and anyone attempting to buy drugs from these undercover officers is arrested. The second type of operation targets known sites of heavy public drug use (such as nightclub parking lots, rock concerts, and recreational areas) for surveillance and arrests. In either case, the operations are infrequent and sporadic events, but their high local visibility and media coverage publicly reinforce the "Do Drugs. Do Time" message.

Uniformed Patrol Officers

Uniformed patrol officers, who encounter the largest number of users through routine traffic stops and field calls, are the backbone of the program. Officially, of course, full enforcement of drug (and all other) laws has been the policy and practice for all uniformed patrol officers. Unofficially, however, the reactions of these officers are known to vary—sometimes enforcing the law, sometimes confiscating the substance without filing charges against the offender, and sometimes just overlooking the infraction altogether. In general, the officers' practices are thought to reflect their view of the likelihood of prosecution, and

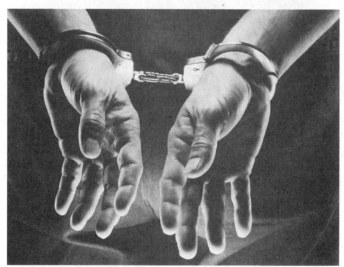

FIGURE 23.2.
Reprinted with permission of the Maricopa County, Arizona Demand Reduction Program.

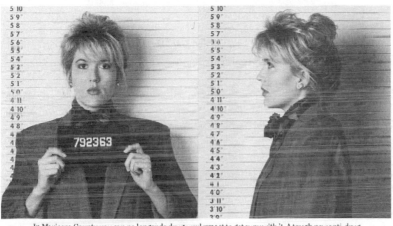

FIGURE 23.3.
Reprinted with permission of the Maricopa county, Arizona Demand Reduction Program.

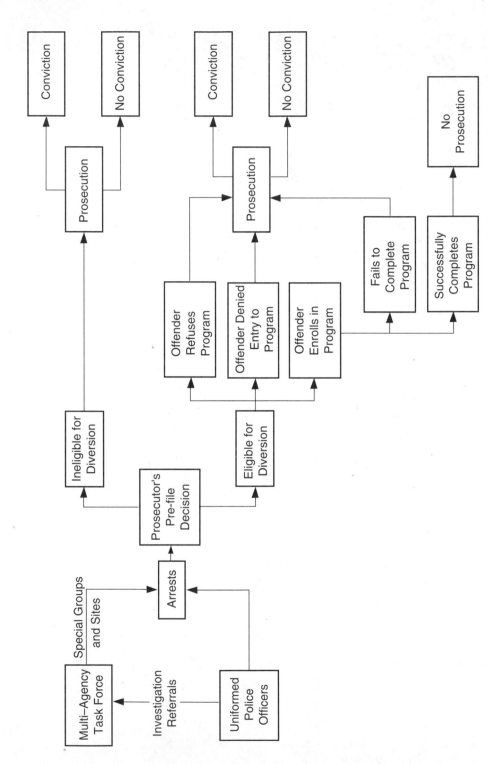

FIGURE 23.4. Demand Reduction Program: Components and Process

arrests are unlikely when subsequent prosecution is unlikely.

In recognition of the crucial role played by uniformed patrol officers, each participating agency directed its uniformed patrol force to take strong enforcement action against users encountered during the normal course of their duties. Patrol officers were assured that the county attorney's office would prosecute or divert each case that was properly founded and documented.

County Attorney

The Maricopa County Attorney's Office prosecutes virtually all offenders who don't qualify for, accept, or successfully complete the diversion program. Qualifications vary somewhat by the nature of the drug possessed, but their general purpose is to offer diversion to only casual users with no prior criminal history. For possession of marijuana, for instance, eligibility for diversion is limited to offenders who do not have either a referral for any other felony charges or any other felony charges presently pending, a prior drug or marijuana felony conviction, a prior drug or marijuana misdemeanor conviction within the past year, felony probation or parole status, prior participation in a felony or misdemeanor diversion program, or transient status.

Eligible offenders may reject the diversion program, but those who enter the program must agree to certain conditions. Random urinalysis tests are required, for example, as is attendance at all seminars, lectures, and counseling sessions. Most controversial, perhaps, is the requirement that all offenders, other than those charged with possession of marijuana, must provide a written statement of facts admitting the instant offense and agreeing that this statement will be admissible in a court of law should the offender fail to complete the diversion program.

Adult Deferred Prosecution Drug Program

This program by Treatment Alternatives to Street Crimes (TASC, a national consortium of treatment programs) removes first-time felony offenders from the prosecutor's caseload and the court's calendar and provides them with a community-based treatment program designed to reduce subsequent drug use. There are four drug-specific treatment programs, which vary in duration, objectives, and methods used to achieve those objectives. Each program involves some combination of random urine testing and an educational seminar, and all but the program for marijuana possession involve some degree of individual or group counseling sessions.

In addition to meeting all requirements of the diversion program, successful completion requires full payment of all fees assessed the offender. Each offender booked and held at the county jail must pay a jailhouse processing fee of $50. The offender also must pay an Arizona Drug Enforcement Fund fee, which varies by drug type from $500 for possession of marijuana to $1,200 for possession of cocaine. Finally, the offender is assessed a fee equal to the costs of the diversion program, which range from $135 for the 120-day possession of marijuana program to more than $1,600 per year for the 12–24 month programs for either cocaine or illegal prescription drugs. A sliding schedule of fees is used for lower-income offenders, and a total waiver of all fees is available for indigent cases. Because total fees may amount to $685–$5,000, the payment of fees may be stretched over 24 months.

Critical Components of the Maricopa County Program

This brief overview of the Maricopa County Demand Reduction Program highlights the features that distinguish it from other demand reduction programs. In general, the uniqueness of the program can be reduced to six components, each of which is critical to its success.

First and foremost, this is a comprehensive program. Whereas other programs rely on a single approach, the Maricopa County program integrates education, law enforcement, and treatment into a unified campaign against casual drug use. Preventive education is targeted to schools, churches, and civic groups, and employers are singled out for special information about establishing a drug-free workplace. Attempts to deter drug use rely on placards, billboards, and televised public service announcements to spread the message that drug users are criminals who will be arrested and prosecuted, and by frequent media coverage of high-profile task force stings and sweeps designed to reinforce this perception by the public. Deterrence also is the objective of increased law enforcement by uniformed police officers. Finally, treatment is available for those who meet the eligibility criteria.

Another critical component is the complete participation of all law enforcement agencies in the affected area. Anything less than a united effort by all local police departments, it was felt, would send a mixed message to the community and may result in gaps in coverage, with a subsequent displacement effect on drug sellers and users. It also provides a singular voice and a unified program plan and creates a pool of personnel, equipment, information, and other resources designed specifically for this program.

Third, the program is distinguished by a high level of community support. Public opinion favored increased education about drugs and tough actions against drug users. In Maricopa County, even casual drug use is viewed as psychologically and morally harmful and public opinion supports severe sanctions for even casual users. Local media have lent their support by extensive news coverage and favorable editorials. Most unusual, perhaps, is the high level of financial support received from the private sector, which provided more than $500,000 in donated time, equipment, and materials to produce and distribute the "Do Drugs. Do Time." posters and television announcements during the first nine months of the program. In 1991, the private sector prepared and financed a more narrowly focused "Put Drugs Out of Work" advertising campaign to promote a drug-free workplace.

Fourth, the Maricopa County program is aided by tough laws. In Arizona, any illicit drug use is a felony. Use or possession of even the smallest amount of marijuana, for instance, is a Class 6 felony (the lowest level), and anyone convicted of this offense may be sentenced to prison for up to 18 months and/or fined the greater amount of $750 or three times the value of the marijuana possessed. The threat of a felony conviction provides more latitude to the prosecutor and increases the likelihood that offenders will accept diversion to the treatment program.

The fifth feature is the program's ability to generate revenues to offset some of its financial costs. Such funds are collected only from those who enter the diversionary treatment program, and then the amounts vary according to the offender's ability to pay. Nonetheless, during the first 24 months of operation, a total of $39,342 was collected in jailhouse processing fees and $850,411 was collected in the Arizona Drug Enforcement Fund. These funds are independent of the fees assessed to cover the costs of the user's participation in the treatment program.

Finally, the program is characterized by close monitoring of all cases. To be credible and effective, the program must keep the inevitable attrition of cases to a minimum: People on bond must appear, treatment staff must chart the progress of each offender, offenders who reject or fail treatment must be prosecuted, and prosecutors must bring all cases to a timely resolution. An automated case management system tracks each case through the system and identifies problem areas as they develop.

Implementation Decisions in Community Programs

No single user accountability program can be packaged for easy adoption elsewhere. In considering such a program, each community must openly discuss and debate the desired nature, scope, and intensity of the program. Will it include education, treatment, and law enforcement, or will it be solely a program of law enforcement? Within the law enforcement component, discussion must focus on the amount of resources to be allocated, the type of actions (such as reversals or sweeps) to be taken, and the implications for meeting the community's other demands on the criminal justice system. Furthermore, this discussion must address the nature of the community's unique drug problem and drug laws in weighing the ability of a user accountability program to have the desired impact.

The option of diversion to treatment must be examined. If diversion is an option, who is to be eligible for this alternative to legal sanction? Should it be reserved for only the truly casual users of certain drugs (such as marijuana) who have no criminal history or should it be made available to heavy users and addicts, to users of any illicit drug, or to people with a criminal history? What about users who also are sellers?

A voluntary diversion program also raises the question of the incentives for participation, which are considerably reduced if possession is not a felony or if the fees and costs approach or exceed those likely to result from conviction. These criteria and incentives for diversion are important for two reasons. First, the more restrictive the criteria and the lower the incentives for diversion, the greater the proportion of offenders who require prosecution and court resources. Second, the criteria and incentives must not create unequal treatment on the basis of socioeconomic status.

THE DEBATE OVER USER ACCOUNTABILITY

The appropriate response to drug use has been discussed and debated for decades. The Harrison Narcotic Act of 1914 and the Marijuana Tax Act of 1937 are two of the most visible mileposts in this ongoing, often heated, debate, but it also is punctuated with numerous court rulings, state and municipal laws, and pronouncements by medical professionals, law enforcement officials, and citizen groups. User accountability programs rekindle this debate.

Changing Social Definitions

Through the 1960s and 1970s, the debate centered on the physiological and psychological harmfulness of drug use, on the addictive characteristics of various drugs, and on the likelihood that marijuana use would inevitably lead to the use of cocaine and heroin (Skolnick, 1968; Mor-

ris & Hawkins, 1970; Goode, 1972). Viewed in that context, there was little impetus to bring strong criminal sanctions against users. By the mid-1980s, however, the context of the debate was altered substantially.

A new social definition of drug users was promoted widely by the White House and major law enforcement officials in an effort to create a public climate of intolerance to drug users. The debate over the harmfulness of drugs to the users was abandoned as unproductive, and the debate was recast in terms of the moral harm to society. Drug users were defined as a moral problem—as a threat to our way of life—and as co-conspirators with the drug suppliers in far-ranging criminal activities.

Gerald Vaughn, executive director of the International Association of Chiefs of Police, for example, argued that drug users share the responsibility for far more serious crimes committed by those who market drugs. "Drug users are co-conspirators in criminal cartels that deal in death, corruption and extreme violence. It is the user who supplies the reason for the trafficker and producer to exist. Users cannot escape responsibility for their actions that are wreaking havoc on our society" (Vaughn, 1988, p. 18).

John Lawn, administrator of the Drug Enforcement Administration, articulated a similar view (1989, p. 49): "Although users would deny their culpability, they must be made to realize that through their collective purchases *they* bankroll every drug murder that is committed. *They* contribute to the bribery. *They* contribute to the subversion and ruin of communities—indeed, whole nations. *They* trigger their own destruction, often pulling loved ones down with them" (italics original).

The Debate Continues

For simplicity, the debate about the legitimate response to illicit drug use can be organized around three questions. The answer to each question varies substantially, however, depending on which social definition of drug use prevails.

Is drug use a legal problem? Not all undesirable behaviors can be regulated by law, Packer

(1968) argues, and criminal law should be reserved for behaviors that cannot be regulated by alternative means. Since before the Harrison Narcotic Act of 1914, critics have argued that drug use should not be treated as a legal problem (Skolnick, 1968; Duster, 1970; Beyerstein & Hadaway, 1990). As Morris and Hawkins bluntly state in their book *The Honest Politician's Guide to Crime Control,* "the invocation of the criminal process is wholly inappropriate. . . . Neither the acquisition nor the purchase nor the possession nor the use of drugs should be a criminal offense" (1970, p. 8).

One popular alternative is to regard drug use as a public health problem (Goode, 1972; Erickson, 1990). Potential users should be dissuaded by educational campaigns, not the threat of arrest; current users need medical care, not criminal punishment. From this perspective, criminal laws are counterproductive because they amplify the problems of users and inhibit the opportunities for successful treatment. An effective response to drug use requires decriminalization or, preferably, legalization of drug use (Geis, 1972; Walker, 1985; Aldrich, 1990).

The conception of drug users as a dangerous class of people justifies law enforcement efforts in the name of demand reduction. Because users contribute to the criminal conspiracy of traffickers, it is argued, their containment and control requires legal sanctions rather than medical treatment. It is noteworthy that this shift also redirects attention from drug addicts to casual drug users. Compared to addicts, casual users are less questionably a legal problem than a public health problem, and casual users are more likely than addicts to be deterred by the threat of criminal sanctions. Accordingly, criminal sanctions against casual users are both justified and effective. At minimum, arresting the previously immune casual users should disrupt and destabilize the illegal drug market.

Is drug use a serious problem? Criminologists distinguish two general types of offenses. *Mala in se* offenses are natural wrongs, or acts that are judged to be wrong by the moral senti-

ments of the society, such as murder, rape, and robbery. In comparison, *mala prohibitum* offenses are regulatory wrongs, or acts that are wrong because they are legislated rather than because they evoke strong moral feelings. Drug use, especially casual drug use, has no inherent moral evil; it is a *mala prohibitum* offense (Walker, 1985; Skolnick, 1990). Advocates of user accountability, however, seek to create a collective sense of moral outrage against drug users.

The seriousness of the problem also can be measured in terms of its magnitude in society. Casual drug use is prevalent among young adults, but available evidence suggests that the number of casual users has decreased rather dramatically throughout the 1980s. The National Institute of Drug Abuse (NIDA) reports that the use of marijuana and most other illicit drugs by high school seniors peaked in 1980, and that use of cocaine peaked in 1985. Because supply has remained rather constant, this reduction in use among high school seniors is attributed to a significant reduction in the social approval of drug use. NIDA's National Household Survey also reports a decrease in casual use among adults throughout the 1980s, although the decrease among adults has not been as dramatic as that among high school seniors.

Although large numbers of people report having used illegal drugs at least once in their life, most drugs are consumed by a very small percentage of the population. NIDA reports that only one-half of those who have ever used marijuana and only one-third of those who have ever used cocaine went on to use these drugs 11 or more times in their lifetime. Relatedly, the National Narcotics Intelligence Consumer Committee reports that heavy users and addicts make up less than 7% of the user population but consume three-fifths of the cocaine in the United States (Falco, 1989; Skolnick, 1990).

Is this the best use of criminal justice resources? Law enforcement activities against users often raise questions about arbitrary policing practices and the relative merits of expending the resources of police and courts on users. In the broader war against crime, what priority is assigned to drugs relative to such *mala in se* crimes as homicide, rape, robbery, and theft? Within the scope of those resources committed to the war on drugs, how many resources should be allocated to users? On one hand, if one defines drug use as a rather benign and victimless crime, then drug-fighting resources should be consolidated against drug sellers and traffickers, popularly viewed as parasites and profiteers. If, on the other hand, users are a part of the problem, then they should receive part of the resources.

At a time when rates of other crimes are increasing and court dockets, jails, and prisons are overcrowded, user accountability has the potential to further strain the criminal justice system with this new class of criminals. At a time of diminished resources, the use of criminal sanctions against drug users—either with or without some program to divert offenders from prosecution or incarceration—is a net widening strategy that will place a greater burden on the resources that do exist.

What's at Stake?

It is interesting that this redefinition of drug users should occur when it did. As noted, the incidence of casual drug use was in decline. Courts and prisons already were overcrowded. Education and prevention programs appeared to be reducing the demand for illegal drugs. Less successful, however, were law enforcement efforts directed at the supply side. Interdiction efforts were judged a failure, and little or no additional benefit was expected from allocating increased resources to the battle against traffickers and sellers (Reuter & Kleiman, 1986; Moore, 1990).

Once casual use is redefined as a threat to our way of life and a new moral consensus is created, law enforcement becomes a means of demand reduction. The severity of the threat justifies a policy of zero tolerance and opens the political door to the possibility of increasingly more repressive measures. The goal is not to merely lower the amount of casual use, but to achieve a "drug-free America."

THE EFFECTIVENESS OF USER ACCOUNTABILITY STRATEGIES

Like any program, user accountability can be evaluated in terms of both process and outcome. The process evaluation must determine the fit between the program as designed and the program as implemented and identify needed program changes. The outcome evaluation will assess the program's ability to achieve stated goals. The Drug Enforcement Administration (n.d.), for example, suggests that user accountability can be evaluated in terms of recidivism rates, cost-effectiveness, and community support. The evaluation of the Maricopa County Demand Reduction Program (Hepburn, Johnston, & Rogers, 1991) focused on the integrity of the program as implemented, recidivism among offenders diverted to the drug treatment program, and changes over time in the arrest and conviction of drug users and sellers. The evaluation concluded that the program had achieved most of its goals, but the evaluation was not able to address the major question of the extent to which such programs actually lower (deter) the level of casual use of drugs.

In fact, there is reason to believe that user accountability programs will have only limited success in reducing the demand for illicit drugs among casual users. User accountability is a single-strategy approach being applied to a very complex problem involving a very heterogeneous user population.

The user's demand for drugs can be expressed as a function of causes, supports, and costs:

Demand = Causes + Supports + Costs

Causes is the complex array of psychological, medical, and socioeconomic background factors that are thought to increase one's desire for or susceptibility to illicit drugs. Although the etiology of drug use is not clear, it is evident that increased law enforcement efforts do not address this element of demand.

Supports are the social acceptance of drugs among both the broader community and one's significant others, association with people who use drugs, and the informal social organization that arises among drug users to provide them with drug-using occasions. The educational efforts of demand reduction programs attempt to reduce social acceptability, and heightened and visible law enforcement efforts also provide a public definition that casual drug use is unacceptable. For the most part, however, law enforcement operations are not designed to reduce the level of supports for causal drug use.

The final component in the demand equation is *costs*. Indeed, the argument that increased enforcement deters casual users is premised on the assumption that people behave rationally, choosing their course of action on the basis of anticipated costs and rewards. It appears that law enforcement activities can have their greatest impact on casual drug users by affecting the costs of drug use.

There are two types of costs. Typically, cost is conceptualized in terms of legal sanctions, or the probability of detection, arrest, and conviction for use of illicit drugs. Vigilant reactive and aggressive proactive policing, proponents of user accountability argue, deter casual drug use by substantially increasing the likelihood of legal sanctions (Zimmer, 1990). However, heightened enforcement efforts also increase a second type of cost to the drug user—the inconvenience encountered in casual use of illegal drugs. Increases in the price and scarcity of drugs are an inconvenience because they require the user to expend increased time and energy to obtain the desired drugs (Moore, 1977; Kleiman, 1989). Disruptions of the drug market also inconvenience the user by making more problematic the certainty of the source, the quality of the drugs, and the reliability of the connection (Manning & Redlinger, 1983).

Just how viable is a strategy of law enforcement to deter casual drug users? Although in theory police activities can deter drug users by increasing the costs of legal sanction and inconvenience, the impact of police activities on casual users is limited in practice. Indeed, these limitations raise important questions about the viability of user accountability programs as a strategy to reduce casual drug use.

The casual user enjoys a certain amount of impunity from detection. There is no complaining victim, for instance, to expose the offender to authorities. In addition, exposure is minimized because casual drug use is episodic in nature rather than of sustained duration, is spontaneous and sporadic rather than predictable and regular, and occurs in private places with restricted access to complainant witnesses and police. Sweeps occur in public places, but drug users learn to reduce their exposure by moving to the privacy of their homes for such illegal activities. Reversals target curbside service, but casual users reduce their exposure to risk because they often have friends or associates who deal, because they conduct these business transactions in private places, and because they reduce the number of transactions by purchasing larger amounts in a single transaction.

Can user accountability succeed in reducing the demand for illicit drugs by casual users? Yes. It will not affect the social causes or supports, but active enforcement that results in increased arrests, prosecutions, and convictions should measurably increase the costs of drug use. Perhaps the major impact of a user accountability program is more symbolic than instrumental, however. That is, because user accountability programs rely on the deterrent effect of increased risk of arrest and sanction, what is essential to the success of such a program is its high visibility in the community. The mere implementation of such a program, together with publicized activities and arrests, alerts casual users that the costs of continued drug use have been increased.

However, because user accountability is largely irrelevant to the social causes and supports of drug use, its overall impact on demand is minimal. Furthermore, because the effect of a user accountability program on costs depends on the level of enforcement activity, it seems unlikely that a user accountability program will have an impact on demand that outlives the program.

SUMMARY

Americans have fought a nationwide war on drugs throughout the twentieth century. User accountability is the newest campaign in this war, deploying the armies of law enforcement in the theater of demand reduction. Those who conduct the war struggle to define the enemy as a threat to our way of life. The battle is just, the enemy immoral, and victory occurs only when the last of the infidels is driven out or taken as a prisoner of war. Only then will we achieve our goal of a drug-free America.

The analogy to war can be taken only so far, despite the similarities in public rhetoric. More properly, use of illicit drugs is viewed as a social problem in need of a solution, and the debate centers on the best strategy to ameliorate this problem. Those who struggle for control of the definition of the problem know that the prize is the prescription for the solution. If drug use is a public health problem, then the solution resides in education, prevention, and treatment. If, however, it is a legal problem, then the criminal justice system must intervene.

The concept of user accountability asserts a new rationale for treating casual users as a serious legal problem. Redirecting discussion away from the long-standing debate over the harmfulness of drugs to their users, user accountability is based on the argument that users must be seen as a legal threat because they provide the customer base for the criminogenic suppliers of illegal drugs. Criminal co-conspirators call for legal remedies, and these remedies should affect both the supply side and the demand side of this conspiracy.

The concept of user accountability has been developed at the national level, but its survival depends on local implementation. The Maricopa County Demand Reduction Program contains a rather comprehensive and integrated user accountability program, and it illustrates the general principles and criteria of such a program. Programs will vary by locale, however, to reflect local conditions and objectives. Without external funds, few communities will be able to initiate intensive programs. Without tough laws, the advisability of any program is questionable.

To date, the ability of user accountability programs to reduce demand is untested. Tighter enforcement may visibly reduce the use of drugs, or at least reduce the visible use of drugs, but the effect will last only as long as the heightened police activities.

The greater promise of user accountability is its symbolic statement. With little effort beyond what currently is expended locally, each community can publicly endorse the concept that casual users contribute to the legal problems of fighting drug suppliers, announce its intentions to get tough with users, and showcase any subsequent arrests of users as signs of the new get-tough policy. The effect will be threefold. First, the endorsement becomes a part of the broader education program to potential and current users, thus inhibiting demand. Second, the endorsement removes social support for drug users by creating a community definition of drug use as an unacceptable behavior. Third, a publicized get-tough policy announces that the risk of arrest has been increased, thereby gaining whatever deterrent benefit accrues when increased certainty of sanction is communicated to potential offenders.

Finally, we must not lose sight of the fact that user accountability must be a temporary approach to the problem of drug use. At best, it is a stopgap measure to stem the tide until the demand is significantly reduced by education programs, especially those directed to young people. At worst, it is but another of a long list of proposals and programs that have been tried and discarded, some because interest wanes, some because they are replaced by newer ideas, and some because they fail.

REFERENCES

Aldrich, M. (1990). Legalize the lesser to minimize the greater. *Journal of Drug Issues, 20,* 543–553.

Barron, B. (June 1988). Texans' war on drugs—A national model. *The Police Chief,* 37, 41.

Beyerstein, B., & Hadaway, P. (1990). On avoiding folly. *Journal of Drug Issues, 20,* 689–700.

Carter, L., & Knowles, L. (1987). The narcotics reverse sting: You can't trust anyone these days. *Journal of California Law Enforcement, 21,* 77–83.

DEA sets up new section to reduce demand for drugs (1986). *Narcotics Control Digest, 16,* 4.

Dickson, C. (1988). Drug stings in Miami. *FBI Law Enforcement Bulletin, 57,* 1–6.

Drug Enforcement Administration (n.d). *User accountability: A compilation of information including actions by several law enforcement agencies.* Washington, DC: Drug Enforcement Administration.

Duster, T. (1970). *The legislation of morality.* New York: Free Press.

Erickson, P. (1990). A public health approach to demand reduction. *Journal of Drug Issues, 20,* 563–575.

Falco, M. (1989). *Winning the drug war.* New York: Priority Press.

Gates, D. (Oct. 1986). Drug Abuse Resistance Education: A police officer-taught drug prevention program. *The Police Chief,* 54.

Geis, G. (1972). *Not the law's business.* Washington, DC: National Institute of Mental Health, Center for the Study of Crime and Delinquency.

Goode, E. (1972). *Drugs in American society.* New York: Alfred Knopf.

Hepburn, J., Johnston, C. W., & Rogers, S. (1991). *The Maricopa County demand reduction program: An evaluation report.* A report submitted to the National Institute of Justice, U.S. Department of Justice, Washington, DC.

IDL update: Drugs and the law (1985). *Inside Drug Law, 2,* 7.

International Association of Chiefs of Police Board of Officers (Oct. 1986). IACP renews its efforts in war against drugs. *The Police Chief,* 21.

Justice Department to begin arresting and prosecuting drug users (1988). *Drug Law Report, 2,* 20–22.

Kleiman, M. (1989). *Marijuana: Costs of abuse, costs of control.* New York: Greenwood Press.

Knapp, E. S. (Oct. 1989). Fighting back against drugs. *State Government News,* 6–9.

Koven, S. G. (1989). Fighting the drug wars: Rhetoric and reality. *Public Administration Review, 49,* 580–583.

Lawn, J. C. (Oct. 1986). Law enforcement's other role: Drug demand reduction. *The Police Chief,* 35–36.

Lawn, J. C. (Aug. 1989). User accountability: A long-overdue concept. *The Police Chief,* 49–50.

Manning, P., & Redlinger, L. (1983). Drugs as work. In *Research in sociology of work: Peripheral workers,* vol. 2. New York: JAI Press, 275–301.

Moore, M. (1977). *Buy and bust.* Lexington, MA: DC Heath.

Moore, M. (1990). Supply reduction and drug law enforcement. In M. Tonry & J. Wilson (Eds.), *Drugs and crime.* Chicago: University of Chicago Press, 109–158.

Morris, N., & Hawkins, G. (1970). *The honest politician's guide to crime control.* Chicago: University of Chicago Press.

O'Connell, R. (1987). White House's "arrest the user" policy causes heated debate at House hearing. *Narcotics Control Digest, 17,* 1, 8–10.

Office of National Drug Control Policy (1989). *National drug control strategy.* Washington, DC: USGPO.

Packer, H. (1968). *The limits of the criminal sanction.* Stanford, CA: Stanford University Press.

Reuter, P., & Kleiman, M. (1986). Risks and prices: An economic analysis of drug enforcement. In M. Tonry & N. Morris (Eds.), *Crime and justice,* Volume 7. Chicago: University of Chicago Press, 289–340.

Skolnick, J. (1968). Coercion to virtue: The enforcement of morals. *Southern California Law Review, 41,* 588–641.

Skolnick, J. (1990). A critical look at the national drug control strategy. *Yale Law and Policy Review, 8,* 75–116.

Stahl, M. B. (1992). Asset forfeiture, burdens of proof and the war on drugs. *Journal of Criminal Law and Criminology, 83,* 274–337.

Vaughn, G. (Oct. 1988). Combatting the drug problem in the United States. *The Police Chief,* 17–20.

Wadman, R. C., & Crowley, J. M. (June 1986). Omaha, NE: Controlling supply and demand. *The Police Chief,* 44–45.

Walker, S. (1985). *Sense and nonsense about crime.* Monterey, CA: Brooks/Cole.

Webster, W. (Oct. 1986). Federal response to drug threat: Eliminating supply and demand. *The Police Chief,* 43–46.

Zimmer, L. (1990). Proactive policing against street-level drug trafficking. *American Journal of Police, 9,* 43–73.

CHAPTER 24

LEGALIZING/DECRIMINALIZING DRUG USE

RICHARD S. SANDOR

Brer Fox mixed up a big batch of tar and made it into the shape of a baby. Then he took his Tar Baby down to the road, the very road Brer Rabbit walked along every morning. He sat the Tar Baby in the road, put a hat on it, and then hid in a ditch.

from "Brer Rabbit and the Tar Baby,"
adapted from the *Tales of Uncle Remus,*
as told by Julius Lester.

In the Anti Drug Abuse Act of 1988, the United States Congress announced its intention to control illicit drugs:

It is the declared policy of the United States Government to create a Drug-Free America by 1995.

The Congress finds that legalization of illegal drugs, on the Federal or State level, is an unconscionable surrender in a war in which, for the future of our country and the lives of our children, there can be no substitute for total victory.

1. Proposals to combat sale and use of illicit drugs by legalization should be rejected.

2. Consideration should be given only to proposals to attack directly the supply of and demand for illicit drugs, such as proposals to strengthen and expand penalties for sale and use, proposals to encourage greater multinational cooperation in eradication and interdiction, and proposals to promote educational awareness programs for young people.

In order to implement its policy, Congress created a special Office of National Drug Control Policy in the White House (with the "drug czar" as its head), established more severe penalties for drug users and dealers (including the death penalty in some cases), denied specific federal benefits to convicted drug users, brought new precursor chemicals and drug manufacturing devices under regulation, directed foreign aid officials to distinguish between friendly and uncooperative countries, and much more. The complete package was budgeted at more than $5 billion.

The new spending called for in this measure came on top of a previous tripling of federal spending to curb the use of and trade in illicit drugs—from less than $1 billion in 1981 to more than $3 billion in 1987 (Cooper, 1990). This same seven years saw the DEA's budget grow from $200 to $500 million. In 1986, the drug war consumed one-fifth of all state and local law enforcement investigative resources, and in 1987, total government drug control expenditures (federal, state, and local) totaled about $10 billion (Nadelmann, 1989). Since 1980, most of these resources (70% of the 1990 drug control budget, for example) have been spent on what is now called supply-side reduction. In plain English, this strategy has translated into the following tactics:

- Suppression of opium, marijuana, and coca cultivation (domestic and foreign crop eradication and substitution)
- Destruction of clandestine processing laboratories
- Interruption of drug smuggling cartels
- Blockade of the borders against smuggling
- Crippling domestic drug distribution networks

One of the major arguments made by those who want to abandon the war on drugs is that these measures have failed to reduce drug use. In fiscal year 1988, for example, interdiction efforts aimed at keeping drugs from crossing our borders cost $1 billion (accounting for about 25% of that year's program), but instead of reducing supply and raising prices (and, by extension, decreasing use), the street cost of cocaine fell by over 50% (Reuter, 1988). In the same year, a NIDA study estimated that 33% of all Americans had used marijuana (6% used regularly), 11% cocaine (2% regularly), 7% hallucinogens or stimulants, and 5% tranquilizers or sedatives (DHHS report cited in Cooper, 1990).

In addition to their criticism of ineffectiveness, however, drug war dissenters make the more damaging claim that the policy of escalating prohibition has fostered the development of a whole new set of problems worse than the ones it was supposed to solve. Writing for The Drug Policy Foundation, a Washington-based group dedicated to the search for responsible drug law reform, Kevin B. Zeese (Zeese, 1989) asserts that the government's prohibition of drugs has contributed to the following developments:

- Severe overcrowding of the criminal justice system
- Climbing crime rates driven by exorbitant black market drug prices
- Aggressive drug marketing to expand customer bases
- The discovery and spread of more concentrated substances that are easier to conceal and more potent
- Police and governmental corruption, both domestic and international
- Encroachments on privacy and civil liberties protections
- Random drug testing without due cause
- Summary forfeitures (loss of entitlements) in the prosecution of crimes lacking a complaining witness
- Destabilization of foreign countries and skewing of U.S. foreign policy
- The spread of AIDS and other infectious diseases through the sharing of outlawed hypodermic syringes

Ethan Nadelmann, writing in the influential journal *Science,* adds statistical details to some of these points (Nadelmann, 1989):

- Drug law violators account for 10% of 550,000 inmates in state prisons and more than one-third of federal prison inmates.
- Drug trafficking and drug possession offenses accounted for 135,000 (23%) of the 583,000 individuals convicted of felonies in state courts in 1986.
- Police arrested 750,000 people for violations of drug laws each of the last few years. Slightly more than 75% of these were not for manufacturing or dealing, but for possession of an illicit drug (especially marijuana).
- In New York City, drug law violations in 1987 accounted for more than 40% of all felony indictments, up from 25% in 1985; in Washington, D.C., the figure was 50% in 1986, up from 13% in 1981.
- More than half of organized crime revenues are believed to come from the illicit drug business—$10 to $50 billion per year.
- 25% of all AIDS cases result from IV drug use, and the number is growing rapidly. 50% of deaths from AIDS in New York City from 1981 to 1986 were among IV drug users.

There is also the puzzling behavior of government officials who alternately declare victory but then later, citing new evidence of epidemic use, call for redoubled efforts against the burgeoning danger. In 1958, for example, Harry Anslinger, head of the Federal Bureau of Narcotics (FBN) from 1930 to 1962, declared that "cocaine has disappeared," but by 1985, it was reported that fully 40% of all graduating high school seniors had tried cocaine at least once, and interdicted imports of the drug were being measured in tons, not pounds. In 1973, President Nixon proclaimed that the nation had "turned the corner on drug addiction," (King, 1990); however, that same year, official surveys revealed that fully 50% of college students had used marijuana—a fivefold increase from six years earlier. Finally, in 1986, noting statistical evidence of a decline in cocaine and marijuana use among high school seniors (Monitoring the Future Study, 1989), President Reagan stated that his antidrug campaign was "an untold American success story . . . our students are just saying 'no' to drugs" (Reagan, 1987). However, only a few years later, President Bush declared that "the gravest domestic threat facing our nation is drugs" (Lapham, 1989). The American public was convinced and polls conducted in early 1990 revealed that the public regarded drugs as the number-one problem (*New York Times* CBS Poll, 1990).

In the face of the staggering costs of drug prohibition and contradictory governmental communications, a growing and remarkably varied group of public figures has called for a re-examination of the idea of making war on drugs. Long-time liberal critics of narcotics prohibition such as Arnold Trebach and Rufus King have now been joined by some well-known conservatives (William Buckley, George Shultz, and Milton Friedman), a federal judge (Robert Sweet), elected officials (Baltimore Mayor Kurt Schmoke, New York State Senator Joseph Galiber), physicians, academics, and writers.

Not surprisingly, these calls for policy reform have provoked an angry response from those charged with carrying out the congressional mandate. William Bennett, Bush's first White House drug policy advisor, called talk of drug legalization both "stupid" and "morally scandalous"; nevertheless, drug law reform is hotly debated on television, radio, and in the press.

Extreme libertarian critiques notwithstanding (Szasz, 1974), there is no question that the drug problem really is a problem. If nothing else, it is a problem because an enormous mass of people think it is. Beyond this simplistic level, really significant questions, both practical and theoretical, must be asked. Reduced to the bare bones they are these: What kinds of problems does drug prohibition solve? What problems does it create? Is the goal of a "drug-free America" attainable? If so, what means will be required to achieve it? Are these means compatible with democratic values? If the goal is not achievable, what are the consequences of dedicating vast resources to an impossible task?

Henry Ford, prophet of mechanization, once proclaimed that "History is bunk." But because Ford himself is now history, and thus, by his very own standards, also bunk, we might do well to pause a moment and reflect on how we came to be where we are.

A BRIEF HISTORY OF U.S. DRUG POLICY

Brer Fox had scarcely gotten comfortable before Brer Rabbit came strutting along like he owned the world and was collecting rent from everybody in it. Seeing the Tar Baby, Brer Rabbit tipped his hat . . . but Tar Baby didn't say a word.

The evolution of American drug policy cannot be understood without considering the larger historical trends of which it was a part. Up to the end of nineteenth century, an ever-expanding frontier absorbed wave after wave of immigrants—religious, political, and economic refugees who gave the American character its form through the common values of hard work, inventiveness, and self-reliance. During this stage of national expansion (roughly 1750 to 1900), "doctoring" was also a matter of self reliance and most illnesses were treated in the context of one's own family. Organized medicine was nothing like the highly regarded profession it is today—many physicians were poorly educated and their methods (not to mention fees!) incurred as much fear and loathing as gratitude. The violent treatment methods of "approved" medical practice—purgings, bloodlettings, amputations, and so on—gave the "Heroic Age" of American medicine its name, and drove patients into the hands of all kinds of nonphysician healers. Of this period, Oliver Wendell Holmes, Sr., made his famous remark (Holmes, 1891): "I firmly believe that if the whole *materia medica,* as now used, could be sunk to the bottom of the sea, it would be so much the better for mankind—and all the worse for the fishes."

In considering the history of narcotic control, however, it is significant that Holmes did not include the widely used opium in this wholesale condemnation. On the contrary, he noted that "the Creator himself seems to prescribe" it. In addition to being the only really effective sedative and anodyne available, opium was one of the few drugs that alleviated the diarrhea of dysentery and cholera—endemic and epidemic diseases that devastated nineteenth-century Americans.

Following the closing of the frontier, the industrial and transportation revolutions stimulated new influxes of immigrant labor—in the West, Chinese laborers to build the railroads and work in the mines; in the East, European arrivals to labor in the mills and factories. Periods of economic instability sharpened the competition between "foreigners" and those who now regarded themselves as "natives" and gave rise to conflicts with distinctly racist overtones. Some of the first antinarcotic legislation appeared in this context and was simply a legitimized attempt to set the perceived interlopers apart. Thus, in 1878, the city of San Francisco banned opium smoking establishments. The law was clearly intended to make life unpleasant for the Chinese because the city fathers did not deem it necessary to protect the populace from whiskey saloons, where whites did the same things Chinese did in their "dens"—became intoxicated, gambled away wages, and consorted with prostitutes. In any case, there is little doubt that foreign, cheap laborers were resented and that some drug laws were a covert expression of that dislike.

In addition to economic and racist influences on the development of drug control laws, nineteenth-century attitudes towards drugs and drug taking in general were more tolerant (if innocent) than they are today. The spread of basic literacy, coupled with the proliferation of newspapers and unregulated advertising, resulted in the widespread promotion and use of unlabeled "patent" medicines. Many of the most popular of these secret formulations (such as Godfrey's Cordial, Mrs. Winslow's Soothing Syrup, Ayer's Cherry Pectoral; see Brecher, 1972) contained the same opium (or morphine) municipal authorities found so harmful when smoked by Chinese. All of them were widely available without a doctor's prescription. Coca Cola®, labeled the "intellectual beverage," really did contain cocaine when it was first produced. Ironically, it was advertised as a "temperance drink"—an alternative to the

popular *Vin Mariani (Coca de Perou)* for those who eschewed alcohol! By 1906, the furor over the widespread use of these unlabeled medical concoctions rose to such a pitch (fueled by a series of articles written by Samuel Hopkins Adams for *Colliers Magazine*) that Congress was able to pass the Pure Food and Drug Act.

This same period saw the rise of scientific medicine as a sovereign profession (Starr, 1982). Gradually, proprietary medical schools were replaced by accredited, university-affiliated institutions where Pasteur's germ theory and Virchow's doctrine of cellular pathology were taught. Practical application of these discoveries, primarily in the form of sanitary municipal water works and waste disposal systems, benefitted the collective health of Americans enormously. Progress in antisepsis and anesthesia paved the way for modern surgery, and purification of pharmacologic agents made rational and uniform prescribing possible. These advances in the general state of medicine indirectly contributed to an increasing intolerance of indiscriminate narcotics use.

For a long time, physicians had little of real benefit to offer their patients but morphine, and the demographics of narcotic addiction reflect it. Before about 1900, the majority of opiate addicts were white, upper- or middle-class women who received their drugs from their physicians. Significant numbers found relief from various ailments through self-medication with patent medicines. Astonishingly, many of them may not even have known they were addicted (Lindesmith, 1965)—all they knew was that their "illness" returned if they failed to take their medicine. Of course, those who became dependent on subcutaneous morphine injections (the hypodermic syringe was invented in 1853) must have had a clearer notion of what the real problem was. Not surprisingly, the next largest group of narcotics addicts at this time was physicians themselves.

As medicine advanced, however, the treatment of mere symptoms became synonymous with bad medical practice; moreover, as awareness of the addicting properties of the opiates grew, physicians became reluctant to dispense opiates as liberally as their predecessors had, and the number of medical addicts declined.

At the same time, however, an apparently growing number of nonmedical or pleasure (or, as we would say now, recreational) narcotics users emerged (Courtwright, 1982). By and large, these new addicts were male, urban, and poor—the unsupervised offspring of impoverished immigrant or black laborers. Many of these young men also became involved with various "deviant" (at least in terms of the mainstream values) or criminal enterprises associated with the brothels, saloons, and gambling houses. Narcotics use became increasingly associated with the criminal subculture and fear among the general population added new fuel to the fires of narcotic prohibition.

American political aspirations in the international arena also played a role in shaping our narcotics control regulations. Beginning in the eighteenth century, the English colonials in India took over the lucrative trade in opium to China from the Great Mogul. Despite years of protest by Chinese rulers, this commerce grew to enormous proportions by the mid-nineteenth century (partly because it balanced money lost to the English in the purchase of silk and tea from China). The Chinese had even engaged in two brief and humiliating military conflicts (the so-called Opium Wars) against the English.

In 1898, the Spanish–American War gave the United States possession of the Philippine Islands and, with it, responsibility for a large number of ethnic Chinese addicted to smoking opium. That problem and the dazzling prospects of commercial access to China—long dominated by the great European powers—stimulated American interest in a vigorous attack on international narcotics problems. Eager to establish the United States as a friend of China, Episcopal Bishop Charles H. Brent and Hamilton Wright (a physician with substantial political ambitions) prevailed on Theodore Roosevelt's administration to sponsor several international opium conferences aimed at helping the Chinese combat the debilitating importation of Anglo-Indian opium.

But American ambitions at these conferences (Shanghai, 1909, and the Hague, 1912–13) were frustrated by lack of a domestic narcotics policy, so in 1909, Wright developed the Foster Bill and lobbied Congress to adopt it (Musto, 1987). This first attempt to pass a federal narcotic control law failed, but five years later, resurrected as the Harrison Narcotic Act, it was enacted. Although some legislators (notably the populist William Jennings Bryan) certainly had narcotic prohibition in mind, the 1914 statute contained specific language protecting the right of the medical profession to prescribe these drugs: "Nothing contained in this section shall apply . . . to the dispensing or distribution of any of the aforesaid drugs to a patient by a physician, dentist, or a veterinary surgeon registered under this Act in the course of his professional practice only" (Brecher, 1972).

Nevertheless, within a few years, agents of the Treasury Department, who would soon become responsible for enforcing alcohol prohibition (the Volstead Act of 1920), began to seek out and prosecute physicians who provided narcotics "merely to maintain addicts." Several Supreme Court decisions upholding these convictions followed (*Jin Fuey Moy*, 1915; *Webb and Doremus*, 1919; *Behrman*, 1922), and, despite a later reversal of interpretation (the 1925 case against Charles Lindner), enforcement practices remained unchanged.

In an attempt to preserve medical supervision of opiate addicts, public health officials in Los Angeles, New York City, St. Petersburg, and Shreveport established narcotics maintenance clinics, but few achieved any success. Poor organization, lack of a clear purpose, and the pressure of federal harassment eventually undid them all. When the Louisiana facility, under the direction of Willis P. Butler, stopped maintenance treatment in 1923, it marked the end of an era. Over a period of approximately 25 years, the use of opiates had been transformed from a medically sanctioned response to illness to a despised criminal enterprise.

The idea that treatment of narcotic addiction should be a part of federal policy did not entirely disappear, but without effective medical advocacy, it took the federal government more than 10 years to build two rehabilitation "farms"—the first in Lexington, Kentucky (1935) and the second in Houston, Texas (1938). About a quarter of the patients admitted to these facilities were involuntary (O'Donnell, 1969) and the places were a kind of hybrid between a prison and a hospital. The Lexington institution in particular also served as a major training and research center.

Following a 1929 scandal involving the leadership of the Federal Bureau of Prohibition, Congress created the Federal Bureau of Narcotics and assigned it the task of enforcing the continuing prohibition of "narcotics"—opium, morphine, heroin, and cocaine—even though the Eighteenth Amendment banning alcohol was repealed. Harry Anslinger, its chief from 1930 to 1962, launched an unrelenting campaign against marijuana, and in 1937 succeeded in having the Marijuana Tax Act adopted by Congress. This federal statute followed several state actions against the use of marijuana (just as the Eighteenth Amendment followed the creation of several "dry" states), and some of the sentiment against marijuana originated in exactly the same kind of racism (this time against Mexicans) that had produced the California anti-opium ordinances 60 years earlier. This newspaper account describes the deliberations of the Montana State Legislature in 1929:

> There was fun in the House Health Committee during the week when the Marihuana bill came up for consideration. Marihuana is Mexican opium, a plant used by Mexicans and cultivated for sale by Indians. "When some beet field peon takes a few rares of this stuff," explained Dr. Fred Fulsher of Mineral County, "he thinks he has just been elected president of Mexico so he starts to execute all of his political enemies." Everybody laughed and the bill was recommended for passage. (Inciardi, 1986)

In addition to these racist and economic fears (again, the concern over the prospect of cheap alien labor), the FBN circulated ghastly stories designed to arouse public intolerance of the drug:

> The sprawled body of a young girl lay crushed on the sidewalk the other day after a plunge from the fifth story of a Chicago apartment house. Everyone called it suicide, but actually it was murder. The killer was a narcotic known to America as marijuana, and to history as hashish. It is a narcotic used in the form of cigarettes, comparatively new to the United States and as dangerous as a coiled rattlesnake. (Inciardi, 1986)

Having added control of the "evil weed" to his domain, Anslinger resumed his combat with opiates and cocaine. Opiate supplies were scarce and smuggling severely restricted during World War II, but "The Man," as he was known, continued to use the press to advance the cause of his agency. Sometimes his methods were something less than forthright. In a 1953 publication, for example, he wrote:

> The bright side . . . is the Lexington story. From 1935 to 1952, 18,000 addicts were admitted for treatment. Of these 64% never returned for treatment, 21% returned a second time, 6% a third time, and 9% four or more times. These figures should give everyone confidence that the U.S. Public Health Service Hospitals can secure good results in one of medicine's most tremendously difficult tasks. (Anslinger & Tomkins, 1953)

Anslinger was far too intelligent a man not to have known that the number of addicts *not* returning to treatment facilities was a poor measure of treatment efficacy. In actuality, properly conducted follow-up of Lexington graduates revealed dismal results: One analysis showed that only 6.6% remained abstinent after discharge (Hunt & Odoroff, 1962), and another found an even lower success rate of 3% (Duvall, Locke, & Brill, 1963).

Narcotic control legislation enacted after World War II has been, for the most part, increasingly punitive while at the same time laws have broadened the scope of activities and substances controlled. The Hale–Boggs Bill of 1951 and the Narcotic Drug Control Act of 1956 established mandatory minimum sentences for narcotics violations with escalating sentences for repeat offenders (including the death penalty for some). Although these acts were hailed by law enforcement professionals (who could control punishment by manipulating charges), they also severely increased the workload of the judicial system. Without hope of lenient sentencing from a judge, more defendants opted to take their chances with a time-consuming and expensive jury trial (Platt, 1986).

In the early 1960s, California laws had the effect of making addiction itself a crime, and the Supreme Court declared such statutes to be a violation of the Eighth Amendment's prohibition of cruel and unusual punishment (*Robinson v. California*, 1962). The result, in combination with the conclusions of a White House conference on addiction in the same year, was a new interest in treatment, by means of civil commitment, if necessary. The Narcotic Addict Rehabilitation Act of 1966 called for the development of in- and outpatient treatment in mental health centers under the direction of the National Institute of Mental Health. In 1967, however, another presidential commission was critical of both the concept and cost-effectiveness of civil commitment, and in time, it was abandoned.

The current outline of American narcotics control policy stems from the Drug Abuse Prevention and Control Act of 1970. This law replaced all preceding statutes, proclaimed that federal law superseded all state and local laws, transferred authority for enforcement from the Treasury Department to the Bureau of Narcotics and Dangerous Drugs under the Department of Justice, and created a schedule of drugs reflecting their potential for abuse. Supervision of treatment programs was shifted to the Department of Health and Human Services in the National Addict Treatment Act of 1974.

In conjunction with the increased emphasis on addiction treatment during the 1960s and early '70s, and following the federal example set in the Controlled Substances Act of 1970, eight states joined Oregon in making minor marijuana offenses comparable to parking tickets—punishable by a fine without arrest or criminal record. This decriminalization was endorsed by the American Bar Association, the National Council

of Churches, the National Education Association, the Governing Board of the American Medical Association, and others (Grinspoon, 1977). Culminating this trend of liberalizing drug policy, the State Supreme Court of Alaska made home cultivation of marijuana for personal use legal (Bakalar, 1984).

The "Reagan revolution" of the 1980s, however, rededicated government resources to narcotics prohibition, up to and including the declaration of war against drugs in the bill cited at the beginning of this chapter. Opposing drugs has always been a safe political stance, but in the current era, where uncontested issues seem increasingly rare, political leaders seem interested only in outdoing one another's "toughness" on drugs, and the hyperbolic language of the 1988 Anti-Drug Abuse Act reflects it.

The history of U.S. narcotics policy reveals that the prohibitionist enforcement of a law that originated in international politics left narcotics addicts, regardless of the origin of their difficulties, at the mercy of an expanding and unregulated black market. The change in prescribing practices over the same period of time also shaped the perceived character of the typical narcotic addict. It is an oversimplification, however, to assert that prohibition *caused* this transformation. Individual medical addicts did not become street criminals en masse; rather, over a number of years, one population replaced another.

This is not to say that criminalization of narcotic use (addictive or otherwise) has not played a role in the development of many of our current drug problems. Because the illegal market placed a premium on drugs that were most easily smuggled, traffickers gradually switched from dealing in smoking opium (a bulky product) to the more easily handled and more potent heroin. With the departure of the laid-back (and relaxed, if debauched) opium smoker of the early 1900s, the stage was set for the entrance of the street-hustling, strung-out junkie of the inner cities.

For 10 or 15 years after the Harrison Act, heroin supplies were still relatively plentiful. Street supplies were also fairly pure, and snorting was the preferred method of use. However, as the unregulated market developed, unscrupulous suppliers found it increasingly profitable to "step on" (dilute) their wares while at the same time increasing prices. Confronted with dope of decreasing potency and increasing expense, many addicts turned to intravenous injection despite its terrible hazards (Courtwright, Herman, & Des Jarlais, 1989). The weaker the heroin, the more time and effort had to be spent obtaining enough of it to stave off withdrawal, and in this fashion, whatever other life the addict might have had was swallowed up. Legitimate work, family responsibilities, nutrition, personal hygiene, and dignity—everything was sacrificed in becoming a twentieth-century American heroin addict.

Other drugs have come and gone over the years—cocaine in the 1920s, amphetamines in the '30s, barbiturates in the '50s, marijuana and the psychedelics in the '60s, and minor tranquilizers in the '70s. Now cocaine is back again, and smokable methamphetamine ("ice") is threatening to become the scourge of the 1990s. Of course, the trade in legal drugs of abuse—tobacco and alcohol—continues essentially unabated.

If there is one lesson to be learned from the history of American drug policy, it is that, for better or worse, we are a drug-using culture. Some have been legal, but now are not. Some have been promoted, and others prohibited. Some are intrinsically dangerous and others relatively harmless, but they are all drugs, and like a long-running musical, although generations of performers have come and gone, the songs and story have remained the same.

THE DEBATE—ARGUMENTS

Brer Rabbit was getting kinda annoyed. "I don't know what's wrong with this young generation. Didn't your parents teach you no manners?" The Tar Baby didn't say nothin'. "Well, I reckon I'll teach you some." So Brer Rabbit hauled off and hit that Tar Baby in the face. BIP! And his fist was stuck.

Having reviewed current drug policy, as well as its consequences and origins, I want to sketch out the basic arguments for and against reforming it. In hopes of clarifying what has become a complex collection of issues, I have divided the arguments into following areas: criminal justice, economic, political, and medical.[1] I leave the question of values to the conclusion section of this chapter because this debate cannot come near resolution without considering the ethical and moral questions it raises.

CRIMINAL JUSTICE CONSIDERATIONS

For Liberalization

Prohibition creates criminals. The bulk of those arrested for drug violations commit "crimes without complaints"—selling or possessing small amounts. More serious crimes against persons and property do not receive the investigative resources they should. Criminals already serving prison terms are set free early to create space for newcomers because the prisons are overflowing with drug law violators. Mandatory sentencing favors plea-bargaining and expensive, time-consuming jury trials. Police control sentencing through selection of charges and weaken the integrity of the system by using informants. Legalization will reduce these numbers and promote returning the criminal justice system to manageable size.

Against Liberalization

The criminal justice system is not crippled, but in fact has played a key role in restricting drug use to current levels. If it is overburdened, it needs additional support, not confused policies. Prohibition does not create criminals. Criminal careers are usually established before the onset of drug use. Mandatory sentencing is necessary because judges are either too liberal or are susceptible to intimidation by the accused. Legalization may actually increase crime because most addicts will be unable to support themselves with regular jobs as a result of being chronically intoxicated. In addition, drug use itself, especially of cocaine, causes violent behavior that must be contained.

ECONOMIC CONSIDERATIONS

For Liberalization

Prohibition maintains high prices essential to the growth of an illegal market. By reducing prices, liberalization will eliminate the incentives that create and maintain a black market. Inner city youth who have turned to the fast profits of the illicit drug business will return to mainstream employment. Gang warfare over drug market territory will diminish. The billions of dollars currently lost to the general economy will be restored to circulation as legitimate industries, markets, and occupations take over drug commerce. Taxation of drug sales and manufacture will be high enough to offset costs associated with higher use (if that occurs), but not so high as to stimulate a black market. The fabulous profits of the unregulated drug market have created corruption at all levels. Hundreds of law enforcement personnel have been convicted of taking bribes, stealing confiscated property, reselling drugs, blocking investigations, and direct smuggling and distribution. Bringing drug profits in line with other businesses will reduce corruption.

Against Liberalization

Liberalization will not eliminate a black market in drugs. Wherever limits are placed on access to drugs, people will find a way of skirting them. Drug prices, particularly if taxed, cannot be reduced to the point of not providing a profit motive for the criminally inclined. Even a legitimate manufacturing and distribution system will be subject to tremendous pressures of corruption and will require extraordinary regulation. The resulting bureaucracy will be extremely expensive. If run by the private sector, drugs will be advertised and promoted just as alcohol and tobacco are now; if run by the federal government, the system will be

so inefficient as to favor the development of black market. Inner-city youths will not have the training for new jobs created by a legitimate commerce in drugs. These jobs will go to more advantaged groups, and the unskilled will be on welfare or will turn to other criminal endeavors. Gangs are an enduring feature of inner-city poverty, and gang members will turn to other methods of obtaining money to sustain themselves.

POLITICAL CONSIDERATIONS

For Liberalization

Total prohibition is not achievable without violating the most fundamental rights of democratic society. Civil liberties are endangered by searches without warrants, searches without probable cause (random urinalysis), wire-taps, informant–police collaboration, and mandated punishment without judicial review. Prohibition of alcohol didn't work and was repealed. No one has the right to decide what forms of consciousness-altering substance another may or may not use. Use may be prohibited only if it leads to harm to another. Foreign countries have been destabilized and corrupted, and their economies have now become dependent on the cultivation and transportation of these drugs.

Against Liberalization

We are fighting for the preservation of our way of life. In dire circumstances, such as war, the majority of the population accepts infringement on constitutional rights. Society has the right to protect itself from intoxicated people. Legalizing drugs will result in more intoxication and therefore more harm to others in the form of lost production, traumatic accidents, and reduced parental supervision of children. Prohibition of alcohol did work, but was undone by poor enforcement and half-hearted federal support. Increased demand for drugs will further weaken foreign economies by shifting cultivation away from food to drug-producing plants.

MEDICAL CONSIDERATIONS

For Liberalization

Prohibition leads to serious health problems among drug users. Unregulated production of illegal drugs results in contamination and uncertain strength. The high cost and difficulty of obtaining illegal drugs drives users toward more and more potent forms of drugs and to the most efficient form of using them (usually smoking or intravenous injection). The need to use drugs quickly and not to be caught with injection equipment has favored sharing needles and syringes at "shooting galleries," thus promoting the spread of AIDS. Antidrug hysteria and misinformation is seen as "fake" by young people, and inadvertently creates interest in experimenting with drugs (the "forbidden fruit" phenomenon). For similar reasons, counterculture or "outlaw" groups identify themselves with use of illegal drugs. "Treatment" of addicts who do not regard themselves as ill is ineffective and corrupts the healthcare system by making it an enforcement instrument of dominant ideology.

Against Liberalization

Drugs are intrinsically dangerous. If they were made more available, more people would be injured or die by overdose and trauma instead of by AIDS. Experience with alcohol shows that, regardless of a drug's legal status, addiction itself leads people to use increasing amounts of drugs. For the same reasons, if drugs were legalized, people would escalate to using the most potent form. In taking drugs, people make a conscious choice that places them at risk for all kinds of harm, including that of illness. By limiting the amount of drugs available, we diminish, not increase, those risks. Children who want to experiment with drugs have not been educated to their dangers or have poor parental models. If they cannot be taught to say no, societal authorities must attach negative consequences to drug use in order to deter them. When science and organized medicine have learned more about addiction, we will find a cure.

THE DEBATE—CONFUSIONS

"You let me go!" Brer Rabbit yelled. "Let me go or I'll really pop you one." He twisted and he turned, but he couldn't get loose. "All right! I warned you!" And he smacked the Tar Baby on the other side of its head. BIP! His other fist was stuck.

One of the most interesting aspects of listing these arguments side by side is the state of confusion they engender—all can be made to seem right or wrong. There are at least two sources of this confusion, one in semantics and the other in faulty reasoning.

Semantic Confusion

It has been observed, and not in jest, that the more people argue about something, the more likely it is that they are using the same words to describe two entirely different things or are using different words to describe the same thing. Alternatively, people who believe they agree with one another may, for the same reasons, actually disagree without realizing it.

There are certainly more profound levels to this observation; however, at a simple level, it does describe the confusion in the debate over the legalization of drugs that originates strictly in semantics.

First, the word *drug* means different things to different people. Among most hard-liners, it describes all illicit substances regardless of their pharmacologic differences, but it does not refer to alcohol or tobacco—not because they aren't psychoactive substances, but simply because they are legal. This sort of inconsistency has resulted in the strange irony of a government making war on the producers, exporters, distributors, and users of one plant—marijuana—while pursuing just the opposite activities for tobacco, all despite scientific consensus that one is as harmful as the other (Coggins, 1976).

Such semantic confusion is not trivial. Many young people who have used both licit and illicit substances find this division of drugs into "good" and "bad" at best foolish, and at worst hypocritical. All psychoactive substances are potentially addicting and harmful. As we have seen, which are legal and which illegal seems largely a matter of history and culture, not biochemistry.

Arbitrary use of the words *addiction* and *abuse*—especially when they are used interchangeably with *use*—contributes to more semantic confusion. Setting aside the word *addiction* for the time being, drug abuse is usually defined as continued use despite adverse consequences. Unfortunately, particularly in the case of illicit substances, this is no definition at all, but rather, a tautology—use of an illicit substance is automatically abuse because it exposes one to the harm of arrest, prosecution, and imprisonment. When *abuse* is then used synonymously with *addiction,* it causes even more confusion. The popular notion that Washington Mayor Marion Barry was unable to resist crack is illustrative. It may well be that Barry is addicted to cocaine, but given the current political climate and Barry's legal troubles, we will never know whether he felt compelled to use that cocaine—but he may not have.

The fact is that for large numbers of people, the use of drugs, whether of the legal or illegal variety, is neither compulsive nor particularly hazardous. Although some alcohol users become severely addicted to it, most do not, and the same holds true for other substances as well—notably marijuana. On the other hand, some drugs (smoking tobacco, for example) show just the opposite pattern—few casual and many addicted users.

The point is that drugs are not equally addicting for all people, and in a prohibitory environment, it is difficult to sort out what is caused by the pharmacologic properties of a substance and what is a result of who uses it and under what circumstances. Recognizing these differences, the National Commission on Marijuana and Drug Abuse (1972) divided drug use into five categories: recreational, social, and situational use (regarded as rarely harmful) and intensive and compulsive use (often harmful). These distinctions, however, rarely enter the policy debate, and their omission causes significant confusion.

Additional semantic chaos accompanies the use of the word *legalization*. Between the extremes of total prohibition and a totally free market lie various forms of partial prohibition. Decriminalization, which makes the sale of a drug a criminal offense while relegating personal use (and possession) to noncriminal sanctions (Gettman, 1989) is not legalization. When the word *legalization* is used as a catch-all, it unfortunately lends itself to the types of distortion that make rational discussion difficult, such as the image of vending-machine access to heroin and cocaine.

Faulty Reasoning

Confusion in the legalization debate also results from various forms of faulty reasoning. First, there is the terrible lack of appreciation of the history of drug problems in the United States. As noted previously, there will never be a "drug-free America," but there never was, right from the start. The first English-speaking colony in the new world (Jamestown, Virginia) was saved from collapse by exporting the intoxicating leaf tobacco. Those who argue that tobacco is not a drug are simply unaware of the degree to which its use was feared and condemned in the early seventeenth century (Corti, 1931). Indeed, if the language of the *Counterblaste to Tobacco* (1604) written by King James I, were modernized a little, he could be George Bush declaiming on cocaine.

The United States also has a long and complex relationship with the intoxicating drug alcohol. In the early nineteenth century, per capita consumption of alcohol in America reached levels that have never been equaled since—some five to ten gallons per person per year (Aaron & Musto, 1981)—and the social consequences were severe. As already noted, nineteenth-century Americans also consumed enormous amounts of patent medicines, many of which contained substantial quantities of opium, cocaine, or alcohol (Young, 1961). From the historical perspective, it seems particularly strange that legalizers should be charged with wishing to perform social experiments, as though that were something new and dreadful. President Hoover himself called the Eighteenth Amendment "an experiment noble in intent."

Simplistic ignorance of the history of narcotics control is also deeply entrenched in the American mind. Thus, in a publicized debate on legalization, we read, "When heroin, cocaine and marijuana were legally available early in this century, the alarming spread of addiction gave rise to legal controls" (Evans, 1990). Aside from being factually wrong—marijuana use was hardly widespread nor was addiction of opiates or cocaine the sole motivation for regulatory legislation—the author's facts come almost exclusively from the *Drug Abuse Update,* a publication of the Families in Action, hardly an impartial source. It should be remembered however, that for years the Federal Bureau of Narcotics deliberately engaged in antidrug propaganda and manipulated the media to spread fear of drugs (Courtwright, 1982).

Clear reasoning does not flourish in a climate of fear and anger, and both sides of legalization argument are guilty of the most basic error of reasoning—inferring causation from association. As discussed earlier, for example, it is simplistic to imagine that narcotic prohibition caused the increase in crime associated with opiate use, and that indiscriminate legalization will restore the *status quo ante.* On the drug war side, the comments of Mitchell Rosenthal, founder of the New York-based Phoenix House organization, demonstrate the same kind of erroneous logic: "There are some 1.5 million teenage runaways now—three times the number there were in 1984—and street workers estimate that 80 percent are drug abusers" (Rosenthal, 1988). The clear—and unsupported—implication is that drug abuse causes teen runaways.

Scientific study has shown that many of the problems associated with drug use—especially the more severe aspects of juvenile delinquency—definitely precede the use of illicit drugs (Clayton, 1981). In addition, moderate drug use does not appear to lead inevitably to more problems among high school (Shedler & Bloch, 1990) or college students (Mellinger et al., 1978).

That otherwise intelligent and compassionate individuals can fall victim to the most funda-mental sorts of tortured thinking is revealed in further congressional testimony given by Rosenthal: "And what I find hardest to understand about the legalization proposal, which has been around for decades, is why it is suddenly being considered—if not seriously—then at least by serious people. It is ironic, I believe, for this notion to resurface at this time. Today, the American public has a better understanding of drug abuse and its dangers than ever before."

Why couldn't more and more Americans be considering liberalization of drug prohibition precisely *because* they have a better understanding of drug abuse than ever before?

More puzzling is the statement of Robert DuPont, former head of NIDA, in a letter to the executive editor of the *Journal of Drug Education* (dated January 24, 1989): "The problem with the idea of legalization of currently illegal drugs is that no proponent of the idea has ever made a serious proposal that opponents like myself can object to." For many years, critics of drug prohibition have pointed to the Dutch (Englesman, 1989) and English (Trebach, 1982) drug policies as models for American reform. Although one may argue over the applicability, benefits, and drawbacks of these systems, it is simply untrue to say that serious proposals for reform do not exist, unless, of course, any such proposition is by definition not serious.

In 1972, the Consumers Union Reports book *Licit and Illicit Drugs* concluded with a series of suggestions for decriminalizing marijuana. A few years later, several states markedly reduced or, in the case of Alaska, eliminated criminal penalties for mere possession of marijuana. Only a week after DuPont's remark, an exceptionally detailed proposal to legalize drugs was put before the New York State Legislature (Senate Bill 1919, introduced by Senator Galiber, Feb. 6, 1989).

As long as congressional policy demands "total victory" in the war on illegal drugs, it is unlikely to welcome or sponsor the sort of conferences and publications that could produce the detailed plans DuPont is calling for. Incidentally, no such demands were ever made of prohibition advocates.

Science also contributes two more sources of confusion in the legalization debate: the volatile nature of scientific information itself and the belief that scientific methods of investigation can be applied to all questions, otherwise known as scientism (Needleman, 1985).

Not long ago, most physicians regarded cocaine as a nonaddicting substance. Obviously, that opinion has changed with further research.

Beyond the discovery of new information, however, it must be recognized that science is not without its prejudices. Current scientific thinking on addicting drugs, for example, is very heavily weighted toward biochemical–pharmacologic conceptualizations. From this perspective, the most important aspect of psychoactive drugs is not the setting in which they are used, but rather to what degree they are "reinforcing." Experiments with captive, restrained laboratory animals are cited as evidence that cocaine is the most addictive substance on earth. Not long ago the same epithet was applied to heroin (Smith & Gay, 1972). There may be something to generalize from the behavior of imprisoned primates—human beings also experience such conditions, both actually and symbolically—but to what extent such experiments warrant generalization to the complex, multifaceted situation of real human beings in a real world is an unanswered question.

A naturalistic study (Zinberg, 1984) of longtime heroin users, for example, demonstrated that a significant number were able to consistently control both the degree and duration of intoxication. Studies purporting to demonstrate that alcoholics could learn controlled drinking in an experimental bar-like situation (Sobell & Sobell, 1973) provide further evidence of imperfect correspondence between the laboratory and the real world. Follow-up studies of these "successful" subjects revealed that several had died, several had returned to heavy drinking, and some found that recovery from alcoholism required total abstinence (Pendery, Waltzman, & West, 1982).

Field studies of drug use and users may be far more important to the drug policy debate than more easily conducted and controlled "bench"

research because the latter tends to fuel the simplistic models of drug abuse favored by the current federal administration and so many of its advisors. As reduced for political consumption, this paradigm is stripped of the critically important ideas of resistance and susceptibility and thus does not adequately describe addictive illness.

During the Vietnam War, for example, very large numbers of American troops used and became addicted to heroin, but on returning home, nearly 90% stopped using it (Robins, 1973). This finding has often been used in the argument against legalization, on the theory that difficulty obtaining the drug was the main reason soldiers discontinued their use, despite their reports that drugs were readily available if they wanted them. But what the military experience may also suggest is that the inception and continuation of compulsive drug use may be less a matter of simplified neurochemistry than the present scientific model would lead us to believe.

CONCLUSIONS AND REFLECTIONS

Then Brer Fox came and said, "You ain't gonna be going around through the community raising commotion anymore, Brer Rabbit. And it's your own fault too. Didn't nobody tell you to be so friendly with the Tar Baby. You stuck yourself on that Tar Baby without so much as an invitation. There you are and there you'll be until I get my fire started and my barbecue sauce ready."

As a relative newcomer to the issues of drug policy, I have found it necessary to aim this chapter at a broad overview while trying not to take sides in what has become a very acrimonious controversy. Each element of the larger question deserves a whole chapter (if not a book) of its own; nevertheless, there is a certain advantage in taking a wide perspective in a fresh way. One sees things before habitual reactions have established themselves.

Perhaps I can best illustrate the value of this sort of naivete by disclosing my confusion on reading the title of a news article: "Drugs: America Looks for the Way Out" (*Los Angles Times,*

1990). To what, I thought, did this headline refer? Was it about why and how Americans use drugs? Or did it deal with the effort to rid ourselves of them? That the title could refer to either makes the first point about current drug policy: The same motivations drive both drug taking and drug warring. Of course, that isn't so surprising. Both, after all, are attempts to escape problems. The oddity is that one seems so bad and the other so good.

David Musto, one of the most knowledgeable students of the history of narcotics control, titled his book *The American Disease.* He didn't mean, of course, that Europeans or Asians don't have drug problems, but rather that there is something about the American character that has made these problems far more terrible for us than for others.

We are a people, perhaps above all others, who believe that through democratic government, we can arrange the conditions of life so as to make possible a perfectly harmonious society. We have led the world into an age of mechanized production, created a nation of enormous wealth, and given ourselves the leisure time to enjoy it. But along the way we have also altered the most fundamental aspects of human life—family and community structure, the meaning and nature of work, and the sense of basic competence to provide for oneself. At the same time, our march of progress has made available extraordinarily potent chemicals for escaping the despair that results from being unable to endure it all.

Confronted by unanticipated and problematic consequences of this way of life, we reaffirm ourselves as can-do people and elect politicians who promise to "get the job done"—never mind exactly what the job is. Unfortunately, as the story of Brer Rabbit's misadventure with the Tar Baby so wonderfully teaches, impatience rarely makes things better.

Just as Brer Rabbit's fighting only entangles him more, it seems that the more strenuously we try to battle the drug problem head on, the less we accomplish. It's entirely analogous to the plight of the drug user who descends into the maelstrom of addiction, searching more and more desperately for next fix to cure the pain of withdrawing from the last.

Does drug prohibition prevent abuse? It does prevent some, but it does so at great cost and creates a host of additional problems that, depending on your point of view, may be even worse. Unfortunately, it seems inevitable that the opposite policy—sweeping drug legalization—although it might solve other drug abuse problems, would probably also create an entirely new set of problems.

No doubt this conclusion begins to sound suspiciously like a grand American heresy—a problem for which there is no solution. Confronted with this unpalatable prospect, some behavioral scientists look once again to technological advances to bail us out. The latest suggested fix for the drug problem is to engineer chemically "ideal intoxicants which would balance optimal positive effects, such as stimulation or pleasure, with minimal or nonexistent toxic consequences" (Seigel, 1989). Can anyone possibly imagine that such a mythical substance would not also be addicting for us mere mortals? While they're at it, perhaps these engineers will also come up with a water substitute that doesn't have the inconvenience of being wet.

It would seem that this consideration of drug policy has embarked us on a voyage into some very deep waters—perhaps to the very foundations of modern culture itself. How else can we explain the multifaceted deterioration of a culture in the midst of unparalleled material bounty?

In his brilliant essay *The Arrogance of Humanism,* David Ehrenfeld exposes the ironic circularity of our naïvely altruistic "wars," be they political (Vietnam), social (poverty), or medical (cancer). Summing up the latter, he writes, "The society clever enough to perform sophisticated research on cancer is the society clever enough to invent the sugar substitutes, children's sleepwear ingredients, food coloring agents, and swimming pool test kits that may cause it" (Ehrenfeld, 1978).

Noting that the untestable assumptions of religion are attacked by humanists as superstitions, he goes on to describe the same sorts of articles of faith held by a humanistic society:

— All problems are soluble by people.
— Many problems are soluble by technology.
— Problems that are not soluble by technology, or by technology alone, have solutions in the social world of politics and economics.
— When the chips are down, we will apply ourselves and work together for a solution before it is too late.

To continue the drug policy debate in ignorance of the despair that accompanies the unexamined assumptions of this pervasive belief system is to fail to recognize how really desperate our situation is. The conclusion of this chapter, then, is based on the suspicion that our drug abuse problems derive from our most fundamental sense of the purpose and meaning of human life. The prevention of drug abuse is a far larger problem than a national drug policy alone can address. The alternative paths mapped out by drug legalizers and prohibitionists differ only in the types of problems they solve and create, not in whether one is better or worse.

Meanwhile, people are dying of AIDS, rotting in prisons, and slaughtering one another while driving intoxicated. We cannot do nothing.

In its annual report for 1990, the California Research Advisory Council broke precedent to make the following policy recommendations concerning drug use and addiction problems:

— Separately consider different drugs involved and not consider that there is one massive drug problem.
— Distinguish between the effects of drugs and the associated criminal activity.
— Design the legislation with the awareness that these are initial efforts subject to change with experience.
— Think of drugs as including alcohol and nicotine, not as being separate substances.

The panel also recommended three possibilities for demonstration legislation:

— Permit the possession of syringes and needles.

— Permit the cultivation of marijuana for personal use.
— As a first step in projecting an attitude of disapproval by all citizens toward all drug use, take a token action in forbidding the sale or consumption of alcohol in state-supported institutions devoted in part or whole to patient care or educational activity.

Sadly, the Attorney General of California rejected the suggestions and refused to pay for publication of the report.

"Do what'nsoever you want to with me, Brer Fox, but please don't throw me in that briar patch" . . . *he snatched him off the Tar Baby and chunked that rabbit smack dab in the middle of the briar patch. Then Brer Rabbit broke into the loudest laughter you ever heard. "I was born and raised in the briar patch, Brer Fox! Born and raised in the briar patch!"*

NOTES

1. I offer no citations for the arguments presented in this section. First, their origins cannot be attributed to specific individuals; second the statistical data marshaled to support them have rarely been interpreted in a value-free way.

REFERENCES

Aaron, P., & Musto, D. (1981). Temperance and prohibition in America: An historical overview. In M. H. Moore & D. R. Gerstein (Eds.), *Alcohol and public policy: Beyond the shadow of prohibition.* Washington, DC: National Academy Press.

Anslinger, H. J., & Tomkins, W. F. (1953). *The traffic in narcotics.* New York: Funk and Wagnalls, 24.

Bakalar, J. B., & Grinspoon, L. (1984). *Drug control in a free society.* Cambridge: Cambridge University Press.

Bensinger, P. B. (1988). *Drug abuse update, 26,* 14–15.

Brecher, E., and the Editors of *Consumer Reports* (1972). *Licit and illicit drugs.* Boston: Little, Brown and Company.

Clayton, R. R. (1981). *Young men and drugs in Manhattan: A causal analysis.* NIDA Research Monograph 39. Washington, DC: USGPO.

Coggins, W., Swenson, E. W., Dawson, W. W., et al. (1976). Health status of chronic heavy cannabis users. *Annals of the New York Academy of Science, 282,* 148–161.

Cooper, M. H. (1990). *The business of drugs.* Washington, DC: Congressional Quarterly, Inc.

Corti, E. C. (1931). A history of smoking, trans. P. England. London: George C. Harrap & Co.

Courtwright, D. (1982). *Dark paradise. Opiate addiction in America before 1940.* Cambridge, MA: Harvard University Press.

Courtwright, D., Joseph, H., & Des Jarlais, D. (1989). *Addicts who survived.* Knoxville: University of Tennessee Press.

Duvall, H., Locke, B., & Brill, L. (1963). Follow-up study of narcotics drug addicts five years after hospitalization. *Public Health Reports, 78,* 185–193.

Ehrenfeld, D. (1978). *The arrogance of humanism.* New York: Oxford University Press.

Englesman, E. L. (1989). Dutch policy on the management of drug-related problems. *British Journal of Addictions, 84,* 211–218.

Evans, D. G. (1990). Legal drugs: More crime, dramatic increase in use. *Addiction Review, 2,* 1–6.

Gettman, J. (1989). Decriminalizing marijuana. *American Behavioral Scientist, 32,* 243–248.

Grinspoon, L. (1977). *Marijuana reconsidered* (second edition). Cambridge, MA: Harvard University Press.

Holmes, O. W., Sr. (1891). *Medical essays: 1842–1882.* Boston: Houghton Mifflin.

Hunt, G. H., & Odoroff, M. E. (1962). Follow-up study of narcotic drug addicts after hospitalization. *Public Health Reports, 77,* 41–54.

Inciardi, J. A. (1986). *The war on drugs. Heroin, cocaine, crime and public policy.* Palo Alto, CA: Mayfield.

King, R. (1990). (Quoted in) A report from an anti-prohibition pioneer. In A. S. Trebach & K. B. Zeese (Eds.), *Drug policy 1989–1990: A reformer's catalogue.* Washington, DC: The Drug Policy Foundation.

Lapham, L. (Dec. 1989). (Cited in) A political opiate. *Harper's Magazine.*

Lindesmith, A. (1965). *The addict and the law.* Bloomington: Indiana University Press.

Los Angeles Times (1990). Drugs: America looks for the way out. March 12–17.

Mellinger, G. D., et al. (1978). *Drug use, academic performance, and career indecision: Longitudinal research on drug use.* New York: Wiley.

Monitoring the Future study (1989). Washington, DC: U.S. Department of Health and Human Services, National Institute of Drug Abuse.

Musto, D. (1987 expanded edition). *The American disease. Origins of narcotic control.* New York: Oxford University Press.

Nadelmann, E. A. (1989). Drug prohibition in the United States: Costs, consequences, and alternatives. *Science, 245,* 939–947.

National Commission on Marijuana and Drug Abuse (1972). *Marijuana: A signal of misunderstanding.* Washington, DC: USGPO.

Needleman, J. (1985). *Sin and scientism.* San Francisco: Robert Briggs Associates.

New York Times CBS Poll, Jan. 15, 1990. (33% regarded drugs as the most important problem facing the United States).

O'Donnell, J. A. (1969). *Narcotic addicts in Kentucky.* Public Health Service Publication no. 1881. Washington, DC: USGPO.

Pendery, M. L., Waltzman, I. M., & West, L. J. (1982). Controlled drinking by alcoholics? New findings and a reevaluation of a major affirmative study. *Science, 117,* 169–175.

Platt, J. J. (1986). *Heroin addiction: Theory, treatment, and research.* Malabar, FL: Robert E. Krieger Publishing Company.

Reagan, R. (1987). State of the Union address.

Reuter, P. (1988). Can the borders be sealed? *Public Interest, 92,* 51–65.

Robins, L. N. (1973). *A follow-up of Vietnam drug users.* Special Action Office Monograph, Series A, No. 1. Washington, DC: Executive Office of the President.

Rosenthal, M. (1988). Address before the Select Committee on Narcotic Abuse and Control, United States House of Representatives, on the issue of drug legalization, Sept. 29, 1988.

Seigel, R. K. (1989). *Intoxication.* New York: E.P. Dutton.

Shedler, J., & Bloch, J. (1990). Adolescent drug use and psychological health: A longitudinal inquiry. *American Psychologist, 45,* 612–630.

Smith, D., & Gay, G. R. (1972). *It's so good, don't even try it once: Heroin in perspective.* Englewood Cliffs, NJ: Prentice Hall.

Sobell, M. B., & Sobell, L. C. (1973). Alcoholics treated by individualized behavior therapy: One year treatment outcome. *Behavior Research and Therapy, 11,* 599–618.

Starr, P. (1982). *The social transformation of American medicine.* New York: Basic Books.

Szasz, T. (1974). *Ceremonial chemistry: The ritual persecution of drugs, addicts and pushers.* Garden City, NY: Anchor Press.

Trebach, A. S. (1982). *The heroin solution.* New Haven: Yale University Press.

Young, J. H. (1961). The toadstool millionaires: A social history of patent medicines in America before federal regulation. Princeton, NJ: Princeton University Press.

Zeese, K. B. (1989). Drug war forever? In A. S. Trebach & K. B. Zeese (Eds.), *Drug policy 1989–1990: A reformer's catalogue.* Washington, DC: The Drug Policy Foundation.

Zinberg, L. (1984). *Drug, set and setting. The basis for controlled intoxicant use.* New Haven: Yale University Press.

EPILOGUE

HERBERT D. KLEBER

Although there will probably be periodic upturns in use of one illicit drug or another, it appears that we may be in the decline phase of a drug epidemic that began about 30 years ago. The sharp decrease in illegal drug use over the past decade, from 24 million current (any use in past 30 days) drug users in 1979 to 11.4 million in 1992, reflects a dramatic cultural shift that is still not as widely appreciated as it should be. Ultimately, the effects of the decline will show up in our schools, workplaces, and neighborhoods as fewer individuals use drugs and fewer become addicts. Progress was a result of a variety of forces, including parent groups, community organizations, the media, drug-free workplace initiatives, better school-based education and prevention efforts, and strong antidrug political leadership, at the national and local levels.

Because of the widespread nature of the drug use, the first major prevention theme and effort had to be denormalization. During the 1960s and 1970s, our society became very tolerant of drug use, a major change from the preceding decades. Large increases in the use of illegal drugs, especially marijuana and psychedelic drugs in the '60s and '70s, and amphetamines and cocaine in the '70s and '80s, resulted. It has been estimated that in the early 1960s, less than 4 million Americans had used illegal drugs; by 1993 that number had climbed to more than 75 million. We cope everyday with the results of that "experiment" in our emergency rooms and dangerous streets.

It is necessary, however, to take the long view about the coming decades and the role of prevention, to realize that ongoing significant progress will take much time and effort and we cannot give in to the same temptation as the drug user—the search for the quick fix. There is neither a painless nor a quick solution to the complex problems that are involved in all aspects of the fight against drug use. Certainly, legalization as proposed by a vocal few would make the problem substantially worse. Furthermore, if we rely solely on the federal government, we are setting ourselves up for certain failure. Substantially reducing drug use requires the nation—states, communities, schools, religious groups, and families—to participate in the struggle.

The ready supply of drugs on our street corners increases demand and makes prevention and treatment activities much more difficult. Law enforcement activities remain necessary, therefore, even if they are not as effective as we would like and take too large a percentage of the drug control budget. Increased demand can lead to increased supply, as happened in the early 1980s when rising demand for cocaine in the United States led to sharply increased production in the Andean countries. In the 1990s, the reverse is likely to happen: As use of cocaine in America diminishes sharply, the glut of cocaine in the world will lead the trafficking organizations to seek new markets, the most likely being Western Europe, Japan, and the South American countries themselves. Thus, in the 1990s, supply will drive demand. In 1989, smokable methamphetamine, or "ice," appeared in Hawaii, and the push on the supply side created a demand market that formerly was not there. A similar situation occurred in 1985 with the introduction of smokable cocaine in a cheap, readily usable form: crack.

The chapters of this book have elucidated in great detail various approaches to prevention. In general, it is not possible to treat our way out of a drug epidemic. Although treatment is vital to helping the casualties of this epidemic, without preventing new cases, the struggle will be a constant uphill effort. Prevention is essential and, as the chapters illustrate, good models are available. The key is to remember that prevention is not a monolithic phenomenon nor adequate by itself.

Prevention must begin with epidemiologic data as to the nature of the problem. It is a common misconception that most drug abuse occurs among the poor and disadvantaged, a notion fostered in part by the media. In newspaper articles and television programs—the "48 Hours on Crack Street" type—one is likely to see primarily black and Hispanic addicts. It is easy to lose sight of the fact that most of the people in those neighborhoods are not using drugs, that most people who use drugs are neither poor nor minority, and that most of the poor do not use illicit drugs. Our epidemiologic studies have been inadequate and must be improved, especially with regard to protection and resilience factors and the move from use to abuse.

Prevention activities necessary to decrease experimentation and casual use may be quite different from those necessary to prevent the transition from use to abuse to dependence. For those who have already begun to use drugs, the goal must be to get them to stop. Ironically, such casual users (the term is inadequate, but *recreational* and *controlled* are no better) may be the vectors of the drug problem and, by definition, these users can usually stop without treatment if faced with appropriate sanctions. This leads to the user accountability strategy.

Observation of how individuals begin drug use shows that a major carrier of this problem is the casual drug user, not the addict. The addict is not the role model; nobody wants to be the falling-down drunk, the burned-out addict, or the psychotic cocaine abuser who has lost health, possessions, and family. The role model is the person who is using drugs at school or work, who sends the message by his or her behavior that you can have it all: You can enjoy the pleasurable effects of drugs and still keep your health, your friends, your possessions, your family, and your job. Most individuals who start on drugs do not buy them the first time. More often they are given drugs by older siblings or friends and acquaintances at school, at work, or at parties.

A second major prevention theme in the 1980s, after denormalization, became user accountability. Denormalization may have helped many nonusers not to start and may also have helped nonaddicted users from going on to heavy use and dependence. User accountability laws and policies provide clear consequences for possession or use of illegal drugs. Examples are laws that lead to the suspension of drivers' licenses and pilots' licenses and drug testing of bus drivers and train engineers. Public housing projects and neighborhood block coalitions have turned free-drug zones into drug-free zones by evicting and forcing out drug abusers and by establishing resident patrols.

Because children and adults spend most of their time either at school or at work, school and workplace policies and procedures were developed to deter drug use. Some school districts adopted a policy stipulating that the first time a student was caught using drugs, parents were notified and the student temporarily suspended. If caught distributing drugs, students were expelled and sent to alternative schools. It would be useful to know whether these policies led to decreased drug use in schools, as they did in the military and the business world.

Businesses, through clear policies, supervisor and employee training, and drug testing, held employees accountable by imposing drug treatment or possible termination of employment on discovery of drug use. However, efforts to compel current users to give up drugs are at best only one part of a comprehensive prevention strategy. Education has an important role in preventing drug use as well, and is the third prevention theme.

Although some individuals use the terms *prevention* and *education* synonymously in regard to alcohol or illicit drug use, it is clear that they are not the same. Education may be a necessary part of prevention, but it is clearly not sufficient. What is needed is a comprehensive approach that includes the family, the faith community, the workplace, and the media, in conjunction with education. Using this comprehensive approach, project STAR (Student-Taught Awareness Resistance) in Kansas City, Missouri showed a decrease in drug use compared with control groups.

School-based education must be conducted in an effective way. There is a consensus that merely providing cognitive knowledge about drugs does not work. Columnist William Raspberry made the point that knowledge is the cure only so far as ignorance is the disease. The most promising approach appears to be refusal skills training or resistance training, and is based on the social influence model. It grew out of previous efforts to teach youngsters how to say "no" to smoking. Resistance training has had success because it correctly recognizes the enormous role peer pressure plays in influencing decisions to try drugs. The training method is summarized in four basic points: identify pressures to use drugs, counter pro-use arguments, learn how to say "no," and provide the motivation to say "no" by explaining present rather than future negative effects on daily life and social relationships and by dispelling the belief that drug use is widespread, desirable, or harmless. The Department of Education gives more than $500 million to local school districts for drug prevention programs, but, unfortunately, there is minimal tracking of how this is spent or how effective the programs are. This increases the likelihood that in times of tight budgets, such a program will be hard to defend.

Prevention is most successful if it is appropriate and targeted and recognizes the diversity of the problem. Such targeting is the fourth prevention theme. One approach to segmentation is to conceptualize four groups: high-risk and low-risk youngsters growing up in high-crime or low-crime areas. A different kind of prevention program is needed for the high-risk youngster in the high-crime areas than for the high-risk youngsters in the low-crime areas. This latter group is often made up of children of alcoholics, children from dysfunctional families, and those with psychological problems. They make up the majority

of drug users. They need attention directed to these psychological issues just as the high-risk youngsters in the high-crime areas may need academic tutoring, adult male role models, and after-school recreational activities. Both of these groups need strategies different from those for low-risk youngsters in low-risk areas, for whom a "just say no" method with appropriate resistance strategies may often be sufficient. Because many risk factors (such as poverty and dysfunctional families) decrease the motivation to say no and are difficult to ameliorate in the short term, increased attention should be placed on programs that attempt to provide possible protective factors. We not only need more drug education, we need to develop better ways of going about it and targeting it more effectively. It is important to learn whether prevention programs that aim at altering high-risk behavior in young children will be effective in reducing substance use a decade later when these children are adolescents.

It is important that institutions of higher learning also adopt clear and systematic approaches to substance use on campus. Institutions that are dedicated to the life of the mind too often do not have, or do not enforce appropriate policies. They often look the other way. Drug use not only extols present over future gratification, it can also interfere with learning via the physiologic effects of the drugs.

As mentioned earlier, for the adult, a key area to target for prevention is the workplace. Federal law requires firms that have government grants or contracts of more than $25,000 a year to develop a drug-free workplace with four components. The first component is clearly enunciated drug-free workplace policies that spell out the company's policy on drug use, including consequences. Workers are often more concerned about losing their jobs than they are about losing their spouses. Drug use in the workplace is also associated with higher absenteeism, more accidents, and poorer quality of work. Thus, the workplace becomes a natural setting on which to focus.

The second component of a workplace program is training and education about drug abuse for supervisors and employees. Someone using drugs is more likely to be known of by co-workers than supervisors. Whether the co-worker puts pressure on his or her colleague to get help, or reports the person to the employee assistance program, is probably a function of what the co-worker thinks will happen. If the perception is that the drug user will be fired immediately, the co-worker will not report the colleague. The co-worker is much more likely to do so, however, if he or she thinks the colleague will get help. Such help benefits not only the drug user but also the co-worker because drug use on the job makes work more dangerous for everyone and makes the company less competitive, which could lead to job layoffs. Firm policies and rehabilitation programs are needed so that individuals can get help.

The third component, therefore, is an employee assistance program. Employee assistance programs can be very effective. A number of such programs have been studied, and they commonly show a success rate for drug and alcohol problems up to 65%. They are a cost-effective and humane way of approaching the problem.

The fourth component is appropriate drug testing. There are essentially four kinds of drug testing: pre-employment, post-accident or for cause, on suspicion, and random. The first three are relatively noncontroversial and businesses find them useful in deterring use and identifying those with drug problems who need help. Random testing is more controversial, but it is encouraged at least for employees in safety-related or sensitive positions; some companies, such as the Motorola Corporation, have found random testing of all employees, from the CEO to line workers, to be effective.

Ultimately, the most important part of the prevention effort may be at the community level. All segments of the community have become involved: parents, law enforcement and health professionals, the faith community, service clubs, businesses, and government officials. Numerous communities have organized for this effort.

The Robert Wood Johnson Foundation sponsored a $26 million "Fighting Back" initiative in which communities with populations between 100,000 and 150,000 had the opportunity to get up to $3 million for community-organized efforts to combat drug use. More than 700 indicated some interest in applying, 300 of these organized themselves enough to send in the demanding application, and 15 received initial grants. This example led the Office of National Drug Control Policy (ONDCP) to the development of the Community Partnership initiative, working together with the Department of Health and Human Services (DHHS). The Office of Substance Abuse Prevention in DHHS has spent more than $200 million to fund such community coalition-building efforts. The use of trained volunteers could markedly improve the work of the community coalitions and better initiatives to do this must be implemented. Volunteers trained as to what has been successful in other communities would bring effective techniques within reach of the millions of Americans who, in poll after poll, indicate their desire and willingness to get involved in the fight against drug abuse.

Intensive and thoughtful media campaigns can work side-by-side with schools and communities to help shape public opinion and attitudes about drugs. The antismoking campaign of the 1970s and the recent emphasis on the dangers of second-hand smoke may have had a great deal to do with the reductions in smoking by adults during the past decade. In the last few years, we have seen similar attention to drugs via the ads produced by the Partnership for a Drug-Free America, created in 1986. They set (and reached) a target in 1989 of raising $1 million a day from the private sector for three years—one billion dollars to continue and enhance this media effort. Not only is the space and time for these ads donated, but the creative work is provided free of charge as well. Surveys have shown that in the areas of higher media saturation by the Partnership, changes in attitudes toward drug use and users have been greater. The campaign recognizes that it is necessary to focus on both potential consumers and influencers—parents, peer groups, healthcare professionals, opinion leaders, and teachers. The primary influencer messages have three components: informational, to arm them with facts so they can discuss the issue credibly with users and potential users; responsibility, inducing the point that control is possible and that it must be exercised; and finally, cost–benefit balance, to communicate to the public the costs of drug abuse on a personal and societal basis. The primary consumer messages also focus on three elements: motivation, dispelling the myth that one can benefit from illegal drug use; the countering of misinformation, highlighting the true negative effects; and values, stressing responsibility to oneself and society. In short, these attempt to influence the decision to use drugs by providing information and moral persuasion to help shape attitudes and desires, as well as by providing information on consequences and penalties.

The Partnership ads are examples of efforts to encourage negative attitudes toward drugs, to denormalize their use. Such efforts are more effective when part of a consistent media approach in which not only ads but the stars of regular television programs, motion pictures, and sports, as well as other role models, convey an unambiguous antidrug message. In a democratic society such efforts will, of course, not be universal (witness the recent pro marijuana and psychedelic use promoted by certain rock and rap groups). As drug use declines, we must avoid the enforced silence about drugs that occurred in earlier decades and is cited by historians as paving the way for the drug use explosion in the 1960s and 1970s.

The federal government must put greater resources into research that will identify the most effective means of preventing drug use. Carefully monitored demonstration projects—with control groups, independent testing, and follow-up research—are necessary to determine what kinds of prevention programs work best, and why. More basic prevention research that examines both biologic factors (serotonin levels, for example) and psychological ones (such as learning and attention disorders) that put individuals at higher risk need more funding, as does the role of psychiatric disorders.

Prevention is neither perfect nor a panacea. The effect of legal availability on use can be examined by comparing adolescent tobacco use to marijuana and cocaine use over the past decade. Despite greatly increased publicity about tobacco's dangers, stepped up prevention programs, and the lack of TV advertising, tobacco use barely declined among adolescents from 1980 to 1990, going from 30% (past 30-day use) only to 29%. At the same time, in contrast, marijuana use declined dramatically from 33% to 14%. Put another way, in 1980 current use of the two substances was almost equal; 10 years later, half as many were using marijuana as cigarettes. The marijuana decrease did not lead to increased alcohol use. Both occasional and heavy alcohol use declined—more than tobacco but much less than marijuana. Cocaine use sharply declined from 1985 to 1990 after rising in the first part of the decade. The legal availability of tobacco and alcohol for adults, and the corresponding societal attitudes, makes preventing their use among adolescents much harder, even though such use is illegal for them.

Our current drug situation follows the historical pattern of earlier drug epidemics. As use has gone from epidemic to endemic, disadvantaged groups are more likely to maintain use, a function of greater availability and fewer alternative opportunities. That is why minority communities not only want treatment facilities, but also call for fair laws, justly applied, to reduce the horrendous toll crime takes in their neighborhoods. The illegal open-air drug bazaars that flourish in southeast Washington, D.C. and the South Bronx would not be tolerated in Georgetown or Scarsdale. Legalizing drugs would hit this group hardest, as has been the case with tobacco and alcohol. This critical factor of availability speaks to the need for continued law enforcement activities even while increasing treatment and prevention. Community policing looks promising but has been unevenly applied to date.

The importance of developing prevention initiatives effective in the decline phase of an epidemic is heightened by reports of increased drug use and decreased perception of risk by eighth and twelfth graders in the 1993 High School Surveys. Both marijuana and LSD use significantly increased. As drug use declines, first-hand knowledge of casualties declines and students tend to become skeptical of the drug education messages they receive.

The major themes that have driven the prevention effort over the end of the 1980s and the beginning of the 1990s are denormalization, user accountability, school-based education, the workplace, the community, and the media. In the coming years, we must examine how effective these have been singly and in combination, and put more emphasis on targeting interventions to specific segments of the at-risk population and better research design and execution.

Although drug policy is never perfect, keeping the pressure on over time in both organized government and private sector effort appears to be the key. The drug problem is still far too big. Too many communities, families, and individuals still suffer the terrible consequences of drug use and drug crime, and progress has been uneven. The drug situation in too many neighborhoods has not improved. Now is definitely not the time to reduce effort, decrease the rhetoric of national leaders, or cut funding. The evidence of the past decade suggests that progress is possible, not that it is inevitable. Continued national and international support of antidrug efforts can make a definitive and lasting difference; lack of such support will lead at best to a stalling at present high levels and at worst to a deterioration. The goal of a drug-free America is an unrealistic one; it is realistic, however, to strive to reduce use to the pre-1960 era when drug use was a small problem in America. Prevention efforts are a critical factor in such an endeavor.

INDEX